Medicinal and Other Uses of North American Plants

A HISTORICAL SURVEY WITH
SPECIAL REFERENCE TO
THE EASTERN INDIAN TRIBES

Charlotte Erichsen-Brown

DOVER PUBLICATIONS, INC.
New York

ACKNOWLEDGEMENTS

I want to thank Dr. J.H. McAndrews of the Royal Ontario Museum for his explanation of the analysis of pollen from archeological sites and for the material and advice he gave me. I want to thank John Riley for making the nomenclature, botanical index, habitat and distribution of the plants discussed in this book technically correct and botanically accurate. The time he has spent and his interest and encouragement have meant much to me. I want to thank Mrs. Norman Endicott for reading the Sources cited in this book and for her useful comments.

I want to thank those who lent me or gave me their family recipe books, manuscripts and books. These are listed in the sources.

For books written in English I wish to thank the librarians in the Science and Medicine, Botany and Pharmacy libraries of the University of Toronto, the Royal Ontario Museum and the inter-library loan service of the public libraries of Canada. Articles written in French and published in Quebec have proven extraordinarily difficult to obtain. This book has not been funded either as to research or publication.

Without the patient understanding of my husband, John Price Erichsen-Brown throughout the years this book never could have been written. His criticism, advice, and comments upon the manuscript were always pertinent and are deeply appreciated.

Published in Canada by General Publishing Company, Ltd., 30 Lesmill Road, Don Mills, Toronto, Ontario.

Published in the United Kingdom by Constable and Company, Ltd., 10 Orange Street, London WC2H 7EG.

This Dover edition, first published in 1989, is an unabridged republication of the work originally published under the title *Use of plants for the past 500 years* by Breezy Creeks Press, Aurora, Ontario, Canada, in 1979.

Manufactured in the United States of America
Dover Publications, Inc., 31 East 2nd Street, Mineola, N.Y. 11501

Library of Congress Cataloging-in-Publication Data

Erichsen-Brown, Charlotte.
      [Use of plants for the past 500 years]
      Medicinal and other uses of North American plants : a historical survey with special reference to the eastern Indian tribes / Charlotte Erichsen-Brown.
            p.   cm.
      Reprint. Originally published: Use of plants for the past 500 years. Aurora, Ont. : Breezy Creeks Press, c1979.
      Bibliography: p.
      Includes indexes.
      ISBN 0-486-25951-X
      1. Ethnobotany—United States. 2. Ethnobotany—Canada. 3. Botany—United States. 4. Botany—Canada. 5. Indians of North America—Ethnobotany. I. Title.
      [GN560.U6E75 1989]
      581.6′1′097—dc19   88-30447
                                                                                        CIP

CONTENTS

PREFACE

Between the conception of a grand idea and its fruition there is an uninviting and barren ground. How many times has the suggestion been made that one of the significant gaps in our knowledge concerns the historical and modern uses of our native flora? How many times have we asked or been asked about the past uses, practical or medicinal, of some wild plant encountered in our travels?

In most cases, we feel sure that the plant was put to good use and that the original peoples of eastern North America were masters in their own home, but often we can't go much further. If we went to the trouble of assembling a small library of articles and books, many of them recent and derivative works, the same difficulties remain. The knowledge hides, like some rare orchids, in unexpected and inaccessible places.

We know that the aboriginal knowledge of plants was communicated to the early explorers and settlers. Much of the material is recorded as the anecdotal asides of gentlemen explorers, traders and missionaries who were chronicling the more pressing details of commerce, transportation and salvation for their profit-wise European sponsors. Professional naturalists and scientists from Europe toured eastern North America a century later, producing volumes of observations. Ethnologists, some of them native, were the recipients and recorders of threatened aboriginal cultures. Upon this scattered and original data base there later flourished, predictably, a field of opportunistic misinformation, often with a pseudo-medical flavour. The popularization of such information, though laudable, often resulted in plagiarism and miscegenation of the original knowledge, confusing much of it.

The purpose of this work was to cull the available sources, explore the earliest and original materials, and to present the chronology of the recorded data in its original form, in such a way that it would serve the needs of the interested public as well as the more specialist needs of historians, ethnologists, botanists, archaeologists and pharmacists. This volume is the first step towards that goal. No synoptic work of this kind can be complete, but it roughs out the trail we have taken out of the past and raises a myriad of questions as to how we might use our native plants in the future.

There are many technical problems in compiling such a sourcebook. Interpreting casual references to plants unknown to Europeans 300 years ago is often difficult at the generic level and sometimes impossible at the species level. The usage of common names varied considerably. Knowledge of the present distributions of the plants and their preferred habitats was often valuable. The decision to order the material in roughly recognizable field groupings created many problems but will make it more useful to those with practical, rather than reference needs.

Charlotte Erichsen-Brown is a noted and inspired student of the ethnobotany of eastern North America. She has completed a study of great imagination and energy. Whether on a library's reference shelf or in a backpack along the trail, her work will inform and educate, and often amaze.

J.L. Riley, Botany Department, Royal Ontario Museum.
March 1979. Toronto.

CAUTION

This book is not intended for prescribing medication or for curing afflictions. Its purpose is not to replace the services of a physician but rather to serve as a reference in matters relating to the use of plants. The use of any of this information for purposes of self-treatment without consulting a physician can be dangerous. The publisher cannot assume any responsibility for any injury resulting from the utilization of information contained in this book.

INTRODUCTION

"Powerful are the things we use." Menomini.

This book is a record of man's use of some of the plants, trees and shrubs that grow in an area bounded by the Atlantic Ocean on the east, the barren lands of the arctic on the north, south down the western boundaries of Minnesota, Iowa and Missouri, and east along the southern boundaries of Missouri, Kentucky and Virginia. Many of these plants also grow as far south as Florida and Texas and as far west as the Pacific coast. They supplied the various Indian peoples with food, fuel, fiber, clothing, shelter, utensils, transportation and medicine.

I first saw the need for this book seven years ago when I was collecting and drying plants that grow around the Georgian Bay of Lake Huron for my personal herbarium.

I found many books on eating wild plants but only a few of these explained how to identify the plant in the field. There were some older books on the medicinal use of native plants but only about a third of the plants I had collected were mentioned in them. Several good accounts of the use of native plants by the different Indian peoples have been written.

It seemed to me that a book that would bring together the reports of the use of our native plants over the past 500 years would be of help to many people.

Dr. Richard Evans Schultes listened to my outline of such a book and encouraged me to write it. He took me over the Oake Ames Library in Harvard and showed me some of the types of sources I should consult.

As the number of different accounts of the use of each plant grew I saw that they would be more valuable if left in their original form and if they were presented in chronological order. Then the contradictory assertions on the use of each plant would be clear to the reader or researcher. The full record of each plant should always be read as there are frequently conflicting reports on the safe use and the dangers of using a plant or parts of a plant.

As a result of my experience in trying to identify plants in the field, I decided that a non botanical description with a line drawing of each plant would ease the task of the amateur collector, as would also the grouping together of plants found in the woods, or in wet open places or in dry open places.

However, as this is primarily a book about the use of plants, where different species, growing in different habitats, were used for the same purpose, I have placed them together. For instance I have done this with the three main fiber plants, milkweed, dogbane and nettle because it is difficult to know to which of these plants the earliest records of Indian use of a plant for fiber refer.

The first written European reports on the use of a plant in America rarely make plain the species or even genus. Here, only by considering subsequent uses, can a reasonable hypothesis as to the identity of the plant be made. Where it has seemed possible to do this I have included the early reports under the most probable species.

A case in point is Cartier's tree "annedda", included in this book under the spruce tree. It could equally as well have been put under the hemlock tree.

The earliest certain record of the use of any species of plant by man is the recovery of its pollen or seeds in a dated archeological site. This indicates that these plants were used by the peoples who occupied that site at that time. It does not tell us how they were used, except in the case where fiber made from a specific plant is found. This book is based on the premise that only when a species is identified by a competent observer, who is told by the user how he uses that particular plant, is there a valid record of use.

The Indians of Virginia, so clearly portrayed in John White's drawings of 1590, the tribes described by Champlain as he explored the Atlantic coast from 1604-07 from Tadoussac to Boston, the Iroquoian peoples of the St. Lawrence and both sides of Lake Ontario as well as some of the Algonquin tribes to the north and west of them, cultivated corn, beans, pumpkins and tobacco. Cartier's description in 1536 of Hochelega (Montreal) where he found a palisaded village of 50 long houses is confirmed by archeological reports from all over eastern north America of similar village sites surrounded by former corn fields.

All these peoples had a sophisticated agriculture and a net work of trade routes. They had brought corn to its northern limit of development by carrying north with them the seeds of frost resistant plants. They had planted the good edible nut trees near their fields for easy harvest, again bringing some of these trees to their northern limits by choosing the nuts from late budding trees for planting. They spread the native apples, choosing the largest and sweetest to plant near their fields. There is some question as whether they knew how to graft as well. They soaked their corn seed in a decoction of plants before sowing it to protect it from slugs and birds. They sprouted their pumpkin seeds in their houses near their fires ready to plant out as soon as danger of frost had passed. They semi-cultivated the raspberry, two kinds of strawberries, grapes, june-berries, milkweeds and the citron or may apple for its delicious yellow fruit. This is another plant they brought to its northern limit of growth.

They burnt the climax forests around them to make large clearings of sixty acres or more in which to plant their corn and to encourage the growth of those plants they semi-cultivated for medicine, fiber and food. They had a complete knowledge of what roots were good to eat and how to prepare them. They gathered the sweet sap of the maples, birch, beech, hickories and other trees. By 400 A.D. they made ceramic pots and so could boil the maple sap down to a syrup and probably a sugar. Their oil they obtained from nuts, from the seeds of the sunflowers they cultivated and from other seeds they gathered.

The plants that the Indians improved by selection and cultivation exist to-day in many different varieties, i.e. the juneberries or *Amelanchier*. The number of varieties of these plants is much greater than that of the flora as a whole. Not all the plants in our area known to be used by the Indians are discussed in this book for reasons of space. Cultivated plants are outside its scope. However tobacco is dealt with at length because the Indians smoked many plants long before they smoked tobacco in our area and they continued to smoke these plants after they could obtain tobacco.

The Indian smoked primarily in order to please the spirits upon whose goodwill his whole existence depended. The smoke ascended as an incense. Their pipes were hollow stone tubes and, later, tiny pipe bowls. They drew the smoke slowly through their mouths and swallowing it, exhaled it through their nostrils. Several of these plants, as well as tobacco, produced for them a narcotic effect when smoked in this manner. The north eastern American Indian did not ferment plants to produce alcohol deliberately. Vinegar may have been produced and used — this is conjecture — but alcoholic drinks they did not know. Instead they were a civilisation that relied upon narcotics whose effects were obtained by smoking, chewing or drinking a decoction of plant material. Sweet flag was one such plant brought north along the trade routes and planted near the villages.

The Indians also smoked many plants for their medicinal properties. They smudged them upon the fire as revivers of consciousness, or to drive away insects, or as purifiers. Tobacco is of course a potent insecticide and bacteriocide.

There is throughout man's recorded history a duality in his approach to disease and the curing of it. Medicines from plants were used to cure a sore and magic spells were intoned as the plant material was applied. This was the usual method of healing all over the world.

This duality in man's approach to the use of plants for medicine and magic is found in his earliest records, the clay tablets of Sumer of 4000 B.C. There are tablets which contain straightforward prescriptions, giving the names, parts of plants, methods of preparation and dose. There are other tablets, such as the one containing the hymn to the patron deity of the art of medicine, naming half a dozen of the demons who were believed to get into a man's body and cause serious illness. This duality has persisted in all accounts that we have of man's treatment of disease for the last 6000 years.

As man's mastery over his environment grew his fear of unseen evil forces around him lessened. He experimented with different parts of plants for different diseases. The Egyptians were sophisticated users of plant drugs, as their mummies testify. The school of medicine founded by Hippocrates in fifth century Greece represents a plateau in man's long climb out of ignorance and superstition. It is the epitome of man's medical knowledge to that date.

Pliny's exclamation "Is there anything more astonishing than the commerce in plants, which from all points of the globe arrive [in Rome] for the aid of mankind," illustrates the part plants played in the Roman economy. Many of those plant drugs are still traded internationally today.

Dioscorides, the Greek physician gathered together in a book the sum of man's knowledge of the use of plants for medicine up to the first century B.C. Galen wrote in the 2nd. century A.D. his textbook on the medical use of plants that was the bible of the medical profession of the western world for the next 1500 years.

That man had been using plants to heal and for magic for a very much longer period of time was dramatically demonstrated by the finding in 1975 by Leroi-Gourhan of concentrated deposits of pollen in some of the earth taken from near a Neanderthal skeleton in a dig in Iraq where

Solecki was excavating a 60,000 year old burial. The pollen in these deposits was from *Achillea* (yarrow), *Senecio* (groundsel), *Centaurea* (knapweed), *Liliaceae* (grape hyacinth), *Althea* (mallows) and *Ephedra*-type plants. These plants still grow in the area of the tomb to-day and are used by the people living there for medicine.

Solecki wrote (1975) "One thing is certain from Leroi-Gourhan's discovery, these flowers were not accidently introduced into the grave and hence represent clumps of flowers purposely laid down with the Shanidar IV burial. One may speculate that Shanidar IV was not only a very important man, a leader, but may also have been a kind of medicine man or shaman in his group." Richard Evans Schultes remarked that the shaman was usually a knowledgeable botanist and probably the oldest professional man in the evolution of human culture.

Artemisia species also grew wild around the tomb and its pollen was found within it, but not concentrated in any one spot. I put forward the hypothesis here that *Artemisia dracunculus*, linear-leaved wormwood, which grows throughout the steppes of Asia, was carried by wandering bands of hunters as they crossed the land bridge to north America. Possibly during the time that Beringia (the land bridge and parts of Yukon and Alaska) was practically cut off from the rest of north America during the last Ice age but open to central Asia where man was slowly mastering his environment.

Artemisia dracunculus grows on the steppes of Asia and then is not found until one reaches southern Alaska and the Yukon (Beringia) where it grows in a few places. Again it is found spottily across the northern plains eastward to Lake Superior. It is also found down the Pacific coast and around the Mesa Verde cave village in Colorado.

Dioscorides wrote that dracunculus checks cancer, is an abortifacient, killing the foetus, cures gangrene, prevents putrefaction, is good for the eye sight and that those who thoroughly rub their hands with the root cannot be stung by vipers. A woman who belonged to a tribe of hunters which had to move as their game moved would be at a disadvantage at times if she carried a foetus. There would be many wounds to be healed. She would need a plant with the supposed properties of dracunculus.

Densmore found *Artemisia dracunculus*, dracunculus, or linear-leaved wormwood, used on the White Earth Chippewa reservation in Minnesota in 1925 where it was regarded as a "chief medicine", the only plant that must be pulled not dug, a sign of its magic power. The women of the Chippewa used it for difficult labor (plants that abort are also useful to bring down the foetus when its term is reached or to bring on the menses). The leaves and flowers were chewed and used as a poultice for wounds. For stoppage of woman's periods and for heart palpitations the dried leaves and tops of the sterile plant were steeped, and the infusion drunk. This was also drunk for dysentery.

My hypothesis is strengthened by the large degree of variation in the plants of *A. dracunculus* in herbaria and presumably in the wild. This is one of the accepted signs that the plant was semi-cultivated by native people. However only the finding of its pollen in a dated archeological site would be real confirmation.

There is a clone of *A. dracunculus* var. *sativa*, called tarragon and propagated only by root divisions or cuttings. It has a strong anise flavor and leaves a biting sensation in the mouth on being chewed. Fascinatingly enough it was listed in a representation made to the Dutch government in 1650 by some of the Dutch settlers in the New Netherlands (New York) as being among the medicinal plants native to the country that they could find with little search.

The simplest explanation is that it was brought over by some settlers from Holland as a medicinal plant and had escaped from their gardens. It is not a spreader and so would not escape very far. Equally it could have been planted before 1600 by Europeans who stopped over on Manhattan while exploring the coast. Alternatively, it might have been the *A. dracunculus* of western America, traded from hand to hand by Indians as a valuable plant.

The introduction of portulaca (*Portulaca oleracea*) from the south into northeastern north America is on much firmer ground. Neiderberger in her excavations of the Playa phase (6000 to 4500 B.C.) in the Basin of Mexico found in a hearth area an assemblage of well manufactured, ground stone tools, relating to the preparation of food plants, including small grinding slabs. The plant remains identified include seeds of portulaca, a plant with edible fleshy leaves. Neiderberger suggests that this points to an experimental cultivation of plants for food on the shores of Lake Chalco from 6000 B.C. onwards. Her find of nettle seeds, *Urtica dioica* indicates human occupation as well. Nettles were one of the important European and Indian fiber plants of the historic period.

Yarnell reported finding portulaca archeologically in north America from 3000-2500 B.C. and considers it spread by Indian use. McAndrews and Boyko found portulaca pollen in Crawford Lake, Ontario near an Indian village of 1380. They postulate that the women came to the lake to wash the portulaca before preparing it for food.

Interestingly portulaca is also mentioned in the Icelandic medical manuscript of 1475 as a medicinal plant good to drink for jaundice, flux of blood from the stomach, crushed and applied to a toothache or to sore eyes, and good for those who spit blood. When the Jesuit fathers found portulaca growing in Huronia in the seventeenth century they scathingly said that the Indians did not use it but that they themselves put it into the drink they gave their sick.

In spite of all this evidence the leading eastern American taxonomic botanists to-day still refuse to recognise portulaca as an indigenous plant.

Besides influences and plants entering our area from the west and south it is possible that they came from the north also. 400-1200 A.D. was a warm period in the climatic history of the world. By the year 800 very little ice remained in the waters around Greenland. A papal bull of 835 mentions Gronland and Christian settlement there. Mowat (1965) suggests that these may have been Celts driven westward by the Vikings. Erik the Red found human habitations, skin boats and stone tools there when he landed in 985. These could be considered Celtic remains. It is all very speculative as yet.

The evidence for the Viking occupation of Greenland from 985 to 1400 is not speculative. Leif Eriksson's 995-96 voyage to Newfoundland and the existence of several Viking camps there from 1004-7 is now established. The small wooden statue recently found under the floor of a Thule house, the figure dressed in a 13th. century Scandinavian long-hooded cassock with a cross incised on his breast, attests to the continuing presence of the norsemen there. That they penetrated into the interior of the continent as far as Lake Nipigon is not yet accepted although Mowat makes a persuasive case.

What is known is that there was a trade route from the St. Lawrence and Lake Ontario to Lake Superior and further north. Furs of the Algonquin tribes of the north were traded to the Huron and Iroquois peoples for corn, tobacco and nets. Crawford Lake village was a thriving community in 1380.

Given the long occupation, almost 400 years, as long as the current European occupation of North America, of the Vikings and norsemen in the north and the trade routes from there to the south, ideas, and the valuable cult objects and medicinal practices of the norsemen could have influenced some of the Indian nations to the south.

The evidence has been accumulating that the Atlantic coast was a busy place from 1400 onwards. It was then that the Bristol merchants sent ships to trade with Iceland and possibly Greenland, as well as to fish and whale. The Basque whalers, who also fished for cod, came over each year to their chosen cove, often on Newfoundland. They would leave some of their men ashore to process the fish and go out to the banks.

These ordinary seamen, while they held firmly to the old European beliefs in demons and charms, also knew that many illnesses could be cured by using the appropriate plant. They certainly did not set out in the early 1400's across the Atlantic without taking with them a few of the plants they would need to cure dysentery, poison, fevers, and other troubles. Nor can it be credited that they did not plant the seeds of those that they considered most efficacious near their temporary summer camps, especially as they seem to have come back year after year to the same spot.

At Quiddy Viddy, near St. John's Newfoundland is found the European plant, Tormentil, one of the very few spots it grows in north America. Tormentil has traditionally been regarded as an antidote for all poisons and good against the venom of any creature. It guards against the plague and is good for pestilential fevers and contagious diseases. Clearly a valuable plant to have by one when long voyages on crowded, unsanitary, small ships bred these pestilential fevers.

That these seamen were trading with the Indians is witnessed by the finding of two copper trade beads in the 1500 A.D. Draper site in Ontario by Finlayson (1975). Few commodities have been regarded by man as more valuable than drugs and these may very well also have been traded.

In 1514 it was stated that the French had been paying a tax on the fish caught off the coast of the new world and other islands for the last 60 years. The St. Lawrence is said to have been explored by Jean Denys in 1506. In 1508 Thomas Aubert brought back Micmac or Boethuk Indians to France where they were used as models for part of a work in bas-relief which is still preserved in the Church of St James in Dieppe. Aubert is said to have ascended the St. Lawrence to a distance of 80 leagues. There was a Portuguese whaling station on Newfoundland 1520–25.

Cartier was told by the Indians who boarded his ship, "as freely as if they had been Frenchmen", along the north shore of the St. Lawrence in 1534, that "the ships had all set sail from the bay laden with fish". Showing that by then the fishing vessels had begun to penetrate beyond the strait of Belle Isle. The crews of some of these fishing boats occasionally may have passed the winter with the Indian bands.

On his second voyage Cartier wintered at Stadacona (Quebec) in 1535–36 and visited the thriving Laurentian Iroquois village of Hochelaga (Montreal). His men sickened of scurvy and were so debilitated by it that he was afraid to let the Indians know of their condition. He saw that his friend dom Agaya, who had been sick with scurvy, was completely cured and asked him what he had taken. Dom Agaya showed Cartier the tree they used and sent some women with branches and instructions as to how to prepare and use them. Some of his men finally drank the decoction of the branches, washed with it and were cured, "an evident miracle."

Cartier's account of this affair is quoted in full in translation from his original French because it is so often repeated in part and at second hand. Also it is the first record of a specific use of a north eastern north American plant to cure a disease.

The Laurentian Iroquois of Cartier's time certainly knew how to cure scurvy, by using a drink made of the branches of a tree very high in vitamin C, almost certainly either the spruce or the hemlock, as the green branches were picked during the winter. This knowledge of the Indians was far in advance of that of the Europeans of that time. Indeed they anticipated by 400 years the European discovery of the correct cure for scurvy. An account of the scourge that scurvy was to the Europeans in America from 1535 to the early 1700's and even later, is also given under spruce in the text. Cartier apparently did not succeed in bringing back to France either the seeds or seedlings of the tree "annedda" that cured his men. As the Laurentian Iroquois of Cartier's time were conquered by Algonquin who did not know of the use of either the spruce or the hemlock to cure scurvy, the secret, so badly needed, was lost.

The Indians, dom Agaya and Taignoagny were taken to France by Cartier on his return from his first voyage in 1534 and returned to Quebec with him in 1535. It was then that dom Agaya told Cartier of the tree annedda. The Chief Donnacona went back with Cartier in 1536 to tell the King of all the marvels to be found in his country, Canada. He obliged by weaving some fantastic tales. Thevet talked to Donnacona while he was in France.

Champlain on his first voyage to America in 1603 tells of DuPont bringing back to Tadoussac two Indians he had taken to France. They told their tribe, who assembled to hear them, how well they had been treated in France and of the castles, palaces, peoples and their manner of living.

Nearly one hundred years earlier in 1509, seven Indians and their birchbark canoe were taken to Rouen. It seems to have been a consistent practice to return from a voyage to the New World with some of the native people. Those who returned to their tribes would have brought knowledge of European medical practice with them as they were treated for their illnesses while in France.

The next reported medical use of a plant was that of Alfonse who wrote of his 1542 voyage to the St. Lawrence that there were "large numbers of cedars. . .arbre de vye which contain medicine, they have a gum that is white as snow. . .also some very large cedars." Here "arbre de vye" best fits the Canada balsam, *Abies balsamea*. The Indians used its gum as medicine. Boucher (1663) reported that the gum was used on wounds like balm and had much virtue. It was in use in English Canada for healing wounds at the end of the 18th. century. It is known today that the gum is antiseptic, another Indian use that we would consider the correct one, if my hypothesis is right.

The next report is that of Thevet in France in 1557, writing of the Gulf of St. Lawrence, which he knew only through Donnacona and Cartier's accounts, that : "when the savages are ill with fever or persecuted with other interior illness they take the leaves of a tree which is very like cedars, and take the juice which they drink. In 24 hours they are not as sick, the drink cures them. Christians have tried this drink and brought the tree to France." White cedar was reported growing in Paris in 1558. Seventy-five years later Father LeJeune reported that the Huron cured dysentery by drinking the juice of the leaves or branches of cedar which they boiled, and that a child had recovered after taking this medicine. Dysentery was endemic for the next 300 years or more in north America. The Huron also used cedar branches as an emetic. One hundred years later the Algonquin were reported to be using cedar branches in an enema for bloody flux.

What was the state of man's knowledge of medicine in Europe in 1534? What did Cartier's surgeons on board his vessels know?

After the fall of Rome the knowledge of medicine summed up by Dioscorides and Galen was kept alive in Egypt at Alexandria, in the Jewish colleges, in Iran (Persia) and in the middle east. Alexander's conquests in Afghanistan had made the amalgamation of Greek and Indian medicine possible, from this the Arabian medicine developed. The monasteries in Europe copied Dioscorides' and Galen's books, and each had their medicinal plant gardens.

But it was the flowering of the Arabian civilisation from 750-1450 A.D. that saw the establishment of medical schools, each with its medicinal plant garden, where material for use and experimentation could be at hand, and foreign medicinal plants collected and grown. These were established wherever the Arabs conquered and ruled. The great Arabian books on medicine were, along with those of Galen and Dioscorides, the foundation of European medicine.

When Salerno was retaken from the Arabs in 1060 Constantine Africanus was made head of the former Arabian medical college there. The teaching at Salerno was based on that of Greece and Rome, with a minimum of magic incorporated. It was on the writings of Constantine Africanus and of Macer, also of the School of Salerno, that the Icelandic medical manuscript of 1475, quoted in this book, is based. This manuscript is valuable in that it gives in clear terms how a particular plant was used from 1000-1600 in European medicine. It is also valuable as it was written by and for norsemen, our first authenticated white settlers.

Cabot was sent by Henry of England in 1494 to north America to look for spices and drugs. Cabot had been to Mecca in a caravan in 1476 and Henry wanted to establish a spice and drug depot in England larger than that at Alexandria through which most of the valuable drugs used in medicine in Europe passed. It was not Cabot who found the drugs but the Spaniards landing much further south.

The medicinal plant gardens of the Aztecs amazed the Spaniards when they first saw them. These gardens had been established in 1467 by Motecuzoma I and were maintained primarily to provide the Aztec medical profession with raw materials for medical formulas and experimentation. The Emperor's envoys had orders to seek out additional species wherever they went.

Some Spaniards had the wit to understand that the Aztecs had a medical knowledge in many respects comparable if not in advance of their own. It was a Spanish axiom that native diseases should be treated by native medicines. Some members of the Franciscan order arrived in Mexico in 1529 just after the conquest and started schools where they taught the sons of Aztec nobles latin as well as other subjects. These schools and a college founded in 1536, were encouraged by Emperor Charles V and funded by his viceroy. In this college, for a short time, these Aztec boys studied science and the medical use of native plants taught them by Aztec physicians. It was here, in 1552, that one such physician wrote what is known as the Badianus manuscript, an illustrated book giving the Aztec medicinal use of many native plants.

The foundation and cherishing of these schools was the work of a Franciscan, Father Sahagun, who himself wrote a book on the Aztec medicinal plants using as his source Aztec physicians. This flowering of tolerance and understanding was brief. The conservative forces in the Church triumphed. It was these forces that ruled when the Jesuit Fathers poured scorn on the medical knowledge of the native peoples among whom they lived in northeastern north America. One can't help speculating how much valuable knowledge of the use by the native peoples of their plants has been lost because a man of Sahagun's calibre did not live in Huronia in the 1630s.

By 1600 there had been about 200 years of European contact with the various Indian tribes on the Atlantic coast from Virginia northwards. The fishing boats did a little buying of furs on the side and came into the natural harbors where the Indians waited for them to obtain the iron pots, hatchets and knives that could save them weeks of work with their stone tools.

Lescarbot wrote (1609) that the Indians from Port Royal to Tadoussac spoke a pidgin Basque and called Frenchmen "Normans" in the Basque language. Various settlements of Europeans, stranded on the Atlantic coast from Tadoussac in the north to Roanoke in the south, had disappeared. The young boys who accompanied all expeditions at that time probably would have been adopted into any Indian tribe that found them alive.

All this long and continuous contact of Indian and white makes it quite possible that the Indians learnt how to use some European medicines from the various ships' surgeons, who, it has been recorded, were not above trading the contents of their medicine chests for furs. The Indians were eager to try European medicine because the white gods were obviously more powerful.

Lescarbot describes in 1609 the Indian medicine man, Membertou, curing a wound by scarifying it, sucking it and then placing slices of the beaver's stones upon it. The Icelandic medical manuscript of 1475 recommended beaver's stones to help all sores and injuries, to ease swelling, pressure and pain.

Beaver's stones are known by the name of castor, or castoreum which is a reddish-brown substance consisting of the preputial follicles of the beaver and their contents, dried and prepared for commercial purposes. It has long had a high repute as a medicine and contains salicin which is antiseptic and eases pain. It is also an important commercial article in perfumery. The beaver used to be a common animal in all the northern parts of the world.

While not a plant the use of castoreum is mentioned because it is a specific medicine cited in one of the earliest written reports and also because it was used for the same purpose, the correct one as we now regard it, by both the Indians and the Europeans in 1600.

The arum is another example of a medicine used for the same purpose both in Europe and by an Indian nation, in this case, by the Huron, as reported by Sagard in 1624. He recommended bringing the plant to France. Obviously he did not know that Galen had prescribed the root of the arum to purge phlegm, the same purpose for which it was used by the Huron.

Pine gum is another such medicine. In England Gerarde in 1633 remarked that the liquid resin issuing from wild pines was good for healing wounds. Boucher in Quebec in 1663 wrote that the savages use pine gum for wounds "for which it is a very sovereign remedy". In all these cases the remedy could and probably was discovered on both sides of the Atlantic independently. These remedies could, on the other hand be very ancient ones going back to a common source. Finally as has been shown, it is entirely possible that some Indian tribes could have learnt of these remedies from the white man during the 200 years of contact before 1600.

There are equally confused reports as to what the whites learnt from the Indians. Fenton (1942) claimed that the Iroquois taught the settlers the virtues of sassafras. The facts are that Monardes in 1577 promoted its value in Europe where it was enthusiastically received as it was hoped it would alleviate syphilis which was rampant there. Boats from 1601 onwards sailed across the Atlantic and returned loaded with sassafras. The Europeans experimented with sassafras for at least 50 years before they had any contact with the Iroquoian nations in what is now New York state. Incidentally, sassafras does not grow naturally at Quebec or Montreal where Cartier first met the Laurentian Iroquois.

The Europeans were reluctant to try Indian medicine. They much preferred their own with a few exceptions such as sassafras. Father Garnier in Huronia in 1641 writes of the "dearth of this country" and asks for some medicinal seeds from France such as purgatives. All around him were excellent purgatives in the native plants. The Huron medicine men and women knew which plants purged. They knew when and what part to collect, the preparation and the dosage. One example is the dogbane *Apocynum androsaemifolium* or *A. cannabinum*, which Clayton in 1687 mentions the Indians of Virginia using as a purge. Millspaugh cites it as an emetic and a cathartic. The Hurons almost certainly used it as such as it was one of their fiber plants, and there is a wide Indian use of these plants in medicine.

Elder root bark was used by the Onondaga in 1809 as the emetic of choice when poisoned by the root of *Cicuta maculata*, the poisonous plant called water hemlock. Sagard mentioned in 1624 that when a Frenchman ate some of this root, becoming very ill, the Hurons immediately gave him emetics, saving his life. Elder has been used in Europe and the middle east since the time of the Egyptians as a purge. The Indians knew it was a strong purge, one to be handled with caution. Elder also grows all over Huronia.

All early European accounts are in agreement that the Indian nations, and this seems to apply to all of them, had better methods of healing wounds than they did. Lescarbot says Membertou when called on to heal a wound, "sucked the bad blood from it." Clayton some 60 years later wrote that the Virginia Indians sucked the nasty matter out of a wound with their mouths until the wound was clean. "A very nasty but no doubt the most effectual way and the best imaginable." This demonstrates the Indian knowledge of poisons, they apparently knew that if the matter was held in the mouth, not swallowed but spat out, there was no danger of poisoning. Morice in 1901 reported that the Carriers of the north have some members of their tribe who are known as "He whose mouth effects cure."

Champlain mentions that his friend Chief Yroquet brought his son, who had been badly mauled by a bear, to the winter camp of the Algonquin near Cahiague (Orillia) in the winter of 1616. The Algonquin, perhaps because of their Medewiwin, or grand medicine lodge, were considered to be great healers.

Cadillac wrote from Detroit (1698) of the Potawatomi and other Algonquin tribes gathered there, "They are very good anatomists and so when they have an arm or any bone broken they treat it very cleverly and with great skill and dexterity and experience shows that they can cure a wounded man better in a week than our surgeons can in a month."

Deliette reported in 1702 that the commander of a Miami war party carried with him on the war path herbs for healing the wounded. The gum of the Canada balsam and that of the pine tree have been mentioned as being used by the Indian tribes to heal wounds. Sagard wrote in 1624 that the Huron chewed the root of a plant called *oscar* to heal all sorts of sores and wounds. This is considered to be American sarsaparilla, *Aralia nudicaulis*. The 1724 memoir on the Miami medicinal plants lists it as used by them for sores and cuts. Zeisberger says the same of the Delaware in 1779. Rafinesque reports the same use by whites and Indians at the beginning of the 19th. century. This plant is a relative of our American ginseng, *Aralia quinquefolia*. Perhaps its chemistry should be fully investigated.

Smartweed juice was sprayed on the wound by the Virginia Indians in 1687. Over one hundred years later Tournefort in Paris found that a decoction of smartweed restrained the progress of gangrene.

Leatherwood (*Dirca palustris*) is an entirely Indian remedy, as is American sarsaparilla. It was a textile plant of importance being found in archeological sites dated 400 B.C.-250 A.D. in Ohio. Sarrazin 1708 wrote that the Indians used the cooked bark of leatherwood to alleviate the pain of old ulcers, hemorrhoids and cancer.

Another area of medical knowledge in which the advanced Indian nations of northeastern north America were ahead of contemporary European practice was in that of childbirth. In Europe bearing a child often meant the loss of both mother and child from infection or botched delivery. The tombstones of our oldest cemeteries tell the same story on this continent several hundred years later. The native peoples had a much better system. The medicine woman of the tribe kept the mother on a special regime for weeks before delivery. She was given a tea made of the root of the blue cohosh (*Caulophyllum thalictroides*) and her delivery was usually easy and swift. The root possesses caulosaponine which provokes strong uterine contractions, intermittent and more successful ones that those provoked by ergot, the plant fungus used by white physicians for the same purpose in childbirth. The Indians also used the blue cohosh root to control profuse menstrual discharge. White women who were settled far from doctors and even other white women were glad to have the help of the Indian midwife. The blue cohosh became widely known and appreciated. It was adopted by the Eclectic doctors. Among other plants used to facilitate childbirth by the Indians were the roots of trilliums, yellow clintonia and wild ginger.

The wild ginger root is known to contain an antibacterial substance against gram positive pus forming bacteria. The Illinois in 1724 used the root, crushed to powder, for putting stop to the pains of women in childbirth. Much later the Algonquin used it in dressing wounds. The Meskwaki put it into any meat they considered might be tainted when cooking it. Warriors were reported to mix it with the rations they carried on the warpath. It was considered to guard food against sorcerers.

Rafinesque reported that the Indians used wild ginger root to abort the foetus and to-day it is considered an oral contraceptive thought to excite temporary sterility. Indian women were experts in methods of birth control. Wandering bands could not afford too many children, everyone would starve if there were more mouths than food to feed them. Bloodroot was mentioned by Sarrazin in 1708 in Quebec as being used by the Indian women there as an abortifacient. Sarrazin did not consider it had this property but used it instead to control the menses. Rafinesque in 1830 considered it an abortifacient but he knew nothing of the previous Indian use. Plants that brought on the menses, could also abort the foetus and were useful when it had grown to full term to help deliver it.

Any woman reading this book would be very foolish to try dosing herself with any of the plants mentioned. Indian medicine women spent years learning to know the plants, the parts of a plant, their preparation and dosage. They learnt of the difficulties and dangers that could arise from taking these medicines. They learnt what to do in such cases. They had a full, practical knowledge of the poisonous properties of the plants that grew around them. In most cases a dose that aborts, if a little too much is given, can kill. The case histories are full of tragedies. The fine line between killing and curing is not learnt by reading any book.

It is in the knowledge the Indians had of the poisonous properties of their plants that they demonstrated their undoubted control of the plant material they used in their medicines.

In 1628 de Rasiere in the New Netherlands describes the training young Indian men were given. "He must go out every morning (in May) with the person who is ordered to take him in hand; he must go into the forest to seek the wild herbs and roots, which they know to be the most poisonous and bitter; these they bruise in water and press the juice out of them, which he must drink, and immediately have ready such herbs as will preserve him from death or vomiting; for if he cannot retain it, he must repeat the dose until he can support it, and until his constitution becomes accustomed to it so that he can retain it."

Father Brebeuf in 1636 wrote of the performance of the curing ceremony in which those who took part gave each other poison. As it had not been practised before among this Huron band it is probable that the neighbouring Algonquin members of the Medewiwin, or grand medicine society, came and performed this dance. Brebeuf says that the members of the society often avenged their injuries and gave poison to their patients instead of medicine.

This knowledge of, and skill with, poisons, was obtained by scientific experiment. Father Biard writes in 1617 that some of the Indians of Gaspesia had bought some arsenic and sublimate from certain French ship's surgeons in order to kill whoever they wished and boasted that they had already experimented upon a captive who died the day after taking the dose they gave him.

Raudot in 1709 wrote that the Indians were prone to commit suicide by taking the root of the poisonous water hemlock, *Cicuta maculata*, or that of the may apple, *Podophyllum peltatum*.

This mastery of the poisonous plants in their environment makes nonsense of claims that the Indian peoples stumbled by chance on the plants they used for medicine. They knew to a nicety the amount needed for a killing dose. They had birchbark measuring spoons to be sure the right dose was taken. They also knew of poisons that killed slowly, taking years to do so according to Zeisberger in 1779 writing of the Delaware.

Narcotic and poisonous plant material was also administered by scarification. This was the scratching of the skin until some blood flowed, the decoction then being rubbed into the scratches. This often left its color in the skin and this was regarded as a charm against the return of the disease. Tatooing and scarification for medical purposes blend into one another in aboriginal practice.

Champlain describes the head of a gar pike, given him on the Atlantic coast by an Indian. He was told that it was used when anyone had a bad headache to scratch the part where the pain was. The use of a decoction of the root of the poisonous water hemlock in scarification by various Indian tribes confirms their knowledge that this plant eases pain when administered in this manner.

Another important method of curing the sick was the sweat bath. Coe (1966) reports the existence in 850 A.D. in the ruins of the Classic Maya site, Piedras Negras in Mexico of eight sweat baths. These were complete with stone built hearths lined with potsherd, masonry benches for the bathers and drains to carry off the water used in the bath. Sweat baths were used in Saxon England. Their value and dangers are discussed in the Icelandic medical manuscript of 1475.

Huron Smith describes how the Ojibwe and Menomini used coils of the branches of Canada balsam, hemlock, white pine, white cedar and American yew in their sweat baths which they took for cleansing, medication or ceremonial reasons. Candidates for degrees in the medicine lodge must undergo a sweat bath in a ceremonial way. He remarks that the methods of taking a sweat bath had not changed much over time.

Lescarbot, writing of the Indians of Acadia in 1606 says, "But yet they have other preservatives which they use very often, that is to say sweats, whereby they prevent sickness." He goes on to describe how they build and use the sweat bath. Capt. John Smith wrote of the Indian sweat baths in Virginia in 1612 and De Vries of those in the New Netherlands. Champlain wrote of the Huron practice when he wintered in Huronia in 1616. "To bring a cure the Oqui will go and sweat himself with several of his friends. For two or three hours they will steam themselves under long strips of bark, wrapped up in skins with stones heated in the fire. They sing the whole time, stopping only to catch their breath or take a drink of water, for of course they get extremely thirsty."

Sagard reports the use of the sweat bath both for preserving health and curing the sick among the Huron. He says some of the French joined the Indians in the bath and was astonished that they could and would support it and that modesty did not persuade them to abstain. Thirty years later Evelyn (Diary 1655) reported seeing at St. Germaine in France some caves walled off and set aside for the sick to sweat in.

Sweat baths were also an important part of that other side of medicine, the magic side. The shaman or medicine man took a sweat bath in order to find the answers to questions such as whether his tribe would win the coming battle, the cause of an epidemic, where the game was, as well as to bring rain or make his medicine more effective.

Another purpose of the sweat bath was ceremonial purification prepatory to initiation into the Medewiwin. The candidate must also fast. Father Brebeuf wrote in 1636 that formerly it was necessary for a candidate for medicine man among the Huron to fast for thirty days in a cabin apart and for his servant who brought him his wood to fast also. The candidate must talk to the spirits during his fast.

The Winnebago shaman told the candidate for initiation, "If you do not possess one of the spirits from whom to obtain this strength and power you will be of no consequence socially and those around you will show you little respect. . .If you are blessed by the spirits and if you then blow your breath upon people who are ill they will become well and thus you will help your fellow man" (Radin 1957). This dual aspect, the spiritual and altruistic on the one hand, and the economic and social on the other, is part and parcel of all shamanism, as it is of society everywhere, even the 20th. century western medical profession.

In the best tradition, the Winnebago medicine man offers tobacco to grandmother earth, and asks her to let him take the herbs he needs. "Make my medicine powerful, grandmother." The two most general theories of the cause of disease were the entry into the body of a foreign object which the shaman must remove before recovery could take place, or the loss of the soul which must be induced by the shaman to return. The practical and indisputable fact that herbs, sweating and purging were also effective did not in the least lessen the need of the tribe for the shaman.

While the shaman owed his power to his control over and ability to talk to the spirits, magic does not owe its power to any supernatural being. Magic forces an object to do what you wish it to do. This act of magic is dangerous and therefore the doer must protect himself by knowing the correct spells, the words, and the correct actions, the rites, so that his own magic does not turn around and harm him. A simple magic act performed by many to-day is spitting on the dice before throwing them, while intoning certain words. We can all think of many others.

Most of the magic charms listed by Densmore as used by the Chippewa were hunting charms. Before the Indian possessed firearms the ability to approach game close enough to kill with a bow and arrow required a magic charm to lure the game towards you. Clayton's account (1687) in this book of the Virginia Indian who used the angelica root to call the deer to him is worth reading in this context. There is the possibility that something about the odor of the plant actually attracts the game sought. The female deer secretes a scent between her toes that attracts the male deer and the hunter tries to mimic this scent with his hunting charm. Sweet flag root was used to scent the nets and ensure a full catch of whitefish.

Love potions were also very important. They sold for the highest prices and few white inquirers were told of all the ingredients. Both the blue and red lobelia roots were used to reconcile quarrelsome couples. Doubtless if both men and women believed such potions worked, they did.

A curing ceremony of the Huron that impressed the Jesuits was described by Father Pijart in 1637. A number of stones about the size of pigeon eggs were placed in a fire hot enough to burn the cabin down. The medicine men placed their hands behind their backs and bending down took the red hot stones in their mouths, holding them well within the mouth for as long as a minute. They walked to the patients and blew on them. When one spat out a stone it fell on the ground and sparks of fire issued from it. Next morning one of the performers' mouth was examined and found to be unmarked, unhurt and whole. Champlain and Sagard also describe such ceremonies where hot coals were taken in the mouth or rubbed by the medicine man's hands. In other ceremonies the hands and arms were plunged into boiling liquid.

Younken (1924) reports that the Zuni of the southwest had secret fraternities who performed with fire. They chewed the flower heads and roots of yarrow beforehand and rubbed this mixture on their limbs. Those who danced in the fire used this same mixture for bathing beforehand. They placed some in their mouths before taking red hot coals in the mouth for as long as a minute. To-day it is known that yarrow stimulated the flow of gastric juices and is useful as a gargle in inflammation of the gums.

Father Lalement in 1641 writes of one Huron who pretended to handle the hot coals with the other medicine men but was very careful not to touch them. One night he dreamed that he was handling fire and heard a song which he remembered perfectly when he awoke. He sang this song at the next fire handling ceremony and found he could take live coals in his mouth and plunge his bare arm in boiling kettles without feeling any pain or being injured. On the contrary he felt a coolness of the hands and mouth.

Alexandra David-Neel (1931) describes the training undergone by anchorites in Tibet in order to learn how to sleep on the ice and snow in the depth of winter without any covering other than a cotton shirt. It was a process of concentrating the mind on warmth. Thinking of heat until finally they became warm. In Tibet power was obtained by learning to concentrate one's energies.

The north American shaman learned by dreaming. All early reports agree that the guiding principle of the Indian's life was the dream. Nothing of consequence could be done without the right dream. Every member of the tribe dreamt, but only those who had had several true dreams would be taken seriously.

The shaman fasted apart to dream of the plant that would cure a particular disease. The account of the dream of the muskrat root as told in the text under sweet flag is typical. Each shaman was therefore a specialist. He would treat only certain diseases. He consulted with other medicine men and was also often at odds with the various other ranks of sorcerers.

The Greek principle of nothing to excess guided the life of the American Indian to the extent that the shaman believed that if he tried to dream of the cures for too many disease, or tried to use his powers too often, they might leave him. When gathering his medicinal plants, only a few could be taken from a patch. The rule was always leave a growing plant.

The Medewiwin or grand medicine lodge of the Algonquin exemplifies the duality of magic rites on the one hand and a solid botanical knowledge of plants and their properties on the other.

The practical knowledge of which environments produced plants having the highest quantity of the desired properties; what parts of the plants to pick and at what time in their growing cycle; how best to preserve them; how to prepare the medicine, knowing whether some plants were spoiled by boiling and should only be infused; what doses to give in different illnesses, all this invaluable tribal knowledge was held by the medewiwin and handed down in their ceremonies and recorded on the mnemonic birch bark scrolls. The giving and taking of poisons and their antidotes was also a part of the ceremonies.

The candidate for initiation had to pay by gifts to the Medewiwin for the right to be initiated. He had to fast and sweat and be instructed by his mentor. Only some of the plants and their properties and methods of use were taught at each level. The costs became progressively larger, the higher the rank the candidate was trying to enter.

The purpose of this insistence throughout the native medicine of north America of payment for the right to learn how to cure a particular disease was to make certain that this hard won knowledge was not lost or adulterated. What is bought at a high price mankind everywhere regards as valuable and to be carefully guarded. Among the Huron, where there was no Medewiwin, this rule also applied. If a man was cured of his sickness and had paid for the cure, then the medicine man told him how he had effected the cure. The patient could then use his knowledge to cure someone else on payment of a fee.

The rites and magic ceremonies had also to be learnt by the initiate. He must know just which ones should be performed with each cure. We now realise that these rites and ceremonies could be as important in effecting a cure as the medicine swallowed. This is the fashionable "placebo effect". The faith that the patient has in the ability of the physician, or in his methods, or medicine will help to relieve even angina pain. Dr. Benson of Boston, in research published in 1979, found that 82% of the patients improved after taking placebos (sugar pills).

It is known now that the brain manufacturers its own pain killer, or opiates called endorphins. Much is being learnt about the chemistry of the brain and its effect upon the body. The curing ceremonies of the Huron described at length by the Jesuits, created the necessary environment in which the placebo effect could operate.

When the Europeans first encountered the Shamanism of the northeastern American Indian during the period 1500-1650, they were in their turn bound by their own mental set, which was as rigid and surprisingly quite like that of the Indians whom they so derided. Europe had been persecuting witches and sorcerers for hundreds of years. Everyone was afraid of sorcery and the persecution of anything that could be suspected to be sorcery was total and unreasoning.

The Church relied on St. Thomas and St. Augustine when they said, "All that happens visibly in this world, can be done by demons." The Papal bull of 1484 gave sanction to this theory and to the persecution. Huizinga could write (1924), "So towards the end of the middle ages this dark system of delusion and cruelty grew slowly to completion. . .transmitted to the coming age like a horrible disease that for a long time neither the classical culture, nor the Protestant reformation, nor the Catholic revival were able or even willing to cure."

Montaigne, the epitome of classical culture, could write in 1595, "All that is over and above simple death appears to me pure cruelty. Our justice cannot hope that the man who is not deterred from wrong doing by fear of being hanged or beheaded will be prevented by the idea of slow fire, or the pincers, or the wheel."

The Jesuit fathers who encountered torture, slow fire and the cruelty of the Huron and other Indian tribes were dealing with social behaviour that they were totally familiar with within their own Church. The Church was rooting out sorcery in Europe and the Jesuits tried to root it out in north America. They ridiculed the shaman, medicine men, sorcerers, good, bad and indifferent whenever they had a chance. In the tribes which came totally under their influence and were dependent on the white man for support, the shamans' power was broken. With him went the tribal pride, its heritage and the knowledge so hardly won over so long a time.

The medical practices of Europe were often similar to those of the Indians. The section on charms in the Icelandic medical manuscript of 1475 advises washing the cross in the church with holy water and then pouring that water over the sick person, giving him some to drink and reciting a special prayer. That would cure him.

The church believed that baptism would cure, they believed in omens, they believed in demons. Marie de l'Incarnation wrote a letter in 1661 that is revealing. She writes of magicians from France that caused a young girl to be persecuted with spectres, flying objects and stones. She writes of the Fathers going to drive away the demons with the prayers of the Church. Then she says, "After this pursuit of sorcerers, all these regions were afflicted with a universal malady, of which it is believed they are the authors. . . .We had never yet seen a like mortality, for the malady terminated in pleurisy accompanied by fever. I do not believe twenty persons in Canada were free from this sickness, which was so universal that there is a strong foundation for the belief that those wretches had poisoned the air."

The apothecaries of Europe used fat in making up many of their pills, apparently even human fat. After the hideous massacre of St. Bartholemew in France in 1572, at a certain signal the populace ran furiously and threw all the bodies into the river, reserving the fattest who they left for the apothecaries.

European medical practice relied almost entirely on purgatives such as rhubarb and aloes from the east and hence expensive, bleeding and treacle. This was called Theriac in French and was a mixture of some 150 plants, animal parts, minerals and precious stones that had been first concocted by Nero's physician and constantly improved since then. It was prepared at Montpellier in France, in Venice, and hence also called Venice treacle, and in Queen Elizabeth's time in London under the superintendance of the College of Physicians. There were great controversies in Europe over its composition and who had the right to make it and sell it. Because Galen had recommended Mithradatum, an earlier name for Theriac, as a cure for all poisons, bites, headaches, vertigo, deafness, epilepsy, dimness of sight, loss of voice, asthma, coughs, spitting of blood, tightness of breath, colic, appendicitis, jaundice, hardening of the spleen, stone, fevers, dropsy, leprosy, and all pestilences, and because Galen's writings dominated medical practice for 1500 years, every physician of note prescribed theriac and also claimed to have made some improvement on the formula. Apothecaries made their own mixtures and pawned them off as the real Venice treacle.

Theriac was carried in every ship's medicine chest, it was at the top of the list of medicines ordered from France for the use of the King's troops in Quebec in 1698. It was in every missionary's and explorer's bag. The Icelandic medical manuscript regarded theriac as an antidote, a counter-poison that "exceedingly helps those to whom it is given." Orvietan was a similar mixture regarded as a panacea and popular in France in the 17th century.

Sarrazin's account of a laborer in Quebec who ate the root of the poisonous water hemlock, *Cicuta maculata*, and feeling ill took some theriac and then died, sums up the difference between Indian and European medicines in 1700. The Huron, as Sagard reported in 1624, knew that strong emetics must be given immediately after eating this root or death followed. Sarrazin and presumably the other physcians in Quebec in 1700 also knew an emetic must be given immediately but the settlers did not. Sarrazin saw 3 people die and he knew of 12 or 15 who had died in the last ten years. Some ate the root cooked and fell into lethargic sleep, they were saved by an emetic. There is no mention of its use externally. Theriac was of no use against the water hemlock. This suggests that the French settlers were not familiar with Indian medicine.

Hennepin (1698) wrote that he kept his orvietan carefully by him in his travels in the interior. He claims to have cured Indians bitten by rattlesnakes by scarifying the bite and sprinkling orvietan on it. He credits it with keeping himself and his companions in good health. Radisson, exploring Hudson Bay, also relied upon orvietan. The anonymous reporter on the medical practices of the Illinois and Miami wrote that they used wild ginger root for the bite of the rattlesnake but that orvietan and treacle had a faster and more certain effect.

It is interesting to speculate that if theriac did have any effect in diseases, and it must have had some to have lasted for 1500 years as a principal medicine, it may have been due to the vipers that were Andromachus's addition to the formula. Moses Charas, the great European physician (1618-1698), whose pharmacopoiea was translated into Chinese by the order of the Emperor of China, gives these directions for making oil of vipers. Take 12 large, fat, shiny, live vipers, put 3 lbs. of the purest olive oil into a glazed earthern pot with a narrow mouth; heat it until too hot for a finger to bear; put in the vipers one by one, and when they are smothered, add 2 ozs. of white wine. Cover the pot and heat until the humidity of the vipers has about disappeared, then cool and express.

Kilmon reported in 1975 that snake venom offers promise in the treatment of a wide variety of nervous, muscular, immunological and metabolic disorders. Cobratoxin from cobra venom is a more effective analgesic than morphine. It works by blocking nerve transmissions and only one daily dose is required. It seems possible that some of the myriad cures claimed for mithradatum, theriac and orvietan, if they contained oil of vipers prepared as Charas recommended, may also have been due to the toxin that might be found in them.

The medical training given in France in the 17th. and 18th. centuries was regarded as the best in Europe. Every ship leaving France was obliged to carry a surgeon for the duration of the voyage who often had to fill the triple role of physician, surgeon and apothecary at sea so he was also taught physiology and anatomy. Champlain had his surgeons perform post mortems on some of those who each year died in New France of scurvy. He wanted to be sure they had all died as the result of the same disease and also to see if any cause could be found for it.

There was a botanical garden attached to the medical school in Paris as well as the King's garden. All French explorers were looking for strange and interesting plants. Boucher in 1663 described some of the trees and plants growing in Quebec. Dr. Michel Sarrazin, who practiced medicine in Quebec following 1698 collected the native plants. He had a herbarium in Quebec of 800 specimens and a library of 178 books. Between 1698 and 1708 he sent each year to Vaillant, at the Jardin des Plantes in Paris, specimens of these plants, occasionally with notes on their use in Quebec and by the Indians.

When de Glassoniere was governor of New France he ordered a young doctor, just arrived in Quebec from Paris, Jean Gaultier, to prepare a questionnaire to be sent to all the officers at the French posts in the interior and given to all missionaries and travellers as well. A number of trees and plants were to be collected, including the senega snakeroot which had created such interest in England 5 years earlier. Other kinds of seeds and roots were to be gathered. The methods of doing so was stated as well as how to preserve them for shipment to Quebec. There Gaultier received them and planted them in the garden of the Superintendant's palace, sending specimens on to France. The Marquis de Glassoniere himself sailed for France in 1749 with a quantity of young trees and plants in boxes full of earth.

The French who settled in Quebec during the hundred years after the return of Quebec to the French by the British in 1632 brought with them from their native province its medical folk lore. The women healed the sore throats, colds, coughs, rheumatism, dysentery, diarrheas, sores and other ordinary ills in New France as they had in the old. They bought their medicines at the apothecaries in Quebec and probably grew some of the European plants around their houses. Their sons who left the settled areas and became coureurs de bois, outlaws most of the time, usually had Indian wives and families. From these they learnt of some medicinal uses of native plants. The Indians who became Christians and were settled near Quebec also told the sisters who ran the hospital and school of some of the Indian remedies.

Over several hundreds of years there was an amalgamation of Indian and French knowledge, a sort of popular folk medicine of Quebec. It was this that Rousseau records on the Isles des

Coudres in 1945. Mockle drew on this knowledge in his detailed work "Contributions to the study of medicinal plants in Canada" in 1955.

Kalm, when he travelled from English speaking north America in 1749 to Quebec, had to go by canoe to the frontier post of Fort Nicholson, then by foot over a no-man's land until he arrived at the first French post, Fort St. Frederic. There he became an honored guest of the French government during his many months in French Canada. There seems to have been a similar no man's land in intellectual circles between the two peoples. Sarrazin could write in 1708 of the Indian use of bloodroot as an abortifacient and of his use of it to regulate the menses, of the Indian use of the bark of leatherwood, *Dirca palustris*, to cure cancers and the Quebec use by Abbé Gendron for the same purpose, although Sarrazin did not believe it had any value for this purpose. Bigelow at Harvard could write a little over one hundred years later that leatherwood had not been applied to any medical purpose of importance and he was merely mentioning the plant because it obviously had medical properties. Rafinesque did not know of the Indian use of bloodroot as an abortifacient. There are other such examples.

The English speaking settlers brought with them from England Gerarde, Culpepper (first reprinted in Boston 1708), Wesley, Buchan and W. Lewis all writing of European plants. They also brought with them their handwritten recipe books containing their tried and true remedies for the common household ills. They brought the seeds of many of the plants they used in Europe and sowed them by their door steps. These are our common weeds in cultivated areas today; catnip, motherwort, mullein, Queen Anne's lace, elecampane and many other. As the Indian tribes were conquered the settlers moved westward taking their books and seeds.

White men with no medical training but some practical common sense, great initiative and sense of commercial opportunity set up as root and herb doctors in the frontier regions. They may have known some Indian medicines but mostly they relied on remedies that had proven themselves by long household use.

George Howard is an example of the settler who set up to practice medicine. He came to Quebec from England in 1820 as a farrier. His medical recipe books were lent me by his great great grandaughter. These handwritten recipes were most likely used by his wife to heal men while he attended to the animals. The plants used were all European ones but some grow on both sides of the Atlantic.

Much confusion exists as to what the white settlers learnt from the Indians. In this book I have quoted from the European medical practice when the same plant or a very similar species of the same genus, is native to both Europe and America.

There were trained physicians who sought out Indian remedies, they called themselves Eclectics open to the practice of all kinds of medicine as opposed to the Allopaths, the medical establishment. The Empirics were men for the most part without any medical training and among them are found the root and herb and botanist physicians.

The medical profession in all parts of northeastern north America fought to control the practice of medicine. They denigrated the "Indian doctors". One of the more respectable of the practitioners of this type was Dr. Samuel Thomson whose practice was based on sweating, purging with *Lobelia inflata* or wild tobacco, a poison and the use of lady's slipper, known in European practice as nervine. Dr. James Richardson in his handwritten reminiscences says that "Thompsonianism prevailed in Toronto as well as over the country and in the neighbouring United States in the early 1830's." Its mainstay was recipe no. 6 consisting of gum myrrh from the middle east, cayenne pepper from south America and brandy.

False elixirs abounded, being sold by white "Indian medicine men" travelling about the country touting their nostrums. The Indian himself was not to be left out of this lucrative trade carried on in his name. He sold quack remedies to the whites as they did to him. Isham saw no harm in the Hudson's Bay company in 1743 carrying the ingredients for this trade and selling them to everyone.

In Upper Canada the candidates for a license to practice medicine had to pass an examination in Materia Medica among other subjects. The author found notes on a course of lectures on materia medica, handwritten on blank pages interleaved in an 1817 Edinburgh pharmacopoiea printed in Latin. The signature of Henry H. Wright, Toronto 1837 appears at the top of the title page. Wright studied medicine in Toronto with Dr. John Rolph, who had the first medical school there, and passed his examinations in materia medica in Toronto in 1839. These lecture notes probably are one of the first text books on this subject used in Upper Canada. Only European plants with a very few exceptions, are considered.

In the United States at the end of the 18th. and beginning of the 19th. centuries the first medical botanies dealing with north American plants were written. Schoepf wrote in German in 1788 but was not translated. Cutler, Bigelow of Harvard, Barton and Rafinesque are the best known. The latter sums up the knowledge obtained to that date and deals with by far the greatest number of plants. He notes that yarrow was exported to Europe as the American plant was considered medicinally stronger. He laments, as do the other medical botanists that the native drug plant material offered for sale was so adulterated. They all had praise for the Shakers at New Lebanon who produced pure plant drugs, gathering as well growing, the native plants. These Shaker drugs were exported to Canada and Europe.

The Shakers illustrate two of the problems of depending on drugs from plant material. They would sometimes lose their whole crop of one plant. This happens in any agricultural crop but there are usually many other growers to fill the gap. The Shakers were almost alone. Secondly they were limited in the amount they could produce, modern large scale agriculture was over one hundred years away.

The gathering of medicinal plants as it has been and is being done all over the world is a rather haphazard procedure. It is an ill paid seasonal occupation so more often than not several different plants are mixed together, or the right parts are not always gathered, or they are not gathered at just the period when the plant is producing the greatest quantity of the wanted chemicals, or not gathered from plants growing in places where the most chemical content will be produced. The result is that the content varies from one batch to another. The science of pharmacognosy and its text books teach the pharmacists how to tell if he has the right part of the right plant and how to test his material.

At the same time, between 1830 and 1900, the medical profession was relying less and less on medicines obtained from plants, with the exception of opium from the opium poppy, grown in the middle and far east. Mercury had been a drug of choice since 1550, especially for syphilis. The chemists were learning how to produce synthetically in the laboratory the chemicals that the plant made in the field. The first was coniine from the poison hemlock, *Conium maculatum*. Salicin from the willow, *Salix* sp., followed soon afterwards. So as the population increased dramatically the fact that the medicines needed could not be had from gathering in the wild or by cultivation spurred on the chemists' research.

The homeopathic physicians however still prescribed some plant drugs and supported a homeopathic pharmaceutical company which prepared plant drugs appreciated by all branches of the medical profession. Millspaugh, a homeopath, wrote his American medical plants in 1892. It is safe to say that more people refer to it to-day than did when it was written.

At this period also, interest in the knowledge the Indian peoples had of the use of their plants increased. Speck (1915) studied the maritime Indian tribes, Densmore (1925-26) lived amongst the Chippewa and Huron Smith (1923-32) with the Menomini, Meskwaki, Ojibwa and Potawatomi. However Huron Smith was generally convinced that no white man would ever get all of the data, names and uses of plants from the Menomini because of the sanctity of their medical knowledge. He was also convinced that they certainly knew what it was in the plant that effected the cure.

Most Indian medicines were mixtures. These mixtures are usually of 7 or 9 plants but may be of a very great many more and include minerals, earths and animal parts. Huron Smith gives some of those made by the Meskwaki in 1928 and Reagan gives some made by an Ojibwa medicine man that same year. He copied the recipes from the medicine man's note book, identifying each plant. Useful medical knowledge may lie unexplored in these mixtures. The chemical structure of plants is so complex that with all our investigative tools we still know only a part of it. Rafinesque wrote, "Plants are compound medicines prepared by the hand of nature."

Digitalis is an example of this complexity. The drug is produced synthetically, seemingly an exact copy of that manufactured by the plant *Digitalis purpurea* or *D. lanata*. Certain heart patients however respond better to the plant drug than to the synthetic one. What that difference is, it is extraordinarily difficult, expensive and time consuming to find out.

Tests of plant material in laboratories are done to look for a certain set of properties. The plant may contain quite other properties but these will not be found by that test. New, different, sets of tests would have to be done to find them. And so on ad infinitum, years of painstaking work. The plants reported to have been used as folk remedies for cancer are being tested but it will take a long time. The most promising ones are given priority.

An example of what has happened to some attempts to test Indian plant remedies is that of

Dr. Sylvia Bensley. She learnt that the Ojibwa of Georgian Bay used a decoction of the leaves of the American yew, *Taxi canadensis*, for arthritis. She managed to get funds for 2 years of research and obtained some promising results. All work ceased when she could not obtain any more money.

Man is living a longer, healthier and happier life thanks to modern scientific research. Heart attacks and strokes are no longer so likely to be fatal as they were such a short time ago. Tuberculosis does not kill inevitably as it did when I was a girl. Smallpox is eliminated from the world, we hope. Pneumonia is not the dreaded killer it once was. These are but a few examples, we can all think of others. The bite of a rabid animal, or of a rattlesnake, and cancer, these we do not know how to cure yet. We can save the life of those bitten if time is not wasted, some cancers seem to be being cured, but as modern medicine is cautious it will not claim victory yet. These are the great and enormous good of our chemical medicine.

There is as always another side to the coin. Because much money is made by pharmaceutical companies, more drugs are created than need be. Rival companies' drugs are copied and time, men and money wasted. Sometimes the drugs are improperly tested, perhaps in order to place them on the market sooner and make more money. Drugs known to be hazardous but selling well are not removed from the market. Tests on suspected hazardous chemical products are being sloppily done. Doctors are being pressured every day and in every way to buy a certain company's pills and to prescribe them. Patients are demanding of their doctor, "Give me a pill to fix this trouble of mine." The harried physician finds it simpler to prescribe a pill than not to.

The results we all know. People dying in hospitals from having been fed too many different pills whose reaction with each other no one understands. Housewives addicted to sleeping pills or amphetamines. Children ruining their lives experimenting with dangerous chemicals. These are but a few of the results of our credulity, ignorance and unwillingness to take care of ourselves.

People, rather than blaming themselves, are turning away from the medical profession. Many people are dosing themselves with plant drugs of whose properties they know nothing, much less what the interaction of these properties are with other medication they are taking.

Plant materials that are poisonous in certain doses are being sold across the counter. This book reports what is known to-day about the deadly, the dangerous or the merely very unpleasant results that will ensue when a particular plant or a part of it is taken internally or externally.

We should return to a study of the properties of our native plants beginning in our schools. We know that our plants, trees and shrubs could provide us with fibers for use in textiles, films and plastics, lignin to replace some of the chemicals used in industrial processes now supplied by chemicals made from oil. Our trees could supply enough protein to feed our cattle and leave our grain for human consumption. The hybrid poplar program in Ontario is an example of what is being done now.

This book is offered as a basis from which to begin a part of this task. Our past history speaks with its own voice in its pages. The legacy left us by our native peoples, by New France, by all the other peoples who have added their knowledge of the use of plants to ours must be preserved and increased.

Charlotte Erichsen-Brown 1979.

EVERGREEN TREES

including the larch which drops its needles

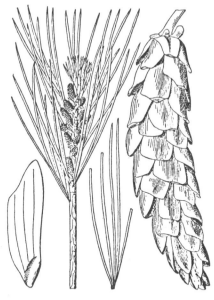

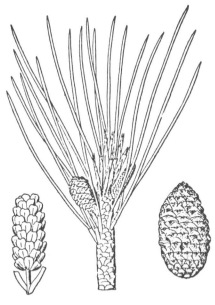

WHITE PINE

RED PINE

WHITE PINE   *Pinus strobus* L. Pinaceae

Tall tree to 70 m with thick furrowed bark. The slender needles, pale green and shiny are 8-13 cm long in bundles of five. The cones, on long stalks, are rarely over 20 cm long, opening at maturity, with seeds much shorter than their wings.

Range. Nfld., N.B., P.E.I., N.S., s. Que., Ont., se. Man., s. to ne. Io., Ky., N. Ga., and nw. S.C., chiefly in sandy soil, many habitats.

Common names. Weymouth pine, northern pine, deal pine.

RED PINE   *Pinus resinosa* Ait. (*P. rubra*)

Tree to 40 m often clear of branches for three quarters of its height with reddish to pinkish scaly bark, on old trunks furrowed. Needles dark green, 9-16 cm long in bundles of two. The stalkless cones are 4-8 cm long.

Range. Nfld., N.B., N.S., P.E.I., s. Que., Ont. to se. Man., s. to Minn., Wisc., Mich., Pa., Conn. and n. Mass. in dry woods or rocky soil.

Common names. Norway pine, Canadian pine, hard pine.

1354 McAndrews & Boyko 1974 Crawford Lake Site s. Ont. 8. "Before the Iroquoians migrated into the Crawford Lake area the forest surrounding the lake consisted mainly of beech and maple with some oak, elm and birch. There was little or no pine. Archeobotanical remains in the nearby village middens, including charred seeds and charcoal, indicate that maize and beans were cultivated and that beech and maple constituted most of the firewood. The pollen diagram parallels this evidence and indicates that white pine and oak succeeded beech and maple on abandoned Indian fields. This explanation seems adequate when archeological and palynological evidence for agriculture are present. However, there are many more sites which show the characteristic white pine increase before European settlement. . .The other possible explanation for white pine increase is proposed, namely, response to the Little Ice Age. . .Crawford Lake lies to-day at the southern boundary of the Great Lakes conifer-hardwood forest. White pine probably would migrate southward in response to climate cooling. . .6. Zone 7 is defined by a rise in white pine pollen and the varve date at Crawford Lake is 580 years ago."

1475 Bjornnson Icelandic mss. Larsen transl. 111. "Pix liquida, tar hot and dry in the third degree. If one takes a full spoon of it and a second of honey, it is good for lung trouble and for heavy breathing. If one adds to it meat of almonds, that dries water in the ears, if it is put into them. If one adds salt to tar, that is good to apply to whatever vermin get into. If it is mixed evenly with wax, it heals impetigines [pimples] and softens what is hard in them. If it is mixed with brimstone, it helps for dandruff. Pitch helps almost all the same and is good to put in plasters and ointments for all sores."

1501 Cantino Lisbon 17th. Oct. to Ferrara transl. "And in all this region, several great rivers flow into the sea; by one of these rivers they penetrated to a place in the interior of the territory where on their arrival they found an abundance of very sweet and different fruits, and trees and pines of a height and diameter so great that they would be too large to be used as masts for the biggest boats that cross the sea."

1501 Pasqualigo 19th October; 209. "They report that the land is thickly peopled and that the houses are built of very long beams of timber, and covered with the skins of fishes. . .210. They have an abundance of timber, principally pine, fitted for masts and yards of ships, on which account his serene majesty [King of Portugal] anticipates the greatest profit from this country, both in providing timber for ships, of which he, at present, stands in great need." [The above two quotations relate to the voyage of Gaspar Corte-Real to the coast of Labrador in 1501 for the King of Portugal, as cited by Rousseau 1937.]

1613 Champlain Fourth Voyage fac. ed. Ottawa transl. 25. "The lands around the Lake were sandy, & covered with pines, which had almost all been burnt by the savages. . .When they want to make the land cultivateable, they burn the trees, & this is very easy, for there is nothing but pines, full of resin."

1633 Gerarde-Johnson 1361. "Out of the Pine trees, especially of the wilde kinds, there issueth forth a liquid, whitish and sweet smelling Rosin. . .very aptly mixed in ointments, commended for the healing up of greene wounds, for they both bring to suppuration, and to also glue and unite them together. . .1362. Gathered out from the Rosins. . .a congealed smoke. . .which serveth for medicines that beautifie the eie lids, and cure the fretting sores of the corners of the eies, and also watering eies, for it drieth without biting. There is made hereof. . .writing inke, but in our age not that which we write withall, but the same which serveth for Printers to print their bookes with, that is to say, of this blacke, or congealed smoke, and other things added."

1663 Boucher Quebec transl. 40-1. "I will commence with one, which is the most used here, which is called Pine, which does not bear fruit as do those of Europe; they are of all sizes and girths; ordinarily they are fifty to sixty feet high without any branches: they are used to make planks, which are good and fine; & it can be said that these trees would be very good to make masts for ships. They are found thin and high enough for this purpose: these trees are very straight: there are large parts of the country where there are none: but the places where they are found are called Pineries. These trees yield a quantity of gum; the Savages use it to mend their canoes, & they also use it happily for woundes, for which it is a sovereign remedy."

1672 Josselyn New Engl. This tree (white pine) "yields a very sovereign turpentine for curing desperate wounds."

1744 Colden to Gronovious Dec. 89-90. "The Indians cure all sorts of wounds without digestion by the Inner bark of Pinus no 192 of the collection I sent you. They soak it so long in water as to make it soft & then apply it. If I be not misinform'd it is effectual even in Gun shot wounds. The Wound keep of a fresh & ruddy colour till it unites without digesting."

1749 Kalm Bay St. Paul Quebec August 30th. 483. "The inhabitants live chiefly upon agriculture and the making of tar, which is sold at Quebec. . .492. Great quantities of tar are made at Bay St. Paul. . .The tar is made solely from *Pin rouge* or red pine. . .People use only the roots which are full of resin, and which they dig out of the ground with about two yards of the trunk, just above the roots, laying aside the rest."

1778 Carver Travels 496. "That species of pine tree peculiar to this part of the continent is the white, the quality of which I need not describe, as the timber of it is so well known under the name of deals. It grows here in great plenty, to an amazing height and size, and yields an excellent turpentine, though not in such quantities as those in the northern parts of Europe."

1779 Cartwright J. Labrador [1770] 1.10. "The arrows are made from Weymouth pine; they are slender, light, perfectly straight, and about three feet long." Lord Weymouth introduced the white pine to England in 1705.]

1799 Lewis Mat. Med. Disp. 208. "Tar, Pix liquida, a thick black unctuous substance obtained from old pines and fir trees by burning them with a close smothering heat, part soluable in water. The water drunk for smallpox, scurvy, ulcers, fistules, rheumatism, asthma, coughs, cutaneous complaints and to cure all symptoms of dispepsy. It promotes urine, promotes perspiration, used also externally for skin diseases mixed with fat."

1809 Hugh Gray 207. "The dock-yard can be supplied with masts of the largest size. Some have been brought down to Quebec, 120 feet in length, and about four feet in diameter. It is the white pine which arrives at this immense size and may be stiled the monarch of the Canadian forest."

1812 Peter Smith. "The bark of the white pine is a great medicine for sores. It should be boiled, and the soft part stript out and beat to a poultice in a mortar, and then sufficiently moistened with the liquor and applied to burns or sores of any kind. Repeat the poultices and wash with the liquor until the sore is well. This will not terrify or smart in its application. A new skin will come on quickly without a scar. The same application is a cure for piles. A little tea of the bark should be drank while the external applications are continued."

1820's Mat. Med. Edinburgh-Toronto mss 54. "Pix liquanda. . .macerated with water it gets the name of Tar Water which operates chiefly as a stimulating Diuretic and Diaphoretic. . .Bitumen Petroleum. . .it is scarcely used."

1830 Rafinesque 25. "White pine. . .The Indian tribes use the bark in a poultice for sores and piles, the boiled root for drawing plaster, the decoction of buds as purgative, the cones in rheumatism, and tar dissolved in spirits as a wash to cure itch, tetters and wens."

1833 Howard Quebec mss 24. "To prevent the cramp. . .Take half a pint of Tar Water night and morning. . .136. To cure Flat Worms.2. Mix a tablespoonful of Norway tar, in a pint of small beer. Take it as soon as you can in the morning fasting. This brought away a Tape worm 36 feet long. . .225. To cure Sores of all sorts in Man. 1 oz. of strained turpentine, 1 oz. of burgundy pitch, 1 oz. bees wax, 2 oz. olive oil mixt all together, rub sores twice a day. Excellent. . .1843. 16. Green ointment to make for all sorts of wounds. Take common corse turpentine and beeswax of each ½ pound, fresh butter without salt ½ pound and 2 ounces of verdigrease. Simmer all together and stir well together then it is ready for use. Never better salve than this."

1840 Gosse Quebec 7. "There is not much [white] pine growing in our neighbourhood; but I have seen some very large logs drawn out to Smith's mill. Moore told me the other day that he was then going in for a pine-log six feet in diameter: he had three yoke of oxen attached to his sled."

1841 Trousseau & Pidoux Paris transl. Use turpentine from pines as the Indians did for terrible pain.

1842 Christison 916-21. "Common turpentine. . .But what is now known by that name comes in great measure from the United States, and is produced by other pines such as the. . .swamp pine [grows south of Va.]. . .Resin. . .in pharmacy it is specially applied to the substance left by the pine-turpentines after removal of their volatile oil. . .Oil of turpentine often called in common speech, spirits of turpentine is obtained, like resin,. . .by distillation. . .The purified oil. . .is the most important of the medicinal agents derived from the natural products of the pines. Its actions are complex. . .According to some it is also in large doses a narcotic, and in small doses a tonic. Therapeutically it is anthelmintic, and, in relation to chronic mucous discharges, an astringent. It acts externally with promptitude as an irritant, producing redness of the skin, and eruption of pimples, and sometimes minute blisters. It is therefor much used as a counter-irritant upon the abdomen in peritonitis, or in the neighbourhood of indolent tumours, and chronic topical inflammations generally. . .and recent burns. . .When given inwardly in large doses, it seems occasionally to produce in man a feeling like that of intoxication, or a state resembling trance; and it causes in animals tetanus, coma, and speedily death. Sometimes it excites in the human subject pain in the stomach, sickness, and vomiting,. . .More frequently it gives rise to symptoms of irritation in the kidneys or bladder. . .In small doses of fifteen to thirty minums frequently repeated, oil of turpentine is a stimulant-quickening the pulse, raising the animal heat, and even producing some degree of exhilaration. . .useful in typhoid stage or form of continued fever. . .good deal employed in chronic rheumatism and neuralgia. . .Its most unequivocal action is that of a vermifuge, in worms generally, but above all in tape-worms. In this variety, which resists most other anthelmintics, oil of turpentine, taken inwardly is the most certain of all remedies, next to pomegranate root-bark. . .In the course of its action it is absorbed; for through whatever channel it enters the body, an odour of turpentine is imparted to the breath and perspiration, and a violet odour is acquired by the urine. . .As a cathartic its best form is that of an emulsion along with castor oil. Six drachms of caster oil and two of oil of turpentine, with an ounce of peppermint-water and twenty minums of Aqua potassae, make a powerful purgative mixture. . .923. Tar (Pix Liquida) has been used immemorially in medicine. . .It is prepared in the northern part of Europe, by digging a hole in the earth near a bank, filling it with the root wood and billets of the branches of the scotch fir [Scotch pine], covering the whole with turf, and kindling the wood at the top so as to let it burn slowly with a smothered heat. During the process tar is formed, which, trickling down to the bottom, is received in an iron pan, Whence it escapes by a pipe in the side of the bank. In other parts of the world, as in India, it is got by fixing in a pit in the earth a large earthern pot with a hole in the bottom, which opens into a smaller pot placed below,—then filling the upper pot with wood and surrounding it with dried cow's dung for fuel,—and collecting in the lower vessel the tar which is produced [see Juniper]. . .It is a very complex substance; nor is its composition yet thoroughly understood. It contains modified resin, modified oil of turpentine, acetic acid, and water, and some kinds of it yield creosote, parrafin, eupion,. . .Tar-water, was employed for some time as a calmative and expectorant in diseases of the chest and of the kidneys. . .it is now abandoned in practice. . .More recently inhalation of tar water was brought into request by Sir Alexander Creighton in catarrhal and phthisical [consumptive] complaints; but this remedy too is already obsolete. The only use now prevalently made of tar is as a local application for some chronic diseases of the skin. . .Oil of tar is poisonous in large doses. . .Pitch. . .is the bituminous matter left after tar has been heated to expel its water, acetic acid, and oil. . .It has been used outwardly in the form [of]. . .black basilicon Ointment, for dressing indolent ulcers, or as an application for porrigo and tinea. Its properties are probably possessed, and in greater energy, by tar."

1846 Bonnycastle. Cited Lower 1936 p. 16. "Bonnycastle described what he called red pine, (he probably mistook white pine for red) that he had seen and measured near Barrie, Ontario in 1846. They were 200 feet high and girthed 26 feet."

1846 Winder Manitoulin Island.9. "Toothache.—Creosote generally affords temporary relief, but the majority return for extraction..' [Remarks in a return of Dr. Darling, the medical officer of the Indian Department.]

1849 Williams, St. p. 921. "Canadian Indians used the bark in poultice for piles and ulcerations, made a drawing plaster by boiling roots, the buds used as tea as a purgative, the cones or strobiles for rheumatism. Tar dissolved in spirits as a wash for burns, tetters, itch. [Compare with Rafinesque above; Williams seems not to have always received his informaton from the Indians.]

1854 Trail Sett. Guide 62. ". . .Grafting fruit trees. . .Some use cobbler.s wax, some apply pitch, and common turpentine from the pines."

1880 Can. Pharm. J. XIII; 348. "Recent advances in organic chemistry. . .Vanilline, the flavoring principle of the vanilla bean, is prepared artificially from coniferine, a glucoside contained in the sap of pine trees. . .and lastly from carbolic acid itself."

1881 Can. Pharm. J. 182. "In a recent paper in the Lancet Prof. Clay says that additional experience confirms his first conclusions as to the use of turpentine in cancer, and in the cases previously reported there has, so far, been no instance of the return of the disease."

1885 Hoffman OJIBWA 198. "The leaves are crushed and applied to relieve a headache; also boiled, after which they are put into a small hole in the ground and hot stone is placed therein to cause a vapor to ascend, which is inhaled to cure backache.2.Gum; chiefly used to cover seams in birch bark canoes. The gum is obtained by cutting a circular band of bark from the trunk, upon which it is then scraped and boiled down to proper consistency. The boiling was formerly done in clay vessels."

1892 Heebner Man. Pharm. Toronto 189. Oil of Turpentine and Oil of Tar listed among the Officinal volatile oils.

1915 Harris Eastern Indians 44. "When suffering from frost bites they applied to the parts affected a resinous plaster made from the sap-pine."

1915 Speck PENOBSCOT 309. "Pitch pine is used as a poultice on boils and abscesses."

1915 Speck MONTAGNAIS 315. "The gum of white pine. . .is boiled and drunk for sore-throat, colds, and consumption. . .317. MICMAC-MONTAGNAIS. The inner bark of white pine boiled for sores, swellings, etc."

1915 Speck-Tantaquidgeon MOHEGAN 308. "White pine bark is steeped and drunk to cure a cold."

1916 Waugh IROQUOIS 47. "Informants at Grand River, Tonawanda and elsewhere mentioned the use of rotten pine or chestnut for the absorption of grease or perspiration, or for dusting babies. This is made into a fine dark red powder. A mohawk name for the material is ohe sa." 117. Extensive use was made [for food] of the vegetative parts of various plants, trees, and shrubs, including pine.

1926-27 Densmore CHIPPEWA 334. "Another use of the knife in surgery was described by Wezawange, who said he had treated a case in which this became necessary. It was a gangrenous wound, and he used the knife, not to remove, but to 'loosen' the affected flesh, which was taken out by the medicine he applied. He said that in a case of this sort everything must be very clean, care being taken especially that the knife or remedies did not come in contact with rust. In this treatment he said that he used a medicine which had been handed down by the Mide and was particularly valued. It consisted of the inner bark of the white pine, the wild plum, and the wild cherry, it being necessary to take the first two from young trees. The writer [Densmore] saw him cut a young pine tree for this purpose and place tobacco in the ground close to the root before doing so. In preparing the medicine he said that the stalk of the pine was cut in short sections and boiled with the green inner bark of the other two trees until all the bark was soft. The water should be renewed when necessary, and the last water saved for later use. The bark was then removed from the pine stems and all the bark mashed with a heavy hammer until it was a pulp. It was then dried, and when needed it was moistened with the water which had been kept for that purpose. He said this medicine was usually prepared when needed, as the materials were so readily at hand. This wet pulp was applied to any wound or to a fresh cut and was a healing remedy, but was especially useful for neglected wounds which had become gangrenous. . .352. The informant stated that he used this successfully in a gunshot wound after gangrene had set in. This would be applied to any form of 'rotten flesh', after which a knife was used to cleanse the wound. . . .In the southern part of the White Earth Reservation the writer witnessed the offering and burying of tobacco by a medicine man who wished to cut pine bark for medicinal use. The remedy was his own and he described several instances of its successful use. . .380. Little figures were made of tufts of the needles of the red pine. . .by cutting across the needles at different lengths to represent the arms and the hem of the dress. These little figures were placed upright on a sheet of birchbark or, better, on a piece of tin, which was gently agitated in such a manner that the figures appeared to dance. Considerable skill could be shown in producing a motion of the figures."

1923 H. Smith MENOMINI 46. "[White pine] The inner bark of the young tree, two feet above the ground is used. The trunk must be smooth and free from cracks. The first incision is made vertically facing the east, then the outer bark is peeled and the inner bark removed. While this is being done, the proper song for gathering this medicine is sung and tobacco is buried about the roots of the sapling. This bark may be steeped to form a drink to cure pain in the chest, or it may be pounded to shreds and used as a poultice for wounds, sores, or ulcers. It is one of the most important Menomini medicines."

1932 H. Smith OJIBWE 379. "[White pine] The bark is. . .gathered in the same manner as by the Menomini. . .The cones, when boiled and likewise the bark of the young tree trunk yield a pitch which is medicine. . .The dried leaves are powdered and used as a reviver or inhalant. . .White pine is a very valuable remedy with all Ojibwe but the Norway pine [red pine] is sometimes substituted for it. . .421. The Flambeau Ojibwe used the pitch from the boiled cones, along with the resin that flows from boxed trees, for caulking and waterproofing purposes. . .407. In the spring the Ojibwe use the young staminate catkins of the pine to cook for food. It is stewed with meat. . .[I was] assured. . .was sweet and had no pitchy flavor." [See balsam for use in the sweat bath.]

1932 H. Smith OJIBWE 379. . ."Red pine was used in all particulars. . .just as the White pine. . . .421. The Flambeau Ojibwe gather resin from the Norway pine just as they do from the White pine, Balsam and Spruce, by chopping a hole into the trunk and collecting the resin as it forms. It is boiled twice, being combined with tallow the second time, to make a serviceable waterproof pitch. This is not only used for caulking canoes, but for mending roof rolls of birch bark and other things. The wood is also utilized."

1933 H. Smith POTAWATOMI 70. "[Red pine] The Forest Potawatomi use the leaves of this pine also as a reviver. . .[White pine] The Forest Potawatomi use the pitch or resin of the wood and the bark as the base of a salve. . .123. Use the pitch rendered from the bark or cone to caulk boats or canoes."

1938 Lower 16. The White pine under the best conditions has been known to reach a height of 250 feet and a diameter of six or more. . .Pine in the township of Barford, Quebec, was spoken of early in the nineteenth century as girthing 15 feet. (Can. Arch. Ser. Q. 96 74.)

1945 Raymond TETE DE BOULE transl. 129. "The inner bark is dipped into boiling water and then applied to the chest for tenacious colds."

1955 Mockle Quebec transl. 21. "White pine. The decoction of the cones in milk makes a drink to which a tonic property is attributed. The bark, rich in turpentine, is used for burns; it is also used in the preparation of sirups for coughs on account of its expectorant properties. . .red pine uses same as jack pine."

The use of pine gum, resin, turpentine for ulcers tumors, etc. goes back at least to the Arabs. Reported from Europe, United States, Germany as a home remedy, folk remedy of Pennsylvania Dutch of 1800, used in commercial remedies since the beginning of the 19th century. (Hartwell 1970).

1976 Antoine King Go-Home Bay personal communication. When at a lumber camp on Green Bass Lake he got a boil on his face. An Indian put pine pitch on it, cured it in a few days.

1977 Rapson 8. "Consider the tree as a combination of carbon, hydrogen and oxygen. With these atoms we can make more than 2 million different substances. We could harvest the trees, put them back into carbon and water, from these make carbon monoxide and hydrogen, and from these make all the chemicals we need. Eventually we will have to do this. . .We used to make vanillin synthetically at a high cost and then Howard Smith at Cornwall, Ont. learned how to make vanillin from sulphite waste liquor. That one mill could supply the world with vanillin."

Cutting pine for masts for the Royal navy in quantity dates from the Napoleonic wars. The difficulty of getting the long pine poles to the sea meant it was the coastal rivers that supplied the bulk of the masts. The prerevolutionary marking of tall pines as reserved for the navy was stopped in the United States but continued in British America. Some Provincial governments still reserve to the Crown the pine on some Crown lands. There are some good yarns of the rafting of tall pines, running the rapids with Iroquois or French Canadian steersmen.

MICMAC and MALECITE of the Maritimes provinces of Canada used the White pine for colds, cough, grippe, hemorrhage, kidney trouble and scurvy. (Chandler, Freeman and Hooper 1979).

Pinosylvine in the heartwood of the scotch pine, *P. sylvestris*, is a bacteriocide. Pyrone found in pine needles is approved by the F.D.A. as an intensifier of the sugar flavor in bread and cakes by 30-300 x. Pine resin contains a substance that is 1600-2000 times sweeter than sugar but its toxicity is unknown (Lewis and Elvin-Lewis 1977).

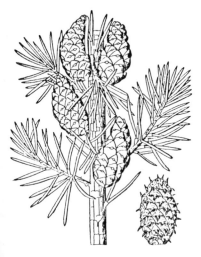

JACK PINE

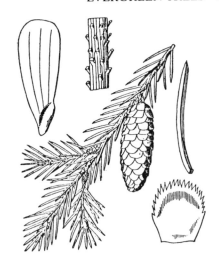

WHITE SPRUCE

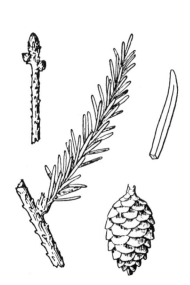

BLACK SPRUCE

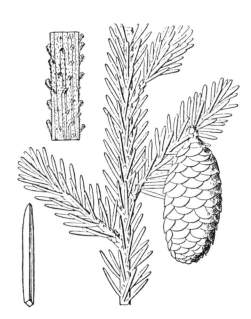

RED SPRUCE

JACK PINE   *Pinus banksiana* Lamb. Pinaceae
Tree to 20 m (25), needles 2-3.5 cm long in bundles of two spread apart, stiff and sharp pointed.
Cones 3-5 cm long commonly twisted without stalks, persistent.
Range. N.B., P.E.I., N.S., Que., n. Ont., Mackenzie s. to c. Alta-Sask. Minn., n. Ill., n. N.Y. and
N. Engl. in barren, sandy or rocky soil.
Common names. Labrador pine, gray pine, Hudson Bay pine, northern scrub pine, Unlucky-tree,
rock pine, Bank's pine.
1923 H. Smith MENOMINI 45. "Every part of the tree is used as a medicine. Even the cone is
boiled to make a sort of medicine. The uses were not divulged."

1932 H. Smith OJIBWE 379. "The leaves are used as a reviver...421. Jack pine roots have ever been esteemed by all Ojibwe as fine sewing material for their canoes and other coarse and durable sewing. They dig the roots with a grub hoe. . .and often find them fifty or sixty feet long. These are split lengthwise into two halves starting at the tree end, and are wrapped in coils. . .They are then sunk in the lake which loosens the bark and enables them to be scraped clean, as well as adding to their flexibility. They are ivory white when used and very tough and flexible."

1933 H. Smith POTAWATOMI 70. "Among the Forest Potawatomi, the pitch is considered medicinal. The pitch is obtained from boiling the cone of the tree and the resultant pitch is the basis for an ointment. The leaves of the jack pine are used as a fumigant,. . .to revive patients who are in coma and to clear the lungs where there is congestion. . .122. For night hunting, the Forest Potawatomi make pine pitch and cedar torches. These torches were placed upon the bow of a canoe when they were hunting down a stream or on a lake. . . .113. They use the root. . .as a heavy sewing material. . .sunk beneath the surface of the lake until the outer bark has loosened from the root. Then they are peeled and split in half, each half being serviceable cord for sewing together canoes and bark strips intended for the roofs of wigwams and for other purposes. The cones of this tree also yield a pitch, which is used to waterproof the seams which they sew."

1955 Mockle Quebec transl. 2. The decoction of the cones is given for obstinate colds. The heart of the wood gives an extract of pinobanksine.

WHITE SPRUCE   *Picea glauca* (Moench) Voss Pinaceae (*P. canadensis, Pinus alba*)
Tree to 25 m, twigs smooth, needles 4 angled 8-18 mm long, winter buds smooth and rounded. Cones 3.5-5 cm pale brown.
Range Lab., Nfld., N.B., P.E.I., N.S., Que. Ungava, to Yukon and Alaska, s. to B.C., Wyo., s. Dak., Minn., Wisc., Mich., n. N.Y. and Me. mostly in rich moist soil.
BLACK SPRUCE   *Picea mariana* (Mill.) BSP. (*Pinus nigra, Abies n., Picea n.*)
Tree to 20 m, twigs hairy, needles 4 angled 10-30 mm bluish green with a white sheen, winter buds pointed. Cones persistent for many years dark purple becoming dull gray brown, 1.5-3.5 cm.
Range. The same as the white spruce; found in bogs except in north range.
RED SPRUCE   *Picea rubens* Sarg. (*P. australis, P. rubra, Pinus r., Abies r.*)
Tree to 25 m (35) twigs covered with orangey-brown dense short hairs, winter buds long pointed with reddish scales longer than bud. Cones 3-4.5 cm long, firm, hanging, opening in autumn and remaining on tree until late summer next year.
Range. N.B., P.E.I., N.S., sw. Que., eastermost Ont., Ottawa, s. to Tenn. and N.C. in woods, loamy moist valleys.

1475 Bjornnson Icelandic mss Larsen transl. 115. "Pinum is spruce. One shall take spruce cones and place upon coals and burn them somewhat. Then one shall throw away the shell and clean the kernels and boil well in water. If one places these kernels thus prepared upon the coals and draws to one's nose the smoke that comes therefrom, that makes a man happy and it moistens his body and is good for that illness where blood passes with the excrements. From these kernels, with other things that belong, an electuary is made which is called Peniteun. These kernels are good food for those who have heavy breathing and are swollen from cold blood and have dry cough. And they increase good blood. These kernels are hot and wet in their nature. If one cuts (?) the bark of this tree during the winter time, a resin runs from it which he can use for incense; and yet it is darker and not equal to that which comes from the Orient."

1534 Cartier Voy. transl. 47. On the north coast of the Bay de Chaleurs. "There are many cedars and spruce, as fine as it is possible to see, for making masts, sufficient to mast boats of 300 tons or more" (y a pluseurs cèdres et pruches, aussi beaulx qu'il soict possible de voir). . .81. "Green tree, Haneda."

1535-6 Cartier Voy. transl. 213-5. "The captain [Cartier] seeing the aforementioned dom Agaya healthy and deliberate, was joyous, hoping to learn from him, how he was cured, so that his men could be given aid and help. So when they had arrived near the fort, the captain asked him how he was cured of his sickness [scurvy]. dom Agaya replied that it was with the juice of the leaves of a tree and the water the leaves were boiled in, that he was cured and that this was the special remedy for the sickness. Then the captain asked him if there were any such trees around there, and asked him to show him one so that he could cure his servant, who had caught the aforesaid sickness in the house of seigneur Donnacona [at Quebec] not wanting to let him know the number of his companions who were sick. Then Agaya sent two women with our captain, to cure him, they brought nine or ten branches; and showed us how the bark must be pulled off and the leaves of these branches, and all put into water to boil; then the water drunk once in two days; and the juice of the leaves and bark pressed out and the water put on the swollen and sick limbs; and he said that the tree will cure all sickness. They call the said tree in their language, *annedda*. Immediately afterwards, the captain had the drink made, so the sick could drink, of these however no one wanted to try it, only one or two, who decided to try it. As soon as they had drunk, they felt better, which they found a true and evident miracle; for of all the sicknesses they had suffered from, after having drunk two or three times, they recovered their health and were cured, so that some of the company who had had syphilis for more than five or six years before getting this sickness [scurvy], by this medicine that a tree, as large and as tall as I have ever seen was used in such a demand for this medicine that a tree, as large and as tall as I have ever seen was used in less than eight days, which made such a cure that if all the doctors of Louvain and Montpellier had tried, with all the drugs of Alexandria, they could not have done as much in one year as this tree did in eight days; For it profited us so much, that all those who wanted to try it, recovered health and were cured, by the Grace of God."

1609 Lescarbot-Erondelle Acadia 34. "Briefly, the unknown sicknesses like to those described unto us by James Cartier, in his relations assailed us. For remedies there was none to be found. In the meanwhile the poor sick creatures did languish, pining away by little and little, for want of sweet meats, as milk or spoon-meat for to sustain their stomachs, which could not receive the hard meats by reason of let proceeding from a rotten flesh, which grew and overabounded within their mouths: when one thought to root it out, it did grow again in one night's space more abundantly than before. As for the tree called annedda, mentioned by the said Cartier, the savages of these lands know it not. . .There died of the sickness 36 and 36 or 40 more that were stricken with it recovered themselves by the help of the spring. . .Monsieur de Monts, being returned into France did consult with our doctors of physic upon the sickness, which. . .they found very new and unknown, for that when we went away [from France], our apothecary [Hebert] was not charged with any order for the cure thereof. . .45. I will not take the physician's office in hand. . .notwithstanding. . .not touching their orders and receipts of agaric, aloes, rhubarb and other ingredients. I will write here that which I think more ready at hand for the poor people which have not the ability and means to send to Alexandria as well as for the preservation of their health as for the remedy of this sickness. . .The young buds of herbs in the springtime be also very sovereign. And besides that reason requireth to believe it, I have tried it, being myself gone away many times to gather some for our sick people, before that those of our garden might be used, which restored them to their taste again and comforted their weak stomachs. . .47. And for the last and sovereign remedy, I send back the patient to the tree of life, (for one may so qualify it), which James Cartier doth call annedda, yet unknown in the coast of Port Royal, unless it be peradventure the sassafras, whereof there is a quantity in certain places. And it is an assured thing that the said tree is very excellent. But Monsieur Champlain who is now in the great river of Canada, passing his winter in the same part where the said Cartier did winter—hath charge to find it out and to make provision thereof."

1613 Champlain fac. ed. Voyages 53-55 transl. [Winter at St. Croix Island 1604-05] "During the winter there was a certain sickness amongst several of our men, called sickness of the country, or Scurvy. . .There died 35. . .We could not find any remedy to cure this sickness. We had several cut open to try and find out the cause of the sickness. . .Our doctors could not do any better for themselves as they were sick like the others. . .One only has salt meat and legumes to eat during the winter, which engenders poor blood: this in my opinion causes in part this annoying sickness. . .65 We passed by a bay [on the Acadian coast] where there are a quantity of islands; and saw large mountains in the west, where is the home of a savage captain called Aneda; which I think is near the Quinibequy river. I was persuaded by this name that here was one of the race who found the herb called Aneda, that Jacque Cartier said had so much power against the sickness called Scurvy. . .which torments these men, savages as well as our own, when they arrive in Canada. The savages knew nothing about this herb, nor know what it is, even though their language contains the name. . .101 [Winter 1605-06 at Port Royal]. We returned to our habitation where we found some of our men ill with the sickness of the country, but not as grievously as at the Island of St. Croix, even then of the 45 we were, 12 died. . .our Doctor, called des Champs, of Honfleur, a man expert in his art, opened several bodies to discover the cause of the sickness. . .could not find a remedy to cure them any more than the others. . .149 [Winter of

1606-07]. There was the sickness of the country amongst our men, but not as sharp as it was the year before, nevertheless 7 died of it. . .Our doctor whose name was Master Estienne, opened several bodies. . .202 [Winter of 1608-09 at Quebec]. The sickness of the country did not commence until February. . .18 became ill and 10 died. I had several opened, to see if they were offensive, the same as the others I had seen at the other habitations. They were the same. . .204 Those who navigate to the West Indies and several other regions, such as Germany and England, have also been stricken as those in New France. A little while ago the Flemish were attacked during their voyages to India, they found a very odd remedy against this sickness, which we could very well use: but we know nothing about it because of no research. Nevertheless I believe it to be evident that having good bread and fresh meats, you will not catch it."

1624 Sagard 264. "It is also said that the Montagnais and Canadians have a tree, called Annedda, with an admirable property; they strip off the bark and leaves of this tree, then boil them all in water and drink the water every other day; they put the dregs upon legs swollen with disease, and they soon get cured of this and of all other kinds of ailments, internal and external."

1631 James Voy. Overwintering in James Bay 137. "We had three sorts of sick men; those that could not move, nor turn themselves in their beds, who must be tended like an infant; others that were, as it were, crippled with scurvy aches; and others, lastly, that were something better. Most of all had sore mouths. You may ask me how these infirm men could work. I will tell you. Our Surgeon (which was diligent, and a sweet conditioned man, as ever I saw) would be up betimes in the mornings, and, whilst he did pick their teeth, and cut away the dead flesh from their gums, they would bathe their own thighs, knees and legs. The manner whereof was this: there was no tree, bud, nor herb but we made trial of it; and this, being first boiled in a kettle, and put in small tubs and basins, they would put it under them, and this would so mollify the grieved parts that, although when they did rise out of their beds they would be so crippled that they could scarce stand, yet after this was done half an hour, they would be able to go (and must go) to the wood through the snow, to the ship, and about their other business. By night they would be as bad again, and then they must be bathed, annointed, and their mouths again dressed, before they went to bed." [See under vetches for account of cure of the men in the Spring. The black and white spruce, the balsam fir and the balsam poplar would have been the trees found by James' crew.]

1632 Champlain Voy. Bourne transl. 14. "But if Cartier could have understood the cause of his sickness, and the beneficial and certain remedy for its prevention, although he and his men did receive some relief from an herb called aneda, just as we did when we were in the same plight, there is no doubt that the King from that time would not have neglected to forward the plan for a colony." [Champlain here trying to play down the bad reputation the 'mal de terre' had given his colony. That the French had no cure for scurvy the following makes plain.]

1969 Bailey 76. "Scurvy was indigenous. It was also prevalent among the natives. . .The remedy with which the Laurentian Iroquois of Stadacona had saved Cartier's crew from destruction in the previous century was not known to the eastern Algonkians of Champlain's time who could do nothing in this respect for the early Quebec and the St. Croix and Port Royal colonies. . .Scurvy or mal de terre ravaged Three Rivers in 1634 and 1635, and the Miscou colony in 1637. . .132. Broke up a mission as in the case of that at Seven Islands in 1764."

1965 Percy Robinson 55. "During the winter of 1688 and 1689 most of the garrison died of scurvy and the post was abandoned." [Niagara River Fort.]

1697 De la Potherie French navy in Hudson Bay. "Suddenly brought about an epidemic of scurvy; and I hardly venture to tell you, Sir, that we were all tormented with vermin to such an extent that some of our scurvy patients, who had become paralytics, actually died from the pest. . .nearly all the sailors took the scurvy. So few escaped that we were obliged to make use of our English prisoners in order to run the ship. . .so many deaths that we threw five or six sailors into the sea every day. . .You will see I have become a great doctor on this voyage. . .the sudden change which takes place in the temperature, after leaving the mildest and most agreeable season of the year, bring about an entire revolution, all at once, in the human body, which contracts a disease peculiar to those regions, called the scurvy. . .The food that one is obliged to take to sea contributes not a little to the malady. . .Lemon juice is very helpful. . .Finally after so many pains, labours, and misfortunes, we arrived at Belle Isle in Newfoundland on November 8. We proceeded to put our scurvied patients in the hospital of Port Louis." [Mowat Ordeal 1976 160-163.]

[This material, showing the prevalence of scurvy and the inability of the French to prevent or cure it, is included because so many confused accounts are current on this subject. There is no agreement among authors as to which tree was the one called annedda by Cartier. It could equally as well have been the hemlock, which has a higher Vitamin C content than the spruce. However these two trees are the ones that do contain the most Vitamin C of all the eastern north American evergreens, and an evergreen 'annedda' surely was if its leaves were picked in winter at Quebec. See the use of hemlock tea by the Iroquois in New York under hemlock. It is interesting that neither Marie de l'Incarnation nor Boucher mention it or spruce beer. Instead the drink of Quebec was 'bouillon' made from fermented yeast and grain.]

1652 Marie de l'Incarnation to her son 204. "The hulled barley is for our beasts; we also make tisanes from it, which serve us as beverage."

1663 Boucher Quebec transl. 43. "There is another sort of tree called Prusse; this usually grows into large trees of thirty or forty feet high without branches; they have a large bark & red: This wood does not decay as easily as others; that is why it is ordinarily used for building. What is bad about this wood, is that one finds a lot of mildew in it, which causes it to be rejected. It grows everywhere, in good and bad soils; it does not produce any gum. . .it grows as well in dry as in moist situations. . .140. What do they drink ordinarily. Wine in the best houses, beer in the others: another beverage that is called 'bouillon, is drunk by everyone in all the houses; the poorest drink water, which is very good & and common in this country."

1672 Josselyn New Engl. 200. "The tops of spruce-boughs, boiled in beer and drunk is assuredly one of the best remedies for the scurvy; restoring the infected party in a short time. They [the Indians] also make a lotion of some of the decoction, adding honey and alum." [The honey bee was imported from Europe].

1709 Raudot Quebec 343. "The Indian women wear their hair full length, tied and enveloped with the skin of an eel or snake; they put on it powder of spruce wood to keep it always very black."

1743-4 Middleton wintering over at Churchill Hudson Bay. (Cited Rich 1949 lvii.) "For the Christmas celebrations, which lasted twelve or fourteen days, Middleton decided to 'give our people strong beer and brandy every day all the time', and when the English beer was all expended by Christmas Eve the issue was changed to 'spruce beer and brandy, the only means used here to prevent scurvy.'. . .By the end of the winter eleven men were dead of scurvy and several others sorely stricken."

1749 Kalm Quebec September 27th. 535. "Wine is almost the only liquor which people above the common class drink. They make a kind of spruce beer of the top of the white fir which they drink in summer; but the use of it is not general and it is seldom drunk by people of quality. . .575. The common man's drink was water. The better class, who had the means, used French wine, mostly red though sometimes white. Some made a drink from the spruce as described before. . .August 21st. 474. They commonly drink red claret at dinner, either with water or clear; and spruce-beer is likewise much in use."

1751 Kalm Swedish in Kong. Vet. Acad. Handl. 190-96. An account of how to prepare spruce beer. (Cited Benson 774.)

1761 Henry Travels 14. "The small roots of the spruce-tree afford the wattup, with which the bark is sewed." [for a canoe].

1779 Cartwright Labrador J. 1; 139. 1771. "They supped with me, and afterwards smoked a few whiffs of tobacco and drank a little callibogus; but they seemed to prefer sugar and water." [Calabogus, a favorite drink of admirals, composed of rum, molasses and spruce beer. Cited Macnutt 1965]

1789 Mackenzie DOG RIB 95. "The vessels in which they cook their victuals are in the shape of a gourd, narrow at the top and wide at the bottom, and of watape (this is a name given to the divided roots of spruce, which the natives weave into a degree of compactness that renders it capable of containing a fluid) which is made to boil by putting a succession of red hot stones into it."

1791 Lewis Mat. Med. ed Aitkin 74. "It is said that when (the ulcers) are very deep and foul, the Indians sprinkle them with powder of the internal bark of the spruce tree."

1793 Mackenzie Voyages Athabasca 26. "I found that one of the young Indians had lost the use of his right hand by the bursting of a gun, and that his thumb had been maimed in such a manner as to hang only by a small strip of flesh. Indeed when he was brought to me, his wound was in such an offensive state, and emitted such a putrid smell, that it required all the resolution I possessed to examine it. His friends had done every thing in their power to relieve him. . .I was rather alarmed at the difficulty of the case, but as the young man's life was in a state of hazard, I was determined to risk my surgical reputation, and accordingly took him under my care. I immediately formed a poultice of bark, stripped from the roots of the spruce-fir, which I applied to the wound, having first washed it with the juice of the bark: this proved a very painful dressing: in a few days, however, the wound was clean, and the proud flesh around it destroyed. . .I perceived that the wound was closing rather faster than I desired. The salve I applied on the occasion was made of the Canadian balsam, wax, and tallow dropped from a burning candle into water. In short, I was so successful, that about Christmas my patient engaged in an hunting party. . .I certainly did not spare my time or attention on the occasion, as I regularly dressed his wound three times a day, during the course of a month."

1793 Simcoe Diary Lake Ontario 209. "An Indian woman came to-day with pitch. . .to gum the canoe."

1809 Hugh Gray 383. "Exports from Quebec 1808. . .Essence of Spruce, 150 casks, 100 shillings each."

1814 Clarke Consp. London 1. "Abietis Resina, Resin of the Spruce fir. Stimulant, diuretic, aperient. . .in gleet [pus discharge from wounds] etc. nephritic cases &c. It is, however, at this time rarely used. . .Externally it is an ingredient in various stimulating ointments and plasters, which are employed in catarrh, asthma, and obstinate rheumatic affections."

1816 Hall Ont. 208. "We stopped to bait our steed, and selves at a solitary log hut in the centre of a forest; where, besides oats, we found excellent spruce beer made on the spot and gingerbread cakes as the sign specified, being underwritten 'Cakes and Beer'."

1820's Materia Medica Edinburgh-Toronto mss, 70. "Pix Burgundica. As a Rubefacient it is used spread upon Leather and applied to the skin & excites a degree of inflammation without producing a blister, used with advantage in Catarrh, Dyspnoe & phthisis."

1829 MacTaggart 1; 97. "The spruce fir is very common, and furnishes materials for spruce-beer, a beverage of high request among the Canadians; and spruce knees, which are the roots of this tree, are found to be good substitutes for crooked oak, in boat and ship building."

1830 Rafinesque 183. "Spruce beer is an American beverage, made by the Indians with twigs and cones of spruces, boiled in maple syrup. Now it is chiefly made with molasses and yeast, when no spruce is put in, it is only molasses beer. The proper spruce beer is a palatable and healthy drink, powerfully antiscorbutic. The first discoverers of Canada were cured of scurvy by it, since which, it has become in common use in Canada, the Northern States, and even in Europe. If the use was still more general, it might destroy the bad effects of the scorbutic habit or land scurvy, so prevalent among those chiefly feeding on salt meat. The essence or extract of spruce, is an article of exportation, used as naval stores; spruce beer may be made of it in a short time, and any where. . . .The inner bark is used by empirics in powder and tea for bowel and stomach complaints, rheumatism, and gravel. The timber is valuable for masts, spars, rafters, and boards. The resin exuding from the trees is nearly like frankincense. Josselyn says that it is very good in powder over wounds, to re-produce the flesh; but the resin of the European fir is used in plaster to produce itching, rubefaction, and blistering, the resin of all the firs must be heating and irritating."

1832 McGregor 1; 221. "Spirits are frequently mixed with spruce beer to make a drink called Callibogus."

1842 Christison 914. "Many other pines besides these yield articles which are more or less known in commerce, and which are also probably applied to medical use. . .*Abies nigra* [*Picea mariana*], the Black Spruce-fir of North America. . .such as Essence of spruce, familiarly used for making spruce beer, are got by exhausting the leaves. . .by ebullition with water. . .Frankincense is obtained in the form of concrete tears from the. . .Norway spruce-fir *Picea abies*, spontaneously or by incisions. It is firm and brittle, yet slowly takes the form of the vessel which contains it. . .It is not much used in Britain without having undergone a process of preparation, by which it is converted into Burgundy-pitch. . . .916. Burgundy-pitch constitutes the chief ingredient of the. . .pitch plaster, or warm plaster, which is employed as a rubefacient; and it is also sometimes used alone for this purpose."

1859-61 Gunn 760. "Burgundy-pitch. . .makes an excellent strengthening plaster for weak backs, and is also good for pains, rheumatic swellings of the joints, pains in the chest; and in hooping-cough, it is very good applied over the breast and stomach of children. To form a plaster, it is to be melted and spread thin on soft, thin leather, and as it cools, thin and smooth it and spread it out with the warm blade of a case knife or spatula. To derive any decided effect from these plasters, they should be made large, so as to cover the breast, back, stomach, abdomen, side, or whatever part they may be applied to. A small pitch plaster is of but little account. They are to be worn for several days at a time—or so long as they will stick!"

1868 Can. Pharm. J. 6; 83-5. "The leaves of the black spruce, *Abies nigra* [*Picea mariana*], included in list of Can. medicinal plants.

1878 Can. Pharm. J. 13-14. "Manhattan spruce beer powder. 16½ ozs. double refined powdered sugar, 3½ ozs. of bicarbonate of soda, 4 ozs. of citric acid, concentrated essence of spruce 1 oz. The soda, acid, and sugar must be very carefully dried, separately, and at a temperature not exceeding 120°. Before drying the sugar, the same must be thoroughly incororated with the essence, to which a small quantity of caramel, as coloring, may be added. Immediately put the mixture into a dry bottle, and cork securely. For use put one teaspoonful into a glass of water and stir until it dissolves."

1885 Hoffman OJIBWA 198. "Black spruce. The leaves and crushed bark are used to make a decoction, and sometimes taken as a substitute in the absence of pines. Wood used in manufacture of spear handles. . .White spruce. . .The split roots—wadob—are used for sewing; the wood for the inside timbers of canoes."

1888 Delamare Island of Miquelon transl. 29. "The wood of black spruce, light, resistant and elastic, is used for the construction of little goelettes [small boats with two masts]. The young shoots make the habitual drink of the country, spruce beer."

1894 Turner Hudson Bay NASKOPIE 301. "Each household is supplied with sundry wooden vessels of various sizes which serve for buckets for holding water and for drinking cups. They are made of strips of thin boards cut from spruce or from larch trees, the wider strips being as much as six inches wide and one third of an inch thick. They are steamed and bent into ovoid or circular forms and the ends of the strip overlapping. Then they are sewed with split roots from those trees. A groove is cut near the lower edge and into it is placed a dish-shaped piece of wood for a bottom. These vessels are identical in shape and function with those manufactured by the Yukon river Indians of Alaska. They also use berry-dishes or baskets. . .made from the bark of the spruce peeled in the spring of the year. At this time the bark is quite flexible and may be bent into the desired shape. The corners are sewed with coarse roots from the same tree and the rim is strengthened by a strip of root sewed over and around it by means of a finer strand. These baskets serve a good purpose when the women are picking berries, of which they are inordinately fond; and during the season it is a rarity to see a woman or man without a mouth stained the peculiar blue color which these berries impart. Baskets of this shape frequently have a top of buckskin sewed to them, closed with a drawstring. . .303. The stem of the pipe is of spruce wood and is prepared by boring a small hole through the stick lengthwise and whittling it down to the required size. It is from 4 to 8 inches long and is often ornamented with a band of many colored beads. . .The pipes used for smoking are made of stone obtained from river pebbles, usually a fine-grained compact sandstone. . . .The best of all the pipes and those most valued are of greenish sandstone having strata of darker colors which appear as beautiful graining when the pipe is cut into form and polished."

1892 Millspaugh 163. "Spruce beer may be made from the extract as follows: Take one part of essence of spruce and seventy-six parts of water, boil, strain, allow to cool, and add ninety-six parts warm water, seven parts molasses and one part of yeast. Allow the mixture to ferment, and bottle strongly while fermenting."

1897 Handbook of Canada John Macoun 279. "The black spruce in the east prefers the boggy ground, but as it approaches its northern limit it seems to enjoy drier ground and vies with the white spruce in occupying the last oases before the forest ceases altogether and the continuous barren grounds commence."

1901 Morice DENE 27. "The most common form of ophthalmic trouble among the Northern Dene is snow blindness and its resulting whitening of the affected pupil. A persistent haziness in the atmosphere and the refraction of a strong light on the water will sometimes have the same effect on persons of a delicate constitution. If allowed to develop itself unhindered, this deterioration of the pupil will completely destroy the sight. The Carriers' great remedy against the complaint, as in all cases of soreness resulting from accidental blows or tearings, is the balsam of young spruce tops (*Abies nigra*) [*Picea mariana*]. The upper shoots once cut off the sapling are bent and split in two and then left by the fireside. After the resinous liquid they contain has been heated out, the ball of the eye is gently coated therewith by means of a bird quill."

1915 Harris HURON 54. "To burns they applied a poultice of boiled spruce."

1915 Speck PENOBSCOT 309. *Picea* sp. in a soft state, or else pine pitch is used as a poultice on boils and abscesses. Spruce gum is chewed extensively by the Indians as a pastime.

1915 Speck MONTAGNAIS 314. Twigs of black spruce are boiled to make a broth that is good for a cough. For generally beneficial effects the twigs of white spruce. . .are steeped for a beverage. . .315. Bark of red spruce is boiled with root of sour grass and the liquid drunk for lung and throat trouble.

1926-7 Densmore CHIPPEWA 317. *Picea rubra*, red spruce; the leaves used to make a tea. . .362. The twigs of White spruce with the moss of ground-pine and chips cut from the 'heart' of ironwood are made in a decoction used for steaming stiff joints in rheumatism. . .379. Spruce gum was considered best for use in calking canoes and birch-bark pails. It was prepared by boiling the gum in a wide-meshed bag which retained the bits of wood and bark, allowing the gum to pass into the water. It was skimmed from the surface and stored until a convenient time when it was mixed with charcoal from cedar. . .377. The roots were used in sewing canoes.

1923 H. Smith MENOMINI 45. "White spruce. The inner bark is used to make a tea which is described as good for inward troubles for either man or woman. The half cooked, beaten, inner bark is used as a poultice placed on a rag and applied to a wound, cut or swelling."

1932 H. Smith OJIBWE 379. White spruce.The leaves are used in the same manner as larch, an inhalant or fumigator. . .Black spruce. The bark. . .as a medicinal salt. . .the leaves. . .a reviver. . .421. Black spruce. . .used these roots to sew canoes, and from incisions in the bark gathered the resin to be boiled with tallow to make pitch for calking canoes.

1933 H. Smith POTAWATOMI 70. "The Forest Potawatomi make poultices from the inner bark of this swamp tree to apply to inflammations where infection is suspected."

1945 Rousseau Quebec transl. 83. "White spruce; the bark is used to start a fire, 'the bark is easy to peel when the sap is running. . .when it is between the bark and the trunk, it is easy to lift off'. The gum is used as chewing gum, as a digestive. The branches used to be used as brooms; they evidently were only used once. 'One had no regret, there was plenty.'"

1945 Raymond TÊTE DE BOULE transl. 129. "White and red spruce; the roots were used to sew canoes, baskets, or snow shoes. Curiously enough the Tete de Boule have only one name for both the spruce and the balsam. The gum of the spruce, like that of the pine is applied to sores."

1955 Mockle Quebec transl. 23. "White spruce; The branches in decoction are an antiscorbutic drink by reason of the high content of ascorbic acid. It was this species, called by the Indians 'Anedda' that was drunk by the men in Cartier's command who were cured of scurvy; nevertheless historians hold the most diverse opinions on the exact identity of Anedda. . .24. Black spruce; an infusion of the leaves makes an antiscorbutic drink; those of the branches are used to cure colds. This species furnishes the spruce gum of commerce. From the young shoots the spruce beer is made that is well known and appreciated in Canada."

1975 Chem. Abstr. 83. 203741d Chemical composition of coniferous needles and their uses. Usova N.P. USSR 1973 in Russian M. Ticha-Karlova. The dynamics of ascorbic acid (I) and carotiene (II) chlorophyll and essential oil in needles of fir (*Abies*) and spruce (*Picea*) was investigated. The highest amount of (I) (427 mg/) was found in fir needles, of (II) (23 mg/) in spruce needles. The maximum of (I) and (II) both in spruce and fir needles was found in 3 year needles and with further growth their content decreased. Decreased exposure of needles to light was accompanied by a decrease of the (I) level. Needles of fir and spruce contained from 1-4.5% essential oils.

The MICMAC and MALECITE of the Maritime provinces of Canada used the White spruce for stomach trouble, scabs and sores, as a salve for cuts and wounds and the tea for scurvy. The Black spruce was used as a cough remedy. (Chandler, Freeman and Hooper 1979).

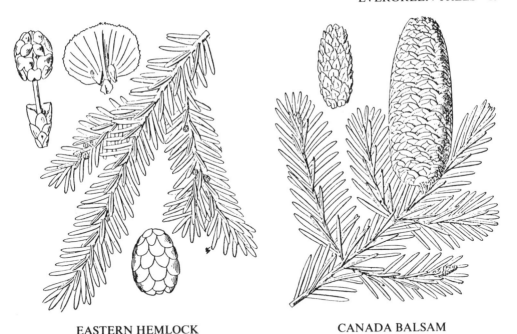

EASTERN HEMLOCK   CANADA BALSAM

EASTERN HEMLOCK   *Tsuga canadensis* (L.) Carr. Pinaceae (*T. americana, Abies c.*)
Tree up to 30 m tall furrows run the length of the bark. The needles all essentially equal in
length, 8-15 mm, with rounded ends and two white lines on the undersides. They join their hairy
twigs in a little cup, and do not fall when a branch is picked. The cones are 12-20 mm long, their
main scales rounded, pale green turning red brown.
Range. N.B., P.E.I., N.S., Que., s. Ont., n. to ne. end L. Superior, ne. Minn., s. to Ala., Ga. and
N.C. in the mts. on rocky ridges, cool hillsides and moist soil. Beauchamp translates the Onondaga name for the hemlock, O-Ne-Tah, as meaning 'greens on a stick'. Cartier 1534 translated
the Laurentian Iroquois word 'haneda' as 'greens on a stick' and gave the name 'annedda' to the
tree that cured his crew of scurvy. See under spruce for a full account. It is possible that the hemlock, a tree unknown to Europeans, was this 'annedda'. It seems probable it was either the hemlock or the spruce. There is no agreement on this subject; see cedar also.
1637 Le Mercier HURON Jes. Rel. 13;261. When smallpox was rampant in the village of Ossosane the Huron medicine man ordered the chief to take: "The bark of the ash, the spruce, the
hemlock and the wild cherry, boiling them together well in a great kettle and washing the whole
body therewith, and that care should be taken not to go out of their cabins barefooted, in the
evening. He added that his remedies were not for women in their courses."
1663 Boucher Quebec transl. 43. "There is another sort of tree called 'Epinette:' it is almost like
the balsam, except that it is better for making masts for small vessels, such as chalouppes & bar-
ques, being stronger than the balsam. I speak of the green epinette: for there are two sorts, one
green, & the other red."
1672 Josselyn New Engl. 200. "The Indians break and heal their swellings and sores with it;
boyling the inner bark of young hemlock very well; then knocking of it betwixt two stones to a
playster; and anointing or soaking it in the soyls' oyl, they apply it to the sore. It will break a sore
swelling speedily."
1698 Hennepin Lake Ontario 73. "Their Forests are replenished with the prettiest trees in the
world, Pines, Cedars and Epinettes (a sort of Firr-tree very common in the country)."
1749 Kalm Ft. St. Frederic Oct. 18th. 589. "The hemlock spruce which was used in brewing."
1778 Carver 498. "The Hemlock tree grows in every part of America in a greater or less degree. It
is an evergreen of a very large growth, and has leaves somewhat like that of the yew; it is how-

ever quite useless, and only an incumbrance to the ground, the wood being of a very coarse grain and full of wind-shakes or cracks."

1796 Simcoe Diary 598. "Mr. McGill drinks a tea made of hemlock pine."

1821 Howison 184. "Here I enjoyed all the comforts that are usually met with in Canadian hotels; and after supping on bread and *hemlock tea*, and supplying my horse with buck wheat and wild hay, I went to bed at an early hour."

1836 Trail Backwoods 54. "Our stock of tea was exhausted, and we were unable to procure more. . .so we agreed to try a Yankee tea hemlock sprigs boiled. This proved to my taste, a vile decoction; though I recognised some herb in the tea that was sold in London at five shillings a pound, which I am certain was nothing better than dried hemlock leaves reduced to a coarse powder. S——— laughed at our wry faces declaring the potation was excellent; and he set us all an example by drinking six cups of the truly sylvan beverage."

1840 Gosse Quebec 8. "The hemlock, as you are aware is a majestic tree, though of very little use. Yet it is sometimes sawn into board and plank; the former though rough grained, answers for undercovering of roofs and for fencing; and the latter, from its solidity, is well enough adapted for the flooring of barns. . .stripped of its bark which is bought at a good price by the tanners."

1855 Trail Settlers Guide 138. "The tops of the hemlock are used by some persons as tea, but I think very few would drink hemlock tea if they could get a more palatable beverage. As a remedy for a severe cold, I believe a cup of hemlock-tea, drunk quite warm in bed, is excellent, as well as suderific. . .The hemlock is very hard to cut down, and difficult to burn up."

1859-61 Gunn 804-5. "This is a large tree, growing in some of the most northern States and in the Canadas, the bark of which is used extensively for tanning. . .There is a sort of pitch, or gummy juice, which exudes from this tree, which is gathered, purified by boiling, and is sold for medicinal purposes. It is hard, brittle, of a dark brown color, and easily softens by heat. . .Is mostly used for plasters;. . .An excellent strengthening plaster for weak backs. . .Oil of Hemlock. This is a valuable essential or volatile oil, obtained by distilling the gum. . .is useful as an external application in rheumatism, croup, and in all cases requiring a stimulating lotion. . .A strong decoction of the Hemlock bark is a valuable injection in chronic leucorrhea, and for falling of the womb; and is also often used internally as a remedy for diarrhea."

1868 Can. Pharm. J. 6; 83-5. Hemlock, *Abies Canadensis*, the bark and essential oil included in list of Can. medicinal plants.

1879 Can. Pharm. J. April 302. "A series of experiments by Mr. W. McMurtrie, of Washington, to determine the tannin value of various vegetable substances. . .gave amongst others, the following results. . .hemlock bark, N.Y., 9.5 per cent."

1885 Hoffman OJIBWA 198. "Raven tree. . .Outer bark powdered and crushed and taken internally for the cure of diarrhea. Usually mixed with other plants not named."

1897 Handbook of Canada Mavor 404. "The presence of tanning barks, principally hemlock, in large quantities in Canada, has brought about the establishment of tanneries in close proximity to the sources of supply of tanning agents". . .Ellis 324. "The bark of the hemlock which abounds throughout most of the Dominion, contains much tannin, and is largely used by tanners. In New Brunswick and Quebec; extract is made from the bark for use in tanning, the yearly value of which is put at $120,000. There were in 1891, 802 tanneries whose output is valued at $11,422,860."

1892 Millspaugh 164. "The stimulating effect of hemlock is well known and greatly utilized. A tired hunter arises fresh and invigorated from his bed of hemlock boughs, and the patient of the city physician, seeking health in our northern interiors, finds supreme comfort in a bath, in which hemlock leaves have been slowly steeping for some hours before his ablutions, and quiet, refreshing slumber awaits him upon his couch of soft branches. A strong decoction of hemlock bark has received the praise of empirics and the laity as an astringent enema in diarrhoea and in injection for leucorrhoea, prolapsus uteri, etc.; the oil as a liniment in croup, rheumatismus, and other disorders requiring stimulant action; and the essence as a diuretic and a remedy to allay gastric irritation and colic, and to correct acidity of the stomach. A decoction of the bark has been used to produce abortion with dangerous effects, tending towards serious peritonitis. Pregnant ewes are said to lose their lambs from gnawing the bark of hemlock. . . .Pix Canadensis (Hemlock pitch, Hemlock gum, Canada pitch). This substance, the prepared resinous exudation from the trunk of the hemlock. . .contains a resin and a volatile oil, uninvestigated, but supposed to be similar to the turpentine obtained from *Abies balsamea*, balsam. Oil of Hemlock (oil of spruce). This essential oil is obtained on distillation of the leaves, a process carried on to a large extent in some portions of the State of New York."

1916 Waugh IROQUOIS 68. "Decoctions of hemlock bark and roots, also the bark of the alder, are used in colouring spoons and other wooden articles a deep red. These become further darkened and polished by usage. . .147. Hemlock, ona da uw. Take the leaves, steep, sweeten with maple sugar, and eat with corn bread or at meals."

1919 Sturtevant 582. "The Indians of Maine prepare a tea from the leaves of hemlock and this tea is relished as a drink. The spray is also used in New England and elsewhere to a limited extent in the domestic manufacture of spruce beer."

1924 Youngken 498. "The Penobscot tribe used finely powdered hemlock bark to relieve and prevent chafing."

1926-7 Densmore CHIPPEWA 356. The inner bark pulverized and applied dry, externally for wounds. This is also used in many combinations. . .371. Dyes. Hemlock bark and a little grindstone dust and hot water. . .gives a mahogany color. . .317. Beverages. Fresh leaves were tied in a packet with a thin strip of basswood bark before being put in the water. . .The quantity was usually about a heaping handful to a quart of water. Beverages were usually sweetened with maple sugar and drunk while hot. . .Hemlock leaves were among those used.

1928 Parker SENECA 10. "It was the tea made from hemlock needles that cured Cartier's crew of scurvy. It was prepared in so mysterious a manner, no doubt, that Cartier did not know what it was, and later he laments that he did not have it. He left, as a clue, however, the Iroquoian word *onetda*, which enables the linguist to make a translation and establish its identity. Hemlock tea was the common table tea of the Iroquois people, especially in winter when the diet was largely restricted to dried foods.". .11. Materia Medica, as a febrifuge, hemlock.

1923 H. Smith MENOMINI 46. "The inner bark is used to make a tea to heal pains in the abdomen. One quart of tea is drunk to cure a cold. The leaves are used in the sudatory [sweat bath], of which ground hemlock [*Taxus canadensis*, yew] is the principal medicine. . .78. Boiled hemlock bark is the source of the dark red coloring of the Menomini."

1928 H. Smith MESKWAKI 197. "An ingredient in a medicine for sore gums, pyorrhoea, stomach troubles. . .the bark of hemlock with the inner bark of the smooth alder, and the root of ginseng mixed with alum."

1932 H. Smith OJIBWE 380. "The bark is used for healing cuts and wounds, and for stopping the flow of blood from a wound. The bark is rich in tannin and naturally quite astringent. . .408. The Flambeau Ojibwe use the leaves of Hemlock to make a beverage tea. This sort of tea is often times used by the Indian Medicine man to carry his medicaments and disguise the fact that the patient is taking medicine. . .422. Hemlock bark was used by the Flambeau Ojibwe for fuel, when boiling their pitch the second time, because the heat from it was more easily regulated than that from a wood fire. . .426. Use the bark together with a little rock dust to set the color, to dye materials a dark red brown."

1933 H. Smith POTATWATOMI 71. "The Forest Potawatomi use the leaves of the Hemlock to brew a tea which causes the patient to break out with copious perspiration and is valuable for breaking up a cold. The inner bark of the hemlock is mixed with other medicaments to cure the Flux."

1942 Fenton IROQUOIS 506. "Until recent times hemlock tea has been a favorite winter beverage with the Iroquoian tribes whose names for hemlock, or evergreen, are clearly cognate with the term given Cartier, 'Anneda'. Curiously enough Cartier says that this decoction brought miraculous relief in longstanding cases of venereal disease among the sailors, and modern Iroquois herbalists employ the hemlock as an ingredient in formulae for boils and venereal disease. This is an interesting fact historically, whether or not the plant is a specific for the disease. Seventeenth century travelers were unable to rediscover the famous tree, because the Laurentians had abandoned their Quebec towns in the intervening decades and the succeeding Algonquians did not employ it as an antiscorbutic."

1945 Rousseau MOHAWK transl. 36. "The young branches are used as a tea."

1950 Wintemberg 11. "Blood purifier. . .Tea made from the leaves of the hemlock spruce."

1952 A.C. Shaw in the preparation and composition of some Canadian coniferous oils, states that the composition of the oils from spruce and hemlock is quite similar. . .they are rich sources of bornyl acetate, hemlock contains 43.4% and black spruce 37%. As well hemlock contains 17.6% a-pinene and 11.5% camphene.

1955 Mockle Quebec transl. 21. The bark is astringent containing 7-12% tannins. The leaves are considered abortificants.

1968 Androsko 41. "Hemlock bark provided the settlers of Eastern United States with another good source of reddish-brown dye. . .This dye was applied to both wool and cotton and employed in tanning leather in Nova Scotia. When combined with an alum mordant it resulted in a durable bright reddish brown hue on wool and an impermanent nankeen (brownish yellow) on cotton. Copperas mordant produced dark drab and slate colors."

1970 Bye IROQUOIS Onondago county N.Y. mss. Boughs used to line storage pits for corn and other vegetables and to make primitive brooms. The bark for poulticing sores and wounds, the leaves as tea for colds, coughs, rheumatism, antiscorbutic, used with pine bark as a poultice. Bark and roots used to stain carved utensils deep red. Mythological tea to sweat.

1973 Su, Staba & Abul-Hajj L1. March 85. "Tannic acid was noted for its antiseptic action as early as 1927. At a concentration of 0.03%, tannic acid has been reported to be bacteriostatic against three strains of *E. coli*, a 10 to 20% tannin solution completely destroyed *E. coli*, *S. albua* and *S. citreus*. . .Tannic acid causes liver damage and is toxic to mice and rats when given intravenously."

ALGONQUIN Indians use the needles to spice wild meat such as bear or porcupine. They drink the tea of the needles. (Assiniwi 1972)

The MICMAC and MALECITE of the maritime provinces of Canada are said to have used the hemlock for:—bowel and internal troubles, cold in bladder, cold in kidneys, cough, chapped skin, diarrhea, scurvy, stomach troubles, grippe. (Chandler, Freeman and Hooper 1979.)

CANADA BALSAM   *Abies balsamea* (L.) Mill. Pinaceae (*Pinus balsamea*)
Trees to 25 m tall, the gray bark eventually becoming scaly, with blisters full of resin on the bark in places. The twigs minutely hairy, the needles 12-15 mm long with white lines on the undersides, the ends rounded, twisted at their base and attached directly to the twigs. The cones 5-10 cm long with rounded scales that fall off.

Range. Ungava-Labrador, Nfld., P.E.I., N.B., N.S., Que., Ont. to Alta., Mackenzie valley, s. to N.Y., Mich., Minn. and in the mts. to Va. and W. Va., n. Io. in moist woods and swamps.

Common names. Balm-of-gilead fir, Canada fir tree, Canada balsam, balsam spruce.

1475 Bjornnson Icelandic mss transl. Larsen 132. "Thus, incense. Hot and dry in the second degree. If one crushes incense and tempers it with white of egg or with warm breast milk, that brightens the eyes. If one crushes incense and tempers it with vinegar and resin and milk, it heals new wounds. If one tempers it with fat pork or with suet of a wether, its good for burns. If one tempers it with warm wine, it is to be put in the ears for earache. If one tempers it with oil of roses and chalk, it is good for swollen nipples. If one tempers incense with wine or vinegar it is good to drink for dysentery. If one crushes incense in breast-milk and applies to pustules which come below upon a man's anus, that helps. If one crushes incense and aloes with whites of eggs till it becomes thick and applies it for fractures or to wounds that bleed much, then he shall leave the application there until he believes the bone to be bound or the wound healed; and he shall use the same leechdom until fully cured. Incense is good for a flux, and its smell strengthens a man's memory. Whoever eats it with the herb called origanum, he will spit forth every illness from his head; and the same is good for illness of the tongue. If one crushes incense with paunch-fat of goose or with suet of wether, it is good for whatever is burned or what fire has injured."

1542 Alfonse Cosmog. transl. 298-9. "And in all that country [the banks of the St. Lawrence near Quebec] there are a large number of trees and of many kinds, such as oaks, cedars (cèdres).. 'arbre de vye,' which contain medicine; they have a gum white as snow; familiar pines, with which are made the masts for the navy. . .And there are some very large cedars." [See white and red cedar, their gum was not used by the Indians as balsam gum was.]

1609 Lescarbot-Erondelle Acadia 305. "Good profit may be drawn from the fir and spruce trees, because they yield abundance of gum; and they die very often through over-much liquor. This gum is very fair, like the turpentine of Venice, and very sovereign for medicines. I have given some to some churches of Paris for frankincense [incense], which hath been found very good. . .123. We had no pitch to caulk our vessels. . .Monsieur de Poutrincourt advised himself to gather in the woods quantity of the gum issuing from fir-trees. Which he did with much labour, going thither himself, most often with a boy or two; so that in the end he got some hundred pounds weight of it. Now after these labours, it was not yet all, for it was needful to melt and purify the same, which was a necessary point and unknown to our ship master. . .Nevertheless. . .Monsieur de Poutrincourt found the means to draw out the quintessence of these gums and fir-tree barks; and caused a quantity of bricks to be made, with the which he made an open furnace, wherein he put a limbeck [Alembic, an apparatus formerly used in distilling] made with many kettles, joined one in the other, which he filled with these gums and barks: then, being well covered, fire was put around about it, by whose violence the gum enclosed within the said lembeck melted, and dropped down into a basin, but it was needful to be very watchful at it, by reason that, if the fire had taken hold of the gum, all had been lost. That was admirable, especially in a man that never saw any made. Wherof the savages being astonished did say, in words borrowed from the Basques: *Endia chavé Normandia*, that is to say, that the Normans know many things. Now they call all Frenchmen Normans, except the Basques, because the most part of the fishermen that go a-fishing there be of that nation. This remedy came very fitly unto us, for those which came to seek us were fallen into the same want that we were. . .245. Canoes. . .made of barks of trees. . .And to the end they leak not, they cover the seams (which join the said barks together, which they make of roots) with the gum of fir-trees."

1663 Boucher Quebec transl. 42. "There are lots of firs as in France: the only difference that I can see is that there are bubbles on the bark, which are full of a certain liquid gum that is aromatic, and it is used on wounds like balms, and has as much virtue, according to the report of those who have tried it; there are other claims made for it, but I will leave that to the Doctors."

1718 (Richard Can. Arch. 1899) Paris to Quebec 529. The flour sent from Canada to the Islands [French West Indies] is packed in barrels made from Balsam wood, which imparts a disagreeable odour and taste. This must be seen to.

1792 Simcoe Diary Ontario 92. "Mr. (Lieut.) Grey cut his finger, and applied the turpentine from the balm of Gilead fir, a remedy for wounds greatly esteemed."

1793 Mackenzie Voyages 27. "The salve I applied [to the wound] on the occasion was made of the Canadian balsam, wax, and tallow dropped from a burning candle into water." [See spruce.]

1799 Lewis Mat. Med. 252. "Canada fir-tree much superior to common turpentine, one of the purest of turpentines. In distillation with water yields a highly penetrating essential oil. Promotes urine, cleanses the parts concerned in the evacuation thereof, and deterges internal ulcers in general; and at the same time, like other bitter hot substances, strengthen the tone of the vessels; they have an advantage above most other acrid diuretics, that they gently loosen the belly . . produces inflammation in urethra-can be dangerous. . .a few drops of distilled oil are a sufficient dose. This is a most potent, stimulating, detergent diuretic, often greatly heats the constitution, and requires the utmost caution in its exhibition. . .externally for sciatica. . .when turpentine is carried into the blood vessels, it stimulates the whole system; hence its use in chronic rheumatism and in paralysis."

1809 Hugh Gray 172. Statement of exports from Canada. "I have taken the average of five years, ending 1805... Balsam, 1780 lbs. at 6 pence a lb.

1814 Clarke Conspect. 26. "Canadian Turpentine. Stimulant, diuretic. In gleet, leucorrhoea, &c. . .This species of turpentine is reckoned the best, and has the most agreeable flavour: it is not properly a balsam, as it contains no benzoic acid. *Pinus balsamea*."

1820's Materia Medica Edinburgh-Toronto mss 54. "*Pinus Balsamea*, its medical virtues seem to be analogous to those of Copaiba, its dose from 20 to 30 drops. . .Copaiba officinalis acts as a diuretic."

1830 Rafinesque 182. "Firs. Those which have a balsamic smell, produce in small bladders on the branches, the Canada Balsam (wrongly called Balm of Gilead) which is healing, useful in internal and external sores. It is injurious in recent wounds, but good after they begin to heal. It may be taken internally on loaf sugar."

1836 Vindicator Montreal May 6th. "On Thursday, a woman of the name of Dupré, living in the concession of Ste. Rosalie, was occupied boiling gum or Balsam."

1842 Christison 916. "Turpentine differs fundamentally from Frankencense only in so far as it contains more volatile oil, and is consequently more or less liquid at ordinary temperatures. Three varieties have a place in the British Pharmacopoeia, Common turpentine, Venice turpentine, and Canada balsam. . .917. Canada balsam is one of the finest of the pine turpentines. It is produced in North America by the *Abies balsamea* or balm-of-gilead fir, and probably also by the *Abies canadensis* or hemlock spruce [*Tsuga canadensis*]. It is collected sometimes by bursting little bladders on the bark, and sometimes by making deep incisions. The former sort, which is the finer of the two, is occasionally sold as true Balm of Gilead. . .318. The turpentines were at one time used in medicine internally; and Canada balsam is still so employed for the arrestment of chronic mucous discharges, such as dysentery, gleet and catarrh. At present, however, they are little applied to any direct therapeutic purpose, and are chiefly used as furnishing resin and oil of turpentine. . .918. Resin. . .in pharmacy it is specially applied to the substance left by pine turpentine after removal of their volatile oil. . .If the process be continued until the water is all expelled. . .matter remains, which is called Colophony, Black rosin, or Fiddler's rosin. . .It is manufactured, as the Edinburgh Pharmacopoeia indicates, from various kinds of turpentine. . .920. Resin is now used in medicine only as an external agent, partly on account of its own stimulant properties, but chiefly to give due consistence or adhesiveness to various ointments, cerates, liniments, and plaster. It forms a material proportion of the. . .Basilicon ointment, a familiar stimulating application for indolent sores; and it constitutes an essential part of the adhesive plaster. . .which in addition to other ordinary uses in the dressing of wounds and sores, has been for some time employed with great advantage in the form of straps for giving support to limbs in cases of chronic ulcers."

1859-61 Gunn 758. "Balsam of Fir—called also Canada Balsam.—This is an article found in all drug stores. . .In large doses it will act as a cathartic. Internally it is good in coughs, gonorrhea, gleet, whites, affections of the urinary organs, and ulcerations of the bowels. Externally, it is good applied in small wounds, as well as old and indolent ulcers and sores. It also forms an important ingredient in some healing salves."

1868 Can. Pharm. J. 6; 83-5. The Balsam of the balsam spruce included in the list of Can. medicinal plants.

1884 Holmes-Haydon CREE Hudson Bay 302. "Wyakash?—This is the fiber of the bark of *Abies Balsamea*, Marshall, freed from the periderm and leaving exposed the numerous vesicles in which the Canada balsam is secreted. The bark is about one line thick, has a short fracture, and is of a white colour when broken; the inner surface is pale brown and the exterior reddish brown. The taste is astringent and bitter, with a flavour of Canada balsam." [Does not indicate use. See H. Smith Potawatomi for Cree usage.]

1885 Hoffman OJIBWA 198. "The bark is scraped from the trunk and a decoction thereof is used to induce diaphoresis. 2 The gum, which is obtained from the vesicles upon the bark, and also by skimming it from the surface of the water in which the crushed bark is boiled, is carried in small vessels and taken internally as a remedy for gonorrhea and for soreness of the chest resulting from colds. Applied externally to sores and cuts."

1888 Delamare Island of Miquelon transl. 29. "The turpentine, called Balsam of Canada is not used in the colony."

1894 Household Guide Toronto 112. "Turpentine has almost as many uses as borax. It is good for rheumatism, and mixed with camphorated oil and rubbed on the chest, it is one of the best remedies for bronchial colds."

1915 Harris HURON 48. "The cough root or Indian balsam was included among their most valuable remedies for colds and incipient consumption and swellings. They stripped from the tree the outer bark, using only the inner. The juice was deemed by them to be helpful in bowel complaints. The inner bark when chewed and swallowed helped to support life when periods of famine visited the tribe."

1915 Speck PENOBSCOT 309. Fir sap is smeared over burns, sores and cuts as a healer. . .312. Fir twigs, one of the seven herbs taken as a sudorific before entering the sweat bath.

1915 Speck MONTAGNAIS 313. Inner bark is grated and eaten as beneficial to diet at times. . .314. Fir twigs are soaked in hot water, made into a mash and put on the skin to draw out inflammation in case of pain.

1926-7 Densmore CHIPPEWA 338. Gum placed on hot stones until it melts; fumes inhaled for convulsions. . .350. Gum combined with bear's grease as an ointment for the hair. . .362. Decoction of the root sprinkled on hot stones, the decoction being very hot. This was used to 'steam' rheumatic joints, especially those of the knees, the patient being covered closely and letting the steam warm the knees.

1923 H. Smith MENOMINI 45. "There are two remedies from this tree. The liquid balsam which is pressed from the trunk blisters is used for colds and pulmonary troubles. The inner bark is also gathered observing the same rules as in the gathering of white pine bark, with, of course, the particular song and a deposit of tobacco in the ground that accompanies all medicines. It is a very valuable remedy with the Menomini. The inner bark is steeped and the tea is drunk for pains in the chest. It is also used fresh for poultices. It is further used as a seasoner for other medicines. Inquiry as to whether the Menomini gathered the bark with the oil vesicles intact and used it as the Hudson Bay Indians do under the name of 'wayakosh' for wounds, developed that they did not know this use. Yet the same effect would probably be produced by the inner bark used as poultices, which the Menomini did."

1932 H. Smith OJIBWE 378. "The Flambeau Ojibwe. . .claim that the liquid balsam is used direct from the bark blisters upon the eyes, for sore eyes. The leaves are a reviver. . .and are also used in combinations as a wash. The Pillager Ojibwe. . .use the balsam gum for colds and to heal sores. This corresponds to the way the Hudson Bay Indians use the bark. The needle like leaves are placed upon live coals and the smoke is inhaled for colds. They also are used as a part of the medicine for the sweat bath. The sweat bath is taken in a small hemispherical wigwam, like the regular abode, but entirely covered with mats or nowadays with canvas. The medicines are coiled into wreaths to fit into large iron kettles. Water is added and finally hot rocks which cause steam. The Indian taking the sweat bath may be taking it for ceremonial reasons, for cleansing, but most likely as a medicated steam bath. He sits naked within until there is no more steam and his body is entirely dried again. He then puts on clean clothes and will not wear the discarded clothes until they have been thoroughly washed. The candidate for degrees in the medicine lodge, must undergo the sweat bath in a ceremonial way. Usual plants employed to medicate the steam are white pine leaves, hemlock leaves, arbor vitae leaves. . .Balsam needles. . .They are undoubtedly very beneficial to the health. . .420. The Ojibwe chop a hole in the trunk and allow the resin to accumulate and harden. When gathered and boiled it becomes a canoe pitch. It is usually boiled a second time with the addition of suet or fat to make a canoe pitch of the proper consistency."

1933 H. Smith POTAWATOMI 68. "The Forest Potawatomi gather the resinous exudate from the blisters on the trunk of the balsam fir, and use it, just as it comes from the blisters, for colds. Although they sometimes gather it in a bottle, it is more often that they go to the trees, open the blister with their thumb nail and pick out the drops of balsam to swallow fresh to cure a cold. Where it is gathered, it is saved in a bottle and used as a salve to heal sores. Perhaps the cure results as much from the exclusion of air from the sore surface as it does from the medicinal qualities of the balsam. They also make an infusion of the bark to drink for curing consumption and other internal affections. . . .The [National] Dispensatory [1916] records the practice of the Hudson Bay Indians who peel the bark, leaving the resin vessels exposed and dry it. They call this 'weakoc' and apply it to wounds. . . .121. The Forest Potawatomi use the Balsam fir needles to make pillows, believing, as does the white man, that the aroma keeps one from having a cold."

1945 Rousseau MOHAWK transl. 37. "During the full moon, the gum runs from the tree, which is gathered by a spoon. It is a remarkable antiseptic with numerous uses. For a cold by adding several drops to a cup of hot water. For cancer make a plaster with the gum of the balsam and the kidneys of a beaver, dried. . . .The plaster 'draws' the sickness. After using, take great care not to burn the plaster; otherwise the sickness will disperse in the smoke in the neighbourhood. It must be wrapped in the skin of a muskrat and buried. The opinion that the gum secretes in the tree during the full moon rests on no foundation. All the Indians of the region use this gum, the balm of Canada. The Potawatomis use it for colds and ulcerations. The Algonquins of Temiscaming, for burns, abscesses, etc. The modern charlatans of Montreal, for the treatment of cancer, use a plaster with apparently the same composition."

1945 Raymond TETE DE BOULE transl. 118. "The mashed gum is used for colds. It is also applied to sores. The branches, thrown on the floor of the tent, as well as those of the spruce, act as mats and bedding."

1950 Creighton Lunenburg N.S. 91. "White balsam is made into a drink and used for fever."

1952 A.C. Shaw Pulp and Paper Mag. Canada. Essential oils in Canada Balsam; Bornyl acetate 14.6%; b-pinene 36.1%; 3-carene 11.1%; limonene 11.1%; camphene 6.8%; a-pinene 8.4%.

1955 Mockle Quebec transl. 22. "The bark is strewn with numerous vesicles filled with turpentine with an agreeable odor known as Balm of Canada, gum of the balsam fir, and wrongly as Balm of Gilead. The gum is used as an antiseptic, resolvant, cicatrisant against certain mucus catarrhs, and as a plaster for burns. The tops of the tree mashed in water are used as an antiscorbutic on account of their richness in ascorbic acid. A great part of the production is used to mount microscope slides and to assemble optical lenses. The Balm of Canada is in effect considered as a substitute for Balm of Gilead or that of Mecca. . .furnished by the *Commiphora Opobalsamum*."

1957 Wallis & Wallis MALECITE Maritime Prov. of Canada 5. Frozen limbs were treated with an application of balsam, prepared by boiling Canada fir in a clam shell. Small hoops similar to snowshoes were made and were fastened to frozen feet. Gyles, (1736) who was thus treated and equipped, says that as a result of these measures he was able to follow his master on the winter hunt, and a year later 'hardly a trace of injury could be seen.'

It is interesting to compare the list of illnesses that the MicMac Malecite Indians of the Maritime Provinces of Canada are said to have used the balsam fir for: bruises, burns, colds, colic, diarrhea, fractures, gonorrhea, as a laxative, sores and wounds (Chandler, Freeman and Hooper 1979) with those listed in the 1475 Icelandic mss as being cured by incense.

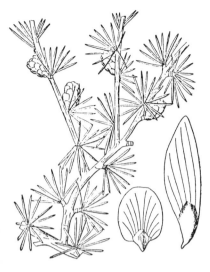
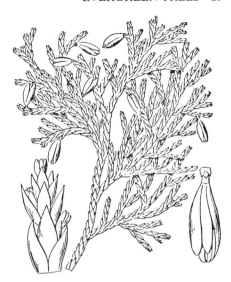

LARCH TAMARACK   WHITE CEDAR

LARCH TAMARACK   *Larix laricina* (Du Roi) Koch Pinaceae (*L. americana, Abies larix, Pinus l.*)
Tree to 20 m tall, not evergreen. Leaves pale blue green, soft, thin, 10-25 mm long in tufts. Female flowers bright red, cone like, male, yellow on the same tree. Cones sit on leafless branches of last year's growth.
Range. Lab., Nfld., N.B., P.E.I., N.S., to Alaska, n. Yukon, Mackenzie delta, s. to N.J., Ill., Minn., W. Va., O. in swamps and bogs.
Common names. Hackmatack, is the Abnaki 'Akemantak' meaning wood for snowshoes; black or red larch, american larch, juniper cypress. Not an 'evergreen'.
1663 Boucher Quebec transl. 43. "Epinette, the red has a firmer and heavier wood, very good for building; it drops its leaves in the autumn, & puts them out again in the Spring: which does not happen with the other firs. The bark is red; it does not give gum, quite the con rary from that of the green epinette, which gives a quantity."
1672 Josselyn New England. I cured once a desperate bruise. . .with an unguent made with the leaves of a larch tree and hogs grease, but the larch gum is best.
1749 Kalm Lake St. George October the 23rd. 594. "The red American larch, which is used in making a beverage, grew here."
1820's Materia Medica Edinburgh-Toronto mss 24-5. "*Pinus Larix* [the European larch]. The tincture of these trees is powerfully stimulant. Has been used in Gleet in the dose of 5 to 20 drops to follow opium, more may be given at the end of an hour. The combination with antimony is not so powerful as with Ipecacuanha."
1830 Rafinesque 235. "Producing a fine balsamic turpentine, good for wounds."
1832 Samuel Thomson used the bark in a tea for bowel complaints. [Riddell 1928; 112.]
1842 Christison 917. "Venice Turpentine is now scarcely ever found of genuine quality in British trade, and is seldom seen even in French commerce. The London College has therefore, not without reason, omitted it in the list of officinal turpentines. It is obtained from the *Abies Larix*, or larch. . .by boring the trees with an auger, and thrusting into the wound a little wooden spout for the juice to pass along."
1868 Can. Pharm J. 6; 83-5. The bark of *Larix americana*, the tamarack, included in list of Can. medicinal plants.
1880 Can. Horticulturist 117. "Mr. Beall stated that at Lindsay he had noted the following facts: Larch was used for poles, ladders, and sometimes for flooring, and was worth $12 per thousand."

1885 Hoffman OJIBWA 198. "1. Crushed leaves and bark used as *Pinus strobus* or white pine. 2. Gum used in mending boats. 3. Bark used for covering wigwams."

1888 Delamare Island of Miquelon transl. 29. "Rare in Miquelon. . .it is used in decoction to treat open sores." Common name is violin wood.

1926 Youngken 180. "Plasters were made by the Penobscot tribe of Maine by evaporating a decoction of the barks of this tree and the American Beech *Fagus americana* to the consistency of an extract and incorporating the pitch of the Norway spruce (*Picea excelsa* Link). The latter was obtained by stripping the bark from the trunk of the standing tree and scorching the wood. The Ojibwa used the crushed leaves and bark as an application for headache. The fumes yielded by placing these on hot stones were inhaled for the same purpose."

1926-7 Densmore CHIPPEWA 352. Inner bark, fresh or dried, chop fine and apply to a burn. Apply in morning, wash off partially at night, and renew. . .377. Roots used in weaving bags, Etc. . .379. Tamarack roots were used in sewing the edges of canoes and in making woven bags.

1928 Reagan OJIBWA 244. Made a tea from the roots.

1923 H. Smith MENOMINI 45. "The bark from both the trunk and the root is described by the Menomini as being pitchy and as equaling one man as a medicine alone, without any help from any other. It is used as a poultice when fresh and is steeped to make a tea. This tea drives out inflammation and generates heat. The water is also given to horses to better their condition from distemper."

1932 H. Smith OJIBWE 378. "The Flambeau Ojibwe use the dried leaves as an inhalant and fumigator. Larch roots are used as sewing material. . .to sew canoes with them. They also make bags from the root fibers, which are considered especially durable."

1933 H. Smith POTAWATOMI 69. "The Forest Potawatomi use the bark and leaves of the Tamarack in just the same manner as the Menomini do. They gather bark from both the root and the trunk. The fresh inner bark is used for poulticing wounds and inflammation while the steeped bark becomes a medicinal tea. . .The Forest Potawatomi also use it as a horse medicine. They mix the shredded inner bark with oats which are fed to the animal and this makes his hide loose so that it slips around when you pinch it. . .The Dispensatory 1916 states that the bark is used to make a tamarack extract or tamarack tincture which is valuable in treating bronchitis and cronic inflammation of the urinary passages, etc."

1938 Lower 25. "The tamarack or hackmatack has been an excellent timber much used for ships. It is practically indestructible under water and stands very well even where exposed. It used to be the colonial substitute for the 'compass timber' of English oak used in the ships of the Royal Navy, its roots furnishing the natural knees and other curved pieces so precious to the early ship-builders. Unfortunately the tamarack as a commercial timber is no more, for some years ago an insect pest swept the country and destroyed all trees of any size. Their gaunt skeletons, bare, grey and dry as tinder, may still be seen standing in northern bogs and muskegs, a tribute to the species durability. Fortunately new growth is rapidly coming on."

1945 Raymond TETE DE BOULE transl. 129. "A tea is made of the young branches as a laxative.

1970 Bye Onondaga county N.Y. IROQUOIS mss. Used bark for tanning.

MICMAC and MALECITE of the maritime provinces of Canada used the bark for suppurating wounds, colds, physical weakness, gonorrhea and consumption (Chandler, Freeman and Hooper 1979).

WHITE CEDAR   *Thuja occidentalis* L. Pinaceae

Tree to 20 m with widely spreading branches. The leaves are soft and flat, sticky when rubbed. They consist of 2-4 mm long scales lying closely one upon the other. Cones to 1 cm with outer scales nearly as long as the inner ones.

Range. N.S., P.E.I., N.B., Que., James Bay, Ont. se. Man., to Minn., s. to Tenn. and N.C. in moist soils and swamps.

Common names. Arbor vitae.

1523 Cartier Voyage Chaleur Bay St. Lawrence transl. 47. "There are several cedars (cèdres) as fine as can be seen to make masts, sufficient to mast boats of 300 tons or more."

1535-6 Cartier voyage transl. 126-7. "There are many fine trees. . .such as cedars (seddrez).

1557-58 Thevet Gulf of St. Lawrence transl. 404-405. "Also one must not omit what is singular, that when the aforesaid savages are ill with fever or persecuted with other interior sicknesses, they take the leaves of a tree which is very like the cedars, which are found around the mountain of Tarare and at Lyonnois; and take the juice which they drink. And it is not to be doubted that in twenty four hours, they are not as sick, even if it is inveterate within the body, that this drink cures them: as many times the Christians have tried, and have brought the plant from there." In the margin of the text is written 'Sovereign drink which they use in their sickness.'. . .1014. 'The country of Canada is beautiful. . .There are many trees and of many kinds, some of which we do not know here and which are of great use: and many plants and trees were brought from here which one can see to-day in the royal garden at Fontainbleau."

1558 Ewan (1978:25). "By my latest count thirty north American plants were known in Europe before 1600. Four of these originated in New France; the oldest American tree is the arbor vitae, *Thuja occidentalis*, mentioned by Belon in 1558."

1590 Harriot Virginia 9. "Cedar, a very sweet wood & fine timber; whereof if nests of chests be there made, or timber therof fitted for sweet & fine bedsteads, tables, deskes, lutes, virginales & many things else, (of which there have beene proofe made already) to make up fraite [freight] with other principle commodities will yeeld profits. . .23. Some of our company which have wandered in some places where I have not bene, have made certain affirmation of *Cyprus* which for such and other excellent uses, is also a wood of price and no small estimation."

1601 Clusius Rarior Pl. Hist. White cedar, a figure and description under the name of arbor vitae after he had seen it in the Royal garden of Fontainbleau.

1603 Champlain-Purchas Tadoussac 155. "Full of woods of Pines, Cypresses, Fir-trees, Burch and some other sorts of trees of small price. . .161. For they [canoes] are made of the bark of a Birch tree strengthened within with little circles of wood well & handsomely framed." [Note below 1613 where Champlain says white cedar used.]

1609 Lescarbot-Erondelle Nova Francia 302. "In the river St. John and Sainte Croix, there is store of cedar-trees besides those that I have named. . .305. Of exquisite woods I know none there, but the cedar and the sassafras."

1612 Capt. John Smith Virginia 92. "There are also Cedars and Saxafras trees. they also yeeld gummes in a small proportion of themselves. We tryed conclusions to extract it out of the wood, but nature afforded more than our arts." [Ships returning from Virginia to England carried cargoes of cedar wood.]

1613 Champlain fac. ed. transl. 169. Tadoussac. "Their canoes are made of birch bark, reinforced within with little circles of white cedar, very well arranged. (renforcez le dedans de petits cercles de cèdre blanc)". . .19. fourth voyage Ottawa River. "Several islands here and there which are covered with pines and white cedars (couvertes de pins & cèdre blancs)". . .23 Ottawa. "And before leaving I made a cross of white cedar, which I placed on a high point, with the arms of France. (une croix de cèdre blanc)." [Champlain in his own text of 1613 speaks only of cedars and distinguishes the white and the red, for the latter he uses the word 'cypre'. He never uses the word 'arbre de vie' nor does Cartier or Lescarbot. None of them mention using cedar in the many bouts of scurvy their men endured. See under spruce.]

1624 Sagard TOBACCO INDIANS 192-93. "Have the body and face engraved in sections, with figures of snakes, lizards, squirrels, and other animals; almost all have the body thus figured, which renders them frightful and hideous to those who are not accustomed to it; it is pricked and made in the same way that are made and graven in the surface of the flesh the crosses which those who return from Jerusalem have on their arms, and it is forever. . .prickings cause them great pains, and they often fall sick from them." [see Densmore, below].

1633 Gerarde-Johnson 1369. "Of the Tree of Life. . .branches surcharged with very oilaeous and ponderous leaves. . .which being rubbed in the hands do yeeld an aromatick, spicie, or gummie savor, very pleasant and comfortable. . .The branches of this tree laid downe in the earth will very easily take root. . .which I have often proved, and thereby have greatly multiplied these trees. . .Groweth not wilde in England, but it groweth in my garden very plentifully. . .Theophrastus and Pliny, as some thinke, have called this sweet and aromatical tree *Thuia*, or *Thya*. . .the new writers do terme it *Arbor vitae*: in English, the tree of life, I do not meane that whereof mention is made, Gen.3.22. . . .Among the plants of the New-found-land, this tree. . .is the most principal, and best agreeing unto the nature of man, as an excellent cordial, and of a very pleasant smell."

1637 Le Jeune HURON Jes. Rel. 13; 25. "Dysentery is cured by drinking the juice of the leaves or branches of the cedar which have been boiled. Father Bouteaux says he saw a child recover soon after taking this medicine."

1642 Jes. Rel. 22; 293. "Barthelemy Vimont reported that natural medicines might be classed as internal and external. The internal consisted of potions obtained from simples, without compounding or mixing them. For instance, he explained, from a species of fir, small branches were stripped, which were then boiled and the sap or juice drunk as an emetic. Branches of cedar. . .were used for the same purpose."

1644 Marie de l'Incarnation Quebec 1st August to her son 134. Postscript. "There are many cedars here—they provide us with brooms."

1653 Bressani HURON Jes. Rel. 38; 251-53. "But those who paint themselves permanently do so with extreme pain, using, for this purpose, needles, sharp awls, or piercing thorns, with which they perforate, or have others perforate, the skin. Thus they form on the face, the neck, the breast, or some other part of the body, some animal or monster,. . .then, tracing over the fresh and bloody design some powdered charcoal, or other black coloring matter, which becomes mixed with the blood and penetrates within these perforations, they imprint indelibly upon the living skin the designed figures. And this in some nations is so common that in the one which we call the Tobacco, and. . .Neutral, I know not whether a single individual was found who was not painted in this manner, on some part of the body. . .it has caused the death of more than one. . ." [See Densmore, below]

1663 Boucher Quebec transl. 41. "There are also cedars, they have flat leaves, the wood is very tender, &. . .almost incorruptible: that is why it is used to enclose the gardens, & for supports in the cellars: it smells very good; but ordinarily the trees are not healthy, nevertheless there can be found several large ones that could be used to make furniture: the gum from them can be burnt, has a very good scent like incense. I do not know that it has any other quality. . .100. The best cabins of the Indians are covered with the bark of cedar, but they are rare. . .146. Charcoal made from cedar is without comparison much better than any other kind, for the composition of powder and artifices."

1709 Raudot Quebec 392. "This fire stick is made of two pieces of wood, one of which is white cedar; near the edge of it the savages made little holes which do not go through the wood, with a notch from each hole through the edge. They have a piece of hard wood that they turn very fast with both hands in these holes, so that you see immediately a dust which throws out smoke and which falling through the notch on rotten wood or well crushed dry grass makes a fire very rapidly."

1744 Charlevoix J. 1; 162. "In the northern parts they [Indians] made much use of glisters [enemas], a bladder was their instrument for this purpose. They have a remedy for bloody flux which seldom or never fails; this is the juice expressed from the extremities of cedar branches after they have been well boiled."

1749 Kalm Quebec Aug. 16th. 467-69. "The occidental *Arbor vitae* (*Thuja occidentalis* L.) is a tree which grows very plentifully in Canada but not much further south. . .The French all over Canada, call it *cèdre blanc*. The English and Dutch in Albany also call it the white cedar. . .Thuja wood. The Canadians generally use this tree for the following purposes. Since it is thought the most durable wood in Canada, and that which best withstands rotting, so as to remain undamaged for over a man's age, fences of all kinds are scarcely made of any other than this wood. All the posts which are driven into the ground are made of Thuja wood. The palisades round the forts in Canada are likewise made of the same material. The beams in the houses are made of it; and the thin narrow pieces of wood which form both the ribs and the bottom of the bark boats commonly used here are taken from this wood, because it is pliant enough for the purpose, especially while it is fresh. It is also very light. The Thuja wood is reckoned one of the best for the use in limekilns. Its branches are used all over Canada for brooms, and the twigs and leaves of its being naturally bent together seem to be very proper for the purpose. The Indians make such brooms and bring them to town to sell, nor do I remember having seen any made of any other wood. The fresh branches have a peculiar agreeable scent which is pretty strongly smelled in houses where they make use of brooms of this kind. . .This Thuja is used for several medicinal purposes. The commandant of Fort St. Frederic, M. de Lusignan, could never sufficiently praise its excellence for rheumatic pains. He told me he had often seen it tried with remarkable success upon several persons in the following manner. The fresh leaves are pounded in a mortar and mixed with hog's grease or any other grease. This is boiled together till it becomes a salve, which is spread on linen and applied to the part where the pain is. This salve gives certain relief in a short time. Against violent pains which move up and down in the thighs and sometimes spread all over the body, they recommend the following remedy. Take of the leaves of a kind of polypody [fern] four-fifths and of the cones of Thuja one fifth, both reduced to a coarse powder by themselves, and mixed together afterwards. Then pour milkwarm water on it so as to make a poultice, spread it on linen, and wrap it round the body; but as the poultice burns like fire, they commonly lay a cloth between it and the body, otherwise it would burn and scorch the skin. I have heard this remedy praised beyond measure, by people who said they had experienced good effects. Among these was a woman who said that she had applied such a poultice for three days, after which her severe pain passed away entirely. An Iroquois Indian told me that a decoction of Thuja leaves was used as a remedy for a cough. In the neighbourhood of Saratoga, they use this decoction in intermittent fevers."

1807 Heriot Niagara Falls 165. "About half a mile from thence [Table Rock] in descending the course of the river, and behind some trees which grow upon the lower bank, is placed the Indian ladder, composed of a tall cedar-tree, whose boughs have been lopped off to within three inches of the trunk, and whose upper end is attached by a cord of bark to the root of a living tree; the lower end is planted amid stones. It is upwards of forty feet in length, and trembles and bends under the weight of a person upon it. As this is the nearest way to the riverside, many people descend by the ladder, led either by curiosity, or for the purpose of spearing fish, which in the summer are found in great abundance in this vicinity. . .proceeding along the beach to the basin of the Table rock. . .The projection of the Table Rock,. . .is fifty feet, and between it and the falls a lofty and irregular arch is formed,. . .to enter this cavern,. . .and to turn and view the falls. . .astonish the mind."

1840 Gosse Quebec 12. "One of majestic size, and of no little importance. . .the white cedar. . .From the facility with which it is split, but chiefly from its great durability, almost incorruptibility, it is in great request for the rails that compose those unsightly zigzag fences, so offensive to the eye of one accustomed to the verdant and blooming hedgerows of England. Cedar rails may be exposed to every vicissitude of weather for a man's lifetime, without manifesting any symptom of decay, except perhaps the separation of the bark. It chiefly grows in marshes, and so densely as to render them almost impenetrable. A cedar swamp is a valuable addition to a Canadian farm; and with us they are already getting scarce, and no providence seems to be manifested for the future."

1842 Christison 272. "Vegetable charcoal when pulverized is dark brownish-black. Wood charcoal has at different times been extensively employed in medical practice, both internally and externally. . .As an external agent it is antiseptic. Internally it is held by some to be a febrifuge, antiseptic, cathartic, anthelmintic, and sedative,—its antiseptic properties as an external application are undeniable. It is serviceable for destroying fetor. . .as in fetid ulcers of the mouth, natural fetor of the breath, caries of the bones, gangrenous sores. . .It is probably the best of all dentifrices. It removes encrustations of the teeth, whitens them, and corrects fetor of the mouth; nor is its employment attended with any risk of injury to the teeth. . .been maintained by some to be a laxative in habitual constipation, a sedative in diarrhoea, a febrifuge in ague, and antiseptic tonic in typhus. . ."

1857 Daniel Wilson CREE 337. "In the grave ceremony of opening the medicine pipe-stem, the Crees make use of a novel addition to the tobacco. It is procured from the leaves or fibers of a species of cedar or spruce, which, when dried and burnt, yields a very pleasing fragrance. A handful of this was thrown on the fire in the middle of the room, and filled it with the fragrant smoke, and some of the same was sprinkled on the top of the tobacco each time one of the medicine pipe-stems was used."

1868 Can. Pharm. J. 6; 83-5. The leaves of *Arbor Vitae*, white cedar, included in list of Can. medicinal plants.

1880 Can. Horticulturist 117. "Mr. Beall stated that at Lindsay he had noted the following facts: White Cedar sold for fence posts, railway ties, telegraph poles, canoes, &c. at from $16 to 20 per thousand feet."

1884 Holmes-Haydon CREE Hudson Bay. "As a diuretic. . .*J. virginiana*?". [The red cedar is not found north of southern Quebec so could not have been used by the Cree of Hudson Bay unless they obtained it by trade. It seems likely they used white cedar or juniper some of which more closely resembles the red cedar].

1892 Millspaugh 165. "Main action of Thuja is on the genito-urinary organs, copious and frequent urination. . .the sexual appetite supressed."

1915 Speck PENOBSCOT 309. "Leaves are made into a poultice for swollen hands or feet. . .311. Several more elaborate cures are as follows: Lambkill [Kalmia]. . .cedar bark. . .and salt used to

be pounded together and made into a poultice. . .By means of a scratching instrument scars were cut into the skin directly over the part affected with pain and the poultice smeared over and rubbed in. This was the nostrum used in olden times for all kinds of trouble. . .312. A concoction of seven herbs is taken as a sudorific before entering the sudatory. . .cedar boughs are one of them."
1915 Speck MONTAGNAIS 315. "The twigs of cedar are bruised and steeped to make a sweat drink."
1918 Anon Arch. Rep. Ont. 42. "The Indians wore armor and helmets that they made themselves from light wood such as cedar or basswood."
1926-27 Densmore CHIPPEWA 333. "An instrument for applying medicine beneath the skin consisted of several needles fastened to the end of a wooden handle. This was used in treating 'dizzy headache,' neuralgia, or rheumatism in any part of the body. . .The remedy used most often in this manner was made as follows: Hazel stalks or cedar wood was burned to a charcoal and a small quantity of the charcoal (or ash) was mixed with an equal quantity of the dried gall of a bear. It was mixed well and placed in a birch bark dish. When used it was moistened a little with water and stirred, after which a little was taken on the blade at the end of the wooden instrument and laid on the affected part. It was then 'worked in' with the needles. The dark spots seen on the temples of many Indians are left by the charcoal in this medicine. [This is also a close description of native tattooing]. . .334. The treatment of a fractured arm. . .Bind with a thin cedar splint. . .386. Cedar was needed for parts of canoes and for numerous other uses. In old times the procuring of birch bark and cedar bark was an event in which all participated. A number of families went to the vicinity of these trees and made a camp. A gathering was held, at which a venerable man, speaking for the entire company, expressed gratitude to the spirit of the trees and woods saying they had come to gather a supply which they needed, and asking permission to do this. . .385. Legend of Winabojo and the Cedar Tree. . .There they found Winabojo. He was too old to travel, and on his head was a beautiful cedar tree. Winabojo wore the cedar tree as an ornament and its roots were all around him. Beside him was a great stone. One of the men asked if he could live always, as Winabojo was doing. Winabojo replied, 'No. You can only live your alloted years. The only way you can become perpetual is by becoming a stone'. . .Winabojo gave each of them a 'snake chain' and told them to be sure not to untie these chains from around their waists." Note by Densmore. "This is a plaited chain worn as a protection against replies or other harm." [She does not say what it is made of].
1923 H. Smith MENOMINI 46. Cedar bark used in the sudatory [sweat bath], the inner bark is also used. It is gathered, dried and steeped to make a tea to treat suppressed menstruation. When a patient contracts a cold and there is a cessation of menses, then the tea is drunk to make the flow easy again. The leaves are used in the smudge for reviving lost consciousness. The inner bark is a seasoner for other medicines."
1932 H. Smith OJIBWE 380. "The Flambeau Ojibwe use the leaves as a perfume. . .and also as a tea for headache. During the ceremonies of the medicine lodge, if it is necessary to purify sacred objects and the hands and persons of participants, a plate of live coals is used and dried Arbor Vitae leaves placed upon them. The servitor wafts the incense over sacred objects by fanning the smoke with his hands. Others hold their hands over and in the smoke, waving it upon their persons. The Pillager Ojibwe. . .also use it as a purifying incense, and as an ingredient for the sweat bath with White Pine, Balsam, Hemlock and other plants. They drink the boiled leaves claiming that the steam goes through the blood and purifies it. This treatment cures coughs. . . .421. The Ojibwe worship the Arbor Vitae or white cedar and the Paper or Canoe Birch, as the two most useful trees in the forest. The pungent fragrance of the leaves and wood of Arbor Vitae are always an acceptable incense to Winabojo, and the wood is their choice for light, strong, straight grained canoe frames and ribs. In earlier times, the tough stringy bark was used in making fibre bags, but these are scarcely ever seen today."
1933 H. Smith POTAWATOMI 70. "The Forest Potawatomi use the leaves in making poultices and also in many combinations with other roots and leaves as medicines. It serves also as a seasoner for other compounds. It is smudged upon coals as a purifier and is supposed to exorcise evil spirits that are inimical to recovery. . .122. The leaves are preserved or may be used fresh. . .to purify sacred objects. . .The Cedar bark is also sometimes rolled into torches which are used for hunting at night."
1935 Jenness Parry Island Lake Huron OJIBWA 50. "To avoid any consequences from a rejected dream, he often scraped his son's tongue with a knife of cedar, and handing him the knife, bade him throw it into the fire. Thus the lad annulled, as it were, the unfavourable dream

and remained to fast for a better. . .84. Should a man who possesses a powerful hunting medicine cross your trail when you are hunting your legs will become so weary and sore that you will perforce give up the chase and return home. In such a contingency Jonas King rubs his legs vigorously with cedar twigs; and other Indians have their own special remedies. . .90. She carried it [the baby] on her back within a cradle of basswood or cedar. . .for its mattress she gathered either sphagnum moss or rotten cedar. . .she crooned it to sleep within a hammock made from twisted cedar bark or basswood twine. . .112. Types of bark lodges. . .Cedar bark was occasionally substituted for birch bark when the latter was difficult to procure. . .113. Some bags were woven of cedar bark. . .occasionally cedar bark was used in mat-making."

1945 Rousseau MOHAWK transl. 35. "They distinguish two kinds of cedar tree: one which produces cones, and the other sterile. They have the same name. The women during the 40 days that follow birth, drink an infusion of the leaves. It is tonic and diaphoretic. The greater the perspiration, the greater the secretion of milk. The hunters use it for the sweat baths. They boil, in a narrow pot, the branches of cedar without fruit. By throwing stones, heated red hot, into the pot they obtain a large amount of steam. For paralysis a preparation is used made of the tips of cedar branches (about one inch long) boiled in milk. For one gallon of liquid there is added half a pound of grease. A woolen cloth is soaked in this mixture and laid over the part that is paralysed. The application must be repeated nine times. Marie-Victorin says the Algonquins of Temiscaming also distinguish two kinds of cedars, the ordinary cedars without cones and a male cedar, with cones."

1633 Gerarde-Johnson 1368 Cypresse. "Of this divers make two kindes, the female and the male, the female barren, and the male fruitful."

1945 Rousseau Quebec transl. 83. "Twigs are placed with lingerie and in the cupboards containing furs to keep away moths."

1945 Raymond TETE DE BOULE transl. 132. "The cedar is used to build the skeleton of the canoe. It is bent by steaming."

1952 A.C. Shaw. The most valuable constituent of cedar oil is thujone. Thujone is also present in oil of hemlock, but in unimportant amounts. Cedar; thujone 56.7%, bornyl acetate 5.9%, fenchone 7.8%, limonene 3.6%. In contrast black spruce contains 37% bornyl acetate and no thujone; hemlock 43.4% bornyl acetate, 1.3% thujone.

1955 Mockle Quebec transl. 24. "The leaves are given as a diaphoretic and galactogene; in steam baths for treating pulmonary complaints; crushed and mixed with pork grease, they make an ointment used in rheumatism; boiled they are used for local application to prevent paralysis of movement. The essence has vermicidal properties."

1970 Hartwell Plants Cancer L1. Sept. 349-50. Lists 25 references to the use of *Thuja* for venereal warts starting with Hahnemann in 1826-7 and ending in the 1950's.

Yarnell (1964) states that Stowe (1940) claims the Chippewa used white cedar as a dye. Densmore, in her section on the Chippewa dye plants, does not mention the use of white cedar as a dye but does give formulas for using the red cedar.

MICMAC and MALECITE of Maritime provinces of Canada used the white cedar for burns, consumption, cough, headache, swollen feet and hands and toothache (Chandler, Freeman and Hooper 1979).

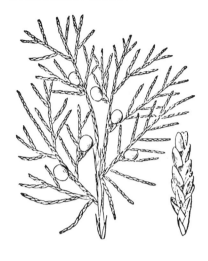

RED CEDAR

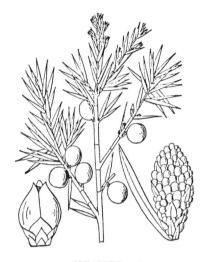

JUNIPER

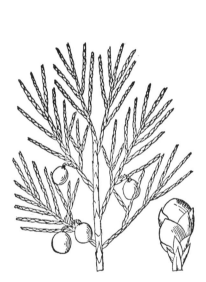

CREEPING CEDAR SAVIN

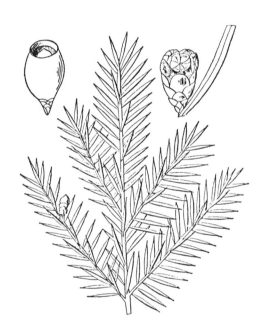

GROUND HEMLOCK AMERICAN YEW

RED CEDAR *Juniperus virginiana* L. Pinaceae
A shrub or tree to 20 m tall, dense, the young leaves each 5-7 mm in whorls of three. The branches spreading or ascending, the adult leaves scale-like, 2-4 mm long, their backs convex. The small, roundish berries containing 2 or 3 pitted seeds grow on straight stems. They are covered with a bright blue, powdery sheen.
Range. sw. Que. and s. Ont., N.H. and Me. s. to Tex.and Fla. in a variety of soils.
CREEPING CEDAR OR SAVIN *Juniperus horizontalis* Moench
Branches creep over the ground, the leaves mostly scale like. The berries contain mostly 3-5

unpitted seeds and are on curved stems.

Range. Nfld., N.B., P.E.I., N.S., Que., James Bay, northernmost Ont., Mckenzie, Athabaska, Yukon, Alaska, s. to B.C., Wyo., Kans., Io., to N.H. and N.Y. in rocky, sandy or boggy places.

1475 Bjornnson Icelandic mss transl. Larsen 128. "[The European *J. Sabina*] Sabina is hot and dry in the third degree. If one mixes it with honey it dries dangerous wounds and swellings and cleanses their foulness. If crushed and applied to a woman's member or if a woman drinks it with wine, then it will draw from her a miscarried foetus. If mixed with white wine, it makes the skin clear, and it is good for all the diseases that come from the cold. If the head is washed with its broth or it is applied to the temples, it is good for headache."

1613 Champlain Voyages fac. ed. Acadia 1605 transl. 83. "The woods are full of oaks, nut trees & very beautiful 'cypres' which are reddish, & have a strong and good perfume". . .Fourth voyage Ottawa river 25. "I saw several beautiful red cedars, the first I have seen in this country, with which I made a cross which I placed at the end of one of the islands on a high point, and in full view, with the arms of France as I had done in the other places we have been." (vismes plusieurs beaux cypres rouge). [Champlain used 'cèdres blanc' for white cedar and 'cypres rouges' for red cedar].

1625 Wassanaer New Netherlands 81. "There is a red wood which, being burned, smells very agreeably; when men sit by the fire on benches made from it, the whole house is perfumed by it."

1633 Gerarde-Johnson 1378. "The leaves of [the European] Savin boyled in Wine and drunke provoke urine, bring down the menses with force, draw away the after-birth, expell the dead childe, and kill the quicke: it hath the like vertue received under the body in a perfume. The leaves stamped with honey and applied, cure ulcers, stay spreading and creeping ulcers, scoure and take away all spots and freckles from the face or body of man or woman. The leaves boyled in oyle Olive, and kept therein, kill the wormes in children, if you anoint their bellies therewith: and the leaves powdered and given in milke or Muscadell do the same. The leaves dried and beate into fine powder, and strewed upon those kindes of excrescences sub praeputio, called Caroles, and such like, gotten by dealings with uncleane women, take them away perfectly, curing and healing them: but if they be inveterate and old, and have been much tampered withall, it shall be necessarie to adde unto the same a small quantity of Auripigmentum [mercury] in fine powder, and use it with discretion, because the force of the medicine is greatly increased thereby and made more corrosive."

1749 Kalm Salem May 5th. 301. "The red juniper is another tree which I have mentioned very frequently in the course of my account. . .The English call it red cedar, and the French *Cedre rouge*. . .Of all the woods in this country this is without exception the most durable, and withstands weathering longer than any other. . .The best canoes, consisting of a single piece of wood, are made of red cedar; for they last far longer than any other and are very light. In New York I have seen quite large yachts built of this wood,. . .The heart of this cedar is of a fine red color, and whatever is made of it looks very fine, and has a very agreeable and wholesome smell. But the color fades by degrees, or the wood would be very suitable for cabinet work. I saw a parlor. . .wainscotted many years ago with boards of red cedar. . .quite faded. . .wood will keep its color if a thin varnish is put upon it while it is fresh. . .Some people put the shavings and chips of it among their linen to secure it against being worm eaten. . .October 7th. Montreal. . .I also talked to the commandent of Fort Frontenac, who informed me that on the plain was found. . .red cedar and herbs, the medicinal value of which he praised most highly. Besides, he knew them well and promised to show them to me when I came there. . .635. The savin (*Juniperus sabina*) is said to grow as a common thing on the banks of the Delaware."

1807 Heriot Kingston Lake Ontario 1; 132. "The number of vessels [to sail across Lake Ontario] in the employ of the merchants is considerable. These are usually built about ten miles below Kingston, and the timber used for their construction is red cedar or oak."

1817-20 Bigelow 52. "The leaves of Red cedar have a strong disagreeable taste, with some pungency and bitterness. The peculiar taste and odour reside, no doubt, in a volatile oil, which however, is not readily separated by distillations in a small way. . .The botanical similarity of this tree to the *Savin*,. . .an European shrub. . .In their sensible and medicinal properties, they are equally allied. . .The American tree is frequently known throughout the country by the name of Savin, our apothecaries have been led to presume upon its identity with that medicine, and it has long been used in cases where the true Savin is recommended. Its most frequent use, however, is in the composition of the cerate employed for keeping up the irritation and discharge of blisters. . .When properly prepared by boiling the fresh leaves for a short time in about twice their weight of lard with the addition of a little wax, a cerate is formed of peculiar efficacy as a perpetual epipastic. When applied as a dressing to a newly vesicated surface, and afterwards repeated twice a day, it rarely fails to keep up the discharge for an indefinite length of time. . . .Internally the leaves of *Juniperus Virginiana* have been found to exert effects very similar to those of Savin. They have proved useful as an emmenagogue, and as a general stimulant and diaphoretic in rheumatism. They have also had some reputation as a diuretic in dropsy. The wood of the red cedar is smooth, light and very durable. . .It is principally employed for posts in fences, in which capacity it proves more durable than almost any species of wood used for that purpose."

1820's Materia Medica Edinburgh-Toronto mss 51. Emmenagogues from the class of Cathartics. *Juniperus Sabina* is a stimulant and from this effect has been supposed to act upon the uterine system but it is scarcely ever used internally. . .73. Escharotics are substances which erode or dissolve animal solids. . .They are employed chiefly to remove excrescences, to establish an ulcer, or to change the surface of an ulcerated part converting it to a simple sore. . .Juniper Sabina possesses an acrid power, when it has been employed by application to old ulcers. . .and some cutaneous disorders."

1830 Rafinesque 16. "The leaves of Savin are the officinal parts. Those of our Cedars are used as equivalents with us, under the name of Savin; but they are weaker than the European Savin, and often fail as emmenagogues, because the doses are regulated upon the European prescriptions. They all have the properties of the Junipers in a higher and even violent degree; they increase all the secretions, but may produce hemorrhagy and abortion, acting chiefly on the uterus, pregnant women ought never to use them, but they are very useful in dropsical complaints, menstrual suppressions, also in rheumatism, gout, worms, &c. in powder, conserve or tincture. None but experienced physicians ought to prescribe them. Farriers use them frequently in diseases of the horse. Externally the powdered leaves may be applied to warts, venereal excrescenses, ulcers, carious bones, psora, tinea, and gangrenous sores, to heal them."

1842 Christison 808. "Savin is sometimes confounded with the tops of *Juniperus Virginiana* of North America, a plant which possess the same properties and in its native country is used for the same purposes. . . .Savin. . .as an irritant it is in large doses a powerful poison. . .six drachms will kill a dog if retained in the stomach. . .employed externally. . .for destroying venereal warts. . .Savin is not now much used as an internal remedy in regular practice; nevertheless its anthelmintic and emmenagogue virtues deserve attention. . .This drug is believed by the vulgar to possess the power of inducing miscarriage, and is sometimes used by them for perpetrating this crime. . . .bringing life into extreme danger."

1859-61 Gunn 852. "Savin. . .This is an evergreen shrub, or small tree,. . .a native of Europe, but found growing wild in Canada and some portions of our Northern States. The small twigs, leaves, and ends of the branches are the parts used in medicine. Savin is a powerful emmenagogue. . .Care must be taken in using it, especially the Oil. . .Oil of Savin is much used for the purpose of producing abortion, in doses of ten to fifteen drops two or three times a day, and is probably the most certain article for that purpose known; but if continued long is apt to occasion inflammation of the stomach and bowels."

1885 Hoffman OJIBWA 198. "Red Cedar, the bruised leaves and berries are used internally to remove headache."

1888 Delamare Island of Miquelon transl. 30. "The special properties of *Juniperus virginiana* are completely ignored by the inhabitants."

1892 Millspaugh 166. "This tree is noted above all others in this country, for the durability of its wood, no matter how exposed to changes of weather. . .The highly colored and fragrant heartwood is largely used in the manufacture of lead pencils, pails, tubs, and various household utensils. . .Sir William Hooker considers *Juniperus Virginiana* identical with the European *J. Sabina*. . .The leaves of *J. Virginiana* are much less rich in oil. . .The oil is largely used as an application in arthritic. . .affections. . .The excrescences (cedar apples), often found upon the branchlets, are quite extensively used in domestic practice in doses of from ten to thirty grains every four hours, as an anthelmintic. . .Case of a woman who took an ounce of the oil to produce an abortion. . .great purging, with stupor without being able to regain consciousness, and death. . .Many other cases of poisoning by the oil taken in doses of from one drachm to an ounce, for the purpose of abortion or as an emmenagogue, show *Juniperus Virginiana* to cause severe venous congestion throughout the body."

1924 Youngken 495. "The Plains tribes boiled together the fruits and leaves and drank the decoction for a cough. For colds in the head and nervousness the twigs were burned and the smoke inhaled."

1926-7 Densmore CHIPPEWA 362. The little twigs of red cedar and of Canadian yew were boiled together and the decoction sprinkled on hot stones or taken internally for rheumatism. The informant, a woman of advanced years, said this remedy came from her great-grandmother. . .371. Red cedar; the bark of this tree was used by Chippewa women in Ontario for coloring the strips of cedar used in their mats. A decoction was made of the dark red inner bark and the strips were boiled in it for a mahogany color. . .377. Red cedar used to make mats.

1928 H. Smith MESKWAKI 194. Inner wood of red cedar one of seven ingredients in an inhalant for catarrh. . .The berries of red cedar with those of the winterberry and the roots of white vervain mixed to make a healing poultice for large external sores. . .234. This is a medicine made by boiling the leaves of the red cedar. It is drunk for weakness and as a convalescent medicine. . .The wood mixed with other undetermined materials. . .is used as a seasoner for other medicines. It is prepared in warm water and is stirred with the fingers during preparation.

1935 Jenness Parry Island OJIBWA Lake Huron 114. "A very deep red dye was obtained by boiling the bark of the red cedar."

1955 Mockle Quebec transl. 23. "A perfumed essence, cedrol is extracted from the wood and leaves and is used as a cicatrisant, the essence of the fruits is said to be an abortifacient for animals."

J. virginiana contains podophyllotoxin [see mayapple] and its activity as a cancer chemotherapeutic agent is being examined (Lewis and Elvin-Lewis 1977:133).

JUNIPER *Juniperus communis* L. var. *depressa* Pursh Pinaceae

Shrubs that grow flat on sand or rock or upright to 1 m tall in patches 10 to 12 m across. Leaves in whorls of threes, jointed at the base, 6-18 mm long, with a white stripe down the middle of the top of the leaf. Strongly scented. The berries without stems, green through to blue black maturing in three years, 1-13 mm thick mostly with 3 seeds.

Range. Circumboreal, with 3 indistinct varieties usually recognised in n. Am. mostly on dry, rocky, poor soil. In our range s. to Me., n. N.H., Pa. and Ill.

1475 Bjornnson Icelandic mss transl. Larsen 72. "Juniper. Is called fire-tree in Greek; for if the fire is covered with its ashes, it will keep alive for almost a whole year. But the berries are hot and dry. And they shall be gathered in the spring. If one boils juniper with rain-water, the broth is good to drink for diarrhoea. But boiled with wine, they are good to drink for disease of the small intestines and it loosens after-birth. From the dry juniper wood one may make an oil in this fashion: one shall dig into the ground an earthenware pot and over it set another which shall have a hole in the bottom. This one shall fill with dry juniper wood, so split as for tar burning, and cover it over with a flat stone and clay so that no smoke may get out therefrom. Then one shall kindle a great fire about it, and while the wood burns within the pot, the oil runs down through the hole into the pot hid in the ground. With that it is good to rub the groins for pain in them. If one eats it, that is good for ——— and if a man gets ——— (note almost certainly mental troubles, for which juniper is well-known remedy.) The spine and back one shall rub with this for epilepsy. . .s16. Here begins many experiments. . .Item for growth of hair, take juniper and oil and boil much, and afterward cool it and rub upon the head, then the hair will grow. . .s 21. Item for teeth. Take the root from in under the elm or juniper; that drives off the ache and fastens the teeth."

1546 Frascatorius Riddell 30. "Others, again, have cured many with the wood of juniper alone." [of syphilis]

1741 Farriers Disp. 220. "Juniper berries detergent & cleansing to the viscera, good in Yellows, all obstructions of Liver, Spleen, have Turpentine in them; they also scour the kidneys and urinary passages, are very serviceable in all disorders proceeding from Wind and Flatulence in the bowels."

1791 Lewis Mat. Med ed Aitkin. The berries of *Juniperus communis* tinge rectified spirits a bright orange colour. Add carroway or fennel seeds to improve flavour. The wood has been recommended as a sudorific and by some accounted similar to sassafras.

1799 Lewis Disp. Mat. Med. 166. "The fresh berries yield, on expression, a rich, sweet, honey-like, aromatic juice; if previously pounded so as to break the seeds, the juice proves tart and bitter. These berries are useful carminatives and stomachics; are chiefly used for their diuretic effects; and are considered also as diaphoretics. The liquor remaining after the distillation of the oil, passed through a strainer, and gently exhaled to the consistence of a rob, proves likewise a medicine of great utility, and in many cases perhaps preferable to the oil, or the berry itself. Hoffman. . .strongly recommends it in debility of the stomach and intestines and says it is particularly of service to old people who are subject to those disorders, or labour under a difficulty with urinary excretions: this rob is of a dark, brownish yellow colour, a balsamic sweet taste, with a little of the bitter, according as to the seeds in the berry have been more or less bruised. Cullen is of a very different opinion. He thinks this rob is an inert substance, and that the berries derive all their properties from the essential oil, which is like that of turpentine, but with a more agreeable odour."

1817-20 Bigelow 46. "The berries of Juniper have long been employed. . .as a diuretic, particularly in dropsy. . .The stronger preparations have been found useful in uterine obstructions. Linnaeus informs us. . .that a fermented decoction of Juniper berries is used in Sweden as a common drink."

1820's Materia Medica Edinburgh-Toronto mss 54. "*Juniperus communis*, the infusion of the berries proved diuretic in the spirit of Juniper mixed with diluted alcohol to form a spirituous liquor known by the name of Gin, prescribed as a cordial diuretic in dropsy."

1830 Rafinesque 15. "The berries, leaves, and wood may be used; the berries have a strong, pungent, aromatic smell and taste, somewhat sweet and bitter, containing an essential oil, tannin, and a sweet mucilage. The leaves and wood contain some of the oil also, in which resides the active properties. The leaves are more acrid and bitter than the berries. . .The Oil of Juniper is chiefly distilled from the berries. . .They impart their flavor to alcoholic liquors, and form the well known gin, which acquires some diuretic properties. The oil us useful in dropsy, in debility of the stomach and intestines, palsy of the bladder, and uterine obstructions. The doses must be minute; or a decoction of the berries and leaves substituted. A kind of beer is made with the berries in Lapland; they improve also the spruce beer."

1833 Howard Quebec mss 147. "To give a cleansing drench for a cow after calving. 3 oz of Juniper berries, 2 oz of round Birth Wort, 1 oz of Fenugreek, 8 oz. of spermacetti, 1 oz. of flower of sulphur, 1 oz. of common antimony, 8 oz. of treacle and ½ oz. of saffron. . .201. To cure a Pain in the Loins of Man. 2 drams oil of juniper, 2 of Powder of Nitre, 5 of oil of Turpentine and 1 of spirits of red Lavender. Mix all together. Take inwardly from 15 to 25 drops in a tablespoon full of water and sugar 3 times a day."

1841 Trousseaux & Pidoux Paris transl. Ferment juniper berries in brandy, distil the volatile oil as an extract for infusion or decoction, an energetic tonic. Also burn juniper to fumigate the sick room.

1842 Christison 573. "Juniper, its berries, and its oil are stimulant, carminative, and diuretic; and large doses are said to irritate the urinary organs and cause strangury."

1868 Can. Pharm. J. 6; 83-5. Berries of *Juniperus communis* included in list of Can. medicinal plants.

1881 Can. Pharm. J. Oct. 88. "The antiseptic properties of oil of juniper have been taken advantage of by Dr. Kocher, of Berne, for the preparation of antiseptic catgut and silk. Lister uses for the same purpose a solution of carbolic acid in an exceedingly dilute solution of chromic acid."

1884 Holmes-Haydon CREE Hudson Bay 302. "Wakinakim, the bark of *Juniperus communis* L. This is used to make a poultice for wounds. According to Mr. Haydon it is prepared for use by taking a stick and cutting it into pieces about four inches long, boiling it until the outer bark comes off easily, scraping off the inner bark and beating it between two stones into a pulpy mass, which is applied to the wound. Mr. Haydon has seen it so used, and remarks, 'It certainly seems to clear a foul wound well, and is the usual remedy employed by Indians for wounds of all kinds.' The beneficial action of the bark is doubtless due to its great astringency, and to the volatile oil present in it, which would naturally be antiseptic."

1888 Delamare Island of Miquelon transl. 30. "The decoction of the plant reduced to the consistency of an extract is applied externally for rheumatism under the name of Cirrouenne or Cirrhoene."

1908 Henderson & Lusk Mat. Med. Toronto 76. "Oil of juniper distilled from field grown, unripe green fruit of *J. communus*..'

1919 Sturtevant 320. ". . .formerly used ripe berries in England as a substitute for pepper."

1924 Youngken 179. "*J. communis* var. *depressa*. The Penobscot employed the fruits as a remedy for colds. . .The leaves used by Cheyenne for cough and irritation of the throat. In case of a bad cough, they chewed the berries and swallowed the juice. . .The Indians regarded the juniper as 'hot' and used almost every part of it for 'cold' constitutions."

1928 Reagan OJIBWA 245. Bark used for weaving mats and house building.

1933 Gilmore OJIBWA 124. Used as a medicine.

1933 H. Smith POTAWATOMI 69. "The Forest Potawatomi use the berries of the Common Juniper in combination with either the American Fly Honeysuckle. . .bark or the root of the Bush Honeysuckle. . .as a cure for various diseases of the urinary tract."

1945 Rousseau Quebec transl. 83. "A tea of the branches is drunk as a tonic for kidney troubles."

1950 Creighton N.S. 89. "Drink juniper tea for colds."

1955 Mockle Quebec transl. 23. "The decoction of the berries is diuretic and sudorific. The leaves and tops of the branches are used as a purgative; the essence of the fruits as a soporific and stupefier; in alcohol as an exterior stimulant. The maceration of the fruits in alcohol, gives after distillation, a tonic alcoholic drink known as 'Gin'."

MICMAC and MALECITE of the Maritime provinces of Canada used juniper for sprains, wounds, tuberculosis, ulcers, consumption, rheumatism and as a hairwash and tonic. (Chandler, Freeman and Hooper 1979)

GROUND HEMLOCK   AMERICAN YEW   *Taxus canadensis* Marsh. Taxaceae
Shrub with upright and straggling branches to 2 m. Leaves 1-2 cm x 1-2 mm with a sharp pointed end, dark green on both sides, they stay on the twig as it dries, when picked. The berries are bright red, pulpy with one seed. no cones. Seed poisonous, the red flesh edible but not recommended, leaves dangerous.

Range. Nfld. and N.S., Que., Hudson Bay, Ont., se. Man., s. to Io., Va., and Ken. in rich woods and thickets, bogs and coniferous woods.

1822 Cormack Nfld. 88. "The soil and shelter are so good here that the ground hemlock, bearing its red berries, constitutes the chief underground wood as in the forests of Canada and Nova Scotia."

1830 Rafinesque 267. "Wood hard, red, useful. Leaves baneful to cattle and sheep. Berries edible, contain sugar, gum, malic and phosphoric acids, a red fat; but seeds acrid, pernicious, oily, the oil of it used for lamps in Japan."

1915 Speck PENOBSCOT 309. "Twigs are steeped to make a kind of tea which is not only beneficial for colds but serves also as a beverage."

1915 Speck MONTAGNAIS 315. "Mixed with ground pine (*Lycopodiums* including *clavatum*) it is used as a brew for weakness and fever. . .317. A very strong decoction of the leaves used to dye green."

1926-7 Densmore CHIPPEWA 362. Little twigs mixed with those of red cedar, boiled and the decoction sprinkled on hot stones or taken internally for rheumatism. The informant, a woman of advanced age, said that this remedy came from her great grandmother.

1923 H. Smith MENOMINI 54. "Branches of this, with white cedar leaves and hemlock leaves, form the medicines of the sudatory [sweat bath] to cure rheumatism, numbness and paralysis. Taxus is pulled on a long string from the ground, and coiled into a circle to fit inside an iron pot. The lateral twigs are tied down to the main circle. Hemlock and Arbor vitae are likewise coiled. Equal quantities of each are put into the pot with water. Then additional sprays of each are placed on top of the pot to keep the steam and the medicine confined. While this is boiling, four stones as big as the fist are heating on the stove. A cabinet is made of canvas or cloth and the naked patient is covered completely with the pot placed in front of the knees. The four stones are then put in and the medicated steam treats the ailment. The sudatory is called 'asapaki'tci.' The patient remains in this tent until dry again, then puts on fresh clothing. The old clothes are washed before wearing again. This is, of course, a modern form of sudatory. The aboriginal one consisted of a small wigwam, with the stones heated in the open fire, and the treatment in general was probably taken with much more ceremony."

1928 H. Smith MESKWAKI 196. A universal remedy for all sickness consisting of nine ingredients, one of which was the leaves of ground hemlock.

1933 H. Smith POTAWATOMI 84. "Use leaves to make a tea used as a diuretic. Usually combined with the root bark of *Deirvilla lonicera* (honeysuckle) for treatment of gonorrhea. Nickell [white] credits the leaves with sedative properties said to act much the same as digitalis."

1945 Rousseau MOHAWK transl. 34. "Used in making of a 'little beer'. The berries and leaves are put into cold water, maple sap is added and it is left to ferment for one week. . .The Mohawk and Onondaga name translates 'hemlock that lies down'. The plant of choice amongst the French Canadians for a little beer is the spruce."

1945 Raymond TETE DE BOULE transl. 132. "The young branches, alone or mixed with those of the ash, *Fraxinus pennsylvanica*, make a tisane [little tea] that is sovereign for stomach pains or menstrual irregularities. Curiously enough, the ground hemlock has always been considered a powerful abortificant rather than an emmenagogue. The Old People warned pregnant women of its shadow."

1955 Mockle Quebec transl. 24. "'If du Canada', American yew, ground hemlock. The leaves are toxic and eating them brings on symptoms of poisoning; vomiting, pains in the stomach, vertigo, irregularity of the heart and breathing. A neighbouring species, the European *Taxus baccata* contains the alkaloids, taxine, ephedrine and a glucoside, taxicatoside, but no work has been done to our knowledge on the chemical composition of the 'if du Canada'."

1957 Wallis and Wallis MALECITE Maritime Provinces of Canada 29. "Steeped ground-hemlock brings out clots and alleviates afterbirth pain."

MICMAC of the Maritime provinces of Canada used ground hemlock for bowel and internal trouble and for fever and scurvy. (Chandler, Freeman and Hooper 1979.)

Both Kingsbury in the United States 1964 and Forsyth in England 1968 warn that the European yew is poisonous. The seed in the red berry is also poisonous but the red flesh can be eaten in small amounts. Both the English yew and the ground hemlock contain taxine, an alkaloid which weakens and eventually stops the heart, death is sudden with few warning signs.

DECIDUOUS TREES

including shrubby willows

DECIDUOUS TREES

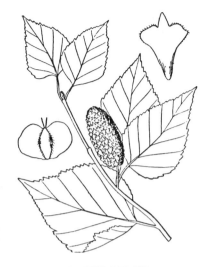

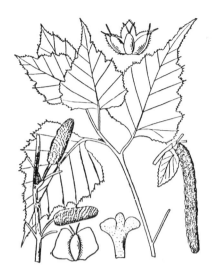

PAPER BIRCH   AMERICAN WHITE BIRCH

PAPER BIRCH   *Betula papyrifera* Marsh. Betulaceae (*B. papyracea*)
A small tree occasionally to 30 m the bark white with black markings, easily pulled off in large pieces. Leaves 5-10 cm long, single teeth, hairy on veins beneath where the 5-8 pairs of side veins meet the centre vein. Wings twice as wide as the seed in their middle. The catkins on stalks, smooth, 3-5 cm long.
Range. Nfld., Lab., N.B., P.E.I., N.S., Que., Ungava Bay, Ont., Great Bear L., Yukon and Alaska, s. to Wash., Mont., Colo., Nebr., Minn., Pa. and N.Y. Woods and rocky slopes. Gleason and Cronquist 1963 consider it perhaps a circumboreal species with European *B. alba*.
Common names. Canoe birch, white birch, spool wood.
835-1320 Juntunen site Yarnell 1964, 188. Bark found archeologically at twenty-seven locations throughout the Juntunen site on Bois Blanc Island, Michigan.

AMERICAN WHITE BIRCH   *Betula populifolia* Marsh. (*B. alba* var. *populifolia*)
Small tree to 10 m with smooth pure white bark that is difficult to separate into thin sheets. The leaves with two sets of teeth, smooth beneath when old, bright green above, paler beneath. Catkins on stalks 13-30 mm.
Range. N.B., P.E.I., N.S., Que. City, Ont. n. to Ottawa, s. to n. Del., Pa., O., nw. Ind. in woods and old fields. Unless this tree is specifically named references below are to the paper birch.
Common names. Gray, poverty, old field, broom or pin birch.
1509 Eusebii 1512 Weise 1884:299. Newfoundland. "Seven wild men were brought from that island (which is called the New Land) to Rouen with their canoe. . .Their canoe is bark, which a man can lift on his shoulders with one hand."
1534 Cartier voyage St. Lawrence transl. 23. "They [the Indians met near Blanc-Sablon] have boats in which they go to sea, that are made of the bark of the birch, from which they catch many fish."
1535-6 Cartier Quebec transl. 144. "There are many birches". . .155-58 Hochelaga (Montreal). "There is in this city about 50 houses, each about 50 paces long or more, and 12 or 15 wide, all made of wood, covered with large pieces of the bark of the said wood, as big as tables, very well sewn, after their manner." [Could be bark of other trees].
1551-68 Turner Herbal England. "Birch. . .Fisherers in Northumberland England pull off the uttermost bark and put it in the clyft of a sticke and set in fyre and hold it at the water side and make fish come thether, which if they se they stryke with theyr leysters or sammon speres. The same is good to make hoopes of and twigges for baskettes, it is so bowings." [Rhodes 1922:89.]

1603 Champlain-Purchas Tadoussac 161. "Their canoewes are some eight or nine pases [paces] long, and a pase, or a pase & a half broad in the middest, and grow sharper & sharper toward both ends. They are very subject to overturning, if one knows not how to guide them; for they are made of the barke of a Birch tree, strengthened within with little circles of wood well & handsomely framed and are so light, that one man will carry one of them easily; and every canowe is able to carry the weight of a Pipe: when they would pass over any land to goe to some River where they have business, they carry them with them. . .198. But with the canoas of the Savages a man may travell freely and readily into all countries, as well in the small as in the great Rivers: So that directing himselfe by the meanes of the said Savages and their canoas, a man may well see all that is to be seene, good and bad, within the space of a yere or two. . .Their cabins are low like their tents, covered with the said barke of a tree. . .159. The men sat on both sides of the house. . .[each] with his dish made of the barke of a tree."

1613 Champlain Voyages fac.ed. Thatcher Island New England coast 1605 transl. 74. "After having stayed some two hours to consider this people, who have their canoes made of birch bark like the Canadians, Souriquois & Etchemins, we raised anchor. . .Having gone 7 or 8 leagues we dropped ancher [Boston Harbour]. . .lots of savages who ran to see us. . .their canoes are made all in one piece, very hard to turn, if you are not very adroit in steering them: & we had never seen any made in this fashion before. . .138. HURONS Then they take a sweat and call their friends to take one, too; for they think it the true cure by which to recover health. They cover themselves with their robes and some big pieces of bark of trees, and have in their midst a good many stones which have been heated red-hot in the fire. While they are in the sweat, they sing all the time."

1609 Lescarbot-Erondelle Acadia 301. "As for the trees of the forests, the most common in Port Royal be. . .birch (very good for joiner's work). . .247. If they be pressed with thirst, they have the skill to suck the trees, from whence do trickle down a sweet and very pleasant liquor, as I myself have tried is sometimes." [See beech].

1620 Whitbourne Newfoundland 1579 72. "Cannowes are. . .made with the rind of birch trees; which they sowe very artificially and close together, and overlay every seam with turpentine."

1624 Sagard HURON 99. "If they have an urgent thirst and no water they know how to suck it from birch trees. . .Torches made of little horn-shaped rolls of birch bark were used. . .122-25. At each end of the houses there is a porch, and these porches serve them principally for holding their vats and tuns of bark, in which they store the corn, after it is very dry and shelled. . .As for the fish of which they make provision for winter, after it is smoked they store it in bark vats called Acha. . .For fear of fire, to which they are subject, they often put whatever they have that is most precious into vats and bury them in deep holes dug in their cabins and then cover them with the same earth; this gives protection not only from fire but also from the hands of thieves for they have no other chest nor closet in all their household but these little casks. . .102. The women made the baskets, both of reeds and birchbark, to hold the beans, corn, peas, meat, fish and other foods, and the bark bowls used for drinking and eating". . .57-60. While on a journey with the Hurons the shelter was made of two pieces of birchbark laid against four small poles stuck into the ground. . .Sagamite was served in bowls of birchbark that each man carried with him, together with a large spoon. . ."The bowls could hardly have a pleasant smell, for when they were under necessity of making water in their canoe they usually used the bowl for that purpose; but on land they stoop down in some place apart with a decency and modesty that were anything but savage.". . .28. Burial. "when all have arrived there [cemetery] each keeps silent, some standing, others seated, as it pleases them, while they raise the corpse on high and arrange it in its coffin, made and prepared expressly for it; for each corpse is put into a coffin apart. It is made of thick bark and is raised on four big wooden pillars, painted a little, about nine or ten feet high; my guess is that in raising my hand, I could not touch the top by more than a foot or two. The corpse being put up, with the bread, oil, hatchets, and other things that they wish to put there, they close it.". . .251-252. Each town or village of the Hurons had its special coat of arms which the travellers erected along the route when they wished it known that they had passed there. In one case, the coat of arms of the town of Quieunonascaran was painted on a piece of birchbark as large as a sheet of paper. It consisted of a roughly outlined canoe, drawn in it were as many black strokes as there were men on the trip. To indicate that Sagard was with them, the Indians roughly drew a man in the middle above the strokes. At the bottom of the piece of bark, they tied with a shred of bark, a piece of dry wood about half a foot long and three fingers thick. Then this coat of arms was hung on the top of a pole struck in the ground so that it leaned over a little. . .283-84. "They also sow many native pumpkins and raise them with great ease by this invention: The Huron women in season go to the neighbouring forests to gather a quantity of rotten wood powder around old stumps; then having prepared a large bark box they make a layer in it of this powder on which they sow the pumpkin seeds; afterward, they cover it with another layer of the same dust and again sow seeds, up to two, three, and four times, as much as they wish in such a way nevertheless that there still remains four or five good fingers of empty space in the box, in order to leave room for the shoots of the seeds. Afterwards they cover the box with a large piece of bark and put it on two poles suspended in the smoke of the fire, which heats gradually the powder and then the seeds so much that they sprout in a very few days; being well grown and ready for planting they take them in bunches with their powder, separate them, then plant them in the places prepared, from whence they afterward gather the fruit in season."

1634 HURON Jes. Rel. 7; 129. "Up to the present I have observed three natural remedies among the savages. . .the third of these medicines is composed of the scrapings of the inside bark of the birch, at least it seems to be this tree. They boil these scrapings in water, which they afterwards drink to make them vomit."

1639 LeJeune Jes. Rel. 17; 29. Granaries or chests of corn in use among the Hurons. . .both elm and birchbark were used for such utensils, as well as for many other household purposes. [Remains of birchbark boxes or storage receptacles have been found on Huron and other villages sites, according to an explanatory note by Waugh 1916].

1643 Lalement Jes. Rel. 26; 113. The French who dwelt far from settled areas around Quebec were often forced to rely upon Indian implements and utensils since the difficulty of obtaining an adequate supply in remote places was sometimes great. Bark containers were in frequent and widespread use at Tadoussac.

1672 Josselyn New England. Birch bark was boiled and pounded into a poultice and applied to wounds and cuts. The exudation of birch gum was used as 'touch wood' for the treatment of sciatica, an all too common colonial complaint. [See elder for its use by the Indians to burn their skin, the pain of this burn being worse than that of the sciatica, it was relieved].

1680 Bacqueville de la Potherie Michilimackinac. "Refuge of all the savages who trade their peltries. . .when they choose to work, they make canoes of birch bark which they sell two at three hundred livres each. They get a shirt for two sheets of bark for cabins" (Blair 1911 1:282).

1691 LeClercq 2; 96. Besides the canoe and snowshoe, industries which were developed by such peoples as the Abenaki, Huron and Micmac, an export trade in curios, ornamental canoes and such trinkets sprang up in Acadia at that time.

1698 Hennepin Fort Frontenac 580. "Our Spanish wine failing us, we made more of wild Grapes, which were very good; we put it into a little Barrel, in which our Wine was kept that we brought with us, and some bottles. A wooden-Mortar and an Alter-Towel was our Press. The fat [vat] was a Bucket of Bark. Our candle was chips of the Bark of the Birch-Tree, which lasted a small while."

1703 Lahontan 1:370. "There are some little Baskets made of the young Birches, that are much esteemed in France; and Books made of 'em, the leaves of which will be as fine as Paper. . .I have frequently made use of 'em for want of Paper, in writing the Journal of my Voyages."

1743 Isham Hudson Bay 136. "Their grow's here Large Berch tree, which they call (wursequatick), on the Root of the branches of the said tree, grow's Large Knops of wood of Different form's which they style (posogan) which posogan is of great service to the Natives, they using itt to strike Light to, as we do touch wood, itts very soft & spunge and Very Light when Dryed., itts substance Resembles Spunge, some being soft, some hard, according to the time geather'd, and is of a Yellowish Colour, some of which pieces is as big as a peck,—and this posogan when once Light is Very Difficult to put out, if not tak'n in time, and if not put out will Clow and Bur'n tell quite Consum'd to ashes and never Blaze."

1749 Kalm Quebec 551. "Birch-bark is said to be quite scarce in Canada and birch-bark canoes daily more expensive. Birch-bark Canoes. All the strips and ribs in them are made of white cedar (*Thuja*); the space between the latter varying in breadth between that of a palm and the width of three digits. The strips are placed so close to one another that one cannot see the birch-bark between them. All seams are held together by spruce roots or ropes made of the same material split. In all the seams the birch-bark has been turned in double. The seams are made like a tailor's cross-stitch. In place of pitch they use melted resin on the outside seams. If there is a small hole in the birch bark, resin is melted over it. The inside of the bark or that nearest the tree always becomes the outer side of the boat. The whole canoe consists ordinarily of six pieces of birch-bark only, of which two are located underneath and two on either side. The bark strip directly underneath is sometimes so long that it covers three fourths of the canoe's length. I have not yet seen a boat whose bottom consisted of one piece only. Birch-bark canoes are dangerous to navigate, because if the sail is forced down in stormy weather, it may splinter the bottom of the boat."

1770 Hearne Coppermine Journey 45. "Lake of the Little Fish. Our numbers had now increased to not less than seventy people, who. . .were employed. . .in making small staves of birch-wood about one and a quarter inches square and seven or eight feet long. These were to serve as tent poles all the summer on the barren ground, and would then be converted into snowshoe frames. Birch bark, together with wood for building canoes, was also gathered at this place. . .1771 Dubawnt river. . .[had encountered strange Indians] The people of this family. . .abode in some woods which are situated so far out in the barren grounds as to be quite out of the track of other Indians [Thelon River]. This place is some hundreds of miles distant both from the main woods and from the sea. . .their woods containing few, if any, birch trees, they had come so far to procure birch bark for canoes, as well as some of the fungus that grows on the birch tree and is used for tinder."

1770 Cartwright J. Labrador 20. "Where any open places intervened in a fence built to catch deer, they made use of a sort of sewell, made of narrow strips of birch rind, tied together in the form of a wing of a paper kite."

1778 Carver Travels St. Pierre River 84. "They draw with a piece of burnt coal, taken from the hearth, upon the inside bark of the birch tree; which is as smooth as paper, and answers the same purpose, notwithstanding it is of a yellow cast. Their sketches are made in a rude manner, but they seem to give a just idea of the country; although the plan is not so exact as a more experienced draughtsman could do. . .124. [Medicine lodge ceremony] The tent was perfectly illuminated by a great number of torches made of splinters cut from the pine or birch tree, which the Indians held in their hands."

1779 Zeizberger DELAWARE 52. "The bark of stone birch trees (*Betula nigra*) as of many others, the Indians pound fine, mix with water and use as a medicine. . .114. If a party of Indians have spent the night in the woods, it may be easily known, not only by the structure of their sleeping huts but also by the marks on the trees, to what tribe they belong. For they always leave a mark behind made either with red pigment or charcoal. Such marks are understood by the Indians who know how to read their meaning. Some markings point out places where a company of Indians have been hunting, showing the number of nights they spent there, the number of deer, bears and other game killed during the hunt. The warriors sometimes paint their own deeds and adventures, the number of prisoners or scalps taken, the number of troops they commanded and how many fell in battle. . .145. Of writing they know nothing except the painting of hieroglyphics, already referred to, which they very well know how to interpret. These drawings in red by the warriors may be legible for fifty years. After a hero has died, his deeds may therefore, be kept in mind for many years by these markings." [see Jameson below]

1799 Lewis Mat. Med. 109. "Birch sap recommended in scorbutic disorders and other foulness of the blood. Its most sensible effect is to promote urinary discharge."

1807 Heriot 1:98. "Sillery Quebec. . .In this vicinity, the Algonquins once had a village; several of their tumili, or burying-places, are still discoverable in the woods, and hieroglyphics cut on the trees, remain in some situations, yet uneffaced."

1820 Sansom Travels in Lower Canada Quebec Hotel Dieu 22. "Where a superieure and twenty-seven sisters take care of the sick poor of both sexes. . .The sisters. . .employ or amuse themselves in making ornaments for altars, and embroidering with fruit and flowers a variety of trinkets, such as pocket-books and work-bags, which visitors take home with them for presents to children or mementos of their journey. They are made of thin, smooth, and pliable bark of a tree, which is common here (The French call it Boulotte;) it will bear writing on as well as paper, the ink not spreading in the least. I brought away a specimen of it from the Falls of Montmorency, which I intend to present to Peale's museum." [Sansom was from Philadelphia and spoke French]

1829 Head Lake Simcoe Ontario 283. "All was then divided into shares, one for the Indian, another for the squaw, and the third for the child. . .put into a small vessel made of birch bark. . .The great utility of the bark of the birch is very remarkable. Not only are the canoes. . .made of it, but also all sorts of small cups and dishes. Besides it burns like pitch; splits into threads which serve for twine; and the filmy part, near the outside, may be written upon in pencil, making no bad substitute for paper. . .265-68. The evening turned out remarkabley fine, and the water was as smooth as a looking-glass. Everything was ready for my fish-spearing expedition. . .The birch-bark, for the purpose of light, was prepared in pieces three or four double, each the size of a large quarto book; and one at a time of these was stuck in a cleft pole five or six feet long, placed at the head of the canoe, overhanging the water in such a manner that the blazing bark might shine upon it. . .kindled the birch-bark. . .Crackling like soft fat, the unctuous matter produced a clear flame, which lighted up the watery depth beneath us to the brightness of day. . .At a depth of ten feet every thing was clear and resplendent. The slightest form was distinctly visible. . .We had regularly replenished our lights, which burnt out every five minutes or thereabouts. . .Saw two other lights proceeding from the canoes of Indians."

1838 Anna Jameson Georgian Bay Lake Huron 161. "We came again upon lovely groups of Elysian islands, channels winding among rocks and foliage. . .In passing through a beautiful channel, I had an opportunity of seeing the manner in which an Indian communicates with his friends when *en route*. A branch was so arranged as to project far across the water and catch the eye: in a cleft at the extremity a piece of birch-bark was stuck with some hieroglyphic marks scratched with red ochre, of which we could make nothing—one figure, I thought, represented a fish. . . .158. We passed this day two Indian sepulchres, on a point of rock, overshadowed by birch and pine. . .The Indians cannot bury their dead; for there is not sufficiency of earth to cover them from sight, but they lay the body, wrapped up carefully in bark, on the flat rock, and then cover it over with rocks and stones. This was the tomb of a woman and her child, and fragments of the ornaments and other things buried with them were still perceptible."

1840 Gosse Quebec 73. "The birch is often tapped, and the sap, (evaporated by boiling) exposed to the summer's sun, by which it is made into good vinegar. . .The fresh sap of the birch has a pleasant, slightly acid taste. It has a curious property, peculiar to itself, I believe, for I have never observed it in the sap of any tree but the birch; wherever it flows, it leaves a mass of fungus-like, mucilaginous substance, of a delicate pink hue, which probably has some affinity with what is called 'the mother' in vinegar. From the stumps of trees which have been felled during the winter, the sap flows in spring so profusely, that I have seen them covered with this substance, a great resort of insects. . .141. It is considered a sign of poor land where it [birch] is plentiful. The outer bark of the birch is composed of many very thin layers, which may by patience be separated, and can be written on as easily as writing paper. The outer laminae are of a delicate cream colour, but as they approach the ·nner bark they become redder. These layers when separated and divided into narrow strips, make an exceedingly soft and elastic bed, equal, if not superior, to a feather-bed; but great patience is requisite to prepare so large a quantity. The inner bark is about half an inch thick, of a crumbly, somewhat farinaceous nature; it is of a rather pleasant smell and taste, and of a bright orange colour, which readily transfers to water. I have read that in times of scarcity, the rude inhabitants of northern Europe make a kind of apology for bread by pounding the inner bark of the birch. The buds have a similar smell, which is strong but agreeable. For some time after the leaves are disclosed, they are covered with a fine silvery down. . .Probably this down acts as a preservative against the effects of cold. . .The wood of the birch. . .when mature, the heart-wood, or all except the sap-wood, is of a dullish red, which deepens by exposure; and is, when polished in furniture, &c. of considerable beauty. . .There is another tree of this genus, the Paper, or White Birch (*Betula Populifolia?*), which is said to be occasionally found in our woods; for instance near the banks of the Masuippi river, on the west side. . .I have been told that the Indians sometimes travel through the country, making inquiries for this tree, for what purpose I do not know. It has a singular appearance: the bark is perfectly white, not glossy or silky as the common Birch, but exactly like white paper, very smooth, but not shining; it readily peels in thin laminae, but does not look so ragged as our tree. . .The timber of the birch. . .is often sawed into planks for tables, and many other articles of furniture, but it is chiefly used as fuel, as it burns readily, even when green, and makes a hot fire."

1840-41 Phelps Mackinac mss. While exploring the island with a group which included the Ojibway wife of Henry R. Schoolcraft, Mrs. Schoolcraft stripped off the bark from a birch tree and scraped from the trunk a milky substance which is said to be a good remedy for consumption.

1857 Schoolcraft 6; 631. "Amongst the Chippewa of Lake Superior there exists a very ingenious art of dental pictography, or a mode of biting figures on the soft and fine inner layers of the bark of *Betula papyracea*, white birch. . .This pretty art appears to be confined chiefly to young females. The designs presented are imitations of flowers, fancy baskets, and human figures."

1880 Can. Horticulturist Aug. 117. "Mr. Beall stated that at Lindsay he had noted the following facts: Birch was used to some extent in connection with Maple for flooring, also for stair railing, bannisters, &c. and varied from $12 to $20 per thousand."

1884 Holmes-Haydon CREE Hudson Bay 303. "*Betula alba*. The white rotten wood of this tree is boiled in a decoction of *Ledum latifolium* [*L. groenlandicum*, Labrador tea] for an hour. The wood is afterwards dried, rubbed to powder and sifted. In this state it is used for chafed surfaces, the flesh being washed with cold water and the powder then sifted on it. Mr. Haydon speaks highly of its value for this purpose, having had personal experience of its efficacy on chafed feet etc. It is also used as a dusting powder for children."

1885 Hoffman OJIBWA 156. "When Schoolcraft attributed wonderful minuteness, as well as comprehension. . .to the Ojibwa hieroglyphs. . .he told the truth, but with much exaggeration and coloring. . .the general rule with regard to birch-bark rolls was that they were never colored at all. . .199. The record of the Mide-'wiwin, given by Minabo-'zho, was drawn upon this kind of bark. . .158. Bark records as have been observed or recorded. . .after the most careful research and examination extending over the field seasons of three years [were]. . .174. This chart, which was in the possession of the Mille Lacs Minn. chief, Baiedzhek, was copied by him from that belonging to his preceptor at La Pointe about the year 1800. . .186. Two similar and extremely old birch-bark mnemonic songs were found in the possession of a Mide at Red Lake Minn.. . .Figure 6 denotes the power of curing by use of magic plants; it would appear to indicate an older and more appropriate form."

1897 Handbook of Canada John Macoun 281. "The Canada balsam and the paper birch are not very common. . .The birch is the more plentiful tree and has a wide range. . .Besides. using its bark for canoes, the Indians in the English River and Chipweyan districts make, in spring, a very nice syrup from its juice, which before the advent of 'canned goods' served in place of the dried and canned fruits now carried by travellers."

1901 Morice DENE Northern Canada 26. "Cataract is easily discerned by the natives who treat it in this wise. A minute pellicle is torn from a piece of birch bark (*Betula papyracea*), after which it is doubled up and its extremities firmly held between the fingers. One of the sides of the curve thus formed is then used as the edge of a scraper on the corner of the eye next to the bridge the nose, and the thin film-like covering on the eye-ball is worked on till part of it is torn asunder, thereby affording a hold for the grasp of the fingers. These now complete the operation by gently drawing off the whole impediment to vision." [See ninebark for after care].

1915 Speck MONTAGNAIS 313. "The inner bark of the canoe birch. . .is grated and eaten as beneficial to the diet at times."

1916 Waugh IROQUOIS 146. Drank the sap of the birch. The twigs from the small growth were taken, made into a small bundle and steeped to make a drink.

1926-7 Densmore CHIPPEWA 313. "A Chippewa living in Canada where there are few maple trees, said that his people tap the white birch trees and boil the sap into a sirup. He said that the sap of these trees does not run as long as maple sap. . .321. A Canadian Chippewa said that he peeled the outside bark from the poplar and also the white birch, and scraped the inner bark, obtaining a little sap which he put in a small makuk [birch bark box]. He said that it had a sweetish taste and 'would keep quite a while. . .331-32. It is said that the early Chippewa understood the administering of both nourishment and medicine by means of an enema. The apparatus consisted of a syringe, a small birch bark tray on which the syringe was laid, and two measures for the medicine, a larger one for adults and a smaller one for children. The syringe was composed of the bladder of the deer. The proper amount of medicine was put into this bladder, then a short piece of hollow rush was tied to the opening by means of a strip of wet slippery elm, the rush projecting about an inch. This was used only once and then burned. The principal medicines administered in this manner were (a) the inner bark of the common white birch. This was scraped and about a hand-hollow steeped in water; (b) the wood of a tree identified as *Fraxinus* [ash]". . .370. Formulae for red dye, first formula, inner bark of white birch, inner and outer bark of red-osier dogwood, oak bark. Boil the barks in hot water. Prepare the ashes by burning about an armful of scraps of cedar bark. This should make about 2 cups of ashes, which is the correct quantity for about 2 gallons of dye. Sift the ashes through a piece of cheesecloth. Put them in the dye after it has boiled a while, then let it boil up again, and then put in the material to be colored. Do not let a man or any outsider look into the dye. . .381-384. Legend of Winabojo and the Birch Tree. . ."As long as the world stands this tree will be a protection and benefit to the human race. If they want to preserve anything they must wrap it up in birch bark and it will not decay. . . .a birch tree is never struck by lightning and people can safely stand under its branches during a storm. The bark is the last part of the tree to decay, keeping its form after the wood has disintegrated. . .387. It is the rule that all the chopping of a birch tree shall be on one side so that the tree after felling will rest on the stump. This prevents the bark from being soiled by falling on the ground. In removing the bark a vertical cut is made, the bark turned back with the left hand, passed under the trunk of the tree and removed by the right hand. . .First and most important is its varied thickness. The heaviest bark, from large trees, comprises six to nine distinct layers and is so strong that it could be made into canoes carrying many persons. The thinnest birch bark is like tissue paper but so tough that it was used in wrapping small packets tied with a thin strand of basswood fiber. . .A peculiarity of the bark is that it keeps from decay whatever is stored in it. . .Even gummy maple sirup being safely stored for a year. . .Heavy birch bark was wrapped around the bodies of the dead. . .The bark was highly inflammable, being used for tinder and for torches, and yet it was possible to use freshly cut bark as a cooking utensil, the inner surface being exposed to the fire. . .Birch bark can be unrolled only by exposing it to the heat of a fire. When heated it becomes pliable and retains any form in which it is placed when thus softened. . . .334. Splints were placed on fractured limbs. The splints were best when made of very thick birch bark similar to that used for canoes. The birch bark was heated and bent to the proper shape, after which it was as rigid as plaster of Paris. . .388. Makuks [containers]. . .These were of various sorts. . .sewed with split roots, and had a thin piece of basswood bark around the top, sewed over and over with split roots, like the tops of a canoe. . .Storage makuks had no binding around the top and were frequently made with one side higher than the other so it could be lapped over and tied. This sort was used for storing fish. . .389. Funnels or cones. These varied in size from tiny cones filled with hard sugar and hung on a baby's cradle board. . .to the large funnels made of heavy bark and sewed with split roots that were used chiefly for pouring hot fat into bladders for storage. Spoons made of bark were also used. . .The dishes for common use were made of birch bark folded and fastened with one or two stitches at each end. . .The largest trays were those used for winnowing. . .It was possible to make a cooking utensil from green bark in which meat could be cooked. A Canadian Chippewa said that he had done this himself making the container with either side of the bark outward. He said he filled it with water and 'put it right on the fire', that the part above water might burn but the part below water would last so long that the meat would be cooked. . .390. Various forms of torches were made by twisting birch bark into cylinders, some of which would last an entire night, and were used by travellers. Slender torches, which could be stuck on the end of a stick that was upright in the ground, were used by women when working around the camp. . .A variety of figures were cut from birchbark. Some appear to have been for pleasure, while others represent dream symbols and totem marks. . .Every woman who did beadwork had patterns cut from stiff birchbark which she laid on the material to be decorated. . .The most primitive form of Chippewa art is that in which the only material is a broad leaf or thin piece of birch bark and the only tools are human teeth and deft fingers. The leaf or birch bark is folded and indented with the teeth, this process being repeated according to the elaborateness of the design. The result is a transparency, the surface of the leaf or bark forming the background and the tooth marks forming the pattern. . .A woman said that when she unfolded the bark she found the design to be what she expected because she 'had the pattern in her mind before she began to bite it.'"

1928 Parker SENECA 11. Birch used as a carminative.

1932 H. Smith OJIBWE 358. "The root of the paper birch was used in medicine as a seasoner. Its sweetish, aromatic, wintergreen flavor disguised less pleasant doses. The root bark and maple sugar cooked together made a soothing syrup to alleviate cramps in the stomach. . .416. Sheets of bark are sewed together with basswood string and made into birchbark rolls, used as waterproof roofing for wigwams, sticks tied across the end of the roll keep it from splitting and tearing. . .425. The innermost bark of the white birch is boiled to extract a reddish dye by the Flambeau Ojibwe."

1933 H. Smith POTAWATOMI 43. "The Forest Potawatomi gather the twigs and put them to soak to extract the fragrant oil which is used to season other medicines, or to mask disagreeable flavors."

1931 Grieve England 104. "Moxa is made from the yellow, fungous excrescences of the wood, which sometimes swell out from the fissures." [See Isham, Gosse, above, Moxa, lit and burning, is placed on the flesh to counteract pain.]

1935 Jenness Parry Island Lake Huron OJIBWA 16. "They sometimes employed the same method at night also, using a birch-bark torch and dispensing with a lure; but starvation alone could drive them to this extremity, for they dreaded not only the cold and darkness, but the enmity of supernatural powers, who might at any moment send a huge snake to their fishing-hole. . .11. Draw a picture on birchbark and suspend the birch bark to a tree along the trail. Should there be danger of enemies lurking in the vicinity place the birch bark on the ground and partly cover with a stone. Friends will be looking for it but enemies will never suspect it. . .82. If you are prevented by a storm from crossing a lake or bay, make a model of a birch-bark canoe, place a louse and a little tobacco in it and push it out into the water, if it upsets the wind will shortly subside. . .112. A man and wife could make a birch bark canoe from bark stripped from the trees in early July in one week. . .108. Thin strips of birch bark are hung outside the wigwam, the snake like undulations in the breeze frightens the soul of the just dead away. . .75. The Grand Medicine Society [Midewewin] may be quite properly defined as a secret medical organization garbed in the mantle of religion. . .The members. . .specialized in 'botany', in the knowledge and use of plants for curing sickness and fabricating charms. . .On special occasions the medés united to treat a patient whose malady yielded to no other cure. They carried the sick man inside a medicine lodge, consulted over him exactly as would a group of European doctors. [Jenness makes no mention of birch bark rolls containing records of the society, which had only two members on Parry Island, both named King in 1935.]"

1945 Raymond TETE DE BOULE transl. 119. "The relationship of the canoe birch to the Amerindian merits a large book. . .There is a civilisation of birch, out of which a folklore has even developed."

1955 Mockle Quebec transl. 34. "The internal portion of the bark is bitter and astringent. The bark contains 10 to 15% of betuloside. . .The leaves in infusion are used in rheumatism and hydropsy."

1977 King Bay Lake Huron OJIBWA Mrs. King's personal communication. She binds the head with birchbark to cure a headache. [The birch family contains a methyl salicylate see discussion under willow].

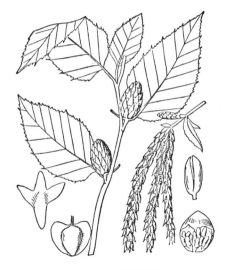

CHERRY BIRCH

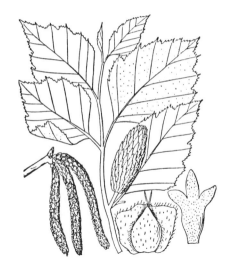

BLACK BIRCH

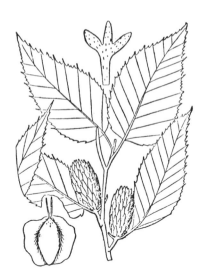

YELLOW BIRCH

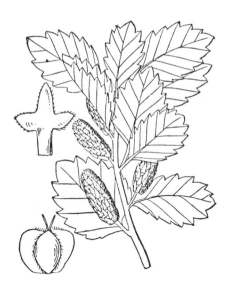

DWARF BIRCH

CHERRY BIRCH   *Betula lenta* L. Betulaceae

Tree to 25 m with reddish brown bark becoming furrowed in age. The twigs when crushed have a strong wintergreen flavor. Leaves 5-10 cm with very fine teeth around their edges and 9-12 pairs of side veins. The catkins have almost no stem and their scales are smooth. The tree much resembles a cherry tree.

Range. Me. to s. Que., s. Ont., s. to Tenn., Ga., Dell. and Ky. in rich moist woods.

1542 Jean Alfonse Gulf of St. Lawrence transl. 298-99. Birch which resembles a cherry tree found there.

1830 Rafinesque 200. "Wood much used by cabinet makers, takes a fine polish; bark with a sweet spicy smell and taste, like *Gautiera*, alterative and anti-scrofulous, pectoral, diaphoretic and depurative. Nelashkih of the Osages, used for colds, coughs, and breast complaints, scrofula and sores. A tea of the bark or twigs commonly used by empirics for obstructions, complaints of the bowels; a syrup of birch bark and peach stones used as a stomachic and restorative after dysentery. A beer is made with the decoction, also with the sap, which is sweet like maple sap and can become syrup and honey by boiling. . .The empyreumatic oil of the distilled wood, gives a peculiar smell to Russian leather, no insects touch it, useful also to preserve furs."

1868 Can. Pharm. J. 6; 83-5. Bark of *B. lenta* included in list Can. medicinal plants.

1882 Can. Pharm. J. 263. "The paper describes a visit to a wintergreen oil distillery, in Pennsylvania, where considerable quantities of the oil (about 30 pounds per week) are turned out, and yield a profit of about fifty dollars. The oil is sometimes obtained from teaberry leaves, but more frequently from the bark of the cherry, sweet or black birch, and from tests made by Mr. Kennedy the products appear to be identical, except in a trifling difference in the boiling point. Small trees, or shoots four or five years old from old stumps, are preferred. The wood is cut up in small pieces by revolving knives, and is placed in a suitable still with water, and subject to distillation. By macerating one night the yield is increased. This appears to be a profitable industry, and might be carried on by some of our country druggists in localities where the birch is plentiful."

1928 Gilmore OJIBWA 118. Bark used as medicine.

1955 Mockle Quebec transl. 34. "The abundant sap, acid and with an agreeable taste, is used as a vulnerary, detersive and antiscorbutic."

1973 Farnsworth ed. Lynn Index VIII; 178. *B. lenta*, gaultherin, methyl salicylate in the oil.

BLACK BIRCH   *Betula nigra* L.

Tree up to 30 m tall, slender, with reddish or greenish-brown bark peeling in very thin layers. The young shoots, undersides of the leaves and their stalks are hairy, there is a double row of teeth. Twigs and leaves not aromatic. Catkins on 5-8 mm stalks.

Range. N.H. to Fla., e. of mts., to s. O., s. Mich., se. Minn., e. Kans. and Tex. in swamps.

Common names. Red birch, river birch, water birch.

1926-7 Densmore CHIPPEWA 342. Bark in decoction for pain in the stomach.

YELLOW BIRCH   *Betula lutea* Michx. (*B. excelsa, B. alleghaniensis*)

Large forest tree up to 30 m tall with yellow or grayish bark, separating in thin layers. Twigs taste of wintergreen. Leaves with single teeth, softly hairy on the veins beneath, 6-10 cm long. Scales of fruits hairy, 6-13 mm long. Catkins without stalks or almost none, 2-3 cm long.

Range. Lab. s. Nfld., N.B., P.E.I., N.S., Que., Ont. to nw. and ne. shores of Lake Superior, s. to ne. Io., n. Ind., Tenn. and N.C., n. O., Pa. and Del. in moist woods.

Common names. Swamp or silver birch, black birch.

1885 Hoffman OJIBWA 199. "Yellow birch (*B. excelsa* Ait.) The inner bark is scraped off, mixed with that of the *Acer saccharinim*, sugar maple and the decoction taken as a diuretic."

1932 H. Smith OJIBWE 397. "The Flambeau and Coudreau Ojibwe tap the Yellow Birch for sap to add to maple sap for a pleasant beverage drink."

1933 H. Smith POTAWATOMI 44. "The twigs are aromatic. . .gathered. . .to extract fragrant oil which is used as a seasoner for other less pleasant medicines. . .112. The Forest Potawatomi recognize the strength of Yellow Birch and it is a preferred material in its sapling stage for wigwam poles. These poles are set up in a circle and then bent down at the tip to meet and overlap in the center where they are tied together in the form of a hemisphere which makes the framework for the wigwam or medicine lodge. It also endures for a fair length of time and when the family moves it is left in position for it is but a matter of half a day to throw together another wigwam."

DWARF BIRCH   *Betula pumila* L. var. *glandulifera* Regel

A shrub up to 2 m tall the young leaves and branches conspicuously dotted with glands containing resin. Leaves with 3-6 pairs of veins. The nut much larger than its wings.

Range. Lab., Que. n. Ungava, Hudson Bay to Yukon and Alaska, (var. *pumila* also in e. Ont., Que., Nfld., N.B., P.E.I., N.S.) s. to Oreg., Wyo., N. Dak., Io., Ind., O. and N.J. in bogs and wooded swamp.

1899 Fernald 147. "*B. glandulosa*. Mainland near Depot Island Hudson Bay used by the natives as a matting between their bedding and the snow."

1932 H. Smith OJIBWE 359. "Low birch (*B. pumila* var. *glandifera*). The Pillager Ojibwe use the tiny cones upon a plate of coals as an incense to cure catarrh. No doubt the resinous covering of the twigs and cones in this variety causes the aromatic incense. Also a tea made from the cones is drunk by women in their menses. Such tea is also accounted strengthening when the patient is enfeebled by childbirth. . .417. Use the twigs. . .for ribs of baskets, where sweet grass is the weaving material."

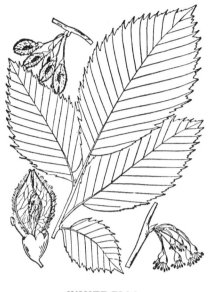

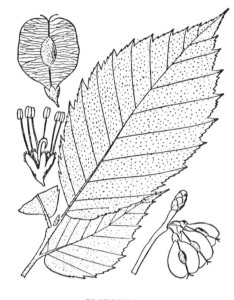

WHITE ELM   SLIPPERY ELM

WHITE ELM

Ulmus americana L. Ulmaceae

Graceful tree to 40 m with dark brown bark, deep ridges, weathering whitish. The twigs smooth or short hairy, leaf buds long, sharp pointed, pale reddish brown, with slightly hairy scales. Leaves smooth or a little rough, 8-14 cm paler green underneath. The flowers appearing before the leaves in hanging bunches on stalks up to 2 cm long. The seed has patterned wings around it that have fine hairy edges, notched at least halfway to the seed.

Range. N.B., N.S., P.E.I., s. Que., Ont., Man. and Sask., s. to Tex., La. and n. Fla. in rich soil, especially along streams and in bottomlands.

SLIPPERY ELM

Ulmus rubra Muhl.

Tree to 20 m with reddish brown bark. Twigs hairy, buds dark brown, blunt and coated at the ends with long rusty hairs. Leaves very rough to the touch, thick and stiff, 10-20 cm, both surfaces hairy. Flowers on tiny stalks or none, not drooping but bunched on the stem, appearing before the leaves. The seed is hairy, surrounded by smooth wings giving a circular effect without any hairs on the margin.

Range. Que. and Ont., Me. to N.D., s. to Fla. and Tex. The English Elm *U. procera* is like this elm.

300 B.C.-500 A.D. *U. rubra*, slippery elm identified in Ohio Hopewell fabrics by Whitford 1941:12. Yarnell 1964:188.

1590 Harriot Virginia 23. "Divers sorts of trees. . .Elme."

1619 Champlain-Macklem Voyage 41. "Cahiague [Orillia Ont. Huronia] There is a lot of oak, elm, beech and spruce."

1633 Gerarde-Johnson 1481-2. "Of the [English] Elme tree. This groweth to be a very great tree. . .the barke on the outside. . .is very tough, so that when there is plenty of sap it will strip or peele from the wood of the boughes from the one end to the other, a dozen foot in length or more, without breaking, whereof are often made cords or ropes: the timber. . .for naves of carts. . .The leaves and barke of the Elme be moderately hot, with an evident clensing facultie; they have in the chewing a certaine clammie and glewing qualitie. . .glew and heale up greene wounds, so doth the barke wrapped and swaddled about the wound like a band. The leaves being stamped with vinegar do take away scurrfe. Dioscorides writeth, that one ounce weight of the thicker barke drunke with wine or water purgeth flegme. The decoction of Elme leaves, as also the barke or root, healeth broken bones very speedily, if they be fomented or bathed therewith."

1634 Journ. to the MOHAWK country 141. "They make canoes and barrels of the bark of trees and sew with bark as well." [Jameson, the editor, notes this is the inner bark of the elm.]

1617-40 IROQUOIS Tooker 1964:23. "During this period the Huron and Algonquin made their canoes of birchbark and the Iroquois made theirs of the bark of the red or slippery elm or of butternut hickory. The Iroquois were forced to use these inferior materials, as birch trees did not grow in their country. Later, however, they did make them out of birchbark. They also used dugout canoes." [See Tulip tree and Basswood.]

1663 Boucher Quebec transl. 46. "There are elms which grow very tall and large, the wood is excellent, & the waggon makers of this country use it much."

1698 Hennepin 184. "They [Indians] pursu'd us in their Pyrogues or Wooden-canows [dugout]; but ours being made of Bark of Birch-Trees, and consequently ten times lighter than theirs, and better fram'd, we laught at their endeavours, and got clear of them."

1699 The Minister, Versailles France to De Villebon Quebec. "The King has had 'Le Nieuport' commanded by De Courbon St. Leger, fitted out to make war upon the pirates. He takes out provisions for Acadia, presents for the Indians, and a party of carpenters to cut timbers: ash, elm and other kinds, for His Majesty's arsenals, to be loaded in a storeship that will be sent out later. . .1700. The Minister to Begon. The report made respecting the quality of the several kinds of wood brought from Acadia, is not encouraging with regard to the young Elm. . .1701. Small elm, M. du Brouillan says, becomes harder in drying." [Richard Can. Arch. 1899.]

1724 Lafitau IROQUOIS 11; 13. Interior sleeping platforms. "The barks which enclose the platforms at the top and which form the canopy of the bed, take the place of a wardrobe or pantry, where they place. . .their dishes and utensils. Between the platforms are placed great boxes of bark in the form of casks and five or six feet high, where they place their corn when it is shelled."

1755-9 James Smith HURON Ohio Kinietz 1965:38. "In this month (February) we began to make sugar. As some of the elm bark strips at this season, the squaws, after finding a tree that will do, cut it down, and with a crooked stick broad and sharp at the end, took the bark off the tree, and of this bark, made vessels in a curious manner, that would hold about two gallons each: they made above one hundred of these kinds of vessels. . .They also made bark vessels for carrying the [maple] water that would hold about four gallons each. They had two brass kettles. . .in which they boiled the [maple] water. But as they could not at all times boil away the water as fast as it was collected, they made vessels of bark that would hold about one hundred gallons each, for retaining the [maple] water; and tho' the sugar trees did not run every day, they had always a sufficient quantity of water to keep them boiling during the whole sugar season. . .69. We had no large kettles with us this year, and they made the frost, in some measure, supply the place of fire, in making the sugar. Their large bark vessels, for holding the [maple] stock-water, they made broad and shallow; and as the weather is very cold here, it frequently freezes at night in sugar time; and the ice they break and cast out of the vessels. . .I observed that after several times freezing, the [maple] water that remained in the vessel, changed its colour and became brown and very sweet."

1778 Carver 499. "The Wickopick or Suckwick appears to be a species of white wood and is distinguished from it by a peculiar quality in the bark, which when pounded and moistened with a little water, instantly becomes a matter of the consistency and nature of size. With this the Indians pay their canoes, and it greatly exceeds pitch or any other material usually appropriated to that purpose; for besides its adhesive quality, it is of so oily a nature, that the water cannot penetrate through it, and its repelling power abates not for a considerable time." [see below]

1779 Zeisberger DELAWARE 23. "If they wish to proceed by water, or having been hunting are anxious to return home heavily laden with meat and skins, they speedily make a canow of bast, load it with their things and go whither they will. These canows are fashioned of one piece of bast bark, the outer side of which is turned inward, both ends sharply pointed and securely sewn with bast, the inside being stretched out by a ribbing of bent wooden rods, which keeps the canoe in its proper form. These canows are so light upon the water that they easily glide away from under the feet of one unaccustomed to them when attempting to stand. Capsize they cannot, because they are very broad and carry heavy burdens. To make one they choose a tree according to the size of canow desired and peel the bark off carefully so that there may be no rent. If a canow gets out of repair. . .the Indians know how to repair it. . .there is a kind of elmwood bast which they crush or pound fine and which is of a sticky consistency, serving them in place of tar, to keep their canows water-tight so that they do not leak. . .At one time they were more used than is the case now. . .For since they have hatchet, axe and other tools they make canows hewn out of trees, using fire also to burn out trunks. . .51. The elme tree already noticed above, is of no particular use, for the wood rots quickly, except that the Mingoes make bast canoes and kettles for boiling sugar of the bark, which is very tough."

1791 Lewis ed. Aitkin Mat. Med. 475. *Ulmus campestris* England. "Tough inner bark applied externally for burns by the common people, it is of use no otherwise than as a simple emmollient. Neither the purgative virtue ascribed by some, nor the astringent by others, appears to have any foundation. A decoction of inner bark, 4 ozs., fresh from the tree, boiled in 2 quarts of water to one is of a beautiful light purple colour when the elm is in flower. It has no purgative effect, rather the contrary. . .It is now in the London Pharmacopoeia."

1800 Haight 1859:186. *U. americana*, white elm. The United Empire Loyalist settlers around Kingston made the roof of their log cabins thus. "This was composed of strips of elm bark, four feet in length, by two or three feet in width in layers overlapping each other, and fastened to the poles by withes. . .with a sufficient slope to the bark this formed a roof which was proof against wind and weather."

1814 Clarke consp. 54. "Decoction of elm bark. . .diuretic, alterative, in incipient dropsies, cutaneous affections, particularly of the herpetic kind, &c. . .it does not. . .appear to possess much efficacy."

1830 Rafinesque 271. "Red, Slippery or Sweet Elm. This sp. is the best officinal Elm. The inner bark is used, it is fulvous [reddish], rather brittle and very mucilaginous. . .Edible, very mild, yet very efficient. . .The powder is a flour making a jelly like arrow root with warm water. Useful in all urinary and bowel complaints. . .sore throat. . .scurvy. . .Beneficial in diarrhea, dysentery, cholera infantum, &c. Very nutritive, but eaten alone produces sour stomach and eructations. Medical doses of the flour a small spoonfull, with as much sugar dissolved in water. Very useful externally in poultice for ulcers, tumors, swellings, shot wounds, (help to extract ball) chillblains, burns,. . .old inveterate sores. . .It allays inflammation, promotes suppuration and heals speedily. . .A specific to procure easy labor to pregnant women by using the tea for 2 months previous, well known to Indian women, whose easy parturition has often been noticed; now becoming in general use. Said to have cured fevers by repeated topical poultices on the abdomen. We have 6 other native Elm trees, all equivalent but less efficient, bark tougher, often bitterish and subastringent. In Norway bread is made with it. The outside bark soaked in water makes ropes. Wood very tough and durable, used for wheels, tools, &c. Seeds are esculent [eatable]. Leaves emollient."

1840 Gosse Quebec 142. "The elm when young, it is often cut and quartered; that is split through the middle into four parts, which are laid by to season. Few farmers have not a number of pieces of elm, white ash and leverwood by them, to be brought into use whenever any small article is wanted, in which hardness must be combined with toughness, such as axe-helves, wheel-spokes, &c. When grown it is not used for anything that I know of, except by those who prepare salts of ley, for the manufacture of potash. As an elm yields a large quantity of ashes when burned, in proportion to other tree, it is often felled by the salts-boilers."

1853 Strickland 11; 49. "The Chippewas, near Goderich, are the only Indians I ever saw use the elm-canoe."

1859-61 Gunn 859. "Slippery Elm, the inner bark of which is one of the most useful medical agents we have. . .is [also] nutritive. . .It is so important an article that it may be had at almost any drug-store now in a finely ground powder. . .I prefer the fresh bark from the tree; a handful of which, bruised a little and allowed to soak overnight in half a gallon of water, will make enough to last as a drink for several days. As a poultice, for all kinds of inflammations, as wounds, sores, scalds and burns, ulcers, swellings, tumors, gatherings, and the like, there is perhaps nothing within the bounds of medical knowledge equal to the Elm bark. . .The fresh bark, pounded soft and covered with hot water and allowed to stand a few hours, and then thickened with a little wheat bran, makes just as good a poultice as the powdered bark. An injection of Elm bark infusion is also very valuable in dysentery, bloody flux, piles and the like."

1868 Can. Pharm. J. 6; 83-5. Inner bark of the slippery elm included in list of Can. medicinal plants.

1879 Can. Pharm. J. 324. "Slippery elm bark is ground up and used for poultices; good to take out fever; its worth ten cents a pound."

1880 Can. Horticurist 116. Mr. Beall stated that at Lindsay he had noted the following facts: Elm was employed in the making of heavy sleighs and cutter work and was worth about $12 per thousand."

1892 Millspaugh 152. "The American Slippery Elm. . .is considered by many anti-syphilitic."

1894 Household Guide Toronto 110. "Slippery elm, the inner bark is a valuable demulcent, possessing very soothing qualities, and is particularly applicable, both as a medicine and injection, in cases of dysentery and other diseases of the bowels. . .It may be used as a poultice in all cases of local inflammation with great benefit."

1915 W.R. Harris 54. The Indians. The wash or lotion used for cleansing wounds was a mucilaginous extract of the slippery elm. . .50. Slippery elm, when boiled, and applied as a poultice or plaster, was prized as a valuable remedy for ulcers."

1915 Speck PENOBSCOT 311. Elm (*U. americana*) bark steeped and drunk is a cure for bleeding at the lungs. This trouble was formerly common among the Indians, but for the last twenty five years it is almost unknown. The bleeding would start suddenly after some exertion and sometimes become very copious. Could elm-bark tea be obtained, they say, relief would be assured."

1915 Speck-Tantaquidgeon MOHEGAN 319. "Elm (*U. americana*) bark is steeped to make cough and cold medicine."

1916 Waugh IROQUOIS 41. "A quite different style of crib or storage receptacle. . .was stated by Chief Gibson to have been used within his recollection. This was round and was sometimes made higher than the ordinary crib. . .It was made by taking small posts up to 6 inches in diameter, for the wall. A hole was next dug about 1½ feet deep and as large around as required. The posts were set closely around the circumference of the hole, the dirt thrown in up to the level of the ground and packed down solidly. This barrel-shaped receptacle was filled with the corn on the cob and poles were laid straight across the top. Over these were placed flat pieces of elm bark, which were removed from the tree in the spring and seasoned during the summer. Another pole was placed on top of the bark and the ends tied down with strips of basswood inner bark. . .55. Squire Johnson, an aged Seneca, remarks that 'they cooked their meat in a bark kettle, which they made by using a flint axe or chisel to separate the bark from an elm tree. They tied the large pieces of bark together at the ends with strips of the inner bark, making a dish large enough to hold the meat, with water enough to boil it. This bark kettle was suspended between two sticks over the fire, and before the kettle was burnt through the meat was cooked. It is said that by protecting the edges of the vessel from the flames it answered this purpose very well. . .64. Large bowls for bread making were frequently made of elm bark. The latter was removed from the tree in the spring or early summer when the sap was up. It was then bent into shape and the edges strengthened with strips of hickory or other material which was bound into position with the inner bark of the elm or basswood. A couple of specimens in the. . .Museum at Ottawa are nearly 2 feet in diameter and 7 or 8 inches deep. . .148-9. It is probable that infusions of many other materials. . .were used from time to time. Slippery elm inner bark is often made into a mucilaginous decoction, considered to have food as well as medicinal value. This was no doubt familiar to the Iroquois."

1926-7 Densmore CHIPPEWA 331. A simple appliance was a strip of slippery elm bark which was often used in place of an emetic, the soft inner bark being used and inserted in the throat. . .342. The bark in decoction gargled for a sore throat, the root dried and chewed for a sore throat. . .379. Slippery elm bark was chewed and used occasionally to calk small containers made of birch bark. . .378. Also used to make fiber.

1928 Parker SENECA 12. For dysentery give plenty of slippery elm solution. . .12. As an expectorant, slippery elm.

1923 H. Smith MENOMINI 56. "Slippery elm, when the inner bark is made into a tea, it is taken as a physic. The inner bark is also used to draw pus out of a wound. A small sliver is forced into the sore and bound up with a poultice to reduce the swelling. After the pus has been drawn out, the sliver is removed, taking the pus with it, and the wound heals readily."

1928 H. Smith MESKWAKI 251. "Slippery elm. The bark is used to make a poultice for old sores. It is pounded, then wet up and put into combinations with other medicines. Speciment 5126 of the Dr. Jones collection is the root of *U. fulva*. . .It is boiled to make a tea for women so that they may deliver a child with ease. . .270. The Meskwaki bark houses are covered with the bark of either the slippery or white elm, preferably the former. Strips six feet long are peeled from old trees, spread out on the ground in piles, and weighted down with stones to flatten out. Then the strips are used to make the sides of the winter wigwam and also to cover them or roof them against the rain. Such houses are often thirty feet long and twelve feet across. . .251. White elm, specimen no 5110 of the Dr. Jones collection is the root bark of this species. . .It is boiled and made into an eye lotion to be applied to sore eyes."

1932 H. Smith OJIBWE 392. "The Pillager Ojibwe use the slippery elm inner bark for sore throat, especially when the throat is apt to be dry."

1933 H. Smith POTAWATOMI 86. "The Forest Potawatomi use the bark of the white elm for cramps and diarrhea. . .They chew the inner bark of the slippery elm and apply the mass to the eye for speedy relief in cases of inflammation. When one has a boil, a splinter of the inner bark is sharpened and thrust into the boil and then a poultice is placed around the splinter. When the boil comes to a head, the splinter is pulled out and with it comes the core. Recovery is complete and permanent. . .One of their women [was] choking upon a chicken bone that could not be dislodged from her throat. Her husband was just about to go for a physician when an Indian medicine woman came along and took a strip of the inner bark of the slippery elm, running it down the patient's throat, past the chicken bone. It was allowed to remain there for an hour and when it was pulled out, it brought the chicken bone with it. . .Among the whites. . .it is the base of rectal and vaginal suppositories. . .115. Made boxes and baskets from elm bark according to Pokagon. . .He also says that the bark of the elm was sometimes used to make the sides of the wigwam. The writer has been in such a wigwam where big strips of elm bark were sewed to the framework with basswood string.'

1935 Jenness Parry Island Lake Huron OJIBWA 14. "The Ottawas were storing their corn, squashes, and beans. . .deposited in the ground inside large, cylindrical boxes made of elm bark, with elm-bark or birch-bark bottoms and covers. . .To keep the food from freezing they then covered these caches with flags from a neighbouring swamp and piled earth over the top. . .112. Nearly all the canoes around Georgian Bay were formerly made of birch bark, stripped from the trees early in July. A man and his wife would make a birch-bark canoe in about a week. For emergencies the Indians occasionally used an elm-bark canoe, which, though heavier. . .was a little stronger and could be made by two men in about half a day. The elm bark, stripped from the tree in a single piece, was drawn round a frame of U-shaped ash ribs, the smooth inner surface of the bark becoming the outer surface of the canoe. Gunwales and ends were stitched with elm root or basswood fibre, and bow and stern stopped with balsam gum or the crushed bark of the balsam. The ordinary elm-bark canoe held two men and lasted two years."

1945 Rousseau MOHAWK transl. 40. "White elm, the twisted bark was used to make a harness for sledge dogs. Mixed with oak bark it was used in infusion for the treatment of ruptures resulting from too great effort. In Quebec the inner bark is used to make chair seats."

1955 Mockle Quebec transl. 35. "Slippery elm, the bark and leaves macerated in water give a mucilage which is used for colds and coughs, and as an emollient to mature wounds, chronic dermatitis and in inflammatory infections."

Slippery elm bark is collected in the spring from the trunk and large branches, deprived of its outer dead portions and dried. Large quantities are collected in the lower peninsula of Michigan. The bark has demulcent and emollient properties. It is used as an external application in the form of a poultice; it is sometimes added to porridge and infants' and invalids' food. (T.E. Wallis 1967:82)

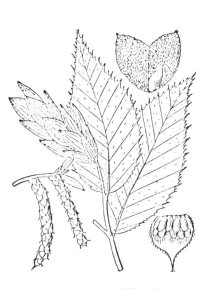

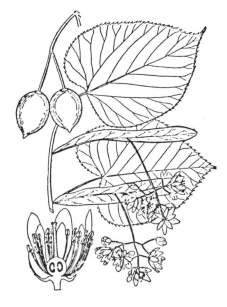

HOP HORNBEAM   BASSWOOD

HOP HORNBEAM   *Ostrya virginiana* (Mill.) Koch Betulaceae (*Carpinus v., C. ostrya*)
Small tree to 20 m, the mature bark breaking into narrow vertical strips loose at both ends. Twigs
and leaf stalks at first hairy, sometimes with glands, then smooth. Leaves like those of the birch
tree but with jagged edges of double teeth, dark greenish yellow above, paler below. Male and
female flowers on same tree. Fruit, a seed at the base of a membrane, these lie one over the other
like the hop strobiles do and identify the fruit bearing tree.
Range. N.B., N.S., s. Que., s. Ont. to se. Man., s. to Tex. and Fla. in rich moist woods.
Common names. Leverwood, ironwood, Indian cedar, black hazel, deer wood, hard hack.
1859-61 Gunn 812. "Iron wood (*Ostrya virginiana*). This is a small tree. . .The young trees are
often used for ox-goads and fishing poles. . .The heart of the wood, or central parts of the
wood—which is of a dark greyish or reddish color—is the portion used. It is said to be a powerful antiperiodic tonic and alterative, and by some regarded as an infallible remedy for ague, and
intermittent fever. Also said to be good in scrofula and dyspepsia. It is used in strong decoction,
made by boiling for a good while a portion of the heart of the tree, cut into chips or small pieces.
Dose, about half a teacupful, three times a day."
1868 Can. Pharm. J. 6; 83-5. The inner wood of the Ironwood, *Ostrya virginiana* included in list
of Can. medicinal plants.
1892 Millspaugh 159. "The fresh heartwood, in coarse powder, is covered with five parts by
weight of alcohol, and allowed to remain eight days in a well-stoppered bottle in a dark, cool
place. The tincture, when separated by filtration, should have a clear, brilliant orange-red color
by transmitted light, a slightly aromatic odor, a peculiar astringent and bitterish taste. . .A decoction of the heart-wood of this tree has long been used by the laity as an antiperiodic in intermittent fever, and as a tonic and alterative in. . .dyspepsia. The wood is very hard, dense and tough,
weighing 48 lbs. 11 oz. per cubic foot. . .It is very valuable to the farmer as a binder for heavy
loads and for use as levers. In the manufactories it has often furnished fine cog-wheels and excellent handles for tools."
1926-7 Densmore CHIPPEWA 340. The inner bark of the chokecherry, the root of the hazel and
white oak and the heart of the wood of the hop hornbeam were steeped together and the liquid
drunk for hemorrhages from the lungs. . .346. The wood at the heart of the branches was cut in
small bits and boiled, making a decoction to be drunk for kidney trouble. . .362. Chips from the
heart of the wood with the twigs of the white spruce and the ground pine were made into a

decoction used for steaming the stiff joints of those suffering from rheumatism. . .340. The leaves of the white cedar and the wood of hop hornbeam were used with other ingredients in making a cough sirup. . .377. The wood used for frames for dwellings, wigwam poles.

1933 H. Smith POTAWATONI 44. "The Potawatomi consider this as one of their so-called cramp barks and infusions of it are used to cure the flux". . .Nat. Dispensatory 1916 U.S. The heartwood and the bark possess a bitter substance that has been used at times as a substitute for quassia.

1950 Wintemberg German-Canadians Ont. 12. "A tea made from the chips of iron wood (*Ostrya virginiana*) is said to be a good cure for dyspepsia. The decoction is prepared from the heartwood, a handful of chips being boiled with 2 pints of water, and the fluid is allowed to boil down to 1 pint, which is then used as a tonic."

1973 Hosie Native Trees of Canada 150. Up to the turn of the century, Hop hornbeam was used for runners on sleighs.

BASSWOOD   *Tilia americana* L. Tiliaceae

Tree to 40 m with many young shoots growing from the roots. Leaves can be very large on young growth, they are distinctly one sided and the main vein beneath usually has a conspicuous tuft of hair on its axils with the side veins. The young leaves can be hairy all over. The flowers are on a long stalk growing from the centre vein of its own long narrow leaflet which helps carry the seeds on the wind later. The white flowers are very fragrant, with five petals each 7-12 mm long. They are followed by hard round balls covered with brown hairs containing 1 or 2 seeds.

Range. N.B., Que., Ottawa, Ont., s. Man. and Sask., s. to Tex., Ala., Tenn., Ark., and Del. in rich woods, moist fertile soil.

Common names. Linden, Lime, whitewood.

1970± 150 B.C. Glacial Kame site Canada; Ritchie 1948 basswood fiber identified in cord in copper beads found at site. Found archeologically in textiles from Ohio Hopewell and rock shelter textiles by Whitford 1941. "Burials were commonly accompanied by necklaces of copper beads strung on cord which was well preserved. The cord was manufactured by twisting strands of fiber from the inner bark of a woody plant. It is quite likely that the fibers are those of the basswood tree. . .but there are other possibilities." (Yarnell 1964:26.)

1612 Capt. John Smith Virginia Indians 103. "Betwixt their hands and thighes, their women use to spin the barks of trees, deare sinews, or a kind of grasse they call Pemmenaw; of these they make a thred very even and readily. This thred serveth for many uses, as about their housing, apparell, as also they make nets for fishing, for the quantity as formally braded as ours. They make also with it lines for angles. . .They use long arrows tyed in a line wherewith they shoote at fish in the rivers." [could be other trees.]

1613 Champlain fac. ed. New England Indians transl. 78. "There came to us 2 or 3 canoes, returning from fishing. . .They fish with tackle made of a piece of wood to which they attach a bone which they shape in the form of an harpoon & tie it properly to make sure it is strong enough; the whole thing is in the form of a little hook: the cord with which they attach it is made from the bark of a tree."

1624 Sagard HURON 240. From the atti tree, [probably the basswood], the Indians tore off long strips of bark. These were boiled to extract hemp from which ropes and bags were made. If the bark was not boiled it was used in place of moose sinews for sewing robes and other articles, for fastening together birchbark dishes and bowls, for tying and holding the planks and poles of houses, and for bandaging sores and wounds.

1633 Gerarde-Johnson 1482-4. "The line or Linden tree. . .The bark is brownish. . .but that which is next to the timber is white, plaine and without knots, yea very soft and gentle in the cutting or handling. Better gunpouder is made of the coles of this wood than of Willow coles. . .The leaves. . .boiled in Smithes water with a piece of allom and a little honey, cure the sores in children's mouthes. The leaves boiled until they be tender, and pouned very small with hogs grease and the pouder of Fenugreeke and line seed, take away hot swellings and bring imposthumes to maturation being applied thereto very hot. The floures are commended by divers against paine of the head. . .against dissinesse, the Apoplexie, and also the falling sicknesse [epilepsy], and not onely the floures but the distilled water thereof. The leaves are very sweet, and be fodder for most kinds of cattle: the fruit can be eaten of none."

1663 Boucher Quebec transl. 48-9. "There are other trees called Bois blanc, which some call Tillot; the wood is white and very tender and rots quickly in water: the bark is used by our Savages in many ways, that of the biggest trees is used to make large casks in which to put their corn and other things. The bark of the young growth is used to tie, & also they make a thread with it which they use for their cordage."

1663 Lalemont Jes. Rel. "The bark of oak, linden or other white wood, and that of other trees 'when well cooked and pounded, and then put into the water in which fish has been boiled, or else mixed with fish-oil, made them excellent stews." (Aller 1958:64)

1695 circ. Cadillac OTTAWA mss. "As to their huts, they are built like arbors. They drive into the ground very long poles as thick as one's leg and join them to one another by making them curve and bend over at the top; they tie and fasten them together with whitewood [basswood?] bark, which they use in the same manner as we do our thread and cordage."

1698 Hennepin ALGONKIAN 527. "The women make Bags of the rind of the Linden tree. . .They make thread of Nettles, and of the Bark of the Line tree."

1709 Raudot ALGONKIAN 369. "The cords used to draw these nets for fishing are made of the bark of basswood or of leather and are very strong and difficult to break. . .390. ILLINOIS. The women do all the housework, cultivate the fields, fetch the wood and water for the cabins, and gather the reeds in which they sew a twine of basswood to make a sort of straw mat which covers their cabins. Two, one over the other, shelter them from the greatest rains."

1724 Anon ILLINOIS-MIAMI 221. "The root of basswood for burns."

1749 Kalm Quebec October the 14th. 564. "The French called the linden 'bois blanc' (white wood). The Indian women used its bark in place of hemp for laces with which to sew their shoes. They were busy during the evening sewing up their footwear with this material and I could have sworn that it was a fine hemp cord they used. They take the bark, boil it in water for a long time, pound it with a wooden club until it becomes soft, fibrous and like swingled hemp. They sat twisting them on their thighs. . .586. The French. . .had with them bags in which they carried their food, which were made by the natives from the bark of this tree. The Indians take the bark, boil it in lye and pound it to make it soft. It becomes like coarse hemp. They weave it in such a manner that the lengthwise threads along the side are broad and scarcely twisted at all, while the crosswise threads which they have twisted on their thighs are about the size of small hemp cords and are not woven in with the lengthwise threads, but wound around as on a hamper."

1778 Carver 499. The Bass or Whitewood. . .the whitest and softest wood that grows; when quite dry it swims on water like a cork; in the settlements the turners make of it bowls, trenchers, and dishes, which wear smooth, and will last a long time; but when applied to any other purpose it is far from durable."

1799 Lewis Mat. Med. 255. The flowers as a tea are antiepileptic, and a specific in all kinds of spasms and pains, as well as an anodyne.

1830 Rafinesque 268. "Linden, Basswood, whitewood, spoonwood, Sucumug, or Sugumuck of Mohegans, Sucuy or Wuckopy of Algic [Algonkian] tribes. Beautiful and useful trees. . .Wood. . .used for canoes, models, spoons, turning, &c. when dry it swims like a cork, makes fine light charcoal for gunpowder. Bark used by Indians for ropes, thread, cloth and tinder, also make of it a hard paste to pitch canoes. Blossoms fragrant, cephalic, sudorific, antispasmodic, useful in tea for headache, epilepsy, spasmodic cough, &c. They contain a peculiar substance Tiline. . .Leaves and bark emolient, flax and paper has been made with the bark. Seeds can make a kind of chocolate."

1840 Gosse Quebec 175. "The outer bark. . .is rough and stringy, the inner bark is viscid and sweet, the twigs and buds are likewise very glutinous when chewed; cattle are fond of them, and in severe winters, when fodder is scarce, it is common for a farmer to drive his stock into the woods of a morning, and cut down a basswood or maple, on which they eagerly browse, and which proves nutritive."

1849 Stephen Williams 880. Basswood bark the best burn remedy he had ever used.

1854 Trail Sett. Guide 62. Grafting fruit trees. . .Some use Bass bark to bind around the grafts.

1859 Haight 227. During the 1797 famine in the Bay of Quinte settlements a grandmother would go away to the woods early in the morning to eat the buds of the basswood and bring an apron-full home to the family.

1860 Kohl Lake Superior 300. "A peculiar Indian mode of cooking turtle is as follows: They trust a piece of 'bois blanc' into the mouth. This wood when young, contains a sweet and pleasantly tasting pith, of which they also make a soup."

1862 C.P. Johnson 61. "Missa, a French chemist found that the fruit of the lime [*T. Europea*] ground up with some of the flowers in a mortar, furnished a substance much resembling chocolate in flavor. Some attempts were made in Prussia to introduce the manufacture of this lime-chocolate but were abandoned on account of the great liability of the paste to decompose. Lime-chocolate contains much nutritious matter and has an agreeable flavor." [Sturtevant 1919:571]

1880 Can. Horticulturist August 117. "Mr. Beall stated that at Lindsay Ontario he had noted the following facts: Basswood was employed in making common chairs, seats, buggy bodies, &c. and was $8 to $12 per thousand."

1915 W.R. Harris ALGONKIAN 54. "Wounds were always kept clean, and when necessary were sutured with threads from the inner bark of basswood, or a fibre from the long tendon of a deer's leg."

1916 Waugh IROQUOIS 87. "Corn and pumpkin were frequently combined in the preparation of foods. For bread making, the corn is hulled and pounded into meal. A quantity of the pumpkin is sliced and boiled to a thin mush. It is then mixed with the cornmeal, to which blackberries or huckleberries have also been added. Basswood leaves are placed on the bottom and sides of a pan, into which the paste is then emptied, covered with more basswood leaves, and placed in the oven to bake. The Iroquoian name for the bread translates 'pumpkin mixed'."

1918 Anon Ont. Ind. 30. "While their spoons were made of a wide variety of material, wood was most frequently used. They were of a large size, much exceeding European utensils of this class. The softer woods, such as basswood, were most commonly employed, and in their manufacture, fire, adze, and scraper were used. At times knots were used, which while more durable, yet were very much harder to bring into shape. The Indians. . .laughed at the white man for using such small [spoons] ones. They even suggested to the newcomers that their arms must get tired carrying such a small quantity to their mouths each time. Their ladles were made in much the same way as spoons, only containing a larger quantity and having a longer handle."

1926-7 Densmore CHIPPEWA 321. "The sap next the bark was used. . .eaten somewhat after the manner of eating corn from the cob. . .334. Old women whose limbs or knees were weak often made supports by taking wide strips of fresh basswood bark and binding it around their limbs in a kind of splint. When dried it was very hard and supported their limbs so that they could travel. . .378. Twine was one of the most important articles in the economic life of the Chippewa. It was made chiefly from the inner bark (fiber) of the basswood, though slippery elm bark was also used for this purpose. The twine was used in the weaving of mats and the tying of large and small packets. For some purposes the fiber was used without twisting, the width of the fiber depending on the strength required; thus a strip of fiber as soft and fine as cotton string could be obtained, or a heavy fiber that would hold a considerable weight. The fiber was boiled to give additional toughness if this was especially desired. In preparing the fiber it was customary to cut the bark from the basswood tree in long strips, put it in the water at the edge of a lake among the rushes, for a few days, after which the soft inner bark could be separated from the outer bark. The fiber thus obtained was separated into strips less than an inch wide and stored in long coils until needed. The twisting of the fiber into twine could be done at any time."

1923 H. Smith MENOMINI 76. "Basswood bast or bark fiber was and is the ready cordage of the Menomini. Balls of the twine are kept in every Menomini household, for tying, sewing, or for weaving bags. The women make this twine and go to the forest to gather the raw material. Saplings are peeled in the spring when the cambium is active and it is readily separable. A long strip of bark is peeled off and the outer cortex is slightly cut. Then the bark is bent at the cut until it projects far enough to get the teeth fastened on the outer rind. This is then pulled off and thrown away. It is now ready for use, except dividing it down to the desired size. Should a ball of twine be wanted, the gathered bark is coiled and bound to keep it in a coil, then boiled in lye water. When the fibers begin to spread, it is taken out, dried and seasoned. Then it is cut three feet long and rolled to break up the fibrovascular bundles. Finally, it is twisted and joined by the Menomini woman against her shins and between her palms. Basswood fibers are used widely in many arts. Matting, baskets, fish nets, and nets for snowshoes are made from it."

1928 H. Smith MESKWAKI 269. "The fiber itself is called 'wikup.' This is the ready Indian string, available at all times in the woods. . .Finally two strands are twisted in opposite directions and allowed to run back together to make a two-ply cord. This twisting is done on the bare leg. It is done in just the same manner that we quadruple a string. . .Meats are hung up to dry in the smoke and a great variety of other uses is found for it. . .248. The inner bark of the basswood is considered medicinal by these Indians, who use it boiled as a poultice to cause boils to open. Specimen 5151 of the Dr. Jones collection is a twig of *Tillia americana*. . .This is boiled to furnish a tea, which is drunk by those having lung trouble. The white man makes no medicinal use of this tree except to express a fixed oil from the seeds."

1932 H. Smith OJIBWE 422. "While they have countless uses for this cordage perhaps the most important is in tying the poles together for the framework of the wigwam or medicine lodge. . .When these crossings of poles are lashed together with wet bark fiber, it is easy to get a tight knot which shrinks when dry and makes an even tighter joint. The bark of elm or a balsam, cut into broad strips is then sewed into place on the framework with basswood string. In olden times, an oak wood awl was used to punch holes in the bark, but at Leech Lake when they made the writer's wigwam, they used an old file end for an awl. The writer lived in this new wigwam all the time he was among the Fillager Ojibwe and scarcely a night passed without a group of them visiting him and sitting around the campfire, telling old time stories."

1933 H. Smith POTAWATOMI 114. "The basswood is perhaps the most important fiber plant that the Forest Potawatomi use. . .Sewing the edge of cattail mats. . .The bast fiber is boiled in an iron kettle to soften the fiber to render it more slender and to increase its strength. . .When they wish to use it. . .it will again be softened in water and made into cords, or rope or bags."

1931 Grieve England 485-6. "European Linden, Lime flowers are used only in infusion as household remedies in indigestion or hysteria, nervous vomiting or palpitation. A prolonged bath prepared with the infused flowers is also good in hysteria. . .If the flowers. . .are too old they may produce symptoms of narcotic intoxication."

1935 Jenness OJIBWA Parry Island Lake Huron 112-3. "Bags were woven. . .of basswood string. . .The rush mats used for covering wigwams were of double thickness, and not pleated but sewn. The reeds were laid parallel and stitched together at top and bottom with thread made from boiled basswood root that had been scraped while soft and then twisted on the leg. These rush mats were heavier and bulkier than rolls of birch bark, but much less brittle. . .Besides the basswood fiber and the roots of tamarck and spruce used for baskets and canoes, and the basswood fiber and occasionally cedar bark used in mat making, the Parry Islanders made an excellent twine from the false [*Boehmeria*] nettle."

1937 Jones 22; 13. "In the Great Lakes region in aboriginal times basswood apparently was the chief source of fibrous material." [Yarnell 1964:190]

1945 Rousseau MOHAWK transl. 51. "Before the birth of a child, the mother drinks an infusion of a handful of the twigs of the basswood each the diameter of the little finger, mixed with the bark from seven pieces taken from a branch of the staghorn sumach. The bark must be peeled from the bottom towards the centre, then from the top towards the centre. The buds are also used. While the infusion is being made the branches must touch each at all times. This remedy is a tonic."

1945 Raymond TETE DE BOULE transl. 132. "Used in basketry and sometimes as the frame for top of birch-bark containers."

1955 Mockle Quebec transl. 51. "The bark and the leaves are emolient; the flowers, infused as a tea, are antispasmodic, sudorific, diaphoretic. They are prescribed for amenorrhea."

1957 Harlow 256. "The Iroquois carved false-face masks on a living tree and, after finishing the outside, cut them off to hollow out the back. The wood has a quality of toughness which makes it the chosen material for honey section boxes. . .The Indians claim that this rope is superior to that of the white man, since it is softer on the hands when wet and does not kink when dry. . .The Indians also used the bark fresh from the tree as an emergency bandage for wounds."

[The European linden, cultivated in n. America, is used as a medicinal plant to-day but *T. americana* our basswood contains a substance that can cause nausea and stomach disorders.]

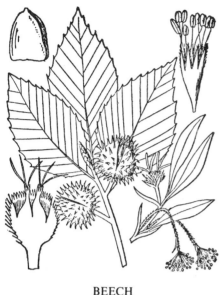

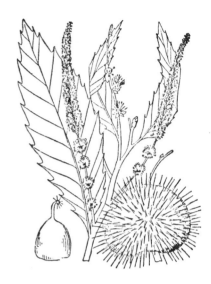

BEECH

CHESTNUT

BEECH

Fagus grandifolia Ehrh. Fagaceae (*F. americana*)

Tree to 30 m with thin, smooth, light bluish grey bark, darker on mature trees. Leaves very silky when young, silky below when old, stalked, of a leathery texture. The buds are long and thin on slender, slightly zigzag twigs. Flowers appear after the leaves unfold, in ball-like clusters on long drooping stalks. The fruit is a prickly husk opening to four parts containing two three sided triangular nuts with sharp points.

Range N.B., P.E.I., N.S., s. Que., s. Ont., s. to Fla. and Tex. in rich woods.

Common names. American beech, red or white beech.

800-1400 A.D. Aylmer site Ontario, IROQUOIAN. Beechnut found archeologically. Juntunen site Michilimackinac Mich. carbonised beechnuts recovered in four locations. "Elderberry, fire cherry, blackberry, acorn, chenopod, beechnut, sumac, acorn and bearberry all occur with each other from 1-10 times each and with corn, hazelnut and birchbark from 1-4 times each. . .It appears then that there is a complex of 9-10 plants, the remains of which tend to be found together in the upper levels of the site." (Yarnell 1964:37)

1380 Crawford Lake site Ont. McAndrews, Byrne and Finlayson 1974:5. Beechnuts, relatively well preserved, occurred in 12.4% of the features.

1541-2 Cartier Voyage St. Lawrence transl. Hakluyt 21. "Besides this there are fairer Arables, Cedars, Beeches and other trees than grown in France."

1619 Champlain-Macklem HURON Orillia 41. "There is a lot of oak, elm, beech."

1624 Sagard HURON 98-9. "If they had no water and were thirsty, they sucked it from trees, particularly the beech tree, which had a sweet and pleasant liquid when in sap."

1633 Gerarde-Johnson 1444. "The leaves of Beech [*F. sylvatica*] are very profitably applied unto hot swellings, blisters, and excoriations and being chewed they are good for chapped lips and paine of the gums. The kernels or mast within are reported to ease the paine of the kidneys proceeding of the stone, if they be eaten, and to cause gravell and sand the easier to come forth. With these, mice and Squirrels are greatly delighted, who mightily encrease by feeding thereon: Swine be fattened herewith, and certaine other beasts; also Deere do feed thereon very greedily: they be likewise pleasant to Thrushes and Pigeons. The ashes of the wood is good to make glasse with. The water that is found in the hollownesse of Beeches cureth the naughty scurfe, tetters, and scabs of men, horses, kine, and sheepe, if they be washed therewith."

1663 Boucher Quebec transl. 45. "There is also beechwood, strong and good, which bears nuts as in France: but it is only used for fuel."

1670 Allouez POTAWATOMI J. Rel. 54; 203. The Potawatomi ate 'fené', this was the nut of the beech tree, roasted and pounded into flour, when hunting and agriculture failed (Kinietz 1965:313).

1724 Lafitau HURON 11; 91-2. They gather beech-nuts with care and crush them.

1749 Kalm Quebec 25th. Sept. 530-1. "Here is an abundance of beech trees in the woods and they now have ripe seeds. The people of Canada collect them in autumn, dry them and keep them till winter, when they eat them instead of walnuts and hazel nuts; and I am told they taste very good."

1778 Carver 501. "The Beech nut. Though this tree grows exactly like that of the same name in Europe; yet it produces nuts equally as good as chestnuts; on which bears, martins, squirrels, partridges, turkies, and many other beasts and birds feed. The nut is contained, whilst growing, in an outside case like that of a chestnut, but not so prickly; and the coat of the inside shell is also smooth like that; only its form is nearly triangular. Vast quantities of them lie scattered about in the woods, and supply with food great numbers of the creatures just mentioned. The leaves, which are white, continue on the trees during the whole winter. A decoction made of them is certain and expeditious cure for wounds which arise from burning or scalding, as well as a restorative for those members that are nipped by the frost."

1830 Rafinesque 220. "Beech trees. Leaves in decoction useful for burns, scalding and frost nipping. Bark also used with oil or butter. Nuts edible, much liked by hogs, contain much sweet oil, proper for all uses. Wood less valuable than chestnut. Ashes good for potash. Beech shavings give much pyrolignic acid."

1840 Gosse Quebec 187. "The wood of the beech. . .is a hard, close-grained, and firm wood, and is used for carpenters' tools, brushes, and many other small articles; but the chief use we make of it is as fuel: a principal part of the firewood used in this country is beech, as it is very abundant, and burns well, and with a strong heat. . .It is heavy in proportion to its bulk. . .This tree grows to a majestic size and height."

1869 Porcher 275. The young leaves used by the common people of the South as a potherb. (Sturtevant 1919:267.)

1916 Waugh IROQUOIS 123. "Nuts used by the Irquois. . .beechnut. . .90. Nut meats of various kinds may be added to corn soup. Beechnuts a popular ingredient at Tonawanda."

1919 Sturtevant 267. "The nuts are esteemed delicious and are found in season in the Boston markets. . .In Maine the buds are eaten by the Indians."

1923 H. Smith MENOMINI 36. "The inner bark of the trunk and of the root are both valuable to the Menomini. They are used in several compounds, but never by themselves alone. . .67. Beechnuts are gathered and stored for winter use. . .Beech and also oaks were used by the Menomini for fencing, for building and for fuel."

1932 H. Smith OJIBWE 401. "All the Ojibwe know and appreciate the sweet nuts of the beech tree. They are never plentiful enough to store for winter, but the Indians like them fresh."

1933 H. Smith POTAWATOMI 58. "In Carver's Travels he tells of the manner of use of the leaves for medicine by the Forest Potawatomi. [see above]. . .100. Forest Potawatomi make good use of beechnuts for food. They are however, apt to rely upon the hidden stores of a small mouse called the deer mouse. . .It will lay up in some safe log or hollow tree from four to eight quarts, which they shell in the most careful manner. The Indians easily find the stores when the snow is on the ground by the refuse in the snow. . .113. Use the beech and one or two other woods to make food or chopping bowls. The kind of beechwood most favored is that with a curly or wavy grain, for the wood is apt to be much harder and resist cutting edges of tools used to chop up foods or meats."

1931 Grieve England 92. "Owing to the capacity of its root system for assisting in the circulation of air throughout the soil, and by the amount of potash in the leaves, Beech trees conserve the productive capacity of the soil better than any other kind of tree, and improve the growth of other trees when planted with them. . .Well-ripened mast yields from 17 to 20 per cent of a non-drying oil similar to hazel and cotton-seed oils and is used in European countries for cooking, as well as burning, and in Silesia as a substitute for butter. The cake left when the oil has been pressed out may be used as a cattle food. During the war an attempt was made in Germany to use beech leaves as a substitute for tobacco, and a mixture was served to the army, but proved a failure. . .Choline is present in the seeds."

1942 Speck RAPPAHANNOCK 34. Rappahannock steeped a handful of beech tree bark from the north side of the tree in a pint of water, to which a little salt was added. This was applied thrice daily to poison ivy sores.

1959 Mechling MALECITE of maritime provinces of Canada used leaves for chancre.

1973 Hosie 176. "The early settlers in southern Ontario often used dried Beech leaves as filling material for mattresses, because the leaves gave a certain springy comfort which was lacking with the universal material, straw."

CHESTNUT   *Castanea dentata* (Marsh.) Borkh. Fagaceae (*C. vesca* var. *americana*)
Tree to 30 m with smooth dark brown bark becoming separated into broad, flat-topped ridges. The short stalked leaves have sharp incurved teeth with bristly points, are yellowish green, almost smooth. Long clusters of male flowers surround a few tiny female ones. The fruit a spiny bur like husk 5-6 cm thick contains usually 2 or 3 nuts, flattened on one or two sides, 1.5-2 cm long, edible.

Range. Me., N.H., Vt., N.Y. to s. Ont. and Minn., s. to Miss., Fla and Ga. in acid upland soils, dry gravelly or rocky. In 1904 there appeared in New York a chestnut bark disease that by 1937 was estimated to have killed 99% of the trees. Fox found in southern Ontario that suckers were common everywhere but "so ubiquitous is the scourge that the odds against a chestnut escaping infection and attaining the size of a normal forest tree are overwhelming." (Fox 1949).

3000-1000 B.C. Holcombe site Mich. Chestnut found archeologically Yarnell 1964:67.

800-1400 A.D. Chestnut found archeologically at the Baum, Gartner sites; Kettle Hill and Canter's Cave sites in Ohio (Yarnell 1964:67) and 1300±200 at the Westfield site N.Y. (Ritchie).

1590 Harriot Virginia Indians 18. "Chestnuts, there are in divers places great store: some they use to eate rawe, some they stampe and boile to make spoonemeate, and with some being sodden they made such a manner of dowebread as they use of their beanes before mentioned. . .14. [beans] Sometimes also being whole sodden, they bruse or pound them in a morter, & thereof make loaves or lumps of dowishe bread [dough], which they use to eat for varietie."

1609 Lescarbot-Erondelle Acadia 302. "Chestnut trees which be not natural as in France." [Were they cultivated by the Indians?]"

1609 Juet-Hudson near Albany 23. "Then wee went on Land, and gathered good store of Chestnuts."

1612 Capt. John Smith Virginia Indians 92. "Of their Chestnuts and Chechinquamens boyled 4 houres, they make both broath and bread for their chiefe men, or at their greatest feasts."

1613 Champlain fac. ed. Lake Champlain transl. 224. "Many chestnut trees, & I had not seen any before except on the borders of this lake."

1619 Champlain-Macklem s. shore L. Ontario 47. "We noticed many vines growing in the wild and thickets of chestnut trees with chestnuts growing in the shell. We tried them and found them small but tasty."

1633 Gerarde-Johnson 1442-3. "This American Chestnut is almost round, but that it is a little flatted on the sides. . .the shell itselfe is brownish, not thick, but tough and hard to breake, smooth and shining on the inside, wherein is contained a kernel of the bignesse and colour of an hares kidney, white within, and sweet in taste like an almond or the common chestnut. Clusius cals this *Castanea Peruana*, or Chestnut of Peru; and hee saith hee had it from the famous Geographer Abraham Ortelius, who had it sent him by Benedictus Arias Montanus [drawing of nut and kernels]. . .Our common [English] Chestnuts are very dry and binding, and be neither hot nor cold, but in a meane between both: yet have in them a certaine windinesse, and by reason of this, unlesse the shell be first cut, they skip suddenly with a cracke out of the fire whilst they be roasting. Of all the Acornes, saith Galen, the Chestnuts are the chiefest, and doe onely of all the wilde fruits yeeld to the body commendable nourishment; but they slowly descend, they be hardly concocted, they make a thicke bloud, and ingender winde: they also stay the belly, especially if they be eaten rawe. Being boiled or rosted they are not of so hard digestion. . .yet they also make the body costive. Some affirme, that of raw chestnuts dried, and afterwards turned into meale, there is made a kinde of bread; yet it must needs be, that this should be dry and brittle, hardly concocted, and verrie slow in passing thorow the belly; but this bread may be good against the laske and bloudy flix. An Electuarie of the meale of Chestnuts and hony is very good against the cough and spitting of bloud. The bark of the Chestnut tree boiled in wine and drunke, stops the laske, the bloudy flix, and all other issues of bloud."

1641 Lalement NEUTRAL Lake Erie J. Rel. 21; 195-7. Chestnuts and wild apples being possibly more abundant than in Huronia.

1642 De Vries New. Neth. 219. "There also grow here. . .chestnuts, which they [Indians] dry to eat."

1650 Representation from New Neth. 295. "The land. . .produces. . .chestnuts, the same as in the Netherlands, growing in the woods without order."

1663 Boucher Quebec transl. 49. "There are chestnut trees. . .which are only found in the country of the Iroquois [s. shore of St. Lawrence]. There they are in abundance, & bear a fruit as good as that in France; the trees are much taller and wider."

1710 Raudot ILLINOIS 384. "The woods are full of horse chestnuts, locusts, oaks, ashes, basswoods, beeches, cottonwoods, maples, pecans, medlars, mulberries, chestnuts and plums. All these trees are almost covered with a vine that bears a handsome grape. . .The medlar [see hawthorn] and the mulberry bear fruits as good as those in France, as does the chestnut, but its nut is smaller."

1794 Loskiel IROQUOIS 70. Chestnuts. "Sometimes they are roasted like coffee-beans, and a kind of beverage made of them, nearly resembling coffee in color and taste, but of a laxative nature."

1830 Rafinesque 205. "The *C. americana* bears chestnuts one fourth the size of the European chestnuts. Valuable tree for timber, posts, staves, hoops, &c. the bark tans and dyes leather red, the Indians use it for deer skins. The sap of old trees is blackish, and can make ink. Chestnuts are flatulent eaten raw, better boiled or roasted: flour, cakes, bread and soap is made with them in Corsica, Italy, Switzerland, &c. The Chincapin has a good fruit, tasting like filberts, and affording a good palatable oil: the wood is as durable as red cedar; the bark is astringent and tonic, used for agues in the South." [The Chinquapin grows to the south of our range].

1882 Can. Horticulturest March 64. "At eight years old a plantation of chestnut timber has begun to pay good profit, in addition to the whole cost, by thinning of the trees for fence posts and rails. While the remaining timber is growing, the cut stumps sprout again, and by the time the former is ready to cut the latter is prepared to occupy the ground, and so an alternate growth may be procured without any planting. A grove of large chestnut trees, with about forty trees to the acre, has paid yearly $120 per acre, for many years, from the fruit alone, which usually sells at $3 a bushel, while trees so grown yield much larger crops than the wild trees. . .1881 April 51 Sweet Chestnut. This tall and handsome tree, the leaf of which much resembles the beech, but is more glossy and attractive, has a still more southerly range. The northern line of growth crosses the Detroit river a little above Windsor, cutting across the Peninsula to Long Point. Taking a northerly direction from this point on Lake Erie, before Port Stanley is reached, the line strikes near St. Thomas, running north of Hamilton and Toronto, curves about forty miles north of Lake Ontario and runs into that lake a little further east than Port Hope. The nut produced by this tree, though frequently sold in stores, has not a very high commercial value as it is smaller than those cultivated in Europe. It however serves to indicate in the same way our wild grapes do, that the better varieties might be easily grown. Its wood is chiefly used for furniture in ladies' boudoirs and bedrooms, as it gives a bright and airy appearance to a room. Its grain is wide and open, and when oiled and varnished has a pretty light yellow color."

1892 Millspaugh 158. "This forest tree, highly esteemed for its timber and edible nuts, attains a growth of from 40 to 80 feet in height. . .there is a specimen on the Nersink Highlands, New York Harbor, called 'elephant', which is said to be fully five hundred years old; Case's Bot. Index, April 1880, mentions an individual near Seymour Ind. measuring 22 feet in diameter, two feet from its base, and 70 feet to its first branch. The nuts when dry are sweet and wholesome, forming an article of merchandise. . .The leaves are official in the U.S. Pharmacopoeia. . .The leaves in decoction have been used for whooping cough. . .Castanea is claimed to have a sedative action upon the nerves of respiration."

1916 Waugh IROQUOIS 122-4. "A considerable variety of edible nuts are met with throughout the Iroquois country and were not only eaten raw, but were also incorporated into other foods. At present they are usually cracked and eaten as a treat during the winter. The gathering of nuts was usually left to the women and children, who gathered the harvest after the frosts had brought it down. . .Nuts used. . .chestnuts. . .A Cayuga informant stated that the older people used to crush the meats of the hickory, walnut, butternut and chestnut, and mix them with the cornmeal for bread. Beans or berries were also added in the usual way."

1928 Parker SENECA 11. Chestnut leaf tea used for whooping cough.

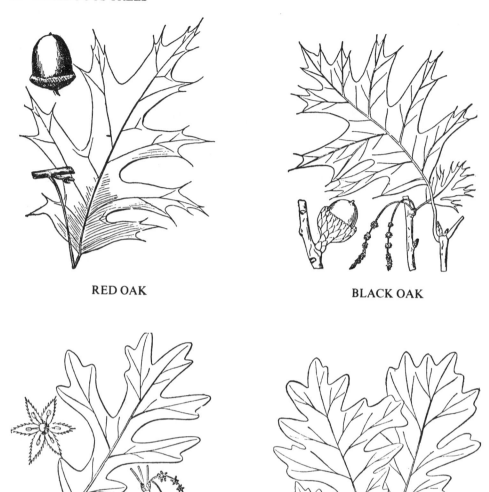

RED OAK

BLACK OAK

WHITE OAK

BUR OAK

Oaks are divided into two kinds. I. Those that have bristles on the tips of their lobed leaves; acorns that mature the year after they are formed and the inner surface of whose shell is furry. The two described here are the Red and Black oak.

RED OAK
Quercus rubra L. Fagaceae (*Quercus borealis*)

A tall tree with dark gray, slightly rough bark. The leaves are shallowly lobed, may have small tufts of hair on veins beneath. The cups of the acorns are more like saucers. The nut is bitter and tannin must be removed before eating. Wood is pourous, take a stem, dip the end in a soapy solution and blow bubbles.

Range. N.B., P.E.I., N.S., Que., Ont., n. to the nw and ne shores of Lake Superior, Mich. Minn., s. to Va., Ala., Miss. and Ark. in dry or upland woods and moist fertile soil.

BLACK OAK
Quercus velutina Lam.

Tree to 40 m with very dark rough bark, the inner bark orange. The winter buds strongly angled or grooved, hairy. Cup of acorn covering half the nut which is as bitter as that of the red oak.
Range. Me. S. Ont. (n. to Huron, Peterborough counties), Mich., Minn., s. to Fla. and Tex.
Common names. Quercitrin, Dyer's oak, yellow-bark oak.

II. Those oaks that have tips of their lobed leaves without bristles and acorns that mature the year they are formed and have a smooth inner surface to their shells. The two most important, the white and bur oaks are described next.

WHITE OAK
Quercus alba L.

Tall trees with light grey scaling bark. The leaves deeply lobed with rounded ends. The acorns with a shallow cup, the fruit sweet and edible raw.
Range. Me., N.S., sw Que., s. Ont. n. to Ottawa dist.; Mich., Minn., s. to Fla. and Tex. in dry woods.

BUR OAK
Quercus macrocarpa Michx.

Low shrub to tall tree with flaky grey bark. The acorn without a stalk, its cup sometimes covering more than half the acorn and fringed. The fruit is sweet and edible raw.
Range. N.B., s. Que., s. Ont. (to Thunder Bay), Man., Sask., s. to Wyo., Tex., Ala., and N.C. in moist woods and bottom lands to dry prairie slopes and sand-hills.
Common names. Mossy-cup oak, blue oak, scrub oak.
3000-1000 B.C. Acorns found archeologically at 6 locations in the Feeheley site Mich; in Fronte-nac Island site Lake Cayuga N.Y. Yarnell 1964:69-70.
1000-300 B.C. Acorns found archeologically in the Vine Valley site N.Y. Yarnell 1966.
300 B.C.-500 A.D. Acorns found archeologically in the McGraw Hopewell site Ohio and Spoon-ville site Mich. Yarnell 1964:69-70.
1000-1430 A.D. Acorns found archeologically in 8 Iroquoian aspect sites, Westfield, Richmond Mills and Silverheels in N.Y. and Alway, Lawson, Sidey-Mackay and Aylmer in Ont. where acorns were prominent for the first time. In Franks, Feurt and Ash Cave sites Ohio; Bates and Castel Creek sites N.Y.; Stroebel, Verchave 11, Moccasin Bluff and in 4 locations in the Juntu-nen site Mich. Yarnell 1964: 69-70.
1500 Draper Site Ontario Finlayson 1975:225. Recovered two acorn fragments.
1535-36 Cartier walking up the path to the top of Mont-Royal [Montreal] tranl. 153. "And we were on the path which we found as well beaten as is possible to see, and the most beautiful country, and even better, full of oaks, as fine as those in the forests of France, and the earth beneath them was covered with acorns."
1541-42 Cartier-Hakluyt third voyage 254-255. "Moreover there are great store of Okes the most excellent that I saw in my life, which were so laden with Mast [acorn] that they cracked againe."
1590 Harriot Virginia 9. "There are also three severall kindes of Berries in the forme of Oke akornes; which also by the experience and use of the inhabitantes, wee finde to yeelde very good and sweete oyle. . .19. Acorne, of which there are five sorts. . .These kind of acorns they use to drie upon hurdles made of reeds with fire underneath almost after the manner as we dry malt in England. When they are to be used they first water them until they be soft & then being sod they make a good victuall, either to eat so simply, or els being also pounded, to make loaves or lumpes of bread. These be also the three kinds of which, I said before, the inhabitants used to make sweet oyle. An other sort is called Sapummener which being boiled or parched doth eate and taste like unto chestnuts. They sometimes also make bread of this sort. The fifth sort is called Mangummenauk, and is the acorne of their kind of oake, the which beeing dried after the man-ner of the first sortes, and afterwards watered they boile them, & their servants or sometimes the chiefs themselves either for variety or for want of bread, doe eate them with their fish or flesh. . .22. Okes, there are as faire, straight, tall, and as good timber as any can be, and also great store, and in some places very great."

1604 Champlain-Purchas 189. Richlieu river. "For their [Indians] Fort is covered with the barke of okes."

1609 Hudson Hudson River N.Y. 49. "I sailed to the shore in one of their canoes. . .I saw there in a house well constructed of oak bark, and circular in shape, with the appearance of having a vaulted ceiling'.. . .Juet on Hudson's voyage 18. "The Countrey is full of great and tall oakes."

1611 Biard ETCHEMIN Acadia Jes. Rel. 1. "For women are everywhere the best managers, they will sometimes make storehouses for the winter, where they will keep smoked meat, roots, shelled acorns, peas, beans etc."

1612 Capt. John Smith Virginia Indians 102. "In May and June they plant their fieldes, and live mostly of Acornes, walnuts, and fish."

1613 Champlain fac. ed. transl. 45. Maine. "I put foot on the earth to see the country: and going to hunt I found the road very pleasant and agreeable. It seemed as if the oaks had been planted for pleasure. I saw few firs, but a good many pines on one side of the river: Nothing but oaks on the other". . .69. Saco river. "The savages have a great cabin surrounded by palisades, made of very big trees side by side where they retire when their enemies come on the warpath. They cover their cabins with oak bark". . .175 Island of Orleans, St. Lawrence. "Where there are a quantity of fine oaks.'. . .Quebec, 6 or 7 leages away. "This is the place where Jacques Cartier wintered, there are still at this place, by the stream, vestiges of a chimney, of which we found the foundation, & the appearance of there having been ditches around their lodging, which was small. We found also some large pieces of squared wood, worm eaten, & some 3 or 4 cannon balls [Possibly pieces of oak to have been large, squared and lasted 70 years]. . .313. I took back to France with me, to try out in France an oak for paths, (chesne de sente)."

1619 Champlain-Macklem 34. "We pushed on another hundred miles or so (up the Ottawa River) until we found ourselves in a barren region where there was nothing to see but spruce and birch and a few scattered oaks. . .[Lake Huron shore.] The north shore of the lake is precipitous in places; elsewhere it is low lying and sparsely wooded, with a scattering of oaks. The whole region is uninhabited. . .40 [Huronia]. Most of the land is cleared of trees. . .41. There is a lot of oak."

1624 Sagard HURON 108. "They also make a dish with acorns, which they boil in several waters to take away the bitter taste, and I found them rather good."

1625 Wassenaer New Neth. 81. "There are oaks of very close grain; yea, harder than any in this country, as thick as three or four men."

1632 Champlain-Bourne 66. Cape La Heve. . .a great tract of oaks. . .145. "Father Biard lived at Port Royal, where he suffered great fatigue and great want during several days, being compelled to collect some acorns and roots for his sustenance."

1650 Representation New Neth. 295. "The indigenous fruit consists principally of acorns, some of which are very sweet."

1663 Boucher Quebec transl. 45. "There are two sorts of oaks; one is more porous than the other. The porous one is best to make furniture, and the other for woodworking and carpentry: it is best for making boats to go on the water: these trees are tall, big, & straight, & are all found near Montreal."

1667 Marie de l'Incarnation Quebec to her son. 331. Father Allouez on Lake Superior. "The Father suffered excessively in this mission. For the space of two years he lived almost entirely upon acorns and moss, which he scraped on rocks. . .To eat this wretched meat, he boiled the acorns in lye to make them less bitter, then mixed in his moss, and this made a sagamite that was as black as ink and as sticky as peas."

1698 Hennepin Quebec 596. "They had a hard winter [1629] of it at Quebec, for they wanted all sorts of Necessaries; and because the Ships which brought Provisions were seized on by the English, they were therefore obliged to divide the small Provision that was left. Our Religious might have had their share as well as others, but they contented themselves with Indian Corn, and the Pulse they had sown. Madame Hebers made them a present of two Barrels of Pease, which are extraordinary good and large in Canada; besides they had Raisins, and had made a provision of Acorns in case of necessity, and they were so happy as to catch some Eeels, which are plentiful in that River."

1710 Raudot PUANT OUTAGAMI MASCOUTIN KICAPOUS 383. "The place where they are is well situated for living and seems to make them more ferocious and more insolent. Although they sow wheat there they often live on acorns and beans."

1718 Quebec, Richard 1899:194. Reserving to His Majesty the right to take and remove, without paying therefor, all such oak timber as it may please him to take from the said lands.

1724 Anon ILLINOIS-MIAMI mss 223. "The bark or the root of white oak boiled for wounds, the leaf of the same tree is also perfectly good. . .The little bark of white oak boiled, for the same soreness of the eyes."

1748 Kalm New York November the 1st. 128. "The bark of the white oak was reckoned the best remedy which had as yet been found against dysentery. It is reduced to a powder; and then taken. Some people assured me that in cases where nothing would help, this remedy had given a certain and speedy relief. The people in this place also make use of the bark (as is usually done in the English colonies) to dye wool brown, which looks like that of Bohea tea, and does not fade by being exposed to the sun. . .221. The millers said that the axle-trees of the mill wheels were made of white oak, that they lasted for three or four years, but that pine did not keep so well."

1794 Loskiel IROQUOIS 1; 68. "If the winter happens to be severe, and the snow prevents them from hunting, a general famine ensues, by which many die of hunger. They are then driven by hunger to dress and eat roots of grass or the inner bark of trees, especially of young oaks."

1799 Lewis Mat. Med. 214. "The astringent effects of the oak bark were sufficiently known to the ancients, by whom different parts of it were used. . .It manifests a taste of strong astringency, accompanied with a moderate bitterness. . .recommended in agues, for restraining hemorrhages, alvine fluxes, and other immoderate evacuations. . .This bark has been supposed by some to be not less efficacious than the Peruvian bark[quinine] especially in the form of an extract; but this is believed by a very few, if any, at present, though it is not doubted but that the bark may have the power of curing some intermittents."

1807 Heriot 128. Kingston, Ont. "The dry lands, which are usually the most elevated, afford growth to oaks and hickory. . .132. The number of vessels in the employ of merchants is considerable. These are usually built about ten miles below Kingston, and the timber used for their construction is red cedar or oak. . .The timber found here and on the south shore of the mainland, is red oak. . .York [Toronto]. . .a part of the town [is a] point of land clothed with spreading oak-trees, gradually receding from the eye, one behind another, until terminated by the buildings of the garrison. . .Lake Simcoe. . .there are plains thinly planted with oak-trees, where the Indians cultivate corn. . .Niagara River. . .A stranger is here struck with sentiments of regret on viewing the numbers of fine oak-trees which are daily consumed by fire, in preparing the land for cultivation."

1820's Mat. Med. Edinburgh-Toronto mss 34. "*Quercus Robur* [an English oak]. The bark of this tree possesses a great degree of astringency which it yields to water. It has been used as a remedy in Hemorrhage, Diarrhoea, Intermittent fever. . .a strong infusion is usually employed as an astringent gargle in Cynanche & Leucorrhoea & profuse hemorrhagy & as a fomentation in Hemorrhisis & prolapsus ani. . .In Medical practice galls though forcefully astringent are seldom internally administered. Its infusion is used for the same purposes as oak bark & its ointment is applied in Hemorrhoidal affections."

1830 Rafinesque 255. "Oak. Nearly 40 sp. All valuable and medical. Useful wood, bark, sap, galls and fruits called acorns. Fine timber used for staves, casks, fences, shingles, boards, houses, ships, &c. Acorns often esculent, taste of chestnuts. . .Indians made oil and bread of them. . .Bark used for tanning, chiefly *Q. rubra* red oak. . .*Q. alba* white oak and other sp. dye brown, contain much tannin, and 18 per cent of a peculiar substance Quercine, insoluble but inflammable. . .Febrifuge, astringent, antiseptic, weak eqw. of Cinchona [quinine] for fevers, very useful in cynanche, ulcers, dysentery, gangrene, hemorrhage, sorethroat, wounds, prolapsus,. . .Use in wash, bath, poultice, decoction &c. Cups and acorns equiv. also in spasmodic cough, asthma, chronic hyseteria, amenorrhea, rheumatism. Dry emanations of oak bark useful in phthisis. . .Oak galls still stronger, used to dye black, make ink, powerful astringent and styptic."

1833 Howard Quebec 26. To cure Dropsy. 3. Take a Decoction of Oak Bough tops. . .100. To Cure a broken skin. Bind a dry oak leaf upon it. . .134. To cure the Whites. Live chastly—Feed sparingly—Constantly use exercise, and never lie on the back and boil 4 or 5 leaves of white noby oak in a pint of milk with a little sugar. Then add a teasspoonful of the Balm of Gilliead. [balsam poplar?] Drink this every morning. **1842** 11. To cure a cancer by free use of potash made from Ashes of Red Oak to the consistence of Molasses. Boil Ashes; Apply as A poultice. Cover all over with a coate of tarr, 2 or 3 applications removes all protubrances. After which it is only necessary to Dress the sore with common ointment or Aney sort of Dressing. This is worth 1000 pounds. . .29. To make good ink; Bruise half pound of Blue nutgalls and boil them half an hour then strain them off and Mix 4 ounces of copperas and 4 ounces of gum arabick in the Boiling liquor, and half an ounce of stone blue and keep it by the fire four hours. When it is cold it is fit for use. . .A Hipp[ed] horse to cure. Make one gallon of strong white oak Bark Water and dissolve one pound of alum in it. Shake well together and wash the horse's hipp with this mixture 3 times a day. This never fails to cure."

1841 Trousseau & Pidoux Paris transl. Use acorns because of natural association of several alimentary substances with a tonic and astringent substance to replace coffee for easy digestion. Roast, grind and make a coffee like substance. Give to infants to drink. Drink powdered oak bark tea for hemorrhage. . .take 64 gr. powdered 12-15 year old oak bark, screened, in 1000 grams of boiling water, infuse 2 hours, screen and use for intermittent fever, chronic diarrhea, veneral diseases, as a vaginal douche and for the eyes and as an antidote to poison.

1842 Christison 765. "Oak bark has been used as an astringent in medicine since the days of the Greek physicians. . .Of late, however, it has been in a great measure abandoned, probably without reason. . .457. Galls were known to the Romans. . .galls are astringent in their action; and all their medicinal applications rest upon this property. . .They constitute the best antidote for poisoning with tartar-emetic."

1855 Trail Sett. Guide Ont. 139. "The acorns of the white-oak, browned and ground, are also used." [As a substitute for coffee]

1859-61 Gunn 881. "Oak bark is a healthy, pure, and very useful astringent, and may be relied on in most cases where astringents are needed; only be careful and do not give too much, or too strong a preparation, and constipate the bowels too much, especially in dysentery."

1868 Can. Pharm. J. 6; 83-5. Bark of the white oak, *Q. alba* and that of the black oak, *Q. Niger* included in list of Can. medicinal plants. [Probably means *Q. velutina*].

1879 Can. Pharm. J. 302. A series of experiments. . .to determine the tannin value of. . .white oak bark 7.85%; red oak bark 5.55%; bur oak bark 7.85%.

1881 Can. Horticulturist 159-161. "White oak. . .most valuable of all. . .It will attain under favorable conditions to the height of eighty feet, with a diameter of from six to seven feet. . .The acorns are oval, large, and sweet. . .The wood is reddish, and similar to that of the European oak and is used for building frames, mill-dams, posts, frames of coaches, baskets, barrels; and ship-building. . .Roots of this species make beautiful furniture. . .being feathered in the most beautiful manner, and taking a polish equal to that of the finest mahogany. . .The red oak. . .is one of the most common in Canada. . .The wood is reddish coarse grained, strong, but not durable, and is principally used for staves. . .Black oak. . .It is one of our loftiest trees. . .From the cellular tissue of this oak is obtained the material known as *quercitrin*, used in dyeing wool, silk and paper hangings."

1885 Hoffman OJIBWA 198. "White oak. 1. The bark of the root and the inner bark scraped from the trunk is boiled and the decoction used internally for diarrhea. 2. Acorns eaten raw by children, and boiled or dried by adults. Red oak. 'Bitter Acorn Tree' Has been used as a substitute for *Q. alba*."

1892 Heebner Pharm. 206. "Gallic acid. Found in nutgalls, sumac, uva ursi, etc. Made by macerating powd. nutgalls with cold water for about a month, then expressing, and rejecting the liquid. Boil the residue with water and filter while hot through animal charcols, and set aside to crystallize. Purified by re-crystallization. By this process, pure tannin, which is degallic acid [is obtained]. . .Officinal Preparation. Ointment of gallic acid. Contains gallic acid (10), incorporated with benzoinated lard (90). Avoid use of iron spatula."

1915 Speck PENOBSCOT 309. "Acorns of the white oak are eaten to induce thirst since it is thought beneficial to drink plenty of water. White oak bark is steeped and drunk for bleeding piles."

1915 Speck-Tantaquidgeon MOHEGAN 319. "White oak bark is steeped and used as a liniment; it is used also for horses."

1916 Waugh IROQUOIS 122-3. "The acorn was used quite commonly, probably more particularly the sweet kinds, such as those of the white oak, the chestnut oak and some others. Even the bitter acorns of the red and black oak were used in times of necessity. . .The Hurons are said to have prepared them by 'first boiling them in a lye made from ashes, in order to take from them their excessive bitterness'."

1926-7 Densmore CHIPPEWA 320. "Bur oak. Sweet acorns were frequently gathered in the late fall and buried for use in the winter or spring, or they could be used as soon as they were gathered. They were cooked in three ways: (1) They were boiled, split open, and eaten like a vegetable; (2) roasted in the ashes; (3) boiled, mashed, and eaten with grease. They were said to be particularly good with duck broth". . .338. The inner bark of the bur and red oaks and the aspen were scraped and dried and equal parts of this mixed with equal parts of the root, bud and blossom of the balsam poplar. The root of the seneca snakeroot dried and powdered was added to the others in a ceremony described under that plant in the Woods section. One swallow was taken as a heart remedy. . .340. For lung trouble the root of the blackberry was made into a decoction with the inner bark of the bur oak and drunk. . .344. A decoction of the root of the bur oak drunk for cramps. . .356. The fresh root of *Quercus*, species doubtful, was chewed and applied to a wound or a poultice made of the dried root. "For a fresh wound, let it bleed a little before applying poultice". . .370. Formulae for dyes; red dye; white birch, red osier dogwood and oak bark boiled in hot water. [see under dogwood]. . .372. Black dye; alder, red osier dogwood and oak barks boiled; bur oak, butternut and green-burs of hazel boiled. . .378. Awls were made of oak.

1928 Parker SENECA 11. As an astringent. . .oak bark.

1923 H. Smith MENOMINI 36. "The bark of the black oak is crushed and boiled to furnish a watery infusion to cure sore eyes. The inner bark of the white oak is also used in compounds, possibly because of its bitter tannic acid content. . .66. Any kind of acorns that were available were eaten in aboriginal times. The hulls were flailed off after parching, and the acorn was boiled till almost cooked. The water was then thrown away. Then to fresh water, two cups of wood ashes were added. The acorns were put into a net and were pulled out of the water after boiling in this. The third time they are simmered to clear them of lye water. Then they are ground into meal with a mortar and pestle, then sifted in a birch-bark sifter. The fourth time the meal is cooked in soup stock of deer meat until finished and ready to eat, or made into mush with bear oil seasoning. The old Indians never made pie, but the Menomini now make pie of them. . .The northern pin oak (Hill's oak) acorns were roasted and ground for coffee. The hulls were removed by flailing."

1928 H. Smith MESKWAKI 221. "White oak. . .The inner bark is boiled and the tea drunk to cause the patient to throw up phlegm from the lungs when they are bound up in the chest. Specimen 3602 of the Dr. Jones collection. . .mixture of the bark of the white oak, flowers of prairie clover and root of *Geranium maculataum*. . .used by one ill with the diarrhea. . .Bur oak used in a mixture with the berries of staghorn sumac and the root of *Euphorbia corollata* to expel pinworms. Both wood and inner bark of the Bur Oak are used. Black oak. The inner bark of this species is mixed with other roots for use in treating lung troubles. . .257. White oak. The acorn of this oak is made into a meal and the mush eaten like cornmeal mush. . .They also made a drink of the ground scorched acorns similar to coffee."

1932 H. Smith OJIBWE 369. "Bur oak. The bark is an astringent medicine to the Pillager Ojibwe. They also use it to bandage a broken foot or leg. . .The Red oak. The bark is a medicine for heart troubles and bronchial affections among the Flambeau Ojibwe. . .401-2. All Ojibwe we encountered told of their former dependence upon acorns for their soup stock. It seems that at least every Algonkian tribe knew and used all species of acorns. . .ground to a coarse mush. . .Blueberries were often cooked with this mush to give it a good flavor and it was seasoned with maple sugar. . .Red oak was so abundant in the Ojibwe territory and so large in size, the acorns were one of their most important starchy foods. They leached the tannic acid flavor with lye and brought them to a par with the sweet acorns of white oak. Black oak. . .Its acorns were equally good as other when the tannin was extracted."

1933 H. Smith POTAWATOMI 58. Red oak. "The Potawatomi used the inner bark as an astringent medicine to cure the flux. . .100. The Forest Potawatomi use all kinds of acorns indiscriminately for their starchy content, as a sort of breadstuff. . .120. Use the leaves of the red oak to furnish a design for their beadwork. Their rushes, which are gathered for mat weaving, are boiled with red oak bark to impart a brownish red dye."

1945 Rousseau MOHAWK transl. 38. "For ruptures caused by violent efforts drink an infusion of the barks of the oak and the white elm."

1955 Mockle Quebec transl. 35. "White oak, the bark astringent and febrifuge. It contains tannin and quercetol."

1958 Aller 70. "Just how important a food was the acorn? [to the Hurons]. . .As discussed, even fairly successful agricultural tribes needed to rely upon the acorn at times. Another interesting fact is that the acorn was used out of what is usually considered the oak belt." [Oaks grew in Huronia from Champlain's time to to-day]

1964 Yarnell 144. "Acorns may have been more important in prehistoric than in historic times in areas where they were rather abundant [for food]."

Unleached acorn flour contains 25.31% fat; 5.44% protein; 59.62% carbohydrates (According to the U.S. Food Administration; cited by Charles Ben Harris 1973:67)

1968 Forsyth England 81-2. "The poisonous quality of oak leaves and acorns for cattle and sheep have been recognized from the earliest times. . .Once they have been eaten by them. . .they acquire a craving for them. . .It is undetermined whether tannic acid alone is responsible for poisoning cattle, or whether there are other unknown substances which may cause some of the symptoms."

1968 Adrosko 33. Black oak. "Dr. Edward Bancroft, who returned from a journey to America [1780's]. . .had learned that black-oak bark yielded an excellent yellow-dye stuff (he named it quercitrin) that he believed could become a cheap substitute for weld. . . . Only after it was introduced to Europe, however, did this indigenous American dystuff take its place among the important vegetable dyes. It remained in commercial use until the second quarter of the 20th. century."

1974 McAndrews and Boyko Crawford Lake site 1380 8. "Before the Iroquoians migrated into the Crawford Lake area the forest surrounding the lake consisted mainly of beech and maple with some oak, elm and birch. . .The pollen diagram. . .indicates that white pine and oak succeeded beech and maple on abandoned Indian fields."

1976 Antoine King Go-Home Lake Huron personal communication. A white oak 3 feet in diameter was cut in the winter by his son on Big Island. When he was lumbering the oak had to be ringed of bark and left to die, so that when it was felled it would float. If this was not done, the oaks could not be held in log booms and towed down the coast to Midland and Penetang to the lumber mills. One result was that many large oaks were not taken at all in lumbering operations.

Personal observation of the author; the red and white oak are common trees in the Go-Home Bay area of the Georgian Bay, Lake Huron, which is well north of the area the Hurons occupied in the first half of the seventeenth century. They reach a good size and bear quantities of acorns. The Bur oak grows to be a big tree at Lake Simcoe.

1977 Varma et al Science 205. "The onset of cataract [in lens of diabetic animals] is effectively delayed when quercitrin is continously administered."

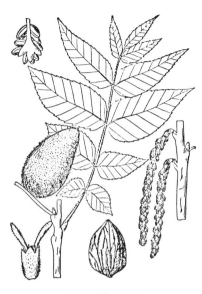

BUTTERNUT

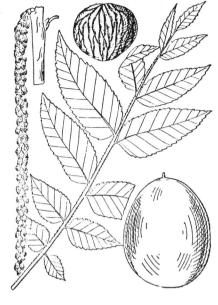

BLACK WALNUT

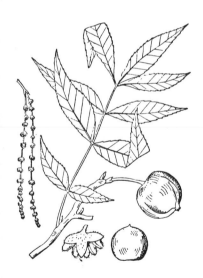

BITTERNUT HICKORY

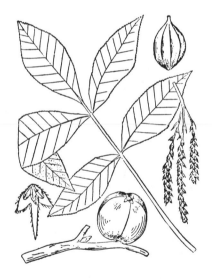

SHAGBARK HICKORY

WALNUTS AND HICKORIES

The native walnuts can be told apart from the native hickories by their nuts whose outer husks do not split apart when mature; their twigs whose pith is divided into chambers with a space between them; and their having leaves with eleven or more leaflets.

BLACK WALNUT   *Juglans nigra* L. Juglandaceae
A medium sized tree up to 40 m with almost black roughly ridged bark when old. Each leaf usually has between 15-23 leaflets. The nuts are in a round, hairy surfaced husk. The surface of the nut is deeply grooved. In the shade of large walnut trees, walnut seedlings and other plants grow poorly probably because of toxic substances produced in the soil by the roots and leaf mould. It is said vegetables will not thrive where there are black walnut roots.
Range. w. Mass., s. Ont. to Minn., s. to Tex. and Fla. in rich moist soil.

BUTTERNUT   WHITE WALNUT   *Juglans cinerea* L.
Small tree to 30 m with ash-gray bark, becoming separated into smooth ridges. Leaves composed of 11 to 17 leaflets. The nut in a sticky hairy husk. The pointed nut longer than thick, very rough, with 2-4 obscure ridges.
Range. N.B., s. Que., s. Ont. to N.D., s. to Ark. and Ga. in rich moist soil but also in dry rocky soil.

BITTERNUT HICKORY   *Carya cordiformis* (Wang.) K. Koch (*Hicoria c., Juglans c.*)
A tall slender tree, the tight-fitting bark smooth until mature then splitting into shallow crevices. Leaves with 7-11 leaflets. The winter buds bright orange. The outer husk of the nuts splits partly towards the middle exposing a thin shelled nut with four wings at its top, flattened, and with a very bitter kernel. The wood of this hickory gives the best flavor to smoked hams and bacon.
Range. N.H., sw Que., s. Ont. (n. to Carleton and Prescott counties), Mich., Minn., se Nebr., s. to Tex. and Fla. in wet or dry woods, streambanks, swamps. Hybridizes with other hickories.

SHAGBARK HICKORY   *Carya ovata* (Mill.) K. Koch (*Hicoria o., Juglans o., Carya alba*)
A tall, slender, straight tree when mature with shaggy bark, in long strips, free at both ends. Leaves with usually 5 leaflets, the end one a third to a half as wide as long. The outer husk thick, woody, splitting to the bottom when the fruit is ripe. The nut has prominent ridges, is sweet and edible.
Range. s. Me., sw Que., s. Ont. (n. to Carleton and Russel co.), Minn., se. Nebr., s. to Tex. and Fla. in rich moist soil.
Common names. Walnut, sweet or white walnut, king-nut, upland or white hickory, red-heart hickory, shell-bark hickory.
2000-1000 B.C. Feeheley site Mich. Butternuts found archeologically at 10 locations, some sp. of hickory at 3 loc. as well as at Frontenac Isl. N.Y. site. along with butternut. Walnut found at Feeheley site. Yarnell 1964.
1000-300 B.C. Some sp. of hickory nut found archeologically at 6 sites in Ohio and one in N.Y. Walnut found in one Ohio site. Yarnell 1964.
300 B.C.-500 A.D. McGraw site Ohio walnut and a sp. of hickory nut found. Muntz Pa. walnut, butternut and hickory found. Spoonville Mich. walnut and butternut found. Schultz Mich. walnut found. Yarnell 1964.
500-1500 A.D. Dutton Ont. butternut and hickory found. Lawson, Roebuck, and Aylmer Ont. butternut found. Sidey-Mackay Ont. walnut and butternut found. Hickory found at 6 N.Y. sites, butternut at 6 and walnut at one. Walnut found at 6 Ohio sites, butternut at 6 and hickory at 10. Walnut at 4 Mich. sites, butternut at 2 and hickory at 4 (Yarnell 1964:23-25).
1380 Crawford Lake site Ont. McAndrews, Byrne and Finlayson 1974 5. "Nut fragments were present in 36% of the features. Three species were found in roughly equal proportions, bitternut hickory, butternut and beech. No acorns were found. . .Bitternut has the widest distribution, occurring in 13.5% of the 78 features sampled. To-day bitternut is the commonest of the nut producers around Crawford Lake and is present throughout the area. . .Butternut was present in 8.9% of the samples."
1590 Harriot Virginia 9. "There are two sortes of Walnuttes both holding oyle, but the one are more plentifull than the other. When there are milles & other devices for the purpose, a commodity of them may be raised because there are infinite store. . .18. In many places where there are very great woods for many miles together, the third part of trees are walnut trees. The one kind is of the same taste and forme or litle differing from ours of England, but they are harder

and thicker shelled: the other is greater and a verie ragged and harde shell: but the kernel great, very oylie and sweete. Besides their [Indians] eating of them after our ordinarie maner, they breake them with stones and pound them in mortars with water to make a milk which they use to put into some sorts of their spoonmeate; also among their sodde wheat, peaze, beanes and pompions which maketh them have a farre more pleasant taste. . .22. Walnut trees, as I have said before very many, some have been seen excellent faire timber of foure & five fathome, & above fourscore foot streight without bough."

1604 Champlain-Purchas near the Richlieu river. "Small islands. . .which are full of Walnut-trees, which are not much different from ours; and I thinke their Walnuts are good when they bee ripe: I saw many of them under the trees, which were of two sorts, the one small, and the other as long as a mans Thumbe, but they were rotten."

1613 Champlain fac. ed. Saco River, New Engl. 1605 transl. 68. "We saw their wheat [corn]. . .They sow 4 or 5 seeds in one spot after which they place around it with the shells of the horseshoe crab a quantity of earth: then farther on they sow more. . .Amongst this corn at each mound they plant 3 or 4 Brazil beans, which come in various colors. When they are full grown they train them around the corn which grows to a height of 5 or 6 feet: and they keep the fields clear of bad weeds. . .We saw a great quantity of nuts, that were small and had several sections. There weren't any on the trees, but we found enough underneath of the year before." [Cultivated by the Indians as their corn, beans, squash and tobacco was?]. . .176. 1608. "From the Island of Orleans to Quebec, it is a league. . .I was looking for the best place for our habitation, but I couldnt find any more suitable, or better situated than the point of Quebec, called this by the savages, it was covered with nut trees."

1609 Lescarbot-Erondelle Acadia 297. "For the most part of the woods of this land be oaks and walnut-trees, bearing small nuts with four or five sides, so sweet and delicate as any thing may be."

1609 Juet Hudson river 23-4. "We went on Land (Athens?) to walke on the West side of the River, and found good ground for Corne and other Garden herbs, with great store of goodly Oakes, and Wal-nut trees."

1611 Champlain-Bourne (Mont Royal) 1632 234-5. "And near this Place Royale there is a little river running back a good way into the interior, all along which there are more than sixty acres of cleared land like meadows, where one might sow grain and make gardens. Formerly savages tilled there, but they abandoned them on account of the usual wars that they had there. There are also a number of other beautiful meadows. . .with a great many walnuts."

1612 Capt. John Smith Virginia Indians 102. "In May and June they plant their fields, and live mostly of Acornes, walnuts, and fish."

1619 Champlain-Macklem HURONIA 1615 40-41. "The soil is good and the savages grow a great deal of Indian corn. . .Sunflowers they grow for their seeds, from which they extract an oil used in anointing their heads. They also grow grapes and plums, raspberries, strawberries, crab-apples and nuts. . .[Canoe route from Sturgeon Lake to Lake Ontario] These lakes, as well as the river which flows from one to the other, abound in fish, and the whole country is very beautiful and attractive. Along the river bank it seemed as if the trees had been planted there in most places for pleasure, and also as if all these regions had once been inhabited by savages who since had been obliged to abandon them for fear of their enemies. The vines and walnuts are very plentiful."

1635 Journey into the MOHAWK country from the New Neth. 155. "Upward of one hundred people came out to welcome me, and showed me a house where I could go. They gave me a white hare to eat that they caught two days ago. They cooked it with walnuts, and gave me a piece of wheaten bread a savage that had arrived here from Fort Orange on the fifteenth of the month had brought with him."

1642 De Vries New Neth. 219. "They [Indians] dry the nuts of trees and use them for food."

1650 Representation New Neth. 295. "It also yields several species of nut wood, such as oil-nuts, large and small; walnuts of different sizes in great abundance, and good for fuel, for which it is much used."

1663 Boucher Quebec transl. 46-7. "There are nut trees of two kinds, which bear nuts: The one kind bears large and hard nuts but the wood of the tree is very tender, & and is never used, except to make sabots, for which it is good: of this kind there are lots growing near Quebec and at Three Rivers: but not many going further up; the other kind of nut trees bear small round nuts with a tender shell like those of France; but the wood is very hard, and red in the middle:

one begins to find them at Mont-Royal, & there are a quantity in the country of the Iroquois. The Savages use them to make an oil, which is excellent."

1698 Hennepin Long Point Lake Erie 109. "The Forests are chiefly made up of Walnut-trees. . .643 [Fox-Wisconsin portage] The River called the [Wisconsin] Mesconsin. The country through which it flows is very fine; The Groves disposed at certain Distances in the Meadows, make a noble Prospect. . .Those Groves are full of Walnut-Trees, as also of Oaks."

1708 Sarrazin-Vaillant, Quebec-Paris, Boivin 1978 transl. 107. "It grows on the Islands. . .This nut is the most common one in Canada. The husk of its fruit is rough and extremely thick. Its shell is so hard that one cannot crack it except by the blows of a hammer and it is deeply chanelled. . .This nut is good to eat fresh and if one takes care it can be kept. There is in Canada a kind of nut tree that without snow gives a kind of thick juice like a sugary sirup, but only in small quantity." [Butternut, according to Boivin 1978.]

1748 Kalm Philadelphia October 14th. 104. "Tanning bark. Woolen and linen cloth is dyed yellow with the bark of hickory". . .1749 27th. March 269. "The Indians. . .likewise prepared a kind of liquor like milk by gathering a great number of hickory and black walnuts, they dried and crushed them. Then they took out the kernels, pounded them as fine as flour, and mixed this with water so that it looked like milk and was almost as sweet. . .June 28th. 363. The boats here were commonly made of the white bark. With the bark of hickory, which was employed as bast, they sewed the elm bark together, and with the bark of the red elm they joined the ends of the boats so close as to keep the water out. . .Aug. 11th. Nunnery some distance from Quebec. . .The dishes were all prepared by the nuns. . .white Canadian walnuts coated with sugar, pears and apples in syrup, apples preserved in spirits of wine, small sugared lemons from the West Indies, strawberry preserves and angelica roots. . .September 26th. The Indians. . .make a delicious meal of several kinds of walnuts, chestnuts, mulberries. . .Dec. 12th. The joiners say that among the trees of this country they use chiefly the black walnut, the wild cherry, and the curled maple. Of the black walnut. . .there is yet a sufficient quantity, but careless people are trying to destroy it, and some peasants even use it as fuel. . . .The cogs of the mill wheel and the pullies were made of the white walnut because it was said to be the hardest which could be found here."

1778 Carver 500-02. "Butternut or Oilnut. . .The inside bark of this tree dyes a good purple; and it is said, varies in its shade, being either darker or lighter according to the month in which it is gathered. . .The Pecan nut. . .This tree grows chiefly near the Illinois river. The Hickory. . .being of a very tough nature, the wood is generally used for the handles of axes. It is also very good fire wood and as it burns an excellent sugar distills from it."

1779 Zeisberger DELAWARE 46. "Of nuts there are found. . .the hickory nut found in great plenty in some years and which the Indians gather in large quantities and use not only as they find them—they have a very sweet taste—but also extract from them a milky juice used in different foods and very nourishing. Sometimes they extract an oil by first roasting the nut in the shell under hot ashes and pounding them to a fine mash, which they boil in water. The oil swimming on the surface is skimmed off and preserved for cooking and other purposes. The walnut of two varieties, the white walnuts. . .the black walnut of which the wood is dark brown, sometimes even shading to violet. . .Very much used by cabinet makers for tables, chests and other things. . .148. For headache they lay a piece of white walnut bark on the temples, toothache is treated by placing the same kind of bark on the cheek over the tooth that gives the trouble. The bark is very heating and burns the skin in a short time, often affording relief. The same bark is applied to any of the limbs that may be afflicted, having the effect at times of driving the pain from one part of the body to another, until there is an eruption somewhere. This bark pounded fine and boiled to the consistency of a strong lye, stops the flow of blood, when applied to a fresh wound, even though an artery may have been ruptured, it prevents swelling and heals the wound rapidly. After this solution has been used for one or two days other roots must be applied, such as the great sarsaparilla and others that have healing powers." [See Spikenard in section on Woods]

1817-1820 Bigelow 118-9. "The sap of the Butternut tree is saccharine, like that of the Maple, and may be procured in large quantities. In the third volume of the Massachusetts Agricultural Repository is an account of an experiment made on this tree by Mr. M.P. Gray. He states that four trees, the trunks of which were only from eight to ten inches in diameter, produced in one day nine quarts of sap, from which was made one pound and a quarter of sugar. . .equal if not superior to that which the maple affords in the same vicinity. The inner bark of this tree, especially that obtained from the root, affords one of the most mild and efficacious laxatives which we possess. It is commonly employed in the form of an extract, which preparation is kept in our druggists' shops. . .During the revolutionary war, when foreign medicines were scarce, this extract was resorted to by many of the army surgeons. . .A patent medicine, long vended in this State under the name of Chamberlain's Bilious Cordial, was a tincture of this bark imbued with various aromatic seeds. The bark is said to be rubefacient when externally applied and even capable of exciting a blister." [See below, 1868 Shakers]

1830 Rafinesque 228. "Hickory tree. Very useful. Good heavy wood, best for fuel. Leaves sweet scented, nervine. Vernal sap sweetish and acid, producing syrup, sugar and beer like Maples. Tendrils of the young roots edible, eaten by Indians when hungry. They made milk, oil and many dishes with the nuts. As good as walnuts, sweeter; some have hard shells, the best. . .The pignut hickories. . .have bitter nuts, their bark is styptic. The inner bark of some is cathartic. . .*Juglans* 233 All valuable trees producing the fine timber, sugar, nuts, oil, medicines &c. *J. nigra*, black walnut, has the finest wood, hard and brown, bark and rind of nuts dye wool brown boiled alone, and black with vitriol. Leaves scented, said to shelter from thunder. Vernal sap sweet, may give sugar. Young green nuts pickled in vinegar, styptic, unwholesome. The green rind rubbed on tetters and ringworm dispels them; their decoction vermifuge and sudorific, also antisyphilitic. Nuts very oily, flatulent; the oil fit for painters and lamps, it is said to expel worms and even tape worms taken with sugar. . .Butternut. . .Fresh outerbark. . .the lint of it used to dress the bites of snakes. Inner bark bitterish, styptic, purgative, that of the root stronger. The pills and extract. . .much used. . .in colds, coughs, hemorrhage in small pills. . .Employed to cure the murrain of cattle and yellow water of horses. The extract ought to be made in the spring, and with care. The nuts are very oily, but pretty good when fresh: the rind and husks dye brown: often pickled when green."

1833 Howard Quebec 22. "To cure a convulsive cough eat preserved Walnuts. . .121. To cure an Ulcer dry and powder a walnut leaf and strew it on and lay another walnut leaf on that or boil walnut leaves in water with a little sugar. Apply a cloth dipt in this—changing it once in two days. This has done Wonders. Foment morning and evenings with a Decoction of walnut leaves and bind the leaves on. This has cured Foul Bones and even the Leprosy."

1840 Gosse Quebec 316. Butternut. "The nut is not in its best condition until it has lain some time to dry, and the frosts of winter have matured it. Then its taste is agreeable; but its shell is hard to break. . .It is best cracked by holding it perpendicularly on a stone, then striking the base with a hammer, when the shell generally flies in pieces without crushing the seed."

1859-61 Gunn 750. "Butternut. . .The way to use it is to boil down a lot of the bark, and reduce it to a thick soft extract, and then make it into pills for use, by mixing, if necessary, a little of any kind of powder. . .even flour will do. Dose, as a purgative, three or four ordinary sized pills; as a laxative. . .one or two pills a day. It is one of the safest and best purgative medicines known. . .762. [Black Walnut] The medical properties of this tree are not very generally known. . .The green leaves and also the green fruit or nut, are the parts used. An infusion or strong sirup of the green leaves is highly recommended as an important remedy in all cases of scrofula. . .Infusing a moderate sized handful, bruised; in a pint of boiling water, allowing them to steep or simmer, awhile, then strain and sweeten with white sugar. . .A grown person should take about one third of this quantity during each day. . .It is said never to cause any unpleasant symptoms. . .no visible effect may be noticed for twenty days. . .It augments the activity of the circulation and digestion and imparts much energy to the functions. It is supposed to act upon the lymphatic system, as under its influence the muscles become firm and the skin acquires a rudier hue. . .A salve made of a strong extract of the leaves mixed with some clean lard and a few drops of the oil of Bergamot, is most excellent for old sores. A strong decoction of the leaves is excellent for washing them. . .A saturated or strong tincture of the green walnuts, is highly recommended by some physicians in the treatment of cramp, or bilious colic. The tincture may be made by slicing the walnuts when green, or before they become much hardened, and adding enough whiskey or dilute alcohol to barely cover them. . .let stand to digest a week or two. . .dose of a teaspoonful or two every half-hour, till relief is obtained. This tincture is also an excellent remedy as an application for ringworm and tetter."

1868 Can. Pharm J. 1; 27. "New Lebanon Shakers by R.W. Elliot. . .We inspected a very complete apparatus for preparing extracts in vacuo. . .the common extracts are made by boiling the crude substance in water, pressing and straining until the whole extractive matter is contained in the liquid portion, which is then boiled down to the proper consistence in iron or copper pans over a fire. Noticing a large pile of spent butternut bark, I was informed that many thousands of pounds of the extract was annually made, Herrick, of Albany, being the largest consumer, in the manufacture of his patent pill."

1868 Can. Pharm. J. 6; 83-5. The bark of the butternut included in list of Can. medicinal plants.

1880 Can. Horticulturist 116-7. "Mr. Beall stated that at Lindsay. . .Butternut was used in the commoner kind of cabinetware, and brought from $10 to $14 per thousand. . .Black walnut was not indigenous about Lindsay, and probably on that account commanded a high price, running from $100 to $120 per thousand. . .1881 49-53. Mr. Bucke read a paper on nut-bearing trees. Can any of our native nut bearing trees be profitably cultivated either for nuts or timber, and where is the northern limit of each? The above question has been put into the hands of every member of the Fruit Growers Association. . .a subject which is awakening a deep interest, not only in Ontario, but in all parts of the Dominion, where the denudation of both the public and private domain is being carried on to an alarming extent. . .We. . .who once had, and are losing our forests. . .The butternut has the most northern limit, which is found to begin at the southern end of Nova Scotia, running north it passes about midway through New Brunswick, crossing the St. Lawrence River at Quebec and extending some thirty miles to the north of the city of Ottawa, and from thence strikes the southern end of the Georgian Bay. . .Every autumn the nuts are sold by the two bushel bag on the Ottawa market. . .With regard to the cultivation of this tree, I speak from practical experience when I state it is one of the very easiest to grow. . .it will produce nuts after ten years planting, and I believe a good saleable tree may be had of 18 inches through, at from twenty-five to thirty years from the nut. . .The bark is also used by farmers' wives for imparting a rich brown to their home-spun yarn, before it is manufactured into stockings or woven into fabrics. . .The black walnut. . .the wood is much more valuable, and its crotches and roots are greatly sought after for cabinet work, gun stock, etc.. . .This tree is only indigenous to a small area, extending from a point near Port Franks, on Lake Huron, running north of London nearly. . .to Toronto, and extending along the Lake shore as far east as Coburg. I am satisfied however these limits could be considerably extended. . .Hickory, The shell bark variety finds its chief home in the woods of the county of Lambton and West Middlesex. The tree is not easily cultivated, as it is a slow grower and difficult of transplantation, but its wood is so valuable where its toughness and elasticity are required that it commands a high price. It is principally used for tool handles, carriage spokes and fellies. . .This tree is usually cut. . .when from four to six inches through at the butt, and consequently could be advantageously grown in plantations between trees used at a more mature age. . .The nut deprived of its shell may be obtained from all itinerant newsboys on boats or cars, as no doubt my hearers can willingly testify. . .Before the white man invaded this continent all the nuts alluded to were used by the North American Indians as an article of diet, and ancient records testify that the quantity consumed at one meal was incredible, and certainly would be unsafe for more civilized stomaches. . .My friend Chief Johnson can supply any amount of either black walnuts or butternuts. . .Chief Johnson said that His Excellency. . .Governor General of Canada had obtained nuts of the black walnut from him to send to Scotland and Hyde Park, England."

1885 Hoffman OJIBWA 199. "Black walnut. Walnuts are highly prized; the green rind of the unripe fruit is sometimes employed in staining or dyeing."

1905 Muldrew 58-9. "Butternut. In Muskoka its northern limits appear to be near the Severn River, where it is very abundant. The large leaves are quite downy, and, like the bark, are fragrant. . .*Carya alba* Shell bark hickory, shag bark, white hickory. I had quite decided from search and inquiry that the Hickories were unknown in Muskoka, when I was handed recently for identification a number of nuts taken from the hollow in a stick of firewood which had been cut within a few miles of Gravenhurst. They evidently belonged to this species, having been discovered and appropriated by that very industrious botanist, the Red Squirrel. I have not yet had an opportunity to determine whether the latter acquired them by honest means."

1915 W.R. Harris 51. "In cases of colic they chewed the rinds or hulls of the black walnut (he-ne-ska)."

1916 Waugh IROQUOIS 123-4. The shell bark hickory, bitternut hickory, walnut and butternut were eaten. "A Cayuga informant stated that the older people used to crush the meats of the hickory, walnut, butternut and chestnut, and mix them with the cornmeal for bread. . .The meats of the hickory, walnut and several others, were pounded, boiled slowly in water, and the oil skimmed off into a bowl. The oil was boiled again and seasoned with salt. This was used with bread, potatoes, pumpkin, squash, and other foods. Nut-meat oil was often added to the mush used by the False-face Societies. The oil was also formerly used (like sunflower oil) for the hair, either alone or mixed with bear's grease. Lafitau remarks that the mixture was used as a preventive of mosquitoes. The meats left after skimming off the oil were often seasoned and mixed with mashed potatoes. Nut-meats were also crushed and added to hominy and corn soup to make it rich. This was described by several informants. . .27. A method for rain-making given by Barber Black, of Tonawanda, was to take a little piece of the bark of a walnut tree where it has been struck by lightening. When the weather is too dry, place this in a cup of water, and leave for a couple of minutes. It will then rain in two days. . .80. Formerly the kernels of walnuts and butternuts were added to boiled corn bread. . .146. Hickory nuts, still plentiful throughout the Iroquois country, formed the basis of a savory beverage. Loskiel observes that 'the Indians gather a great quantity of sweet hickory nuts, which grow in great plenty in some years, and not only eat them raw, but extract a milky juice from them, which tastes well and is nourishing'."

1926-7 Densmore CHIPPEWA 338. *Hicoria alba*, shagbark hickory. The very small shoots that grow beside the leaves gathered fresh and placed on hot stones and the fumes inhaled for convulsions. . .372. Black dye formula, boil together the inner bark of butternut and hazel. . .the inner bark of the bur oak and butternut with a little of the root of the latter, after boiling a little while put in black earth and ocre. The more it is 'boiled down' the blacker will be the dye. . .Butternut inner bark and grindstone dust boiled alone. . .377. Bows were made of the shagbark hickory.

1923 H. Smith MENOMINI 38. "The sap of the butternut is used by the Menomini in the same manner as maple sap, but with the difference that the syrup and sugar from the butternut are a standard Indian physic. . .78. The juice of the husk of this nut was formerly used to dye the Menomini deerskin shirts brown. Butternut bark is used to obtain their black color. . .For a deep black color, the bark is boiled with blue clay."

1928 H. Smith MESKWAKI 196. Hulls of Black walnut one of eight ingredients of a pile medicine. "Cultivated at Tama. . .225. The inner bark of the black walnut is known to be a very strong physic, but it is not used unless imperative, for the Indians have many physics. Specimen 5127 of the Dr. Jones collection is the twig bark and old bark of *Juglans nigra*. . .It is coiled, charred and applied in water for a snake bite. . .Twig bark of the butternut is boiled and drunk as a cathartic, also the wood bark. . .Bitternut hickory, the bark tea of this species yields a beverage for simple sicknesses. It makes the bowels loose and the urine free. . .259. Shellbark hickory gathered and stored for the winter food supply as also the butternut. The black walnut is not so common around Tama and it seems to be there only because it has been planted. . .271. The wood and bark of the black walnut is charred by the Meskwaki to make it give up its best black dye."

1932 H. Smith OJIBWE 405. "Butternut is plentiful in the north and in most Ojibwe territory, while the black walnut is not to be found. They use the nuts for food and the hulls for dye. Hickory trees are scarce in the north, but the Ojibwe appreciate the edible nuts. . .419. The Flambeau Ojibwe use the wood of the Shellbark hickory for making bows. Some are quite particular about the piece of wood they select, choosing a billet from the tree that includes heart wood on one side and sap wood on the other. The heart wood is the front of the bow in use, while the sap wood is nearest the user. It is likewise a wood of general utility. . .425. Butternut. The Ojibwe find this one of their best brown dyes, because they can get from the tree at any time of the year. It is usually used in combinations for brown and black colors."

1933 H. Smith POTAWATOMI 60. Butternut. "The Potawatomi use this bark as a physic and drink infusions of the inner bark for its tonic effect. . .113. Shellbark hickory. The Forest Potawatomi use this strong and elastic wood to make their bows and arrows. Such bows and arrows are still used by their children."

1935 Jenness OJIBWA Parry Island Lake Huron 103. "The weapons of the Lake Huron Ojibwa. . .were the bow and arrow, a knife, a war-club. . .The knobbed club was generally made of hickory, and fitted occasionally with a stone point secured in a socket with pitch."

1945 Rousseau MOHAWK transl. 39. "*Carya cordiformis*, Bitternut hickory. The bark used to make the seats and backs of chairs."

1955 Mockle Quebec transl. 33. "Butternut. The inner bark is purgative and cathartic; it is also used in dysentery, inflammations and ophthalmia. The twigs, leaves and nuts contain juglone. . .Black walnut. The oil of the nut is used as a vermifuge and antisyphilitic. The nut is edible. The plant also contains juglone."

1964 Tooker IROQUOIS 23 ftnt. "During this period [1615-49] the Iroquois made their canoes of the bark of the red or slippery elm or of butternut hickory. The Iroquois were forced to use these inferior materials as birch trees did not grow in their country."

1973 Hosie 142. "Like other hickories, this tree takes up to 200 years to reach maturity. . .Tool handles made of hickory can be identified by their bell-like tone when dropped on end on a hard surface."

The black walnut contains juglone which is active against dermatomycosis. Lewis and Elvin-Lewis 1977:363).

The Norther Nut Growers Association was formed in 1910. Since that time they have greatly increased the numbers of indigenous nut trees, and introduced many hybrid and foreign nut trees to the northern areas of America. Lately they have been carrying out exploratory work seeking to adapt the Pecan to more northern locations. They believe that the species, *Carya illinoensis*, was distributed from its original home in the south throughout the northern part of the continent by the Indians who carried the pecans with them on their canoe trips and deliberately planted the biggest and thinnest shelled nuts at the main portages. As well the nuts were traded by the southern tribes to the northern in exchange for furs. Douglas Campell, Niagara on the Lake, and John Gordon, North Tonawanda N.Y., have found a few scattered trees of native pecans as far north as southern Wisconsin. (Society of Ontario Nut Growers News, Fall 1978.)

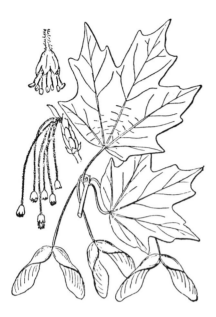

SUGAR MAPLE

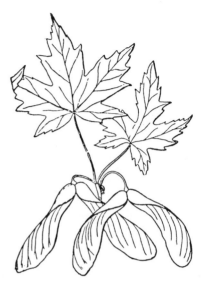

SILVER MAPLE

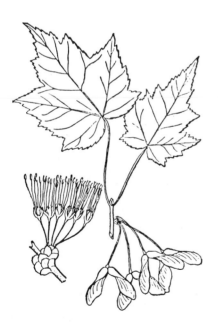

RED MAPLE

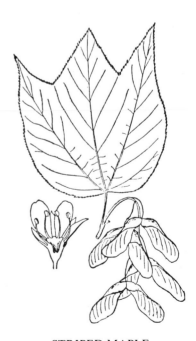

STRIPED MAPLE

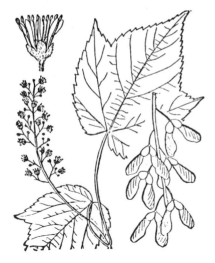

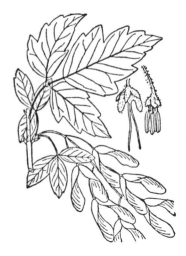

MOUNTAIN MAPLE

BOX ELDER

SUGAR MAPLE   *Acer saccharum* Marsh. Aceraceae
Tree to 40 m with dark gray bark, not conspicuously furrowed. The flat leaves have 3 to 5 lobes, the line from the tip of one lobe to the next is a rounded curve, they are about as wide as long. Flowers droop on slender stalks.
Range. N.B., P.E.I., N.S., s. Que., w. Ont. s. to Tex., Ark., and Ga. in rich rocky or hilly woods. Planted elsewhere.
Common names. Hard maple.

SILVER MAPLE   *Acer sacharinum* L. (*A. dasycarpum, A. eriocarpum*)
Tree to 30 m with light gray bark separating in large scales. The leaves have deep, sharply angled cuts between their lobes, the centre lobe being well over half the length of the leaf. If bent over at its much narrowed base its tip will be on the leaf stalk. The fruit is sparsely hairy.
Range. N.B., Que., s. Ont. to Minn., s. to S. Dak., Okla., Tenn. and Fla. planted eastward and westwards and occasionally escaped. In bottomlands, along streams.
Common names. Soft maple, river maple, white maple.

RED MAPLE   *Acer rubrum* L.
Tree to 35 m with reddish twigs. The leaves with sharply angled cuts between their lobes, the centre lobe broadest at its base and at most only slightly more than half as long as the whole leaf. The flowers red, appearing much before the opening of the leaf buds.
Range. Nfld., N.B., N.S., P.E.I., Que., Ont., s. to Tex. and Fla. in swamps, low ground, moist uplands.
Common names. Water maple, soft maple, swamp maple.

STRIPED MAPLE   *Acer pensylvanicum* L. (*A. striatum*)
Slender tree to 12 m with smooth green bark striped with longtitudinal darker bands. Very large leaves when young shaped like a goosefoot with three sharply pointed shallow lobes with 7-12 sharp teeth per cm around their edges. Flowers droop on their stalks.
Range. N.B., P.E.I., N.S., Que., Ont. to Mich., s. to Ohio, Tenn., and n. Ga. in rich cool woods or rocky woods.
Common names. Moosewood, northern maple, whistle-wood.

MOUNTAIN MAPLE *Acer spicatum* Lam. (*A. montanum*)
Shrub or small tree to 10 m often with a crooked trunk. The leaves on slender red stalks, have a sharp angle between their lobes and 2-3 teeth per cm on their edges. The pale yellowish-green flowers are on a spike that stands upright. They open during or after the unfolding of the leaves.
Range. s. Lab., Nfld., N.B., N.S., P.E.I., Que., Ont., Man., s. Sask., to Io., O., Tenn. and n. Ga. in damp, cool rocky woods.
Common names. Moose, swamp, water, low maple.

BOX ELDER *Acer negundo* L.
Tree to 20 m with light gray smooth bark when young becoming furrowed in narrow ridges in age. The leaves made up of 3-5 leaflets or may be as many as 9. Flowers appear before the leaves.
Range. Que., Ont., Man., Sask., Alta., s. to Mont., Ariz., N. Mex., Tex. and Fla. along rivers.
Common names. Manitoba maple, ash leaved maple, water ash, cut leaved maple. This tree is the source of maple syrup and sugar in the western part of Canada.
1557-58 Thevet Les singularitez transl. 427-9. "There are several trees and fruits which we do not know. Among these there is a tree the size and shape of our large nut trees, which has long been unused and without recognition, until someone wanted to cut it, when the sap poured out, which he found of such a fine and delicate taste, as good as the wine of Orleans, or of Beaune: our men agreed with his judgement when we tasted it: the Captain and the other gentlemen in his company were told, and 4 or 5 large pots of the sap were collected in an hour. I'll leave you to imagine if since then the Canadians [Indians], having tasted this liquor, do not think this a valuable tree because it is such an excellent beverage. This tree is called in their language, *Couton*." [Did Cartier tell Thevet this?]
1575 Thevet Cosmographie transl. 1014. "The country of Canada. . .has many trees. . .several plants and trees have been taken and planted in the Royal Garden at Fontainbleau where you can see them to-day. Among others there is one, which they call *Cotony*, which is the size of a great nut tree here." [Thevet then repeats here what he had written above in 1557-8].
1624 Sagard HURON 275. The women crush their corn in a mortar "made of a big tree trunk of maple or other hard wood, cut to measurements, two feet high, hollowed out little by little with charcoals or burning tinder which they keep on it until it is sufficiently wide and deep; they have sticks six to seven feet long and the thickness of an arm, which as pestles serve better than if they were shorter."
1634 LeJeune MONTAGNAIS Jes. Rel. 6; 272. "When great famine threatened them, they ate the shavings or bark of a certain tree which they called *Michtan*, which they cut in the Spring to draw a sap from it, as sweet as honey, or like sugar; at least that is what some told me, but they do not enjoy much of it so little flows from it." [This could also refer to the birch tree].
1663 Boucher Quebec transl. 44-5. "There is a kind of tree which is called Herable [maple], which grows big and tall; the wood is beautiful even if it is used for nothing except to burn or handles for tools for which it is very good, because it is extremely maleable and hard. When one cuts the maples in the Spring, there runs a quantity of water, which is tastier than water with sugar in it; at least more agreeable to drink."
1672 Nouvel OTTAWA Manatoulin Island Lake Huron J. Rel. 56; 101. "A liquor that runs from the trees towards the end of winter, and which is known as Maple-water, [is collected and drunk by the Indians]."
1684-5 Philos. Trans. Royal Soc. London 1. An Account of a sort of Sugar made of the Juice of the Maple in Canada. . ."The savages have practised this art longer than any now living among them can remember."
1691 LeClercq MICMAC 122. As to the water of the maple which is the sap of that same tree, it is equally delicious to French and Indians, who take their fill of it in the spring. It is true also that it is very pleasing and abundant in Gaspesia, for, through a very little opening which is made with an axe in a maple, ten to a dozen half gallons may run out. A thing which seemed to me very remarkable in the maple water is this, that when by virtue of boiling it is reduced to a third, it becomes a real syrup, which hardens to something like sugar, and takes on a reddish colour. It is formed into little loaves which are sent to France as a curiosity, and which in actual use serve very often as a substitute for French sugar."
1703 Lahontan 1; 366-7. "'Tis but few of the inhabitants that have the patience to make Maple-water. . .so there's scarcely anybody but Children that give themselves the trouble of

gathering these trees". . .1; 169-70 POTAWATOMI. Lahontan attended a feast consisting of four courses. The first was whitefish boiled in water; the second the boiled tongue and breast of a deer, the third two woodhens, the hind feet of a bear, and the tail of a beaver; the fourth a large quantity of broth made of several sorts of meat. For drink he had maple syrup beaten up with water.

1708 Sarrazin-Vaillant, Quebec-Paris, Boivin 1978 transl. 213. "This tree furnishes a great quantity of sugar, which commences to rise from the first days of April and continues until about the 15th May. The north Americans, Indians as well as French, knew that this sap was sugary. They have done and do every year evaporate the sap until it becomes sugar. To do this they make an opening in the trunk of the tree, and do it in such a manner that the sap that runs from that hole falls into a bucket ready to receive it. What is very remarkable is that one of these trees about 2 or 3 feet in circumferance gives, without losing its strength, up to 60-80 pounds (livres) of water in the spring, which will produce about 3 or 4 pounds (livres) of sugar. It is only those who are impatient, who make several holes to take more sap, who shorten the life of the tree. Those who have them growing near their houses, and who keep them just for the water to drink in the spring, only make one hole which they renew each year by cutting out the part that had been dried up by the air that closed the pores. There are others whose sap does not produce very much, finally there are those that are not constant in their production. For a maple to produce sap that will sugar, experience has amply proven that there must be snow at its base. That is why maples in warm countries or cold ones where the wind blows no snow, don't produce any. The reason why some maples don't produce very much, depends on three principal causes, which are, that they have too little snow at their feet, that is to say spread over the earth that covers their roots, or that they are not well exposed to the sun, and thirdly, which seems really extraordinary, that the spring is too warm and it does not freeze at night. This third cause why a maple does not always give a sap that produces the same amount of sugar is when the melting snow turns into a pool at the foot of the tree. This is so true that one must drain off the water and bring in snow to cover the roots, because the sap of those that do not have any is good only to nourish the tree. It is necessary that the snow be melted by the sun, because snow that is melted only by air or warm winds is not productive of sugar either. Finally in order that the snow melted by the sun produce a sap that will make sugar, it must have frozen the night before. Still another factor is the speed with which the melting snow penetrates the earth and enters into the arteries of the tree. That maple that gives sap without snow, but that is not suitable for sugar making, will, if you spread some snow over the earth around it, a half hour or an hour at the most after it has commenced to melt give a sap that is very good [*Acer Saccharum* according to Boivin]. . .3. It is of the sap of this maple that a sugar is made here [Quebec] that has some merit, because syrups, conserves are made with it. It grows in all septentrional America in good soil."

1720-21 Dudley. An account of sugar making in New England in the Phil. Trans. Royal Soc. London.

1724 Lafitau. Describing the method of extracting the sap from the maples by the Indians, adds: "The French women make it [sugar] better than the Indians from whom they learnt how to do it."

1748 Kalm Delaware October 6th. 88. "The red maple, or *Acer rubrum*, is plentiful in these places. . .Out of its wood they make plates, spinning wheels, feet for chairs and beds, and many other kinds of turnery. With the bark they dye both worsted and linen, giving it a dark blue color. For this purpose it is first boiled in water and some copperas. . .is added before the stuff (which is to be dyed) is put into the boiler. This bark likewise yields a good black ink. . .In Canada they make both syrup and sugar of its juice. There is a variety of this tree which they call the curly maple, the wood being as it were marbled within. . .utensils made of this wood are preferable to those of any other kind in this country, and are much dearer. . .The tree is therefore cut very deep before it is felled, to see whether it has veins in every part. . .December 12th. 220. The curled maple is a species of the common red maple, and likewise very difficult to obtain. You may cut down many trees without finding the wood which you want. . .1749 June 12th. Germans of Strasburg (Staatsburg) use a yellow *Agaricus* or fungus, which grows on the maple tree for tinder. That which is found on the red-flowering maple (*Acer rubrum*) is reckoned the best. . .20th. June 340. We lodged with a gunsmith, who told us that. . .the best and most expensive stocks for his muskets were made of wild cherry, and next to these he valued most those of the red maple. . .13th August Quebec 461. . .The sugar maple, the kind of maple which cures scorched wounds (which I have not as yet described). . .13th. Oct. 559. The sugar maples grew in great abundance in the woods here. I call small those which were from 48-60 feet high, as the sugar maple grows to a rather great height in Canada and is amongst the tallest trees in the country."

1756 James Smith HURON 36-37. A captive of the Huron in Ohio. "In this month (February) we began to make sugar. . .On the sugar-tree they cut a notch, sloping down. . .They drove a long chip, in order to carry the water out from the tree, and under this they set their vessel, to receive it." [See under elm for description of making the sugar and that of the following year when, being without brass kettles for boiling they froze the water in shallow elm baskets and threw away the ice every morning, until syrup remained].

1761 Alexander Henry (elder) noted the importance of fish and maple sugar as staples at Michilimackinac. Innis 1956:167.

1772 Ermatinger 14th. May transl. "The letter for M. Hance at Michilimackinac who should give you the following according to his promise to Mr. Oakes. . .4 barrels of 16 pots of Indian sugar (sucre sauvage), if he cannot give them to you he must absolutely buy them for you."

1780 Quebec Gazette 27th. Jan. "There is on it an excellent Maple Sucrerie, capable of producing annually from 300 to 600 w. of Sugar."

1779 Zeisberger 48-51. "From the sap of the tree sugar is boiled. This is done by the Indians in the early part of the year." [Here follows a long description of Indian sugar making]. . ."If the troughs and kettles used for collecting the sap are made of wood that does not give color, the sugar becomes the finer, but if it gives color, as does the white walnut, the sugar becomes black the first year. The Indians very reluctantly make their fields where there are sugar trees, as these are not to be exterminated. . .As the Indians have trees in abundance, their labors are richly rewarded. . .it is possible for him to make several hundreds of pounds of sugar and a quantity of molasses, besides. Sugar boiling is chiefly the employment of the women. . .the men hunt and supply meat. . .generally bear, which they seek in the rocks, hollow trees or thickets in their winter quarters. Bears are at this time generally fat."

1829 MacTaggart 1; 180. "Sugar-maple rum may be made of excellent quality."

1830 Rafinesque 184. "The bark of *A. rubra*, red maple, dies wool and flax of a brown color; the Cherokees use the inner bark boiled for sore eyes. . .The Birch and Hickory have a sweet sap as well as the Maples. The Indians made syrup and sugar from them all, but chiefly from [red maple, silver maple and box elder]. . .Sugar maple and Black maple afford the most. This sugar is equal to cane sugar. . .We could make maple sugar in sufficient quantity for the whole use of our population, and even for exportation. But instead, the trees are wantonly destroyed or neglected. Hardly 100,000 lbs of sugar are made annually, and chiefly in remote settlements. We ought to plant and cultivate these trees instead of destroying them, or leave from 10 to 50 on each acre of cleared land. Whole forests of them have lately been planted in Germany, Hungary, and France. The leaves of *A. striatum* [*A. pensylvanicum*], called Dockmockie maple, are used for topical application for the inflamed breast."

1840 Gosse Quebec 71-2. "Sugar off as it is called. . .boiling the syrup until it will granulate. . .This requires constant attention. . .When it is about half done, it is called maple-honey, from its resemblance to honey in taste, consistence, and appearance. . .less cloying. In this state, the good matrons generally come and take a tribute, and it forms a pleasant addition to the simple fare of our tea-table,. . .They [the sugar makers] take a twig, and bend the end of it into a loop or circle, about an inch wide: dipping this into the kettle, and taking it out, a film of sugar is stretched across the bow; they gently blow on this with their breath; if the breath breaks through, it is not done. . .[when ready] it is immediately baled out of the kettle. . .poured into wooden vessels, the bottoms of which are bored with holes. . .the molasses gradually drains through the bottom, and the sugar is left. . .146. The greater part of our winter fuel is composed of this wood. . .When a tree. . .which has a sudden curve or bend in the trunk is found, it is sawed into plank for the runners of sleds, which are curved up at one end to run on the snow. The wood is handsome, of a bright, changeable, satiny lustre, with many straight lines radiating from the centre outwards, across the grain; these are lustrous, and in one light look darker, and in another lighter than the rest of the wood: these are the medullary rays. It is used for the finer kinds of furniture, and when varnished looks very beautiful; it is hard and heavy but it is not durable. Trees are occasionally found, the wood of which is filled with little knots, or eyes, which make what is called curled, or Bird's-eye Maple, and which is much prized in cabinet work. This appearance is accidental". . .The red maple. . ."The bark of this tree, boiled with copperas, makes a fluid of intense black, which is commonly used in the village schools as ink, but it never dries properly; and in damp weather the writing becomes glutinous and blots, after any length of time: it is also used in domestic dying."

1855 Trail Sett. Guide 142. "Making of maple sugar, though the manufacturing of this Canadian luxury, is no longer considered so important a matter as it used formerly to be: the farmer, considering that his time can be more profitably employed in clearing his land, will not give his attention to it." [Here follows a detailed description of how to tap and boil the sap and make sugar as well as Maple vinegar, beer and wine.]

1885 Hoffman OJIBWA 198. "Sugar maple. 1. Decoction of the inner bark is used for diarrhea. 2. The sap is boiled in making sirup and sugar. 3. The wood valued for making arrow shafts. Black maple, sometimes used as the sugar maple. The sap flows fast from the tree and drunk causes the urine to flow fast also. . . .200. *Acer pensylvanicum*. . .The inner bark scraped from four sticks or branches, each two feet long, is put into a cloth and boiled, the liquid which can subsequently be pressed out of the bag is swallowed to act as an emetic."

1915 Speck PENOBSCOT 310. "Moosewood (*Acer pensylvanicum*) deer wood; bark is steeped and made into a poultice for swelling of the limbs". . .311. One of the ingredients of a gonorrhea remedy. Also used for kidney troubles and spitting of blood.

1916 Waugh IROQUOIS 65. "A favorite material for bowls everywhere was the knot which grows upon the soft maple. The bowls used for playing the peach-stone game [see plums] were made from the knots found on the maple, walnut and other woods. . .70. The wood employed for paddles is usually some variety of maple, though other hardwoods are sometimes used. . .88. Sugar is not used when the food is intended for hunters or for athletes, as it would make them dizzy (the sugar being derived from the maple, the branches of which sway about in the wind). . .119. Bark of the soft maple, *Acer rubra* and *A. saccharinum*. . .is dried beside the fire, then pounded in the mortar, sifted, and made into a bread; said not to taste badly. Bark of the hard or sugar maple. . .is used in the same way. Used also by neighbouring Algonkin tribes, such as the Montagnais. . .140. The sap of the maple, birch and several other trees was employed prehistorically. Besides its use as a beverage, it was boiled and thickened somewhat, though its manufacture into sugar must have been exceedingly difficult, if not impossible, with the crude utensils at hand. . .146. Maple sap is said to have been sometimes fermented and used as an intoxicant, though its use could never have been at all common. This sometimes turned to a vinegar, which was also consumed. The fermentation of sweet liquids and fruit juices takes place so readily that the discovery could not have been readily avoided. . .151. Hoffman remarks that 'Salt is not used by the Menomini during meals, neither does it appear to have a place in the kitchen for cooking or baking. Maple syrup is used instead, and it is singular how soon one may acquire the taste for this substitute for salt, even on meats.'"

1926-7 Densmore CHIPPEWA 308. "The two most important vegetable foods were maple sugar and wild rice. The obtaining of these commodities was attended with much pleasure. . .Each family or group of two or three families had its own sugar bush. . .The odor of balsam and dry sweet birch bark came from the lodge. . .Certain utensils were commonly made of maple, among them being the large wooden spoons used in dipping the sap, the paddles with which the syrup was stirred, and the granulating ladles with the back of which the heavy syrup was worked into sugar. . .The uses of maple sugar were many and varied. It was used in seasoning fruits, vegetables, cereals, and fish. It was dissolved in water as a cooling summer drink and sometimes made into sirup in which medicine was boiled for children. The granulated sugar and the sugar cakes were commonly used as gifts. . .318. A Canadian Chippewa said that in old times his people had no salt and that more maple sugar was used as seasoning than the quantity of salt now used by white people". . .374. Purple dye. The material used to secure this color is rotten maple wood. It is difficult to obtain, as the wood must be very old. Double handful of rotten maple; grindstone dust, single handful; hot water. The material must be boiled in the dye.

1928 Parker SENECA 11. Laxative, maple sap. . .childbirth to contract the womb, use a decoction of maple leaves, a mild astringent.

1923 H. Smith MENOMINI 61. "Maple sugar is one of the most important of Menomini foods and is used in almost every combination of cookery. . .73. Mountain Maple (*Acer spicatum*). From this leaf comes the maple leaf design found in Menomini bead-work and applique work. . .A paper copy of one of these leaves forms a single stencil which is laid down and repeated as often as desired. It is covered with charcoal or flour paste to transfer the design."

1928 H. Smith MESKWAKI 196. The inner bark of the sugar maple is one of eight ingredients in an internal medicine. . .255. "There are not many sugar trees on the Meskwaki reservation; hence but little sugar is made but they recall with considerable longing the sugar they used to make in Wisconsin. Most of their cooking, even of meats in the olden days was done with maple sugar as the seasoning instead of salt. . .200. Box elder (*A. negundo*) inner bark boiled and drunk as an emetic."

1932 H. Smith OJIBWE 395. "Maple sap is saved to drink as it comes from the tree, sometimes with the added sap of the Box Elder or Yellow Birch. Again it is allowed to become sour to make vinegar, used in their cooking of venison, which when afterwards sweetened with maple sugar, corresponds to the German fashion of sweet-sour meat. . .353. The Flambeau Ojibwe boil the bark of the red maple to obtain a tea with which to wash sore eyes. The Pillager Ojibwe reported that the inner bark of the box-elder is steeped to make an emetic. They extract the pith of the twig of the Mountain maple (*A. spicatum*) and pinch off small particles which are put into the eye like flax seed to remove foreign matter. It becomes sticky and holds the foreign matter which can then be removed with the pith. The pith is also soaked in water to make a lotion for treating sore eyes. Among the whites Mountain maple bark is often gathered and sold for Cramp bark (*Viburnum opulus*). In fact it has often been wholly substituted for it, and seems about as effective as a uterine sedative and preventative of abortion. . .413. The three lobed leaf is a great favorite with Ojibwe women for design work for beading, and it is more often seen than any other kind of leaf.

1933 H. Smith POTAWATOMI 92-4. Description of sugar making. "The boiling of sap in birch-bark vessels was quite a difficult thing to do. In those days, the original fire had to be fed with bark of the tamarack tree. . .The flame must never be allowed to come into contact with the birch bark, but the intense heat of the coals made the sap boil. . .The Soft maple [silver or red maple]. . .makes a whiter sugar than the real Sugar maple. . .116. The red maple. The Potawatomi trapper boiled his traps in water with soft maple bark to deodorize them so that the animal would not detect the scent of the previous animal which had been caught in the trap."

1935 Jenness OJIBWA Parry Island Lake Huron 88. "Any man fortunate enough to obtain and chew a little of the earth gathered underground at the base of a maple tree that had a streak of black along the eastern side can not only destroy a sorcerer's medicines but even seize the sorcerer himself on his night of visitation. . .96. When a young couple are married the Parry Islanders used to set a maple log between them the first four nights to please Grandmother Moon and teach them self restraint. . .114. Black dyes were made from barks of oak and soft maple boiled together. . .Children's bows made of maple. . .maple used for arrow shafts."

1942 W.V. Johnston 11. "The great Huron chief, Adario, wrote of fire water about 260 years ago: 'As for the maple-water that we drink, 'tis sweet, well tasted, healthy, and friendly to the stomach, whereas your wine and brandy destroy the natural heat, pall the stomach, inflame the blood, intoxicate and create a thousand disorders.'"

1945 Rousseau MOHAWK transl. 52-3. "Sugar maple. The coureurs des bois who did not have much wind drank an infusion of the entire plant of hepatica and the bark of the sugar maple taken from the side of the tree exposed to the sun. . .They drank a mild beer made of the yew (*Taxus canadensis*) and maple water. This usage could be a very ancient one. . .The wood of the red maple is used in the making of clay pots."

1945 Rousseau Quebec transl. 94. "Mountain maple (*A. spicatum*) popular name 'bois foireux' for diarrhea. Used for intestinal illnesses."

1955 Mockle Quebec transl. 55. "The following maples are used in Canada, the striped, red, silver, sugar and mountain. These maples and particularly the sugar and silver maples, supply the maple sugar and sirup of commerce. The raw sap taken from the collector, contains at least 3% of saccharose. . .Canada and the United States are the only countries that make these products, the Province of Quebec alone produces more then 4/5 of the Canadian production and more than that of the United States. . .The maple sugar industry seems to have been taught the first settlers by the Indians. . .The bark of the maples possesses astringent properties."

The acer-saponin of the box elder, *A. negundo* was scheduled for pharmacological study as a cancer chemotherapeutic agent (Lewis and Elvin-Lewis 1977:133).

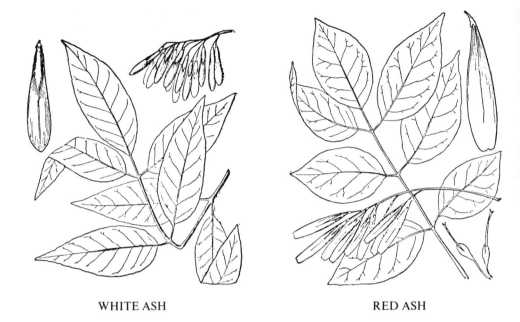

WHITE ASH   RED ASH

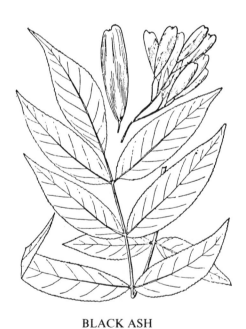

BLACK ASH

WHITE ASH   *Fraxinus americana* L. Oleaceae
Tree to 40 m with gray furrowed bark, often in a diamond pattern. The leaves consist of 5-9
leaflets, most often 7. The seeds have wings attached to them and are called keys. Those of the
white ash have a long wing below the seed.
Range. N.S. to Minn., s. to Fla. and Tex. in rich moist, not wet, soil.

RED ASH   *Fraxinus pennsylvanica* Marsh. (*F. pubescens, F. lanceolata, F. viridis*)
Tree to 25 m the outer bark taken from a branch will be red or cinnamon color on its inner surface when fresh. Leaflets 5-9, their stalks and branchlets of the tree velvety when young. The part of the wing below the seed usually less than half the length of the key.
Range. Que. to Man., s. to Fla. and Tex. in moist soil.
Common names. Green ash (may have smooth twigs), blue or black ash, water, swamp or river ash.

BLACK ASH   *Fraxinus nigra* Marsh. (*F. sambucifolia*)
Tree to 25 m with light gray scaly bark with soft corky ridges easily rubbed off by the hand when mature. Leaflets 7-11 with obvious teeth. The wing covers the flat seed, blunt at both ends. The bruised leaves smell like elder leaves.
Range Nfld., Que., to Man., s. to Del., Ky. and Io. in wet woods and swamps.
Common names. Brown ash, hoop ash, basket, swamp or water ash.
1475 Bjornsson Icelandic mss transl. Larsen 67. "*Fraxinus*, ash. With the ashes that come from burned ash-wood one may make deep brands. If one boils its flowers with vinegar, that is good to rub the genitals and blisters with; and it strengthens wounds. If one crushes young and tender bark of the ash tree, stripped off in small bits, and mixes it with warm wine, it is good to apply to broken bones."
1575 Thevet transl. 1016. "This people. . .fear the fury of lightening, they have been taught. . .that there are trees and animals, on whom this celestial fire never descends. When going to their fishing grounds, a long way from their camps, they put in their boats. . .branches of a tree called Cahené. . .Having this tree with them, they say that neither lightening nor tempest can harm them. . .Furthermore, in those places where the Canadians think there are serpents and venomous beasts, they only have to strew the leaves or branches of this tree cahené, or the bark of the tree, & immediately not a live one among them is left: & it is an undoubted fact that these vipers flee the scent of Cahené, & when the Savages make a fire. . .the serpents prefer to throw themselves into the fire, or to permit themselves to be caught and killed, than to go near the tree they so detest." [Rousseau 1937 suggests that cahené could perhaps be the black ash. See Gerarde below.]
1637 LeMercier HURON Jes. Rel. 13; 261. When smallpox was rampant in the village of Ossosane the Huron medicine man ordered the chief to take: "the bark of the ash, the spruce, the hemlock and the wild cherry, boiling them together well in a great kettle and washing the whole body therewith, and that care should be taken not to go out of their cabins barefooted, in the evening. He added that his remedies were not for women in their courses."
1633 Gerarde-Johnson 1472. "The ash tree, *Fraxinus excelsior*. . .The juice of the leaves or the leaves themselves being applied, or taken with wine, cure the bitings of vipers, as Dioscorides saith. . .Pliny. . .We write (saith he) upon experience, that if the serpent be set within the circle of a fire and the boughes of the ash, the serpent will soone run into the fire than into the boughes. It is a wonderful courtesie in nature, that the ash should floure before the serpents appeare, and not cast his leaves before they begon againe. Both of them, that is to say the leaves and the bark, are reported to stop the belly: and being boiled in vinegar and water, do stay vomiting, if they be laid upon the stomacke. . . .boiled in wine and drunk, do open the stoppings of the liver and spleene, and do greatly comfort them. Three or four leaves of the ash tree taken in wine each morning from time to time, doe make those leane that are fat, and keepeth them from feeding which do begin to wax fat. The seed of Kite-keyes of the ash tree provoke urine, increase naturall seed, and stirre up bodily lust, especially being poudred with nutmegs and drunke. . .The Lee which is made of the Ashes of the barke cureth the white scurfe, and such other roughnesse of the skin."
1724 Lafitau 11; 156. The sap of the ash was drunk by the Indians and although the flow was scanty the taste was delicate.
1724 Anon ILLINOIS-MIAMI mss 225. Some bark of the hybrid ash was chewed and put on felons or sprains.
1744 Charlevoix 1; 84. The Abenaki drank the sap of the ash.
1778 Carver 482. The rattlesnake. . .The bite of this reptile is more or less venomous according to the season of the year in which it is given. . .A decoction made of the buds or bark of the white ash taken internally prevents its pernicious effects. . .485. The gall of this serpent, mixed with

chalk, is formed into little balls, and exported from America for medicinal purposes. They are of the nature of the Gascoign's powders, and are an excellent remedy for complaints incident to children. The flesh of the snake also dried, and made into broth, is much more nutritive than that of vipers, and very efficacious against consumptions."

1799 Lewis Mat. Med. 148. "*F. excelsior* [European ash] bark and seeds. The bark is moderately astringent, the seed aperient. . .All parts of the ash tree have been long neglected."

1830 Rafinesque 221. "Ash trees, many species, valuable wood, compact, elastic, used for implements, screws, wheels, &c. Bark bitter astringent, used for hemorrhages and agues. Leaves for bites of snakes in poultice. Seeds aromatic, dessicative, said to prevent obesity! Ashes diuretic."

1833 Howard Quebec 248. "To cure the greece in a horse. 1 pound of green ash leaves; boil them in 2 gallons of water. Strain off the liquor and wash the legs always rubbing them downwards. It cures if ever so bad."

1846 Dr. Chase 151. "Hydrophobia and snake bites. . .Take the root of the common upland ash, commonly called black ash, peel off the bark, boil it to a strong decoction, and of this, drink freely, dose 1 gill 3 times daily. . .may vomit and purge if taken too freely, Yet a moderate action, either up or down, will not be amiss. . .259. Scours and pin-worms of horses and cattle. White ash bark burnt to ashes and made into a rather a strong lye; then mix ½ pt of it with warm water 1 pt. and give all, 2 or 3 times daily. Whenever it becomes certain that a horse or cow is troubled with pin-worms, by their passing from the bowels, it is best to administer the above."

1862 Provancher Quebec transl. Ash. "It is said that serpents have a very pronounced antipathy to the ash and that one never finds them in the swamps where this tree abounds. Their leaves, put on in the field, stops the effect of their venom when one is bitten."

1868 Can. Pharm. J. 6; 83-5. The bark of the white ash, *F. americana*, and that of the black ash, *F. sambucifolia* (*F. nigra*) included in list of Can. medicinal plants.

1877 Dept. Int. Ann. Rep. Can. 11; 23. "I think that. . .the ash hats, for men and women, manufactured by the Abenaki, will rival in value and quality the Leghorns and Panamas."

1880 Can. Horticulturist 116. "Mr. Beall stated that at Lindsay he had noted the following facts: Black Ash was used for making hoops and in carriage building, and was sold at from $8 to $10 per thousand. White Ash was largely used in manufacture of agricultural implements, and to some extent in house finishing, and sold at $15 to $20 per thousand."

1885 Hoffman OJIBWA 200. "Black or water ash. 1. The inner bark is soaked in warm water and the liquid applied to sore eyes. 2. The wood is employed in making the rims for frames of snow-shoes."

1892 Millspaugh 137. "White ash. The wood is very tough, fine-grained and elastic, and, were it not for its weight, would make fine cabinet material. It weighs 35 lbs., 10 oz. per cubic foot. . .Ash furnished material for the most strained parts of wagons, as well as for all the heavier agricultural implements. An infusion of white ash bark has been much used in cases where an astringent tonic was deemed necessary; it also proved cathartic, and has been found useful in constipation, especially of dropsical subjects. It has received much praise in mastitis, and enlargement of the spleen, as well as in some forms of eczema, and in gouty affections. There is also extant in the south a belief that the seeds prevent accumulation of fat. . .My father relates that among the settlers of Orange Co. N.Y. it was always asserted that the Aborigines used to defend themselves from this snake [rattlesnake] by carrying White Ash leaves about their persons. How much dependence might be placed on this prophylactic, it is hard to tell."

1915 Speck PENOBSCOT 310. "*F. americana*. . .leaves in a very strong, bitter decoction, are given to women after childbirth to cleanse them."

1916 Waugh 61. "The favorite Iroquois basketry material everywhere is black ash. The tree is cut into logs some 6 or 8 feet in length, the bark is removed and the outside pounded with the back of an axe or with a mallet, until the layers can be separated into strips."

1926-7 Densmore CHIPPEWA 364. "Used in an enema a decoction made from a handful of the root of the ash, sp. doubtful. [See under birch for details of administration] The inner bark of the ash was likewise drunk as a tonic in decoction. . .377. Black ash bark used in covering wigwams."

1923 H. Smith MENOMINI 43. "Black Ash. . .The inner bark of the trunk is a valuable Menomini medicine as a seasoner for other medicines. Ancient superstition of the white race accredited the ash with being a charm against serpents. . .Even in our times ash cradle rockers were supposed to shield the baby from snakes. The wine of white ash bark is a remedy of the white man used as a bitter tonic and astringent, and said to be valuable as an antiperiodic. It was also formerly used in the treatment of intermittent fevers. . .75. In aboriginal times, bows and arrows were made of black ash."

1928 H. Smith MESKWAKI 233. "Black Ash. The inner bark of the trunk is considered a remedy for any internal ailment. Specimen 3665 of the Dr. Jones collection is the wood of *F. nigra* together with the root of *Smilacina racemosa* [false solomon's seal]. . .The tea prepared from this mixture is used to loosen the bowels. White Ash. A bark infusion is used on sores and to cure the itch. Itch of the scalp due to vermin is cured in the same way. . .Specimen 5053 of the Dr. Jones collection is the inner bark of a swamp sapling of *F. americana* [white ash] which is cooked into a molasses consistency and used on old sores."

1932 H. Smith OJIBWE 376. "Red ash. The Pillager Ojibwe use the inner bark in combination with other things for a tonic. . .407. The cambium layer is scraped down in long, fluffy layers and cooked. . .They say it tastes like eggs. . .420. Black ash is the wood chosen for basketry splints by the Ojibwe. . .They select a black ash log from a swamp and peel it carefully. Then with a butcher knife, they make a cut about half an inch deep and by pounding with an axe head cause it to split up from the log. . .By inserting wedges, and continually pounding ahead of them, they cause the wood to separate along the annual rings. Then a further cut is made in the centre of the annual ring and the two halves peeled back leaving a glossy surface. These splints are curled up into coils to be immersed in kettles of dye stuff. Then they are woven by the women. All ash wood is quite valuable to the Ojibwe, as they use it for bows and arrows, snow-shoe frames, sleds, and cradle boards. The red ash is not used for the basketry splints when they can get black ash."

1933 Gilmore OJIBWA 139. White ash called spear timber used for fish spears and in canoe and snowshoe manufacture. Black ash was used as a dye.

1935 Jenness Parry Island Lake Huron OJIBWA 83. "For protection against snakes. . .place in the moccasin bark of the white ash. . .114. When tobacco was scarce the Indians substituted. . .the berry like tips of the white ash. . .113. Made baskets of two kinds, from splints of the white ash, and from birch bark."

1945 Rousseau MOHAWK transl. 60. White ash used "to make baskets and sometimes the seats and backs of chairs. . .When large branches of the ash are heated at the center point there escapes from each end a liquid that is used for earache. In the case of deafness, equal parts of this liquid and a rich infusion of the plant of *Coptis groenlandica* [goldthread], is made. Only a few drops are put into the ear which is then closed by a bit of animal skin. The different species of ash are without doubt used in the same manner for medicine as well as basketry. . . .According to Marie-Victorin (1919) the Algonquins of Temiscaming use the water from logs of the white ash to treat ear troubles, also."

1945 Rousseau Quebec transl. 99. "The bark of the ash used to be used to make seats and backs for chairs."

1945 Raymond TETE DE BOULE transl. 128. "*F. pennsylvanica*, red ash. The inner bark is scraped and made into a tea for general fatigue and depression."

1955 Mockle Quebec transl. 73. "White ash bark is bitter and astringent. The seeds are said to prevent obesity. A glucoside, fraxoside is found in the bark, containing coumarin. The black ash has the same properties. The red ash leaves are rubbed on an insect bite to reduce the swelling. There is a belief that they prevent the effects of venomous reptile bites."

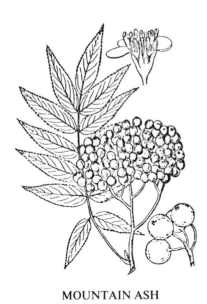

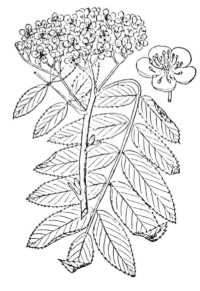

MOUNTAIN ASH   ROWAN

MOUNTAIN ASH   *Sorbus americana* Marsh. Rosaceae (*Pyrus a.*)
Shrub or tree to 10 m, the twigs smooth, the winter buds glutinous. Leaves consist of 9 to 11 leaflets that are 3-5 times as long as wide. The bunch of white flowers is followed by bright orange red berries that are 4-6 mm thick.
Range. Nfld., N.S., N.B., P.E.I., Que., Hudsons Bay, Ont. to Minn., s. to Pa. and Ill. and in the mts. to N.C. in moist woods or wet soil.

ROWAN   *Sorbus decora* (Sarg.) C.K. Schneid. (*S. subvestita, Pyrus d.*)
Shrub or tree to 10 m, leaflets 2-3 times as long as wide, the fruit 8-10 mm thick.
Range. s. Greenland, Lab., Nfld., N.S., N.B., P.E.I., Que., Ont. to Sask., s. to N.Y., Ind., and Io. in dry or rocky soil.
Common names. Dogberry, service tree, Witch wood, wine tree, elder leaved mountain ash or sumach, Indian-mozamize, moose-missy, life-of-man.
1830 Rafinesque 265. "Bark smells and tastes like cherry bark, equal to it, more astringent, fine tonic, antiseptic, contains Prussic acid [hydrocyanic acid] used in fevers and other diseases, like cinchona [quinine]. Fruit very austere, never ripens, becomes mellow and edible when rotten; yields malic acid, makes a very strong cider, and furnishes alcohol."
1884 Holmes-Haydon Hudson Bay CREE 303. "Wetchus-Y-usk-wa, or service tree, (Pyrus sp.?) This is in the form of thin shreds scraped off the young branches. It is of a yellowish-white colour on the inner surface, and of a purplish-brown on the outer. It has a slightly bitter, very astringent taste, and a strong tea like flavour. It is used by the Indians in pleurisy and inflammatory diseases."
1892 Millspaugh 56. "The close botanical and chemical relation of the American and European species render them so closely allied that many botanists consider them identical, and the chemistry of the bark, so far as distinguished, is so much like that of the wild cherry (*Cerasus* [*Prunus*] *serotina*) that its medical uses have been substitutive. The previous use of the bark in medicine has been as a tonic in fevers of supposed malarial types, where it was often substituted for cinchona. The berries were used as an antiscorbutic. . .European species *S. aucuparia*. Amygdalin,—this glucoside occurs in the bark, buds, flowers and kernels of many rosaceous plants [see cherry]. . .Under the action of dilute acids it splits up. . .into Hydrocyanic acid [no

odor but toxic], Benzaldehydé or Oil of Bitter Almonds [odor but not toxic], and Glucose [sugar]. Sorbin is the glucose found in the berries. . .Citric acid. . .occurs together with malic acid in the fruits of both species."

1915 Speck PENOBSCOT 309. "Furnishes a medicine used as an emetic. . .313. MONTAG-NAIS The berries of the mountain ash, 'bear berries', so called because they are a favorite food of bears, are good for people to eat. The bark of the tree is boiled and the decoction drunk to stimulate the appetite and purify the blood. . .317. Bark in infusion as a tea, diuretic. An infusion of the root for colic."

1928 Reagan OJIBWA 236. Used wood for canoe ribs, snowshoe frames, lacrosse racquets because it can be bent into any form.

1933 H. Smith POTAWATOMI 78. "The Forest Potawatomi state that the bear eats the berries of the Mountain ash and that they use the inner bark for a medicine, but we were unable to find out what ailments it was supposed to cure. . .European Mountain Ash. It is rather peculiar to find a Forest Potawatomi using this cultivated tree for medicine. It is very likely that the native Mountain Ash so much resembles the cultivated one that they mistook the identification of this plant. The leaves are used to make a tea for colds. The leaves are steeped in hot water, which causes the patient to vomit and at that time the extra mucous is expelled. This makes it valuable in their estimation for the treatment of pneumonia, diphtheria and croup. . .The 1916 U.S. Dispensatory says that the fruit has been used as an anti-scorbutic."

1945 Rousseau Quebec transl. 91. "The fruits picked in the autumn help digestion."

1945 Raymond TETE DE BOULE transl. 132-2. "The fibers of the inner bark as well as the buds covered with boiling water, are used for a drug that has the reputation of curing general feebleness, moral depression, etc. The fibers are also boiled to make a plaster to put upon the kidneys of women in child-birth."

1955 Mockle Quebec transl. 60. "European mountain ash. The fruits are prescribed for scurvy and in the form of an extract, in the treatment of irritation in the digestive tube and the bile vessels. The alcoholic extract of the fruit, known under the popular name of 'soparine', is used to elevate the prothrombin level of the blood."

European mountain ash, *S. aucuparia* contains parasorbic acid in its fruit which is active against gram bacteria and protozoa. . .A compound shown to cause cancer in animals has been isolated from the mountain ash. Children have been poisoned (Lewis and Elvin-Lewis 1977:41, 362).

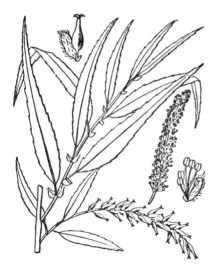

BLACK WILLOW

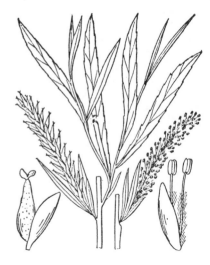

SANDBAR WILLOW

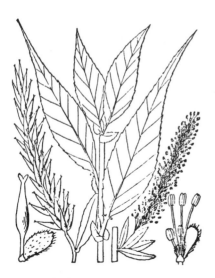

SHINING WILLOW

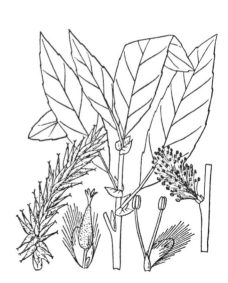

PUSSY WILLOW

BLACK WILLOW   *Salix nigra* Marsh. Salicaceae

Tree to 20 m with rough bark or a shrub with 1-4 leaning trunks to 50 cm thick. The leaves narrow to a long tip, 6-10(12) x 1-1.5(2) cm with fine incurved teeth, often hairy when young then smooth and green on both sides on usually hairy stems 4-10 mm long. Where they grow from the slender twigs there are a pair of leaflets (stipules) which can be minute or to 12 mm in size. The catkins mature with the leaves in this species, slender, loose, 2.57 cm long. The seeds are in a capsule 3-5 mm that is smooth on the outside on a stalk 1-2 mm long.

Range. s. N.B., s. Que., Ont. nw to Thunder Bay, and c. Minn., s to n Mex., Tex. and nw Fla. in moist woods, streambanks and shores, Apr-May.

SANDBAR WILLOW   *Salix interior* Rowlee (A regional ssp. of the more western *S. exigua*; *S. longifolia*)

Many stemmed shrub 2-5 m with reddish-brown smooth twigs. The leaves narrowed at both ends, 5-14 cm x 5-12(18) mm without stems or very short ones, more or less silky when young then smooth and green on both sides with 2-3 teeth to each cm of margin. The catkins appear after the leaves, slender, often 1-3 clustered at the ends of the twigs, 3-6 (8) cm. The capsule 7-10 mm on short stalk, 0.5-1.5 mm.

Range. Nfld.?, N.B., Que., James Bay, northernmost Ontario, Man., to Yukon and Alaska, s. to Va., La. and Tex. Apr.-May in large clumps on sandbars, moist streambanks.

Common names. Red or white willow, Osier or shrub willow, river-bank willow.

SHINING WILLOW   *Salix lucida* Muhl.

Shrub or small tree to 6 m with smooth dark brown bark, the twigs and bud scales chestnut brown, smooth and shining when mature. The leaves shining on both sides as if polished, 5-15(20) x 2-5(8) cm with sharp teeth with glands on their tips; on 5-10(15) mm stalks, with glands near tips. Catkins with the leaves 2-6 cm on 1-2 cm stalks. The capsule straw-color or pale brown or greenish, dull, rounded at the base 4.5-6.5 mm long smooth.

Range. Lab., Nfld., N.B., N.S., P.E.I., Que., James Bay, Ont., Man., Sask., s. to Del., n. Io., and N.D. in moist low ground and swampy places. Plants with twigs and lower leaf surface hairy are occasionally found in the n. part of range.

PUSSY WILLOW   *Salix discolor* Muhl.

Few stemmed shrub or small tree 2-5 (7.5) m with rather stout, reddish to dark brown twigs, hairy when young. The leaf buds large to 1 cm, leaves hairy when young smooth when mature with raised veins beneath, 5-8(10) x 2-3.5 cm, dark shining green above. The catkins, without stalks, thick round, 2-8(10) cm long silvery silky appearing before the leaves. The capsule hairy to 12 mm long on a 1.5-3 mm long stalk.

Range. Lab., Nfld., N.B., N.S., P.E.I., Que., Hudson Bay., Ont. to B.C., s. to Del., Ky., Mo., S.D. and Mont. March-May in swamps or on moist hillsides.

UPLAND WILLOW   *Salix humilis* Marsh.

Shrub 1-3 m with yellowish to brown hairy or smooth twigs. The obovate leaves 3-10(15) x 1-3(3) cm downy becoming smooth above, beneath rough veined and softly wooly with wavy edges, can become smooth in age. The catkins unfold before the leaves appear, 1.5-3 cm long without stalks. The capsule much longer than its stalk, 7-9 mm gray hairy, stalk 1-2 mm, with slender beak.

Range. Lab., Nfld., N.S., P.E.I., N.B., Que., James Bay, Man., s. to N.D., Wisc., Mich., N.Y., and N. Engl. in dry barren places, prairies open woods Apr.-May. The willows interbreed and are very difficult to identify.

1475 Bjornsson Icelandic mss transl. Larsen 131. "Salix, willow. Cold in the second degree and dry in the first. Its juice dripped in the nostrils is good for headache. Willow bark burned and tempered with vinegar removes warts. Willow juice is good for a flux of blood. If one takes milk of willow when it is in bloom, that strengthens the eyes and makes them clear. Juice of willow twigs and of the flowers if drunk prevents the conception of child."

1590 Harriot Virginia Indians 23. "Willows good for the making of weares and weeles to take fish after the English manner although the inhabitants use only reedes."

1633 Gerarde-Johnson 1392. "The leaves and barke of Withy or Willowes do stay the spitting of bloud whatsoever in man or woman, if the said leaves and barke be boiled in wine and drunke. The greene boughes with the leaves may very well be brought into chambers and set about the beds of those that be sicke of fevers, for they do mightily cool the heate of the aire. . .The bark hath like vertues: Dioscorides writeth, this being burnt to ashes, and steeped in vinegar, takes away cornes and other like risings in the feet and toes: divers saith Galen, do slit the barke whilest the Withy is in flouring, and gather a certain juice, with which they use to take away things that hinder the sight, and this is when they are constrained to use a clensing medicine of thin and subtill parts."

1743 Isham Hudson Bay Indians 156. "And when they kill Deer any Distance from the tent, itt's a General rule with them, at their Returning from huntg. to Sticke mawse upon the Bushes or trees, Every 2 or 3 hundd. Yards, or to break a willow, and Lay across his track, by which the women Know's where to find such Deer Killd., if never so many without the men's Going with them. . .137. Pine, Willow, Juniper, Berch and popla'r is the only trees we have Downe this way, of which they make their snow shoes, cannoes and Sleds;—Splitting a tree with their hatchet,—their snow shoes are of Different form's and sizes. . .A hoop nett, which Childn. wears made of willow, when they can not gett Berch or Juniper. . .Another which is round toed, and hee'l, is what Children wears, which they styl' (musquatum). . .It' a little curious how they manage to gett pieces of that Length out of a tree, 14 to 16 inches thro, the frame of the snow shoe not being above one inch thick one way, and one and ½ inch the other way."

1771 Hearne Coppermine Journey 73-4. Indians with him found a young woman alone in a hut where she had spent the winter after escaping from the Athapuscows who had taken her prisoner. She had spent seven months without seeing a human face. During this time she had supported herself very well by snaring partridges, rabbits and squirrels. "Still had a small store of provisions by her when she was discovered. She was in good health and condition, and I think was one of the finest Indian women that I have seen in any part of North America. . .The sinews of rabbits' legs and feet. . .she twisted together for snares. . .Also enough skins to make a warm and neat suit of winter clothing. . .Showed great taste and no little variety of ornament. . .Her leisure hours from hunting had been employed in twisting the inner rind or bark of willow into small-lines, like net-twine, of which she had some hundred fathoms [600 feet]. With this she intended to weave a fishing net as soon as the spring advanced. It is the custom of the Dog-Rib Indians to make their nets in this manner, and they are much preferable to the deer-thong nets of the Northern Indians which, although they appear very good when dry, grow so soft and slippery in the water that the hitches are apt to slip and let the fish escape. They are also liable to rot, unless frequently taken out of the water. . .The poor girl was actually won and lost at wrestling by a half a score of different men that same evening." [Mowat 1973:73-4]

1778 Carver 505. "There are several species of willow, the most remarkable of which is a small sort that grows on the banks of the Mississippi, and some other places adjacent. The bark of this shrub supplies the beaver with its winter food; and where the water has washed the soil from its roots, they appear to consist of fibers interwoven together like thread, the colour of which is an inexpressibly fine scarlet; with this the Indians tinge many of the ornamental parts of their dress."

1785 Cutler. "An Account is given in the Transactions of the Royal Society [England] 1763 by the Rev. Mr. Stone of the great efficacy of white willow bark in curing intermittent fevers. He gathered the bark in summer when it was in full sap, dried it by a gentle heat and gave a dram of it powdered, every four hours betwixt fits. In a few obstinate cases he mixed it with one fifth part of Peruvian bark. Some judicious physicians here [the U.S.], have made trial of the bark of the white willow and recommend it as a valuable substitute for the Peruvian bark. They have used principally the bark of the roots."

1833 Howard Quebec mss 171. "To cure a speck on the horses eye. Dry white willow till the nature is out of it, bruise it to fine powder—blow a little into the eye once a day and wash it with goland water."

1830 Rafinesque 260. "Salix. Valuable prolific genus. . .Twigs used for baskets, wood soft white for chip hats. Bark of all bitter astringent, febrifuge and antiseptic. Eq. of Cinchona [Peruvian bark] in many cases, contains tannin, gluten and salicin similar to Quinine, 3 doses of 6 grains of Salicin have cured agues. . .Schoepf mentions the yellow and swamp willows used with us, roots and barks in bitters. . .Rose willow much used by empirics for fluoralbus, menorrhea, cutaneous eruptions and agues, in tea. The seed wool of some sp. may be spun."

1841 Trousseau & Pidoux Paris transl. Strong decoction of willow for gangrene, bad ulcers.

1842 Christison 816-7. "Willow bark has long been more or less used in medicine as a bitter tonic and astringent. But although undoubtedly so active in these respects. . .it has fallen so entirely into desuetude, that it would scarcely require mention here, except on account of its active principle, Salicin. . .Every botanist knows that willows are very difficult to distinguish from one another,—a circumstance in part explanatory of the opposite opinions that have been given of their virtues. . .There seems little question that the best test for choosing the officinal species is the bitter taste, as Mr. Pereira has suggested; for this quality depends on the salicin. . .[which]

was discovered by Buchnerin 1828. . .concentrated sulphuric acid imparts to it a brilliant red hue, and acts in this way with such delicacy, that it may be used as a test for salicin in willow-bark. . .Willow-bark is to be used as a febrifuge by infusing an ounce of the dried bark in a pint of water, and administering the infusion in the dose of one or two ounces frequently. . .As a tonic stomachic in dyspepsia, it is quite on a par with quina, and it is not apt like quina, to cause congestion in the head when given in large doses."

1859-61 Gunn 763-4. "Black willow, *Salix nigra*. . .is an excellent tonic, as well as a powerful antiseptic. Both the bark and the buds are used. The bark, in powder, or bruised, makes an excellent poultice for foul and indolent ulcers, and in all cases of gangrene or mortification. A decoction, either of the bark or buds, is also good to wash old and gangrenous ulcers, and is also good in such cases taken internally; it may be drank freely. . .There are several species of willow, all of which are more or less tonic. Salicin. . .in many cases, is a good substitute for quinine, especially in intermittent fevers."

1868 Can. Pharm. J. 6; 83-5. *Salix alba* (the European tree brought over to America), white willow, the bark included in list of Can. medicinal plants.

1875 Can. Pharm. J. 389. "Note on Salicylic acid by Edward R. Squibb M.D. Brooklyn N.Y. Salicin is a glucoside or neutral vegetable principle discovered by Leroux in 1830 in the bark of some species of willow, *Salix*, whence its name. It was afterwards found in various species of poplar, and in other trees and plants". . .There was a sudden German interest in salicylic acid in 1875-6.

1885 Hoffman OJIBWA 200. "*Salix candida*, Hoary willow. . .The thick inner bark of the roots is scraped off, boiled, and the docoction taken for cough."

1892 Heebner Pharm. 205. "Salicin, a neutral principle obtained from the bark of *Salix Helix* [European] and other species of *Salix*. . .206. Antifebrine, Dose 20-30 grains. . .Other glucosides (unofficinal) with sources. . .populin (willow)."

1892 Millspaugh 161. "*Salix purpurea*, = *S. helix*, red willow, bitter purple willow [Eurasian, originally introduced for basket making, sparingly escaped from cultivations], we will. . .give the general action and history of willow under this species, in default of specific literature. . .its control over fever was never very satisfactory. Its principle utility has been found to be as an astringent tonic in convalescence from protracted diseases, atony of the digestive tract, chlorosis, diarrhoea, dysentery, leucorrhoea and kindred affections. Salicin itself appears to have a more thorough and effective action than the bark, but still cannot cover the generality of cases like quinine; it is. . .very useful in such cases of hectic fever and of diarrhoea where irritation and inflammation precludes the use of quinine. The bark of *Salix* (various species) is officinal in the U.S. Ph., as is also Salicin. . .This glucoside of the aromatic group is found in the young bark of all species of this order Salicaceae as well as in Castoreum, the preputial follicles of the beaver. . .Salicylous Acid. . .exists naturally in the leaves of the Meadow-sweet (*Spiraea Ulmaria*). It can be obtained from salicin by distillation with dilute sulphuric acid and potassium dichromate. It results as a fragrant, colorless oily liquid having an odor similar to that of almond oil and a burning aromatic taste. . .Salicylic acid is a by-product of the above distillation, and only differs chemically from salicylous acid in having one more atom of oxygen in its composition." [Aspirin, acetylsalicylic acid is chemically related to salicylic acid but not identical to it]

1901 Morice DENE Arctic 22. "Ligature against hemorrhage was unknown. Application of the chewed bark of the aspen root took its place. When the wound or sore manifested a tendency towards decomposition, a sort of blister of the inner bark of the willow (*Salix longifolia*) [*S. interior, S. exigua*] and of the outer bark of the bear berry bush [ninebark] was applied, generally with good results."
In this case, bear berry bush is not *Arctostaphylos uva ursi*, but l'arbe aux sept écorces, though it is not a tree at all. Footnote by Morice.

1913 Hodge & White 40. "The northern Athapascan made long, straight bows of willow or birch, with wooden wrist guards projecting from the belly."

1915 Harris Indians eastern Can. 54. "Arrow-heads or any other foreign substance when deeply imbedded were extracted by a forceps made from split willow."

1915 Speck PENOBSCOT 309. "Willow bark (*S*. sp.) steeped is drunk in quantity for colds. . .Squaw bush (*S. lucida*). . .Bark is smoked to relieve asthma". . .313 MONTAGNAIS "The bark of red willow (*Salix lucida*). . .is scraped and steeped to make a mash to be put in a bandage on the head for headache. The leaves are to be steeped and drunk. The bark is dried and smoked as a substitute for tobacco by the Montagnais, as well as by the other northern tribes". . .317. Speck-Cartwright MICMAC-MONTAGNAIS. "*Salix* sp. root used as a black dye, the leaves bruised in water for sprains and bruises."

1925-6 Tantaquidgeon MOHEGAN 266. Steeped the bark of the red willow (*S. lucida*) and drank the infusion to cure vomiting and remove bile from the stomach.

1925 Wood & Ruddock. *S. nigra*, black willow. When it becomes necessary to supress sexual desire, the buds and twigs made into a tea and drunk freely will accomplish this purpose.

1926-7 Densmore CHIPPEWA 342. The inner bark of *Salix*, sp. doubtful, combined with the bark of other trees in decoction drunk for indigestion. . .344. *Salix* species doubtful, the root used alone or in combination with other roots in decoction drunk for dysentery. . .331. Another method of steaming was used chiefly for rheumatic limbs. . .A medicine frequently used in this connection was identified as willow (species doubtful). The prepared root was put in hot water and allowed to boil a short time. It was usually cooled before using. . .378. *Salix* sp. for smoking and general utility.

1928 Parker SENECA 12. "Septic throat use pussy willow root gargle. . .as an astringent."

1923 H. Smith MENOMINI 52. "Dwarf willow (*S. humilis*). . .The root is used in curing spasmodic colic and to stop dysentery and diarrhoea. The medicinal root is only taken from the shrub that bears insect galls. Other shrubs of the same species are not considered of value medicinally by the Menomini. . .76. One basket woven from willow twigs was observed."

1928 H. Smith MESKWAKI 425. "Dwarf willow (*S. humilis*). . .The root tea of the tree that grew in the lowlands was used in flux and for giving enemas. The upland species. . .McIntosh said that the leaves were used for stopping a hemorrhage. He never used the leaves from the lowland species."

1932 H. Smith OJIBWE 388. "Shining willow (*S. lucida*). The Pillager Ojibwe use the bark of this species as an external remedy for sores. The Ojibwe do not generally distinguish any particular willow with any other name, but Whitefeather, Flambeau Ojibwe, called this species. . .swamp tree and said it was used on a cut to stop bleeding, and that the bark was also a poultice material for sores. . .Bog willow (*S. pedicellaris*). . .[is a] species of the cold bogs and meadows found far up toward the Arctic circle. While the Pillager Ojibwe did not give it a distinctive name, they said it was not used for bark to smoke, but for bark to treat stomach trouble. . .*S. fragilis*. This tree has escaped from cultivation around the water-courses of the Flambeau Reservation and has been accepted by the Ojibwe there as efficacious along with the native willows. The bark is astringent from its salicin content and is used as a styptic and poultice for sores. . .422. *S. lucida*. The Flambeau Ojibwe use this bark for their kinnikinnik or native smoking mixture. It is peeled and toasted over a fire and reduced to flakes."

1933 H. Smith POTAWATOMI 81-2. "Pussy willow (*S. discolor*). Among the Forest Potawatomi the bark is a universal remedy and any species of willow will have approximately the same Indian name. . .The root bark is boiled down to make a tea, which is used in stopping a hemorrhage. We find that the willow galls have no meaning to the Potawatomi whereas they were valuable for medicine to the Menomini, because they were galls rather than because they were from a willow tree. Among the whites [Nickell]. . .The buds have been considered anti-aphrodisiac. . .Slender willow (*S. petiolaris*). . .is used by the Forest Potawatomi in the same manner as others of the willows and particularly just as *Salix discolor* [pussy willow] was used."

1931 Grieve England 846. "Black American willow (*S. nigra*). An aphrodisiac, sedative, and tonic. The bark has been prescribed in gonorrhoea and to relieve ovarian pain; a liquid extract is prepared and used in mixture with other sedatives. Largely used in the treatment of nocturnal emmisions."

1933 Gilmore OJIBWA 126. Sandbar willow (*S. interior*) used for weaving baskets.

1935 Jenness Parry Island OJIBWA Lake Huron 114. "When tobacco was scarce the Indians substituted willow bark."

1941 Whitford ALGONQUIN 11. Fiber of the black willow, (*S. nigra*) used for making bags, pouches, fish nets and cord by the Ojibwa, Menomini, Ottawa and Winnebago. (Yarnell 1964:187.)

1945 Rousseau MOHAWK transl. 39. "*S. interior*. A mixture infused of the twigs of this willow with alder and two other plants which the informer could not show me for a stitch in the side."

1945 Raymond TETE DE BOULE transl. 130-31. "*S. discolor*. The inner bark is reduced to powder and thrown into boiling water to make a paste which is applied to sore throats. The young branches infused for a tea brings on the lactation of young mothers."

1949 Hobart and Melton Pharm. England 28-9. "Salicylic acid [see under Millspaugh] is a tissue solvent and is rarely given by mouth. . .Externally. . .is applied in ointment form to soften hard skin and, dissolved (10%) in collodion, to remove corns and warts. It is a frequent component of ointments intended to remove the horn cells of the epidermis and so promote the penetration of other medicaments. Applied locally it is antiseptic, antipruritic and fungicidal. . .170. Aspirin is partly hydrolysed in the tract but for the most part it is absorbed as sodium acetylsalicylate. The drug exerts the general properties of the salicylates, but the acetyl group confers upon it much more marked analgesic properties." [Without the nausea caused by Salicin.]

1955 Mockle Quebec transl. 32. "*S. alba*. European species escaped in our range. The bark is used as an astringent, tonic and febrifuge. It contains 0.5% salicoside. . .and 3 to 4% tannin. Salicoside has been found in several other species of willow which are found in Canada: *S. discolor*, pussy willow, which contains also piceoside; *S. herbacea, S. nigra, S. pentandra*, which contain also populoside; *S. purpurea*, which contains, salipurposide and populoside, and finally *S. repens* which contains in additon saliperoside."

1966 Campbell, Best, Budd 72. "The willow group contains many different species, most of which are extremely difficult to identify. They have a wide range also, growing on moist slopes and flats, along river banks, and in mountain meadows throughout the northern hemisphere. They may be very small slender shrubs or large trees suitable for lumber. . .Willow and poplar have many characteristics in common and in some instances are hard to distinguish. . .The buds of poplars are covered with several sticky scales, but the buds of willows have a single. . .scale. . .Willows are good browse. Sheep and deer eat the leaves more readily than cattle. . .Chemical analyses show that all willows have higher protein and phosphorus content than grasses and the young growth is lower in crude fiber."

1978 Riley personal communication from G. Fireman of Attawapiskat, James Bay. His Cree mother still uses the live underbark of *S. bebbiana*, the long beaked willow, boiled in water, to stop the bleeding of bad wounds.

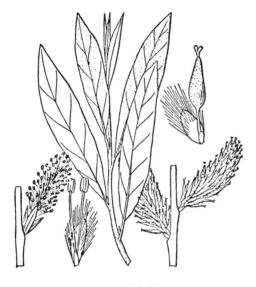

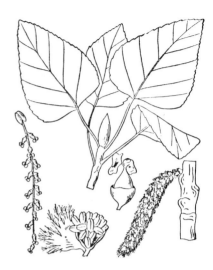

UPLAND WILLOW   BALSAM POPLAR

BALSAM POPLAR   *Populus balsamifera* L. Salicaceae (*P. tacamahacca, P. candicans*)
Tall tree with dark gray furrowed bark with flat topped rough ridges separated by irregular V-shaped crevices on old trees, young trees with smooth greenish brown bark. The twigs smooth or hairy, the terminal bud long, slender, pointed and very sticky with a fragrant gum. Leaves on round stalks have long tapering tips, pale beneath, can be either smooth or hairy. The seed pod on a stout stalk consists of several scales one over the other which split into two parts to let the seeds, on long silky hairs, float out. Male and female catkins on separate trees.
Range. Lab., Nfld., N.B., P.E.I., N.S., Que. Ungava, northernmost Ont., Man., to Yukon, Alaska, s. Oreg., Nev., Colo., Nebr., and Pa. in moist woods, ravines, shores and prairie parklands.
Common names. Taccamahac, hackmatack, balm of Gilead, rough bark poplar.
Here is an excellent example of the confusion common names of plants can cause. "Tacamahac", in many different spellings, is a Nahuatl Indian word for the gum resins of several middle and south American trees. In 1577 Monardes, telling of the gums brought from South America, writes: "Tacamahac is taken out by incision of a tree beyng as greate as a Willowe Tree, and is of a verie sweet smell. . .The Indians use it for swellings in any part of the body and also for toothache." "Balsam", from a tree growing in the Middle east, is a gum from the *Balsamodendron Gileadense* or *B. Opobalsamum* well known since biblical times as Balm of Gilead. The aromatic smell and taste of the gum from the buds of our Balsam poplar apparently earned it the borrowed names of many trees that gave gums to medicine in the seventeenth century. "Hackmatack" comes from an Abenaki Algonkian word meaning "wood for snowshoes", and is the common name for the larch or tamarack. **1774** Robinson & Rispin J. N.S. 34. "This town. . .affords great store of fine timber including tackamahacka, or juniper." There is a further confusion of names compounded by the Balm of Gilead fir, *Abies balsamea*, balsam fir.
1475 Bjornsson Icelandic mss Larsen transl. 116. "Populus, birch. It is of two kinds. One has a leaf on the one side somewhat white but on the other side green; and therefore it is called white. But the one that is called black has leaves green on both sides and buds full of resin on its highest twigs. Those one shall gather in the month of May at the time they are about to burst into leaves, and these one shall crush in unsalted ointment of resin which is made in the month of May. Then boil until all the liquid in the pan is green. Then press it out through a cloth and keep it in an earthen vessel. And that is a very excellent ointment called Populeon. If one rubs the forehead and cheeks with it, it is good for hot headache and lessens heat and puffiness of the limbs, and is good for sores. . .41. It is good for heat and for an epidemic and for sleeplessness. One shall rub the temples and the pulse on both arms and legs and also on the palms and on the soles of the feet."

[Larsen in his notes says that the tree meant here is the White Birch of Europe common throughout Norway and one of the oldest and most general remedies of Norwegian folk-medicine. It seems clear however that the tree with buds full of resin is the European black poplar whose buds were used to make Populeon.]

1633 Gerarde-Johnson 1486-8. "The [European] Black Poplar tree. . .the buds which shew themselves before the leaves spring out, are of a reasonable good savour, of the which is made that profitable ointment called Unguentum Populeon. . .The rosin or clammy substance of the blacke Poplar buds is hot and dry, and of thin parts, attenuating and mollifying. . .The leaves and yong buds. . .doe asswage the paine of the gout in the hands or feet, being made into an ointment with May butter. The ointment of the buds is good against all inflammations, bruses, squats, falls, and such like: this ointment is very well known to the Apothecaries. . .Make an oile also hereof, called Aegyrinum, or oile of blacke Poplar."

1755 Boerhaave Mat. Med. London. Gum of *Populus tacamahaca* for hard swellings.

1789 Edinburgh New Disp. The resin of *P. tacamahaca* used by the Indians for tumors.

1799 Lewis Mat. Med. 249. "Tacamahaca, *Populus balsamifera* the resin. Grows on the continent of America. Best resin is made from exudation from fruit of tree, unctuous pale yellowish or greenish aromatic taste and fragrant delightful smell, approaching that of lavender and ambergris. This sort is very rare, the common sort in shops is from an incision made in trunk of tree, semi-transparant grains or globs of a whitish-yellow-brownish greenish colour and less grateful smell. The resin is said to be employed among the Indians externally, for discussing and maturating tumours, and abating pains and aches of the limbs. From the fragrance of the finer sort, it may probably be applicable to different purposes; but at present it is little used, except as an ingredient in some of the warming plasters."

1830 Rafinesque 252. "Buds tonic, stimulant, sudorific, fragrant and balsamic, good ointment in rheumatism, gout, burns, sores, diseases of the skin, internally for chronic catarrh and diseases of the kidneys. They hold 20 elements, oil, populine, peculiar fat, albumen, resin, &c."

1840 Gosse Quebec 138-9. "*Populus Balsamifera*. . .This tree affords a good example of the perula, or scales, which serve as a sheath to the bud in winter, and which protect the tender, unexpanded leaves within from the cold. That they may better do this, the perules in the Balm of Gilead, and in many other plants, are coated with a thick clammy resinous substance, which may be scraped off with the nail, and which in this species has a fragrant smell. It seems probable that the hive-bee collects the substance call propolis, with which it stops the fissures and crevices of the hive, partly from the resinous perules of plants. Let us examine a bud. . .these two dark-brown convex scales are the perules, they are thick and tough; within them are two more, much thinner and paler. . .here are the leaves: how soft and small they are!, they appear much smaller than they are, for they are so folded up as to occupy the smallest possible space. . .it is found that the young leaves are constantly folded up in the bud in the same way in the same species of plants, but there are many different modes of this arrangement."

1859-61 Gunn 758. "Balm of Gilead buds are expectorant, diuretic, somewhat stimulant and tonic. Useful mainly in coughs, affections of the lungs, and of the kidneys and urinary organs. They are also found useful in rheumatism, scurvy, and in leucorrhea or whites. The manner of using them is in the form of a tincture, which is made by putting an ounce or two of bruised buds into a pint of alcohol or proof spirits and let them digest for a week or two. Dose, from a tea to a table spoonful, three or four times a day. By adding a little honey. . .say one third part honey, it forms an excellent remedy for all ordinary coughs."

1868 Can. Pharm. J. 6; 83-5. Balm of Gilead leaf buds included in list of Can. medicinal plants.

1885 Hoffman OJIBWA 199. "*Populus balsmifera*, the bark is peeled from the branches and the gum collected and eaten. Poles are used in building ordinary shelter lodges, and particularly for the Midewigan."

1892 Millspaugh 162. "Oil of Populus. This body, obtained by aqueous distillation of the leaf buds, is colorless, lighter than water, and has a pleasant balsamic odor. The name Tacamahaca has been improperly applied to this product, to which, it bears no resemblance except, mayhap, in its odor. . .161. The leaf buds of the European Black Poplar are frequently used in the form of Unguentum Populeum as a vulnerary. . .and the buds of the Tacmahac Poplar (*P. Balsamifera*) are considered diuretic and antiscorbutic."

1910 Moody C.H. 43. "The Indians of the Northwest prepare a dressing for burns by cooking deer suet with balm of gilead buds. This is the most effective application for severe burns I have ever seen. If deer suet is not available, any fresh tallow that has been cooked will serve as well.

Throw a handful of the buds into a vessel and cover them with the suet, boil for thirty minutes and strain. When nearly cold apply to the burn and cover with a soft cloth. The pain ceases almost immediately."

1926-7 Densmore CHIPPEWA 304. *Populus balsamifera* constituents: Chrysin, tetrochrysin, salicin, populin, resin and a volatile oil. . .338. Equal amounts of the root, bud and blossom mixed with the inner bark of the aspen, red and bur oaks and the root of seneca snakeroot were made in a curing ceremony, into a decoction for heart trouble [See seneca snakeroot under woods for details]. . .356. The root of the balsam poplar and that of the thistle, equal amounts mixed and a handful put in 1 quart of water, boiled thoroughly and drunk for pain in the back and female weakness. 'take often and freely, about a quart a day'. . .362. For sprain or strained muscles, the buds before they open steeped and used as a poultice. Boiled in grease (about a handful of buds to a cup of grease), strained and kept for use when needed. Deer tallow is not good for this purpose, but bear's grease is excellent.

1923 H. Smith MENOMINI 52. "The resinous buds are boiled in fat to make a salve for dressing wounds and to put up the nostril to cure a cold in the head."

1932 H. Smith OJIBWE 387. "The Pillager Ojibwe cook the buds of the Balsam Poplar in lard or bear fat, and use the cold product for a salve on cuts, wounds or bruises. They also rub it on the inside of the nostrils so that the balsamic odors can course through the respiratory passages and open them in case of congestion from cold, catarrh or bronchitis."

1933 H. Smith POTAWATOMI 81. "The Forest Potawatomi count this one of their most valuable remedies for making salve. The winter buds are melted with mutton or bear tallow to form an ointment for persistent sores and to cure eczema."

1931 Grieve England 79. "The buds of *P. balsamifera*. . .imported into Europe under the name of Tacamahaca. They are covered with a fragrant resinous matter, which may be separated in boiling water, the odour being like incense, and the taste bitter and rather unpleasant. . .A tincture of them is useful for complaints of the chest, stomach, and kidneys, and for rheumatism and scurvy. With lard or oil they are useful as an external application on bruises, swellings, and some cutaneous diseases. . .The bark. . .is tonic and cathartic."

1955 Mockle Quebec transl. 32. "The bark is emetic and cathartic. The buds give a resin known as Balm of Tacamahaca, possessing resolutive and vulnerary properties."

1959 Leising Arctic 91. "Often we found patches of rough-barked poplar, or Balm of Gilead, growing straight to sixty feet with three foot butts."

Bisabolol in the young shoots of *P. tacamahaca* is active against tubercle bacilli (Lewis and Elvin-Lewis 1977:361).

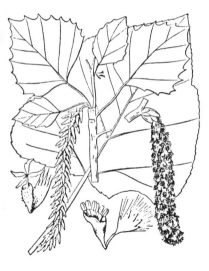 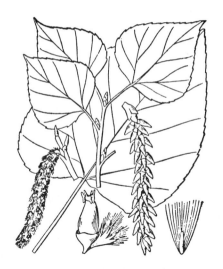

LARGE TOOTHED ASPEN   TREMBLING ASPEN

LARGE TOOTHED ASPEN *Populus grandidentata* Michx.
Tree with light greenish-grey bark when young becoming dark brown grey and furrowed when old. Leaves with not less than 12 large teeth on each side; mostly not more than twice as long as broad on stalks more than a third as long and flattened so that the leaves tremble in the wind. The buds dull brown, finely hairy, not sticky.
Range. N.B., P.E.I., N.S., Que., Ont. and Man., s. to Minn., Mo., Tenn. and N.C. in dry woods, slopes and recently burnt over land.
Common names. White poplar.

ASPEN, TREMBLING *Populus tremuloides* Michx.
A slender tree with smooth pale green almost white waxy bark becoming dark and furrowed when old. Leaves nearly circular with an abrupt short tip, fine teeth on the margin, deep green above, paler below with prominent centre vein, on stalks that are very flat enabling the leaves to tremble even when there appears to be no air movement. The end buds shining brown but not sticky, pointed.
Range. Lab., Nfld., N.B., P.E.I., N.S., Que., northernmost Ont. and Man., to Yukon and Alaska, s. to Baja Calif., n. Mex., Mex., Mo., Tenn., Va. and N.J. in dry or moist soil, especially in cut over land. One of the first trees to grow up and its shade enables other species to gradually establish themselves.
Common names. American aspen, quiver leaf, quaking or mountain aspen, white poplar.
790 ± 200 A.D. Ash and Canter's caves Ohio the bark and bast fiber of *P. tremuloides* found. UMMAEL Rept. 15 Yarnell 1964.
1624 Sagard HURON 13. "They eat also sometimes a certain bark of raw wood, similar to the willow, of which I ate in imitation of the Indians."
1633 Gerarde-Johnson 1488. "The white poplar [*P. alba* of Europe] hath a clensing facultie. . .The barke, as Dioscorides writeth, to the weight of an ounce (or as others say, and that more truly, of little more than a dram) is a good remedie for the Sciatica or ache in the huckle bone, and for the strangurie. . .The same barke is also reported to make a woman barren, if it be drunke with the kidney of a Mule, which thing the leaves likewise are thought to perform, being taken after the floures or reds be ended. The warm juice of the leaves being dropped into the eares doth take away the paine therof. . .in French, Peuplier blanc, Aubeau."
1661 Le Jeune Jes. Rel. In addition to bark, leaves as that of the aspen were also eaten (Aller 1958:64).

1663 Boucher Quebec transl. 48. "One finds here 'Trembles', [trembling aspens and poplars,] of all kinds; that is to say big and little, which serve as food for the beavers, who love their bark."

1710 Raudot ILLINOIS 385. "The black poplar is also a tree of this country. It grows very tall and big and serves these savages in making large canoes for navigating on their rivers and lakes. Formerly, it was an endless task for them to make these canoes; not using iron, it was necessary to set fire to the foot of a tree, to fell it and scrape it with their stone axes, and to remove the charcoal which remained on, in order that the fire penetrate to the center. After felling it they cut it the same way to the length they wish and also hollow it out with fire."

1724 Anon ILLINOIS MIAMI mss 224. "The bark of samelier or Ebeaupin chewed or crushed, for wounds."

1778 Carver 264. "In the spring of the year, the Naudowessies eat the inside bark of a shrub they gather in some part of their country; but I could not learn the name of it, or discover whence they got it. It was of a brittle nature and easily masticated. The taste of it was very agreeable, and they said it was extremely nourishing. In flavour it was not unlike the turnip, and when received into the mouth resembled that root both in its pulpous and frangible nature."

1830 Rafinesque 252. "Poplar. All sp. useful. Wood white, soft, chip hats made with it, cotton of the seeds makes paper and cloth. . .Inner bark used by Indians and empirics in tea or bitters for faintness, hepatic and nephritic diseases. . .Tonic, stomachic, febrifuge."

1859-61 Gunn 845. "Quaking asp (*P. tremuloides*). . .The inner bark. . .is one of our best bitter tonics; in other words, is an excellent ague medicine, useful in all cases of ague and intermittent and bilious fevers, and wherever a good tonic, antiperiodic, and strengthening medicine is needed. . .Be used freely in infusion."

1868 Can. Pharm J. 6; 83-5. The bark of *Populus tremuloides* included in list of Can. medicinal plants.

1884 Holmes-Haydon CREE Hudson Bay 303. "Metoos (*Populus* sp.?) Poplar bark.—This bark is in the form of thin flat strips of fiber about half an inch wide and half a line thick. It has a bitter, slightly mucilaginous taste with some astringency, and a fibrous texture. The colour externally is dull brown and on the inner surface yellowish. Another form of the bark consists of thinner pieces torn into fine shreds. It is used in coughs, half an ounce, in the form of decoction, being the dose. The inner bark of the poplar is eaten in the spring by the Indians, and is considered to act as a mild purgative. Mr. Haydon says he has eaten pounds of it without any effect being produced. It is at that time pleasant in flavour, being sweetish and very tender."

1885 Hoffman OJIBWA 199. "*P. monilifera* cottonwood. The cotton down is applied over open sores as an absorbent."

1892 Millspaugh 162. "*P. tremuloides*. Its wood is light and of an inferior quality except for the lighter household utensils and the manufacture of certain chip hats. . .Populin. This aromatic glucoside was determined by Braconnot in 1830. It exists in company with salicin in the bark and especially in the leaves. . .This body is very similar in its properties and reactions to salicin, from which it seems to differ only in being in intimate combination with benzoic acid."

1894 Household Guide Toronto 113. "The american poplar. This is a good tonic, and is a good remedy for chronic rheumatism, dyspepsia and general debility. Use only the inner part, dried and powdered. Dose a heaping teaspoonful three or four times a day."

1901 Morice DENE Arctic 22. "In no case was amputation resorted to, except when it was self evident that the limb, foot, or finger was too deeply cut to allow of the edges of the wound becoming reunited. In such cases the bark of the aspen root, (*Populus tremuloides*) was much esteemed as an astringent. More than once, too, persons supposed to be endowed with magic powers, and who were on that account styled (he whose mouth affects cure), were in times past asked to suck the blood out of the wound so as to prevent gangrene or any other undesirable result."

1915 Speck PENOBSCOT MALECITE 310. "*P. tremuloides*, poplar bark is steeped for colds, it produces a sweat. . .315. MONTAGNAIS. Bark scraped, dried, and kept until needed, is steeped and given to children suffering from worms. Too much of it however is considered dangerous."

1926-7 Densmore CHIPPEWA 338. The inner bark of *P. tremuloides*, aspen, used in a ceremonially prepared medicine in conjunction with that of the bur and red oaks and the buds, root and blossom of the balsam poplar and the root of seneca snakeroot for heart trouble. [For formula and preparation see seneca snakeroot in woods.]. . .350. For cuts' spit on the cut and draw the edges together, then chew this bark [aspen] and apply thickly like a poultice as soon as possible, dried root may be used in the same manner. . .358. One root of the aspen and one of the balsam poplar are put in a quart of water and steeped, not boiled. Drink about every hour. This is used for excessive flowing during confinement or to prevent premature birth. . .320. Aspen, if the bark of the poplar is cut and turned back from the wood in the early summer there is found between the bark and the wood a sweetish sirup which can be put in birch bark and kept a short time. This is especially liked by children and young people. . .321. A Canadian Chippewa said that he peeled the outside bark from the poplar. . .and scraped the inner bark obtaining a little sap which he put in a small makuk [birch bark box]. He said that it had a sweetish taste and 'would keep quite a while.'

1928 Parker SENECA 11. Poplar bark as a sedative.

1931 Tantaquidgeon CAN. DELAWARE Grand River Reserve [1972] and related Algonkian Indians. *P. tremuloides* leaves used in medicine for infants, the roots in decoction as a tonic for general debility, female weakness, the bark for colds, also antiscorbutic.

1935 Jenness Parry Island Lake Huron OJIBWA 81. "Do not use poplar for any purpose, unless for certain medicines. . .49. A boy who passed through the critical stage without fasting and obtaining a vision became ill likewise, for his soul and shadow lacked guidance and could not work harmoniously with his body, so that blood failed to flow freely through his veins. A tonic brewed with poplar bark would then stimulate the flow of blood, and atune the boy to receive his vision."

1928 H. Smith MESKWAKI 245. "Trembling aspen. The buds are boiled in fat to make a salve or balm for nasal application to cure coughs and colds for children or adults."

1932 H. Smith OJIBWE 387. "Large toothed aspen. The Flambeau Ojibwe use the young roots of this tree in a tea as a hemostatic. Quaking aspen used in the same manner. They use the bark of a young trunk for poulticing cuts and wounds. The astringent salicin in the inner bark undoubtedly draws the cuts together and causes healing. The Pillager Ojibwe. . .use the inner bark for poulticing a sore arm or leg, and make the inner layer of their splints of the inner bark so that a broken limb may heal healthily. . .Externally the whites have used it as a wash for gangrenous wounds, eczema, cancer, burns and body odor. . .410. The Ojibwe scrape the cambium layer of the large toothed aspen to obtain a food which is boiled and is something like eggs."

1933 H. Smith POTAWATOMI 81. "Quaking aspen. The Forest Potawatomi burn the bark and save the ashes to mix with lard which forms a salve to apply to sores upon horses."

1945 Rousseau MOHAWK transl. 39. "*Populus deltoides*, Liard, a little hot water with the bark in it gets rid of intestinal worms. For horses, the bark is dried and reduced to flour, a paste made with a little cold water and applied to the blisters filled with worms on the skin. The bark must be gathered only in the autumn."

1945 Raymond TETE DE BOULE transl. 130. "*Populus tremuloides* the fibrous rootlets are boiled to a consistency of a sirup and applied to rheumatic or painful joints."

1955 Mockle Quebec transl. 32. "*P. tremuloides*, the bark a vermifuge; also the bark of *P. monilifera* [*P. deltoides*]."

1966 Campbell, Best, Budd 71. "*P. tremuloides*, aspen poplar. Nearly all classes of livestock including game will graze upon aspen during all seasons of the year. . .Leaves as well as young twigs will be readily eaten. Chemical analysis of these indicates high protein and phosphorous and extremely low fiber content."

1972 Assiniwi 103. "When you feel tired, boil this inner bark and add some of the syrup that you get to your favorite tonic, or mix it with maple syrup or molasses. You will be surprised how quickly it gives you back your strength."

1978 Dotto Globe and Mail 22 Aug. "Poplar leaves have a taste somewhat like spinach. What's more they are good for you, about 20 to 30 percent of their dry weight is protein (better than some grains) and they contain a higher percentage of the eight amino acids than do oats, wheat, maize or rice, (Amino acids are the building blocks of proteins), according to Dr. Zsuffa, a forest geneticist with the Ontario Ministry of Natural Resources in charge of its poplar breeding program. He is almost positive that protein extracted from poplar leaves could be used as a food for humans. The results of tests have been very encouraging. . .D.M. Roy and Ernest Chen, scientists at the University of Toronto, are mashing up poplar leaves to produce a concentrate that is being used by Canada Packers Ltd. in experimental feeding tests with roosters. Dr. Zsuffa said that the concentrate is almost as nutritional as meat, but can be produced more quickly and cheaply. The Ministry's poplar breeding program is one of its major forest genetic projects. . .In their early years poplar trees can grow as much as 10 feet a year. . .William Raitanen, the forester in charge of the Eastern Ontario Field project, said that poplar can be grown on 'mini-rotation' (harvested every two years as a crop); on 'short rotation (harvested every 10 years for fuel and fiber); or on 'long rotation' (harvested every 30 years for timber). . .Dr. Zsuffa believes that poplar can be a source of food and energy (it can be used to produce methanol) and that it will be used increasingly for timber, and pulp and paper."

[See W.H. Anderson and L. Zsuffa. Yield and Wood quality of Hybrid cottonwood grown in two-year rotation. 1975. It is the hybrid of *P. deltoides* x *nigra* whose clones are used to reproduce the best trees.]

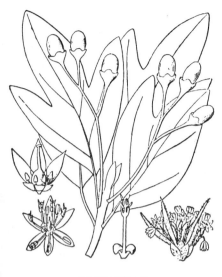

SASSAFRAS

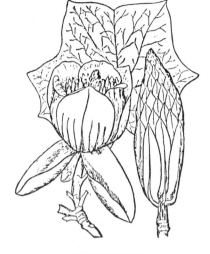

TULIP TREE

SASSAFRAS *Sassafras albidum* (Nutt.) Lauraceae (*S. officinale, Laurus sassafras*)
Shrub in the north or tree to 30 m in the south of its range. Leaves on long stems, silky beneath
when young and of various shapes with 3 main veins. Flowers greenish-yellow with red stems up
to 1 cm long. Berries blue.
Range. sw. Me. to s. Ont. (n. to Peel and York co.), Ill., Io., Kan., s. to Tex. and Fla. in woods
and thickets.
Common names. Saxafras, saloop, ague tree, cinnamon-wood, smelling tree.
1574 Monardes Seville transl. Frampton London 1577. "The Spaniards did begin to cure themselves with the water of this tree and it did in them greate effectes, that it is almost incredible: for
with the naughtie meates and drinkyng of the rawe waters, and slepying in the dewes, the moste
parte of them came to fall into continuall Agues. . .Thei took up the roote of this Tree and tooke
a peece thereof suche as it seemed to theim beste, thei cutte it small into verie thinne and little
peeces and cast them into water at discretion, little more or lesse, and thei sodde it the tyme that
seemed nedefull for to remaine of a good colour, and so thei dranke it in the mornyng fastyng
and in the daie tyme and at dinner and supper, without keeyng any more waight or measure,
than I have saied. . .theie were healed of so many griefes and evill diseases, that to heare of them
what thei suffred and how thei were healed it doeth bryng admiration and thei which were whole
dranke it in place of wine, for it doeth preserve them in healthe. . .[Sailing ships, months on a
voyage, brought seeds and plants to Europe] There came a Packet, as of Letters, inrolled in a
seare clothe [cerecloth-waxed]; so well made that thei might pass to any part beeyng never so farre, the whiche beeyng opened, I found a small cheste made of a little peece of Corke, of a good
thickenesse sette together, which was worthie to be seen, and in the holownesse of it came the
hearbes, and the seeds that the Letter speaketh of, everything written that it was. . .For bicause
that the office of a Souldier is to handle weapons, and to sheed bloud. . .he is much to be
esteemed that he will inquire and searche out herbes, and Plantes and to knowe their properties
and vertue. . .I do esteem much of this Gentlemanne [Who sent me the packet from America]."
1590 Harriot Virginia 9. "Sassafras, called by the inhabitants Winauk, a kinde of wood of most
pleasant and sweet smel: and of most rare vertues in phisick for the cure of many diseases. It is
found by experience to bee farre better and of more uses than the wood which is called Guaiacum [the cure for syphilis at that time]. . .For the description, the manner of using and the mani-
fold vertues thereof, I referre you to the booke of Monardus, translated and entituled in English,
The joyful newes from the West Indies." [Sassafras included by Harriot in the list of Marchanta-
ble commodities found in Virginia].

1609 Lescarbot-Erondelle Acadia 47. "And for the last and sovereign remedy, I send back the patient to the tree of life (for so one may well qualify it), which James Cartier doth call annedda, yet unknown in the coast of Port Royal, unless it be peradventure the sassafras, whereof there is a quantity in certain places. . .297. Sassafras, whose wood is of very good scent and most excellent for curing many diseases, as the pox [syphilis] and the sickness of Canada [scurvy]."

1613 Champlain fac. ed. Mass. Bay 1606 transl. 116. "We saw 200 savages in this place, who are pleasant enough, and there is a quantity of nut trees, red cedar, sassafras, oaks, ashes, and beeches, which are very fine. The chief of this place is called Quiouhamenec." (& y a quantité de noyers, cypres, sasafras, chesnes, fresnes & hestres, qui sont tresbeaux)

1612 Capt. John Smith Virginia 92. "There are also some Cedars and Saxafras trees. They also yield gummes in a small proportion of themselves. Wee tryed conclusions to extract it out of the wood, but nature afforded more then our arts. . .93. There is also Pellitory of Spaine, Sasafrage, and divers other simples." [Sassafras root was gathered on the Massachusetts and Virginia coast for export to England from 1602 onwards. As well, ships bringing supplies to the colonies, returned loaded with sassafras.]

1633 Gerarde-Johnson 1524-5. "Of the Sassafras or Ague tree. . .I have given the figure of a branch taken from a little tree, which grew in the garden of Mr. Wilmot at Bow [England]; who died some few years ago. This tree groweth in most parts of the West Indies. . .and Virginia. . .The best of all the tree is the root, and that worketh the best effect, the which hath the rinde cleaving very fast to the inner part, and is of colour tawnie, and much more sweet of smell than all the tree and his branches. . .The wood hereof cut in smal pieces and boiled in water, to the colour of Claret wine, and drunk for certain daies together, helpeth the dropsie, removeth oppilation or stopping of the liver, cureth quotidian and tertian agues, and long fevers. The root of Sassafras hath power to comfort the liver, and. . .to comfort the weake and feeble stomacke, to cause good appetite, to consume windinesse. . .stay vomiting, and make sweet a stinking breath. It provoketh urine, removeth the impediments that doe cause barrennesse, and maketh women apt to conceive."

1656-57 Le Jeune ONONDAGA Jes. Rel. 43; 259. "But the most common and most wonderful plant in those countries is that which we call the universal plant, because its leaves, when powdered, heal in a short time wounds of all kinds; these leaves which are as broad as one's hand, have the shape of a lily as depicted in heraldry; and its roots have the smell of the laurel. The most vivid scarlet, the brightest green, the most natural yellow and orange of Europe pale before the various colors that our savages procure from its roots."

1687 John Clayton Virginia 8. "The oyl of sassafras leaves may be deservedly considered too, for they will entirely dissolve into an oyle. . .11. And first the Sassafras tree, whose root is well enough known. It shoots forth its blossoms in March, which are yellow and grow in little bunches like grape-flowers. And which when gathered and picked from the husky bud, make a curious preserve. Most Sassafras trees blossom, few bear berrys, but those that do are generally very thick, they are shaped much like those of Dulcamara, but are black of colour and very aromatic, I take them to have considerable virtues."

1748 Kalm Philadelphia October 1st. 78. "The Sassafras tree. . .The people here gather its flowers and use them instead of tea. But the wood itself is of no use in husbandry. . .The bark of this tree is used by the women here in dyeing worsted a fine lasting orange color, which does not fade in the sun. They use urine instead of alum in dyeing, and boil the dye in a fine brass boiler, because in an iron vessel it does not yield so fine a color. Mr. Bartram told me that a woman in Virginia had successfully employed the berries of the sassfras to cure a severe pain in one of her feet, which she had had for three years in such a degree that it almost hindered her from walking. She was advised to boil the berries of sassfras, and to rub the painful parts of her foot with the oil which by this means would be gotten from the berries. She did so, but at the same time it made her vomit; yet this was not sufficient to keep her from following the prescription three more times, though as often as she made use thereof if it always had the same effect. However she was entirely freed from the pain and recovered completely. . .179. Some people peel the root, and boil the peel with the beer which they may be brewing, because they believe it wholesome. The peel is put into brandy, either while it is distilling or after it is made. An old Swede remembered that his mother cured many people of the dropsy with a decoction of the root of sassafras in water drunk every morning. At the same time she used to cup the patient on the feet. The old man assured me he had often seen people cured by this means, who had been brought to his mother wrapped up in sheets. . .Several of the Swedes wash and scour the vessels in which they intend to keep cider, beer, or brandy with water in which the sassfras root or its peel has been boiled, which they think renders all those liquors more wholesome. Some people have their bed-posts made of sassafras wood to expel the bed bugs, for its strong scent it is said, prevents vermin from settling in them. . .Some Englishmen related, that some years ago it had been customary in London, to drink a kind of tea of the flowers of sassafras, because it was looked upon as very healthful, but upon recollecting that the same potion was much used against the venereal disease, it was soon left off, lest those who used it should be looked upon as infected with that disease. In Pennsylvania some people put chips of sassafras into their chests, where they keep woolen stuffs, in order to expel the moths. . .1749 Hudson River 606. Colonel Lydius of Fort Nicholson told me that the natives [Indians] consider the sassafras very valuable in the treatment of diseases of the eyes. They take the young slips, cut them in halves, scrape out the pith or the medulla, put it in water, and after it has been there for some time, wash the eyes with the same water. When the natives from Canada came formerly to his house at the carrying place they were very anxious to hunt for sassafras. They cut the stem in two, took out the piths and preserved it and took it home with them to use as described above. . .Montreal 408. Sassafras is planted here, for it is never found wild in these parts, Fort Anne being the most northerly place where I have found it wild. Those shrubs which were on the island had been planted many years ago; however, they were only small shrubs, from two to three feet high, and scarcely that much. The reason is that the mainstem is killed every winter almost down to the very root, and must produce new shoots every spring, as I have found from my own observations here."

1817-20 Bigelow 146. "The bark and wood of the sassafras were formerly much celebrated in the cure of various complaints, particularly syphilis, rheumatism and dropsy. Its reputation as a specific in those diseases, particularly the first, has fallen into deserved oblivion, it is now recognised only as a warm stimulant and diaphoretic. It is retained by the Dispensatories as an ingredient in several preparations, particularly the compound decoction of guaiacum, formerly called 'decoction of the woods;' and the compound decoction of Sarsaparilla [Mexican], formerly the 'Lisbon diet drink.'. .They derive. . .more of their efficacy from their other ingredients, than from the Sassafras, a principal part of the efficacy of which is dissipated by boiling."

1823 Lamb Elia Chimney Sweeps 128. "There is a composition, the ground work of which I have understood to be the sweet wood 'yclept sassafras'. This wood boiled down to a kind of tea, and tempered with an infusion of milk and sugar, hath to some tastes a delicacy beyond the China luxury. . .I have always found that this composition is surprisingly gratifying to the palate of a young chimney sweeper. . .This is Saloop, the precocious herb-woman's darling—the delight of the early gardner."

1820's Mat. Med. Edinburgh-Toronto mss 59. "*Laurus sassafras*, slightly stimulant & Diaphoretic. Its infusion has been drunk freely in Chronic Rheumatism & Cutaneous diseases. It is often added to the Infusions of Sarsaparilla [Mexican] Quaiacum & Mezereon employed in the treatment of protracted syphilitic affections."

1830 Rafinesque 235. "Roots, bark, leaves, flowers fragrant and spicy. Flavor and smell peculiar, similar to Fennel, sweetish subacid, residing in a volatile oil heavier than water. The *Sassafrine*, a peculiar mucus unalterable by alcohol, found chiefly in the twigs and pith, thickens water, very mild and lubricating, very useful in ophthalmia, dysentery, gravel, catarrh, &c. Wood yellow, hard, durable, soon loses the smell, the roots chiefly exported for use as stimulant, antispasmodic, sudorific and depurative; the oil now often substituted; both useful in rheumatism, cutaneous diseases, secondary syphilis, typhus fevers, &c. Once used in dropsy. The Indians use a strong decoction to purge and clean the body in the spring: we use instead the tea of the blossoms for a vernal purification of the blood. The powder of the leaves used to make glutinous Gombos [soupy stews]. Leaves and buds used to flavor some Beers and Spirits. Also deemed vulnerary and resolvent chewed and applied, or menagogue and corroborant for women in tea; useful in scurvy, cachexy, flatulence, &c. Bowls and cups made of the wood, when fresh it drives bugs and moths. The bark dyes wood of a fine orange color with urine, called *Shikih* by Missouri tribes, and smoked like tobacco."

1859-61 Gunn 853. "A tea made of the root. . .is often used as a beverage at the table, and by many is very much liked. . .is especially good to purify the system in the Spring of the year. As a medicine it is generally used in combination with other alteratives to improve the taste as well as the medicinal virtues. . .There is an essential oil obtained from Sassafras, by distillation, which is often employed with benefit in liniments, embrocations, and external applications; and also used internally with good effect in certain cases, such as painful menstruation, in painful diseases of the kidneys, and the pains which sometimes follow parturition or child-birth."

1868 Can. Pharm. J. 6; 83-5. The bark of the root of sassafras included in list of Can. medicinal plants.

1894 Household Guide Toronto 122. "The bark made into a tea makes a pleasant drink, and will relieve dysentery and inflammation of the bladder. It will also relieve inflammation of the eyes when applied externally."

1915 W.R. Harris 50. "From the roots of the sassafras the Indians made a cooling drink which they used when attacked by fevers or colds. When afflicted with snow or smoke blindness they steeped the pith of the sassafras sprouts or roots in water and with it bathed their eyes. . .56. Sassafras. A moderately sized tree of the laurel family with spicy aromatic bark and roots, common enough around Toronto. It grows from Ontario to the Gulf of Mexico. It is a powerful febrifuge."

1916 Waugh IROQUOIS 148. "Sassafras was widely used. A tea made of the roots. This was frequently employed at weddings on account of its agreeable odor. . .The tree was also highly valued for its medicinal virtues."

1928 Parker SENECA 11. Sassafras leaves used as a laxative. . .as a carminative. . .12. Sassafras tea for coryza [colds], for dyspepsia.

1928 H. Smith MESKWAKI 193. The root of the blue vervain mixed with the root bark of sassafras was a remedy for fits.

1931 Grieve 716. "Oil of Sassafras is chiefly used for flavouring purposes, particularly to conceal the flavour of opium when given to children. . .A teaspoonful of the oil produced dilated pupils, stupor and collapse in a young man. . .Its use has caused abortion in several cases. Dr. Shelby of Huntsville stated that it would both prevent and remove the injurious effects of tobacco. . .The oil can produce marked narcotic poisoning, and death by causing widespread fatty degeneration of the heart, liver, and kidneys, or, in a larger dose, by great depression of the circulation, followed by a centric paralysis of respiration."

1933 Can. Formulary 60. Oil of sassafras, the volatile oil distilled from the root. . .66. Compound syrup of sassafras, includes oil of sassafras and of anise, methyl salicylate, liquorice, syrup and alcohol.

1942 Fenton IROQUOIS 515. "Sassafras serves as an example of how the Iroquois contributed to the introduction of medicines into Europe. Sassafras was. . .employed by all Iroquois as a tonic, created at one time in Europe a stir like that which attended the discovery of. . .vitamins in our own time. . .Since it had been long known among them as a blood purifier, it is not strange that the Iroquois employed it to heal venereal diseases. . .Seneca warriors carried the powdered leaves, women employed it as a tonic after childbirth, it was used in cases of rheumatism, and as a diuretic. . .Iroquois herbalists have regularly peddled the root bark on the doorsteps of their white neighbours."

1955 Mockle Quebec transl. 44. "*Sassafras officinale* in woods and fields of Quebec and Ontario. The bark of the roots is used as a depurative and sudorific. The essence extracted from it is considered as carminative and antiseptic."

Constitutents of Sassafras, about 2% of volatile oil, which contains about 80% safrole, as well as phellandrene and pinene. The wood is used as a diuretic, stimulant and diaphoretic (T.E. Wallis 1967:59).

Safrole is a component of many essential oils such as those of mace, nutmeg, California bay laurel. It was used in root beer. When as much as 0.5 to 1% of their total food was safrole rats developed hepatomas [liver cancers]. The twigs without their bark are antiseptic, they can disinfect the root canals of teeth. Safrole is chemically related to myristicin and asarone and is suspected of being hallucinogenic in large doses. It is carcinogenic (Lewis and Elvin-Lewis 1977).

TULIP TREE   *Liriodendron tulipifera* L. Magnoliaceae

Sturdy tree up to 60 m with brownish bark furrowed into close, interlacing rounded ridges. The leaves are distinctive, 8-14 cm long and about as wide with two points on each side and the top seemingly cut off, on a long stalk, no teeth. The flowers are alone at the end of the shining brown twigs, greenish-yellow 4-5 cm, each petal with a large basal orange blotch within. The seeds are winged nutlets set overlapping each other on the fruit stalk.

Range. Vt., sw. Ont., s. Mich., and Mo., s. to Fla. and La. often cult. May, in rich woods in deep moist soils.

Common names. Yellow poplar, white wood, canoe tree.

1590 Harriot Virginia Indians 23. "Rakiock, a kind of trees so called that are sweet wood of which the inhabitants that were neere unto us doe commonly make their boats or Canoes of the form of trowes, [troughs] only with the helpe of fire, harchets of stones, and shels; we have known some so great being made in that sort of one tree that they have carried well xx men at once, besides much baggage: the timber being great, tal, streight, soft, light, & yet tough enough I thinke (besides other uses) to be fit for masts of ships."

1613 Champlain fac. ed. New England coast 1605 transl. 75. "Those who live here have canoes made from one piece of wood, very difficult to turn, if one is not very adroit in steering it: and we had never seen any made like this before, here is how they make it. After a lot of difficulty and a long time in cutting down the tallest and biggest tree they can find, with hatchets of stone (for they haven't any others, if there are not a few of them who have got some [of iron] from the savages of the coast of Acadia, to whom they bring furs to trade) they lift off the bark and round it, except for one side, where they set fire, little by little all the length of the logs: & taking several red hot stones that they place on it: & when the fire is too sharp they put it out with a little water, not entirely, but from fear that the edge of the canoe might burn. When it is hollowed out enough for their fancy, they scrape all the parts with stones, which they use instead of knives." [Basswood, poplar and elm were also used for dugout canoes].

1612 Capt. John Smith Virginia Indians 103. "Their fishing is much in boats. These they make of one tree by bowing [burning] and scratching away the coles with stone and shels till they have made it in the forme of a Trough. Some of them are an elne deep, and 40 or 50 foot in length, and some will beare 40 men, but the most ordinary are smaller, and will beare 10, 20, or 30, according to their bignes."

1633 De Laet New Neth. 57. "The Indians. . .Their boats are one piece of wood, hollowed out by fire from the solid trunks of trees."

1687 Clayton Virginia Indians 11. "They use much the young buds of the *Populus sive Tulippa arbor*, a vast large tree extraordinary spacious, bearing flowers about April much like Tulips, its leaves are large, smooth and well shaped, which together with the flowers, render the tree exceeding beautifull to behold. It bears its seed coniferous, and is an excellent opener of Obstructions."

1748 Kalm October the 19th. Philadelphia 108. "The tulip tree grows everywhere in the woods in this country. . .The Swedes call it 'canoe tree' for both the Indians and Europeans often made their canoes from its trunk. The Englishmen in Pennsylvania give it the name of poplar. It is considered to grow to the greatest height and thickness of any in North America. . .Its wood is used here for canoes, boards, planks, bowls, dishes, spoons, doorposts, and all sorts of joiners' work. I have seen a barn of considerable size whose walls and roof were made of a single tree of this kind, split into boards. Some joiners reckon this wood better than oak, because the latter frequently is warped, while the former is not, and can easily be worked. . .It is certain that it contracts enough in hot weather to occasion great cracks in the boards, and in wet weather it swells so as to be near bursting. . .The bark. . .is divisible into very thin layers, which are very tough like bast, though I have never seen it employed as such. The leaves when crushed and applied to the forehead are said to be a remedy for headache. When horses are plagued with worms, the bark is pounded and given to them in dry form. Many people believe its roots to be as efficacious against the fever as the Jesuits' bark. The trees grow on all sorts of dry soil". . .1749 26th. November 642. "Leaves held to be a remedy for gout."

1794 Loskiel 1; 115. The fruit and root bark a powerful Indian specific against agues.

1808 Cuming 392. The decoction of the root of this tree an infallible remedy for bite of any snake and "a most powerful alterative and purifier of the blood." [Vogel 1964:386.]

1817-20 Bigelow 112-3. "The disease in which it has been most employed is in intermittent fever. . .As a warm sudorific, this bark seems well adapted to the treatment of chronic rheumatism, and for this purpose it has been employed with success by various medical practitioners in the United States. . .The wood of the Tulip tree is smooth and fine grained, very easily wrought and not liable to split. It is used for various kinds of carving and ornamental work, and for articles of house furniture. In the western States where pine lumber is scarce, Michaux tells us, that the joinery or inside work of houses is most frequently of this material. A common use of it throughout the United States is in the manufacture of carriages to form panels of coach and chaise bodies. For this purpose it is particularly fitted by its smoothness, flexibility and toughness. The true or heart wood of this tree is of a yellowish colour and differs in proportion in different trunks. The Tulip tree has long since been introduced from this country into the forests and fields of Europe. Its use, ornamental appearance, and the facility with which it is raised have rendered it one of the most prominent and interesting objects of forest cultivation."

1830 Rafinesque 239-40. "Tulip tree, poplar, white wood, yellow wood. Valuable, ornamental and medical. Reaching 120 feet high and 30 round. Durable timber, heavy hard and tough, but subject to warp,. . .Espetonga of the Osages, use bark of roots and green seeds as febrifuge and vermifuge for children. Found from Lake Champlain to Texas, in rich soils. Medical. . .Bark must be collected in the winter. Active tonic, antiseptic, stimulant and sudorific, deemed equal to Cinchona in the same doses for intermittent and low fevers, weak stomach, dyspepsia, hysteria, dysentery, chronic rheumatism, gout, &c. Used in powder, infusion, tincture and extract. Contains gum, resin, mucus, fecula, muriatic acid and oil &c. A palliative in phthisis. Sometimes used in cholera infantum and worms, also in the botts of horses. . . .Inner bark of the root most powerful: a fine cordial made with it. Leaves used by Cherokees in poultice for sores and headache, ointment for inflammations and morifications: make the milk of cows bitter. Extract of the root equal to Gentian. Remedy for syphilitic ulcers of the nose. Seeds laxative."

1859-61 Gunn 840. "Poplar (*Liriodendron Tulipifera*). This is the common Poplar tree; known also as the Tulip tree. . .used extensively for lumber. It is sometimes called White and sometimes Yellow poplar, and is one of the finest, as well as most useful trees, of the American forest. . .The bark of the root is the part used. . .There is no root or bark, within my knowledge, that I consider more valuable, and during a long experience it has proved in my hands one of the most valuable of remedies, and may be given in every instance to restore the general health. I have found it superior to the Peruvian Bark, and when administered in equal quantities with Wild Cherry and Dogwood bark, to which may be added, after the decoction is made by boiling, a portion of good French Brandy. . .will prove a certain and speedy remedy in the chills, intermittent fever, worms, hysteria, commonly called hysterics, which generally arises from a diseased womb. In dyspeptic states of the stomach and bowels, this is a valuable remedy, owing to its tonic or stimulating powers. . .The infusion or decoction is made with half an ounce of the powder of the dried root bark to a pint of boiling water. . .boiling as strong as possible and adding as much good spirit as will keep it from getting sour. Dose from half to a wineglassful three times a day, before meals for an adult."

1892 Millspaugh 12. "Tulip tree yields a bark that is at once bitter and aromatic, much valued as a stimulating tonic and diaphoretic in intermittents and chronic rheumatism; it should be proven."

1973 Hosie 212. "In 1886, a popular heart stimulant was first extracted from the inner bark of the root of the Tulip tree." [This bark contains tulipiferine, which supposedly exerts a strong effect on the heart and nerves.]

SHRUBS AND VINES

including cherry and hawthorn trees

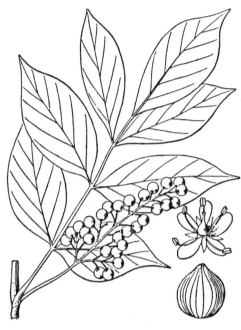

POISON OAK POISON SUMAC

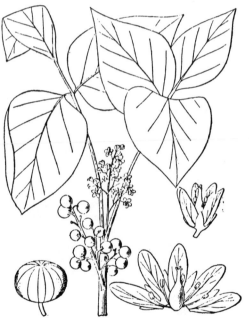

POISON IVY

POISON IVY   *Toxicodendron radicans* (L.) Ktze. Anacardiaceae (*Rhus radicans*)
A plant of many sizes and shapes, but with leaves that always consist of three leaflets with pointed tips, the middle leaflet on a long stalk. The shape of the leaflets varies greatly, oak like, mitten like, plain or with teeth, smooth or lightly hairy. *T. rydbergii* is a northern plant extending south to N.Y. and Ind. or in the mts. to Va. It has a short erect stem, scarcely branched, with a few leaves near the top. *T. radicans* throughout the range has a woody stem, straggling or climbing by aerial rootlets on trees, posts up to 10 m. It rarely has toothed leaves. Both kinds may have leaves that are purplish in the early spring, shining green in summer and vivid red in the fall, unless growing in the shade. All have greenish white flowers growing inconspicuously from the stem where the leaf is attached. These produce clusters of greyish fruit.
Range. Throughout Canada and the U.S. s. to Mex. and the W.Ind.
Common names. Climbing or three leaved ivy, poison oak, climath, mercury.

POISON OAK POISON SUMAC   *Toxicodendron vernix* (L.) Ktze. (*Rhus vernix, R. venenata*)
A shrub to 5 m tall often branched from the base. The leaves with 7-13 leaflets, without teeth, 4-8 cm long each and smooth. The flowering stem to 20 cm with green flowers followed by greyish white fruit. This is the most poisonous sumac.
Range. Along the north shore of Lake Erie, and from Me. to Minn., s. to Ind., Ohio, Fla. and Tex. in swamps.
All the poison ivy or sumac release a white juice when a leaf or stem is broken. This juice turns black on exposure to the air and carries in it the poisonous resin toxicodendrol, that causes the skin of a sensitive person, on contact, to develop allergic symptoms. Burning poison ivy or sumac leaves, twigs, roots, releases this resin in the form of tiny droplets on particles of the ash and dust in the smoke from the fire and can cause severe reactions. There is no cure for the allergic symptoms but there are many treatments.
1557-58 Thevet transl. 422. [The Indians of the St. Lawrence during their wars.] "They also use poisons made from the leaves of trees, herbs, and fruits, which are dried in the sun, and placed amongst the faggots and branches, then they set fire when they see the enemy approaching. . .1575.1012. Or, to fortify themselves, without loosing any of their men, they take a lot of faggots, pieces of small wood tied together, and branches of cedar all greased with seal and other fish oil, & some poisonous composition, & seeing their enemies, try to turn them against the wind, & place their enemy to face it [the wind] : & then they set fire to the faggots, from which comes a smoke so thick, black and dangerous to breathe, as much for the fetid odor as for the poison mixed in these faggots, that several are suffocated."
1635 Cornut 97. Illustration of *Rhus radicans* called "edera trifolia canadensis" drawn from plants in the garden of the Faculty of Medicine, Paris, curator, Robin, sent there from Canada.
1748 Kalm Philadelphia September the 20th. 43. "Poisonous trees. A species of *Rhus*. . .here called the 'poison tree' by both English and Swedes. . .October 9th. 94. Poison Ivy. . .I also know that of two sisters, one could handle the tree without being affected by its poison, and the other immediately felt it as soon as the exhalation of the tree came near her."
1778 Carver 507. "The alder or elder, termed the poisonous elder. . .endowed with a very extraordinary quality, that renders it poisonous to some constitutions. . .others may even chew the leaves or the rind without receiving the least deteriment from them: the poison however is not mortal, though it operates very violently on the infected person, whose body and head swell to an amazing size, and are covered with eruptions, that at their height resemble the confluent small-pox. As it grows in so many provinces, the inhabitants cure its venom by drinking saffron tea, and anointing the external parts with a mixture composed of cream and marsh mallows."
1785 Cutler Boston. A milky juice exudes from the stalk and leaves which will stain linen a deep and unfading black. It is said to have been used by the Indians to stain the hardest substances black.
1788 Dufresnoy France transl. The Properties of the plant called *Rhus Radicans*, its utility and the success obtained with it in curing skin diseases and the paralysis of the lower limbs. [Cited Coulter 1973:64].
1779 Zeisberger DELAWARE 56. "The so-called Poison Vine grows plentifully in the bottoms. It climbs up the trees, much as a grape vine will, the main stem becoming as thick as an arm. Some are affected with swelling in the face and body if they touch it, others, even when the wind blows over it upon them. This is very painful until cured. Others do not suffer from the vine at all. This holds good of Indians as of others."

1791 Lewis Mat. Med. ed. Aitkin 255. "This tree is a native of America though it has been introduced into England ever since the year 1640. People can be poisoned by the smell when the tree is cut down, by the smoke of the tree being burnt, by handling any part of it. Blindness can ensue but it goes off in a few days. Sallal [*Gaultheria shallon*] oil and cream rubbed upon the parts, expedites the removal of its effects. The juice is used to dye linen black. Dr. Alderson has found good effects of its use in paralysis. . .and it is probable that this medicine may produce good effects in other cases of nervous affections."

1814 Clarke Consp. 134. *Rhus Toxicodendron* leaves, Poison Oak or Sumach. Stimulant, aperient. In paralytic affections, herpetic eruptions, &c. Dose of the dried leaves. . .It has been given in larger doses but not with marked success, although it afforded relief; the symptoms are prickling or twitching in the paralytic limb."

1817-20 Bigelow 24. "Dr. Thomas Horsfield writing of. . .various unsuccessful experiments with a view to ascertain the nature of this colouring principle, and the means of fixing it on stuffs. He found that the juice expressed from the pounded leaves, did not produce the black colour, and that strong decoctions of the plant, impregnated with various chemical mordants, produced nothing more than a dull yellow, brownish or fawn colour. The reason of this is, that the colouring principle resides not in the sap. . .but in. . .peculiar juice of the plant, that this juice exists only in small quantity, and is wholly insoluble in water. . .This nigrescent juice, in common with that of *Rhus vernix*, has, perhaps, claims to be considered a distinct proximate principle in vegetable chemistry. . .A person who has been in contact with the Rhus and finds himself poisoned, should immediately examine his hands, clothes, &c. to see if there are no spots of the juice adhering to him. These should be removed, as they will keep up and extend the disorder. . .As washing does not eradicate the stains of this very adhesive juice, it is best to rub them off with some absorbent powder. . .It is to be treated with rest, low diet, evacuations, purging with neutral salts is peculiarly useful, blood letting has been found of service. . .acetate of lead. . .should be used in solution rather than in the ointment, that it may be applied as cold as possible. . .a solution of corrosive sublimate can be externally applied in this disease. . .I have found the lead more beneficial of the two. . .The *Rhus radicans* has been administered internally in certain diseases by a few practioners in Europe and America. Dr. Horsefield. . .administered a strong infusion in the dose of about a teacup full to consumptive and anasarcous [dropsical] patients. . .supposed benefit in pulmonary consumption. . .My own opinion is, that the plant under consideration is too uncertain and hazardous to be employed in medicine, or kept in apothecaries' shops."

1820's Mat. Med. Edinburgh-Toronto mss 3. Advantageous in paralysis, 1 grain 2-3 times a day."

1830 Rafinesque 257. "Poison wood or vines, are poisonous even by handling or exposure to the effluvia in some persons. . .remedy, rest, evacuations and parsley poultice, ice and lead. Acrid milky juice, becomes black in the air, forms indelible ink, inspissated becomes fine black resin and varnish, with cinnabar red varnish of Japan. Root used in chronic asthma, anasarca [dropsy], phthisis, obstinate herpetic eruptions. Extract of leaves chiefly used, a specific in palsy, dose a grain, also for hemiplegia and rheumatism. Contains tannin, gallic acid, green fecula, toxine, resin, & poisonous gas is carbonated hydrogen."

1838 Anna Jameson. Georgian Bay Lake Huron 163-4. "Indians, part of the tribe of Aisence (The Clam). . .Old Solomon asked me once or twice how I felt; and I thought his anxiety for my health was caused by the rain; but no, he told me that on the island where we had dined he had observed a great quantity of a certain plant, which, if only touched, causes a dreadful eruption and ulcer all over the body. I asked why he had not shown it to me, and warned me against it? and he assured me that such warning would only have increased the danger, for when there is any knowledge or apprehension of it existing in the mind, the very air blowing from it sometimes infects the frame. Here I appealed to Mr. Jarvis, who replied, 'All I know is, that I once unconsciously touched a leaf of it, and became one ulcer from head to foot; I could not stir for a fortnight.' I do not know the botanical name of this plant, which resembles a dwarf sumach. . .It is said that formerly the Indians used it to poison their arrows."

1841 Trousseau & Pidout France transl. 184. Americans use powder of dry leaves, 4 grms. in 1000 gr boiling water for paralysis. We have used it, no conclusions, it is dangerous.

1842 Christison 926. "The juice and leaves taken internally are narcotico-irritant in large doses; and in small doses they are held to be diuretic, diaphoretic, laxative, and, in respect to the nervous system, stimulant. The leaves have been used in various diseases, but chiefly in chronic palsy, on account of their stimulating action on the nervous system. Their therapeutic effect is said to be attended with twitches of the paralysed muscles and prickling of the affected limb, like those produced by strychnia and nux-vomica. If this remedy is to be retained in the Pharmacopoeias, the preparation for use ought to be either a tincture of the fresh leaves or an extract from the same prepared in vacuo; for its active part is very volatile."

1868 Can. Pharm. J. 6; 83-5. Leaves of *Rhus Toxicodendron* included in list of Can. medicinal plants.

1881 Burgess Can. Pharm. J. 14; 166-68. "*Rhus Venenata*. . .poison dogwood, poison elder, poison ash, poison sumach, swamp sumach, white sumach and varnish tree. . .masses of fragrant bloom, at the ends of the branches, which attract innumerable swarms of bees. Whether the honey derived from this source possesses any poisonous properties I am unable to say, but, as at various times there have been reports of poisoning by honey, it would be well worthy of investigation whether this form of poison ivy does not also abound there. . .this tree makes one of the handsomest shrubs imaginable when in blossom, but is, unfortunately, one of the most deadly. . .when incisions are made into its bark there is a copious flow of viscid fluid. . .which when boiled makes a fine varnish. . .*Rhus Toxicodendron* was first described in 1635 by Cornutus, in his work on Canadian plants, as a species of ivy. The Indians were well aware of its properties."

1882 Canadian Horticulturist 5; 66. "The *Rhus Toxicodendron*, or poison ivy, is often found as a climber and were it not for its poisonous nature it would be a good thing to plant against painted or brick walls, as it will cling like the English ivy. Its poison is more feared than is needful, for if it affects any part of a person's skin it is instantly neutralized if a little soil and spittle, or a drop of water, with a little ammonia in it, is rubbed on the parts affected. (The writer has collected fifty pounds of leaves at one time, and cut them up fine for medicine, but did not suffer, though all was done with hands bare.) Hoping the reader will excuse him, the writer wishes to say that most vegetable poisons on the skin, the sting of bees or wasps, can be instantly rendered harmless, or the pain removed, by rubbing the parts affected with any kind of soft mud."

1890 Horatio C. Wood Ther. Gaz. 14; 95. "I obtained the homeopathic tincture from a large homeopathic pharmacy; I tried it in all forms and doses, homeopathic, small, and large, and found it exceedingly uncertain in its action and giving no definite good result. I was not able to see that the patients progressed, on the average, any more rapidly when taking it than when left to nature and nursing." [Cited Coulter 1973:64]

1892 Millspaugh 38. "*Rhus Toxicodendron*. . .the plant has rapidly gained a place in general practice, meeting with some success in the treatment of paralysis, rheumatism, amaurosis, [disease of optic nerve] and various forms of chronic and obstinate eruptive diseases. The milky juice. . .[is used as] an indelible ink for marking linen, and as an ingredient of liquid dressings or varnishes for finishing boots and shoes. . . .The plant is more poisonous during the night or at any time in June and July when the sun is not shining upon it. Absence of sunlight, together with dampness, seems to favor the exhalation of the volatile principle. . .Of this Porcher says; 'An acrimonius vapor combined with carburetted hydrogen, exhales from a growing plant of the poison oak during the night. It can be collected in a jar, and is capable of inflaming and blistering the skin of persons of excitable constitution, who plunge their arms in it.' . . .There are almost as many antidotes recommended for *Rhustox.* poisoning as for the bite of the rattlesnake."

1894 Household Guide Toronto 180-85. Rhus tox. recommended for use in:—ague, chicken pox, eczema, erysipelas, rheumatic fever, lumbago, paralysis, remittent fever, rheumatism, ringworm, sciatica, warts. [Under section on how to use all kinds of homeopathic remedies].

1902 Chesnut 364. *Rhus diversiloba—Toxicodendron diversilobum* (T.&.G.) Greene. [This species is closely related to poison ivy. It is found in western North America from southern British Columbia to northern Baja California. . .The poisons have never been studied, but are presumably closely related if not identical, to those of poison ivy. Kingsbury 1964] "It is much less vine-like than the eastern poison ivy, but is equally poisonous to the touch. The older full-blooded Indians are not readily poisoned by it, and in fact several of them use it for various household purposes, and have even been seen to eat a dozen leaves or more without distress, but the half-breeds are often badly affected by handling it. . .Its principal medicinal use is to burn out and remove warts from the hands. The practice is carried out by cutting the wart off to the quick and then applying the juice. I was told that after a few applications the root is totally removed inside one or two days. It is used in a similar manner to remove ringworms. One Indian, a Wailaki, informed me that if the fresh leaves were quickly bound to the wound made by a rattlesnake the effect of the venom would be counteracted. The fresh leaves were formerly used by the older squaws not only to wrap up acorn meal for the baking process, but, as the late Dr. Charles Mohr informed the writer, from personal observation among the Concows near Marysville, to mix with it. The object was not ascertained. The slender stems are still occasionally used for circular withes in basket making. The fresh juice turns rapidly black on exposure to the air, and is some-times used on this account to make temporary tattoo marks on the skin. These disappear as soon as the skin is renewed, but the color, as a rule, is very permanent. Some of the purest black strands seen in the Pomo baskets are produced according to Dr. Hudson, by applying the fresh juice to them."

1928 H. Smith MESKWAKI 201. "*Rhus toxicodendron*. . .Indian name climbs trees. This is a dangerous medicine, according to McIntosh, and is used only by the most skilled medicine men. The root is pounded and made into a poultice to put on a swelling to make it open."

1932 H. Smith OJIBWE 354. "Mukwean (Bearskin), Flambeau medicine man, called this a poi-son to the skin and said that the Ojibwe have no distinctive name for it. John Peper, one of the Bear Island Pillager Indians, gave us the Indian name and said that no one now alive there knew how to use it. Since Kepeosatok, Meskwaki medicine man, at Tama, Iowa, used it in a certain manner for poulticing some kinds of swellings, the writer thinks this may be the use to which John Peper referred."

1955 Mockle Quebec transl. 54. "The leaves rubefacient. This species contains in all its parts a whitish juice, resinous, very bitter, containing a toxic principle. Its touch provokes the appear-ance on the whole body of little pustules, accompanied by a painful inflammation. It is believed that different species of *Pycanthemum* [mountain mint] or impatiens applied fresh by rubbing on the eruptions, cures them. From this point of view, Brookland states that *Hedeoma pulegioides*, [pennyroyal] is much superior to *Pycnanthemum*. The toxic principle seems to be an oil to which the name toxicodendrol is given and which is analogous to cardol, the phenolic principle extracted from Anacarde."

1960 Walpole Island CHIPPEWA mss. Poison ivy is used to prevent infection and heal wounds. The amount of the root used depends on the size of the wound. It is boiled in water until it is soft, drained and the root mashed. A poultice of it is placed over the wound.

1976 Alex Ont. Weeds 100. "The poisonous substance is an oily resin contained in the juice of the plant. Contact with any broken part of the plant, with leaves which have been chewed by insects, or with shoes, clothing, implements, or pets which have touched broken parts of the plant may cause a person with sensitive skin to react. Dry twigs in winter, or dug-up roots in summer can often cause a reaction. . .In cases of suspected contact with the plant, washing the skin and clothing with a strong soap may not prevent a reaction but it will help minimize reinfec-tion to other parts of the body, or to other individuals. If a reaction does develop, one should seek the advice of a physician for proper treatment."

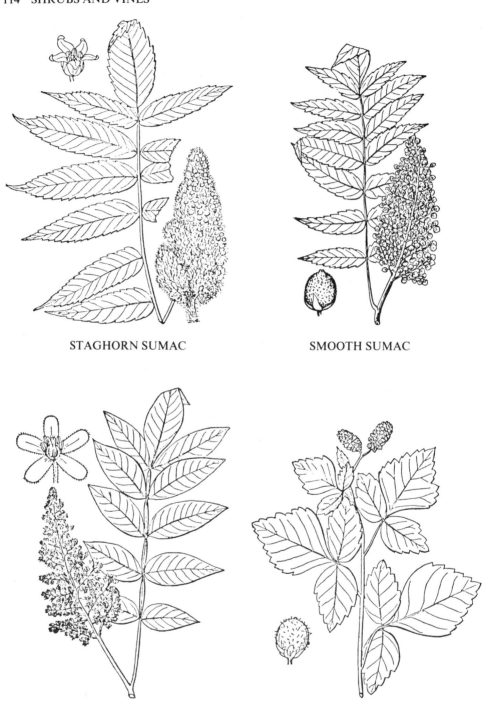

STAGHORN SUMAC

SMOOTH SUMAC

DWARF SUMAC

FRAGRANT SUMAC

STAGHORN SUMAC   *Rhus typhina* L. Anacardiacea (*R. hirta*)
A tall spare shrub or small tree to 10 m, the young branches, stems of leafs thickly covered with

soft hairs. The leaves have 9-29 opposite narrow leaflets, 5-12 cm long. The horn shaped flowering stalk is covered with hairs, the thickly packed greenish flowers are followed by red fruit very densely covered with bright crimson hairs 1-2 mm long.
Range. N.S., s. Que. and Ont. to Minn. s. to W. Va., and Ill. and in the mts. to N.C. in dry soil. May-June.
Common names. Vinegar tree, velvet sumac.

SMOOTH SUMAC   *Rhus glabra* L.
A shrub up to 6 m tall, the young branches and twigs smooth without hairs. The leaves with 11-31 leaflets each 5-10 cm long. The flowering cone up to 20 cm long. The fruit covered with bright red hairs 0.2 mm long.
Range. New Eng. and s. Que. to B.C., s. to Fla., Tex. and Mex. June-July in dry soils. A cross between this and the staghorn sumac is called var. *borealis*.
Common names. Senhalanac, Shoe-make.

DWARF SUMAC   *Rhus copallina* L.
Shrub to 6 m tall, the young branches, twigs, leaf stems densly hairy. The stem to which the 7-21 leaflets is attached has wings on both sides, 1-5 mm wide, except at the spot the leaflets grow. These are 3-8 cm long with few teeth or none. The flowering cone to 15 cm long, the fruit red and hairy.
Range. s. Ont., s. Maine, N.H. to s. Mich. and Mo., s. to Fla. and Tex. June-July in dry soil.
Common names. Smooth or common sumac.

FRAGRANT SUMAC   *Rhus aromatica* Ait.
Bushy shrub to 2 m whose leaves have three leaflets 4-8 cm long usually with 3-6 coarse teeth above the middle of the leaflet. The centre leaflet has no stem or only a very short one. The greenish yellow flowers appear before or with the leaves, in several short, 1-2 cm spikes. The fruits are bright red and very hairy.
Range. Vt., Que., s. Ont. n. to Ottawa river, Man., Sask, s. Alta. s. to Baja Calif. Mex., Miss. and n. Fla.
The leaves and branches of these sumacs exude a milky, juicy, gum when broken. None of these sumacs is poisonous. All have red hairy fruit.
1070-1320 Juntunen site Mich. Sumac seeds found archeologically. Yarnell 1964.
1380 Crawford lake site Ont. McAndrews, Byrne and Finlayson 1974. *Rhus typina*, staghorn sumac seeds made up 15.6% of the wild plant seeds found at the site, they were found in 39.3% of the features examined, pits, ovens, midden etc. These were the only seeds identified to species level.
1500 Draper site Ont. Finlayson 1975 293. Sumac seeds recovered archeologically represented the fourth largest amount of all seeds recovered.
1590 Harriot Virginia Indians 11. "Dyes of divers kindes. There is Shoemake well knowen, and used in England for blacke. . .The inhabitants use them only for the dyeing of hayre; and colour-ing of their faces, and Mantles made of Deare skinnes; and also for the dying of Rushes to make artificiall workes withal in their Mattes and Baskettes."
1633 Gerarde-Johnson 1474-75. "Coriar sumach [*Rhus coriari* European variety] The Arabians name is sumach:. . .The leaves of Sumach boyled in wine and drunken, do stop the laske, the inordinate course of womens sickness, and all other inordinate issues of bloud. The seed of Sumach eaten in sauces with meat, stoppeth all manner of fluxes of the belly, the bloudy flix, and all other issues, especially the whites of women. The decoction of the leaves maketh haires blacke, and is put into stooles to fume upward into the bodies of those that have the Dysenterie, and is to be given them also to drinke. The leaves made into an ointment or plaister with hony and vinegar, staith the spreading nature of Gangrenes. . .The drie leaves sodden in water until the decoction be as thicke as hony, yeeld forth a certaine oilinesse, which performeth all the effects of Linium. The seed is no less effectuall to be strowed in pouder upon their meats which are Coeliaci [diarrhea] or Dysenterici. The seeds pounded, mixed with honie and the powder of Oken coles, healeth the Hemorrhoides. There issueth out of a shrub a gum, which being put into the hollownesse of the teeth, taketh away the paine, as Dioscorides writeth."
1724 MIAMI-ILLINOIS Anon mss 221-3. "For confined women who are not entirely delivered,

they use the leaf of the sumac, with the root of an herb very common in the woods, and which has on its leaves a kind of ball. They call this herb by the generic name of Pallaganghy, [See Bulb-bearing water hemlock] which is to say Ocre; they take an equal quantity of the leaf of sumac and of the root of this herb, they crush the one and the other seperately; and after each is in powder they mix them together and put them in a small kettle on a few embers; they add to it two times as much sumach berries and make the confined women drink the warm water in which the whole is soaked until she is entirely cured. That is to say, the space of two or three days, each day replacing in the kettle a similar dose, and giving some of it to the patient to drink a little before she eats at noon; at four o'clock and in the evening before retiring, the blood comes after the second or third taking, sometimes coagulated and as big as the fist, sometimes purtrid, and at other times drop by drop. Those who have been wounded in the chest, head, or arm, and who lose much blood by the mouth take the same remedy with the same ingredients and are cured in a short time. The dropsical ones find themselves very well from it. They make them swallow the said drug with a little warm water in a spoon. The others above do not eat the medicine, they only drink the water in which it soaked, but they give all together to the dropsical ones. Those who have injured gums, be it from mal du terre, be it from scurvy or other, are cured by holding this medicine on their gums a long time, without adding the sumac berries. . .Besides, those who are burned or frozen or who are attacked by a venereal disease use the same drug, applying it to the affected part without adding the berry of the said sumac. . .for loosenes of the bowels some sumac. . .223. To dye red, there is on the prairie of the Tamarcoua a plant that they name red Micousiouaki [*Lithospermum*], they take the root, dry it, pulverize it in the mortar, and boil it with three times as many sumac berries. The red is very beautiful."

1748 Kalm Philadelphia September 19th. 42. "The sumach. . .*Rhus glabra*. . .Its fruit or berries are red. They are made use of for dyeing [they] afford a color like their own. . .The branches boiled with the berries yield a black ink-like tincture. The boys eat the berries, there being no danger of falling ill after the repast, but they are very sour."

1778 Carver Green Bay Lake Michigan 30. "Sumack likewise grows here in great plenty; the leaf of which, gathered at Michaelmas when it turns red, is much esteemed by the natives. They mix about an equal quantity of it with their tobacco, which causes it to smoke pleasantly [See bearberry and dogwood, the other herbs mentioned by Carver.]. . .358-61. They bear before them the pipe of peace, which I need not inform my readers is of the same nature as a Flag of Truce among the Europeans. . .It is used as an introduction to all treaties, and great ceremony attends the use of it on these occasions. The assistant or aid-du-camp of the great warrior, when the chiefs are assembled and seated, fills it with tobacco mixed with the herbs before mentioned, taking care at the same time that no part of it touches the ground."

1779. Zeisberger DELAWARE 115. "An Indian carries pouch and pipe with him wherever he goes, for they are indispensable. For state occasions they may have an otter skin pouch or a beaver-pouch or one decorated with coral, made by the women. Sometimes they have a buffalo horn, from which a pouch, made possibly of tanned deer-skin, depends. In the pouches they carry tobacco, fire materials, knife and pipe. Sumac is generally mixed with tobacco or sumac smoked without tobacco, for but few can stand smoking pure tobacco. . .The women. . .many of them though not all smoking tobacco."

1791 Lewis Mat. Med. ed Aitkin. Berries of sumach (*R. coriaria*) formerly used for restraining bilious fluxes, and hemorrhages and colliquative [dissolving] hectic sweats; some direct an infusion of half an ounce of the berries, and others two or three drams of an extract made from them for a dose. The leaves and young twigs are strong astringents and have been directed in the same intentions.

1830 Rafinesque 356. "All the sp. medical, two series of them. 1. harmless. 2. poisonous. 1. Series *R. glabrum, typhinum* and *copallinum* eq. Roots antisyphilitic used by Indians, dye wood reddish. Leaves have much tannin, make the Morocco leather, dye wool and silk black, good astringent for all fluxes. Bark and berries make ink. Fresh roots used for rheumatism, spirituous infusion rubbed with flannel. Gum similar to copal [resin from tropical trees] cures toothache put in hollow teeth. Indian flutes made of the stems. Berries used in dysentery, rheumatism, dysuria, sorethroat, putrid fevers, hemorrhage, gangrene, &c. they have an agreeable acid taste, make a cooling drink infused in water. Efflorescence on them used as salt and vinegar: it is malic acid. Seeds in powder used for piles and wounds. The juice removes warts and tetters, is the fine red mordaunt of Indian dyes. Seeds afford oil for lamps. Sacacomi article of trade in Canada, made by drying the berries in ovens after bread, fine substitute for tobacco, those who use it loath tobacco! Kinikah of western tribes is root and leaves, half mixt with their tobacco, used also for drop-sy. Galls of Shumacs lately found equal to Aleppo galls."

1840 Gosse Quebec 289. "That is Sumach (*Rhus Typhinum*): it is somewhat rare here; it keeps its handsome spikes of berries all the winter, whence it is cherished as an ornamental shrub; the berries are extremely acid. Sumach is used in tanning the finer kinds of leather."

1857 Daniel Wilson 254. "The Indians accordingly make use of various herbs to mix with and dilute the tobacco. . .Among the Creeks, Chocktaws, and other Indians in the south, the leaves of the sumach, prepared in a similar manner, answers the like purpose" [See tobacco, bearberry and dogwood.]

1858-61 Gunn 867. "Sumach (*Rhus Glabrum*). . .The Sumach is extensively used in certain districts for making spiles for tapping the Sugar Maple. . .The bark of the Sumach (that of the root preferred) is astringent, antiseptic and tonic; the berries are astringent, refrigerant, antiseptic and diuretic. A decoction of both the bark and the berries is an excellent wash or gargle for the apthous sore mouth and sore throat. . .and a decoction of the bark of the root has been used with advantage in diarrheas, dysentery, leucorrhea, hectic fever and night sweats. The powdered bark of the root forms an excellent poultice, mixed with a little powdered Elm bark, for old, gangrenous ulcers. An ointment made by simmering the bark of the root in lard, is good for scald head, and also for piles. A strong decoction of the bark of the root and White Oak bark, equal parts, is an excellent injection for falling of the womb, for leucorrhea or whites, and as a wash for foul or offensive ulcers. An infusion of the berries is good in diabetes or the excessive flow of urine, in bowel complaints, and as a cooling drink in fevers; and is extremely serviceable in all cases of sore throat and mouth, whether in quinsy, salivation from Mercury, or ordinary sore mouth. The decoction and infusion of Sumach may be used in ordinary doses, of from one to three or four ounces, several times a day."

1868 Can. Pharm. J. 6; 83-5. The bark and root of sumach, *Rhus Glabrum* included in list of Can. medicinal plants.

1871 Can. Pharm. J. 4; 39. "Since the war, and in the reversal of fortunes consequent thereto, many people of the South have turned their attention to other sources of revenue than the former staples of tobacco, corn and cotton. . .Among these new industries, and rising rapidly into importance, are the gathering and manufacturing for market of sumac. This article is used as a dye stuff and for tanning morrocco. Formerly all used was brought from Europe; now the Southern States supply a large quantity. . .The leaves of all these three under discussion are valuable, though we think if care were taken to keep them seperate that the hairy or stag-horn sumac would be found most valuable for dyeing. . .gathering should be done when the flower is in full bloom, not before. . .[the] leaves dried. . . At the mill [the leaves are] ground very fine and screened. The mill is of the usual drug-mill form: an upright wheel revolving on its edge in a circular trough, as the old fashioned mill for grinding clay. It should be tightly enclosed; if not a large quantity of the light, fine, powdered sumac will escape and be lost. . .after grinding it is screened and packed in bags-162 lbs. to the bag. . .To sell well it should be of a light green colour. . .should bring $125 a ton. . .We have stated that sumac is used for tanning and dyeing. For these purposes the user generally makes his own decoctions, and uses them when fresh and warm. It is stated that the liquor injures by standing. For tanning it is valued as it does not discolor the leather. . .In dyeing it is used to produce a fawn and a rich yellow, a black, a peculiar shade of green and a red. The mordants are usually tin or aluminous substances. . . With Brazil wood and tin solution it produces a red. With copperas and logwood a rich permanent black. With a solution of chloride of tin alone, a rich yellow, and this with Prussian blue, shades of green. It is used chiefly as a base, and has the quality of giving great permanency to the colours dyed with it. The leaves of the hairy species called staghorn are considered best to dye yellow. The sumac berries. . .are now used in small quantities by the druggists, and when ripe make a very refreshing and cooling beverage. They should by all means be kept out of the gathered leaves as they contain a red dye, hence would injure the quality of the sumac."

1879 Can. Pharm. J. 12; 302. "A series of experiments. . .to determine the tannin value of various vegetable substances. . .*Rhus glabra*, North Carolina, 26.10%."

1881 Can. Pharm. J. 14; 161-168. [Dr.] Burgess, paper read before Can. Med. Ass. Ottawa. ". . .Genus *Rhus*, a name derived from Greek word. . .'to flow,' so called because it was thought to be useful in stopping hemorrhages. And, truth to tell, the name was not inaptly applied by our forefathers, all the varieties being possessed of more or less astringent properties, some of them in a very marked degree. Fragrant sumac. . .This plant has, during the last two years, whether justly of not I cannot from my own experience say, obtained a high reputation as an astringent, and is at present being lauded in journals devoted to Materia Medica. In haematuria and chronic cystitis, where ordinary remedies—ergot, gallic acid and muriated tincture of iron—have failed, it is said to have been used with the happiest results. In phthisis, though not advanced as at all curative, it has a favorable effect in checking the hemorrhage, night sweats, and diarrhoea, often so exhausting and distressing. Five to twenty drops of the fluid extract may be given every hour in extreme cases of hemorrhage, and lessened as relief is obtained. . .In the diarrhoea of children. . .it is by some regarded as invaluable. Its use is also advocated in menorrhagia, dysentery, and diabetes insipidus, but it is in enuresis (incontinence of urine) that it has gained its highest reputation. . .From the strong testimony to its value, I would urge you. . .to give it a fair trial if you have not already done so. It is given in fifteen drop doses four times a day, the last being administered just before retiring, till improvement takes place, when only the night dose is given, and continued until the habit is cured. At the same time, the patient should strictly adhere to the rules of drinking but little during the evening, and voiding urine just before going to bed. . .Several medical friends, who have been using this drug in various affections, have furnished me with records of cases treated by it,. . .Chronic cystitis one case much improved. . .Menorrhagia 5 cases in all there was a wonderful effect in checking the discharge at the time. In three cases, after use at two menstrual periods the discharge was normal, and has since, now five months, continued so, the fourth case is improving, but the fifth shows no radical change. Enuresis 3 cases two cured; one improved. . . .*Rhus glabra*. . .Excrescences produced on the under surface of the leaves have been used as a substitute for the officinal galls obtained from the oak, *Quercus infectoria*. Like galls, these excrescences are due to the puncture of the young shoots by a hymenopterous insect to deposit its eggs. This irritates the part, and a tumor arises, the result of morbid growth. The eggs enlarge with this growth, and are converted into larvae, which feed on the vegetable matter. Finally the larvae become flies, and escape by eating their way out. For use, these excrescences should be collected when of full size, just before the eggs are hatched. All parts of this plant contain a large amount of gallo-tannic acid. . .The berries. . .owe their acidity to malic acid, which. . .is not contained in the berries themselves, but in the pubescence which covers them. An infusion of the fruit has been used as a refrigerant drink in febrile complaints, and as a detergent astringent gargle in common and ulcerated sore throat. It has been employed with great success in mercurial ptyalism, but for this, an infusion, or still better, a fluid extract of the inner bark of the root, is best adapted. . .staghorn sumach. . .possess properties similar to *R. glabra* and may be substituted for it. . .dwarf sumach. . .possesses similar, but less strongly marked, medicinal properties to *Rhus glabra* and may be used as a substitute therefor."

1885 Hoffman OJIBWA 201. "*Rhus (aromatica)* White Sumac. . .Roots are boiled, with those of the following named plant, and the decoction taken to cure diarrhea. (Gen.et sp.?) 'Big Heart Leaf'."

1892 Millspaugh 36. *Rhus glabra* "An infusion of the berries. . .is said to furnish an unequalled black dye for wool. . .A cold infusion of the berries. . .claimed to be of benefit in diabetes. . .Calcium bimalate. This salt is found clinging to the hairs of the fruit. . .when soaked off the fruits are no longer sour. . .Oil of Rhus—This waxy oil may be extracted from the seeds of this and other species of the genus. It will acquire a tallow like consistence on standing, and can be made into candles, which burn brilliantly, but emit a very annoying pungent smoke. . .During the summer of 1879, while botanizing. . .I came into a swarm of furious mosquitoes; quickly cutting a branch from a sumach bush. . .I used it vigorously to fight off the pests. . .[it was] in constant motion [and I was] perspiring freely during the time. . .also ate of the refreshing berries. On three successive nights following this occurence I flew (!) over the city of New York with a graceful and delicious motion I would give several years of my life to experience in reality. Query: Did I absorb from my perspiring hands sufficient juice of the bark to produce the effect of the drug, or was it from the berries I held in my mouth. I noticed no other symptoms, and never before or since enjoyed a like dream."

1915 Speck Tantaquidgeon MOHEGAN 319. "The berries of 'upland sumac' make a gargle for sore throat. They are also made into a beverage."

1915 W.R. Harris 48. "The root and leaves of the sumac were administered as a decoction for many complaints, but especially for dropsy, which, before European traders visited them, was an uncommon disease among the Indians."

1916 Waugh IROQUOIS 119. "Sumac, *Rhus glabra*, the fresh shoots peeled and eaten raw. . .148. Sumac seed clusters seem also to have been boiled, during the autumn and winter, as a **beverage**."

1926-27 Densmore CHIPPEWA 342. Decoction made from one root of *Heuchera* [Foam flower] sp. doubtful and one sumac blossom, cut when white bloom is on, in a teacup of water, strained and cooled. 'Put it on something soft and wash the child's mouth'. This was used for the sore mouth of a child when teething, and was said to heal the gums quickly. A fungus growing on the sumac was also used for dysentery. . .344. (*Rhus glabra*) This growth was dried and pulverized and drunk in decoction. This remedy was used for obstinate dysentery. *Rhus hirta*, staghorn sumac flowers were used in decoction for pain in the stomach. . .373-4. Dye formulas. . .light yellow; the pulp of the stalk of *Rhus glabra* in hot water.

1923 H. Smith MENOMINI 22. "Staghorn sumac. . .This tree is a very valuable one to the Indians, yielding three distinct kinds of medicines. The root bark, divested of the outer skin and inner wood, yields a tea which is a remedy for 'inward' troubles. It is of course very meagre in quantity compared to the amount of root peeled. The inner bark of the trunk is considered a valuable pile remedy, and is spoken of as being 'puckering' or astringent. The top or twigs, of the smaller shrubs is hairy, and because of this is used in the treatment of various female diseases. The acid flavored berries are used in combination with other herbs like the Greater St. John's Wort for consumption and pulmonary troubles. . .62. The sumac berries are dried and stored for winter use. When they are wanted, an infusion in water produces a drink very similar to lemonade. They are drunk as a beverage. . .77. The roots of the Sumac when boiled yield the Menomini yellow dye."

1928 H. Smith MESKWAKI 197. "One of the eight ingredients of a pile medicine. . . 200. The root bark of the smooth sumac is used to raise a blister on a patient. . .Dr. Wm. Jones collected Smooth Sumac root. . .This is boiled and drunk as an appetizer for an invalid. . .Staghorn sumac mixed with the root of *Euphorbia corollata* [flowering spurge] and the wood and bark of *Quercus macrocarpa* [Bur Oak] as a remedy for pinworms. The sumac berries are the part used in this case. . .271. . .Root of smooth sumac made a yellow dye used on rush and bark mats."

1932 H. Smith OJIBWE 424. "The Flambeau Ojibwe use the inner bark and the central pith of the stem of the Smooth Sumac, mixed with bloodroot, to obtain an orange color. The material is boiled in the mixture. The Pillager Ojibwe use the Staghorn Sumac in the same way. . .354. According to Jack Doud and other Flambeau Ojibwe all parts of the Smooth Sumac are suitable for medicine, the root bark, trunk bark, twig bark, leaves, flowers and fruit. The root bark tea is used as a hemostatic. [to stop blood]. Trunk and twigs inner bark are used in combination with other medicine for their astringent qualities. Blossoms are sometimes steeped for sore eyes, leaves are used in poultices, and the fruit is considered a throat cleanser as well as being the basis of a beverage. . . .The Pillager Ojibwe only use the root as a medicine to stop a hemorrhage (staghorn sumac). They suggested that they had heard of it being used in medicinal combinations but did not know how to make or use them. . .397. They stored the dried seed heads for winter use. . .The Flambeau Ojibwe gather the berries to make a pleasant beverage much like lemonade. The berries are tart and are sweetened with maple syrup, soaked in water until required for use. The dried berries are cooked in water with maple sugar, and form a hot drink, instead of a cooling one, as used in the summer and fall.

1933 H. Smith POTAWATOMI 38. "Most of our Wisconsin Indian tribes make use of the staghorn sumac for medicine and use various parts of the shrub. . .The root bark is used as a hemostatic. The leaves are steeped to make a tea, used in gargling a sore throat, tonsilitis and erysipelas. The berries are used to make a medicinal tea. They are also often mixed with other plant medicines to expel worms. It is quite likely that the abundant hairs upon the fruit, irritate the stomach lining and cause worms to be expelled. . .95. The berries. . .satisfy a natural craving for something acid or tart, among the Forest Potawatomi, who sometimes eat the berries, but none of them knew about its use as a beverage."

1935 Jenness Parry Island OJIBWA Lake Huron 114. "Yellow dye from boiled shavings of the sumac."

1945 Rousseau MOHAWK transl. 51. "Staghorn sumac. . . for women who loose their water easily, an infusion of the bark and flowers with felix-femina fern and a plant with blue grape-like fruit. The infusion is drunk every fifteen minutes 9 times, a ½ cupful at a time. The terminal shoots in spring are cut in fragments and eaten by young mothers, it makes their milk better."

1946 Harris, Seale 179. Dr. Frederick Banting, the co-discoverer of insulin, so greatly admired the Indians that when he heard a report that the Indians had used sumac leaves in the successful treatment of diabetes, he experimented with several bushels of leaves in an unsuccessful attempt to learn the secret of their reputed cure. (Vogel 1963. 199) [Research on the value of sumac for diabetes is going on in the Province of Ontario currently; personal communication.]

1955 Mockle Quebec transl. 54. "Fragrant sumac; the extract of the plant is used in incontinence of urine. Smooth Sumac; the fruits with a sugary and astringent flavor are infused in water, making a refreshing drink. Their decoction is used as a gargle in sore throat. The Staghorn Sumac; leaves and bark are given as an astringent. The fruits are refreshing."

1960 Walpole Island OJIBWAY mss. Three or four cups of the berries of the smooth sumac put into boiling water and boiled one minute. Drink one cup every hour to stop diarrhoea. Gather in August and store for next year.

1970 Bye IROQUOIS mss. Sumac wood used for darts and javelins. The red leaves in the fall smoked with or without tobacco. The inner bark of the root used for wounds. The new shoots as an alterative, eaten raw when peeled, berries used as a gargle for sore throat, ulcer, inflammation, in decoction. The bark and berries astringent used in dyeing and tanning.

1970 Jolicoeur Quebec 5. Sumach used for whooping cough.

1976 Antoine King Go-Home Bay Lake Huron personal communication. Gathered heads of berries in fall and put a quart basket full into a quart of water, boiled it, then strained and added sugar. Kept for the winter; a tablespoonful of this syrup as a cough medicine.

The twigs of *Rhus glabra* when chewed reduces the growth of caries causing bacteria in the mouth. *Rhus typhina* has shown experimental hypoglycemic activity (Lewis and Elvin-Lewis 1977:218,238).

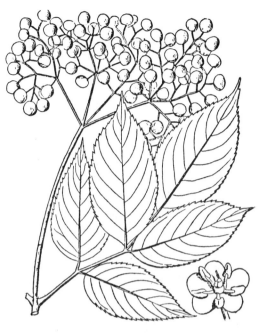

ELDER

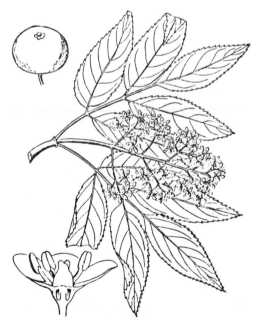

RED-BERRIED ELDER

ELDER
Sambucus canadensis L. Caprifoliaceae

Shrub to 3 m, spreading underground and eventually forming thickets, many young stems from the roots, scarcely woody, with large white pith. Leaves consist of 5-11 leaflets, usually 7, pointed at the tips, toothed, smooth or more often hairy beneath. The bunches of flowers on usually a few stems only. The many white flowers on their stalks have petals 3-5 mm wide. The fruit purple black, juicy, rarely red or green or yellow.

Range. N.S. and Que. to Man. and S.D., s. to Mex. and W. Ind. in woods, fields, moist places.
Common names. Elder-blow, elderberry.

RED BERRIED ELDER
Sambucus racemosa L. var. *pubens*

Shrub to 3 m the younger parts usually finely hairy, their pith is brown. There are 5-7 leaflets, finely toothed, usually soft hairy beneath. The many flowers on stalks up each side of a stem are yellowish white with 3-4 mm wide petals. Fruit red, seldom yellow or white.

Range. Nfdl. to B.C. s. to Pa., Ind. and Ill. and in the mts. to N.C. in rich woods.
Common names. Poison elder, boutry, boor tree, mountain elder, stinking elder.

1070-1320 Juntunen site Mich. Yarnell 1964. Stinking elder seeds found archeologically at seven locations.

1380 Crawford lake site Ontario, McAndrews, Byrne and Finlayson 1974 3. "The genus *Sambucus* is third largest in number of seeds (8.2% 185) identified from the samples. . .Natural depressions contained most of the Sambucus seeds."

1500 Draper site Ontario Finlayson 1975 225. "An examination of 200 samples. . .70 elderberry seeds found."

1475 Bjornsson Icelandic mss transl. Larsen 130. "Sambucus. . .elder. [European elder, *S. nigra*] Hot in the first degree and dry in the second. It makes the tendons soft and also the stomach. And it lets a man spew. If one boils elder leaves, it is good to apply to swollen nipples. An oil made of elder cleanses scabies and opens ill-grown wounds and eases earache. Its juice is good for intestinal worms; and it cleanses that illness which comes below in a man from cold and wet nature."

1624 Sagard HURON 197 "I wondered to see them burn themselves on their bare arms with the pith of the elder tree, for the pleasure of it, letting it burn away and smoulder on them, in such wise that the wounds, scars and cicatrices remained there indelibly." [See Morice below]

1633 Gerarde-Johnson 1423. European elder, *S. nigra*. The leaves and tender crops of common elder taken in some broth or pottage open the belly, purging both slimie phlegme and cholericke humors; the middle barke is of the same nature, but stronger, and purgeth the said humors more violently. The seeds. . .dried are good for. . .such as are too fat, and would faine be leaner, if they be taken in the morning to the quantity of a dram with wine for a certaine space. . .The greene leaves pouned with Deeres suet or Bulls tallow are good to be laid to hot swellings and tumors, and doth asswage the paine of the gout. The inner and greene bark doth more forcibly purge. . .being stamped, and liquor pressed out and drunke with wine or whay. Of like operation are also the fresh flouers. . .being dried they lose their purging qualitie. . .The vinegar in which the dried flouers are steeped are wholesome for the stomache. . .The gelly of the Elder, otherwise called Jewes eare, hath a binding and drying qualitie: the infusion thereof, in which it hath been steeped a few houres, taketh away inflammations of the mouth. . .the throat. . .Dioscorides saith, that the tender and greene leaves of the Elder tree, with barley meale parched do remove hot swellings, and are good for those that are burnt or scalded, and for such as be bitten with a mad dog, and that they glue and heale up hollow ulcers. The pith of the young boughes is without qualitie."

1724 Anon ILLINOIS-MIAMI mss Kin. 224. "The root and bark of elder for a person failing in his limbs, it is necessary to boil it and put it in a little soup, drinking about a pint of it."

1748 Kalm Philadelphia December 31st. 228. "I have seen the Iroquois boil the inner bark of the *Sambucus Canadensis*, or Canada elder, and put it on the part of the cheek in which the pain was most violent from toothache. This I am told, often diminishes the pain."

1785 Cutler. "If sheep that have the rot are placed in a situation where they can get at the bark and young shoots, they will soon cure themselves. The leaves are purgative like the bark but more nauseous. The inner bark and leaves are ingredients in several cooling ointments. A decoction of the flowers taken internally is said to promote expectoration in pleurisies. If the flowers are fresh gathered, they loosen the belly. Externally they are used in fomentations to ease pain and abate inflammations. They will give a flavor to vinegar. A rob prepared from the berries is a gentle opener, and promotes perspiration. An infusion of the dried berries is given to children. The flowers kill turkeys, and the berries are poisonous to poultry. The fresh leaves laid round young cucumbers, melons or cabbages, are a good preservative against worms and insects. It is said, if turnips, cabbages, fruit trees or corn (which are subject to blight from a variety of insects) are whipped with the green leaves and branches of Elder, the insects will not attack them. The green leaves are said to drive away mice."

1799 Lewis Materia Medica 229. "Common black elder *S. nigra.* Inner green bark of the trunk is strongly cathartic. . .Three handfuls boiled in one quart of milk and water to a pint, of which one half is to be taken at night, and the other in the morning, and repeated for several days, usually operates both upwards and downwards, and from these evacuations its utility is derived. . .The young buds or rudiments of leaves, are strongly purgative, and act with so much violence as to be deservedly accounted unsafe. The Flowers are very different in quality; these have an agreeable aromatic flavour. . .imparted by infusion to vinous and spirituous liquors. . .When dry they are supposed to be diaphoretic: and are particularly useful in erysipelatous and cuticular disorders."

1807 Pursh ONONDAGA July 18th. Indians when poisoned by *Cicuta* [Poison Water hemlock] eat elder bark as an emetic.

1830 Rafinesque 260. "*Sambucus canadensis.* . .afford Wine, Alcohol and Oil. Shade deemed baneful, leaves being subnarcotic, said to cure the rot of sheep. . .Bark dyes black, boiled and applied to cheeks cures toothache. . .Elder flowers. . .give a fine flavor to vinegar and wine. Red berried elder equivalent."

1833 Howard Quebec. 1. "St. Anthony's Fire. Take a decoction of Elder leaves as a sweat. . .49. To cure the Gout on the limbs. Drink a pint of the infusion of Elder buds, dry or green, morning and evenings. . .65. To cure Running or Sore legs. Wash them with brandy and apply elder leaves, changing then twice a day."

1842 Christison 818. "*Sambucus nigra.* . .The inner bark, and probably also the leaves, produce both vomiting and brisk purging; and I have known the leaves cause severe irritant poisoning in a child. The source of its properties has not yet been traced. Unless the elder possesses more energetic properties that it is at present believed to have, it may be expunged without detriment from the Pharmacopoeias."

1857-61 Gunn 789. "*Sambucus canadensis.* . .The stalk is jointed, containing a large spongy pith, and is often used for spiles in tapping sugar trees, and for pop-guns by the boys. . .The tea of Elder flowers is good for children, in all derangements of the bowels and liver, and in eruptive diseases, erysipelas, and the like. The juice of the berries, evaporated down till it is about as thick as molasses and given in doses of one or two tablespoonfuls, and repeated, acts as a valuable laxative and alterative: and in large doses as a cathartic. . .An excellent salve or ointment may be made by stewing the inner fresh bark in lard, excellent in cases of burns and scalds, and by melting a little rosin and beeswax with it, makes a good salve for cuts, sores, and ulcers."

1868 Can. Pharm J. 6; 83-5 The flowers and berries of elder, *Sambucus canadensis*, included in list of Can. medicinal plants.

1881 Can. Pharm J. 15; 55. "From an examination of the bark of *Sambucus Canadensis* Mr. C.G. Traub. . .finds the constituents to be valerianic acid, volatile oil, fat, resin, tannin, sugar and coloring matter, besides several compounds, the nature of which was not ascertained. Its composition is, therefore, very similar to that of the bark of the European elder."

1892 Millspaugh 75. "*Sambucus canadensis.* . .Our species is not sufficiently distinct from the European *S. nigra.* . .The pith of the Elder has many offices to fill in the arts and manufacturers; the berries make a really pleasant wine; and, among the poorer class of people (it must be more from necessity than choice), they are made into pies, like huckleberries. In domestic medicine this plant forms almost a pharmacy in itself. . .A decoction of the flowers and leaves, or an ointment containing them, was used as an application to large wounds to prevent deleterious consequences from flies; the leaf buds proved themselves a violent and unsafe cathartic."

1894 Toronto Household Guide 114. "Black elder. . .An ointment made by stirring the fresh flowers into clean melted lard, and subsequently straining it, is an excellent remedy for burns, scalds, wounds and old obstinate sores. The berries are laxative and are good in rheumatism, gout, skin diseases and habitual constipation. The berries can be preserved by canning the same as any other fruit, or they may be dried."

1901 Morice CARRIER Arctic 20. "When an Indian had resolved to get rid of an aching pain that had become too acute for patient bearing, he took a round piece of tinder perhaps one third of an inch in diameter, wetted with his saliva that part of its surface that was to come in contact with the flesh, and then pressed it firmly on the joint the healing of which was deemed most likely to ensure the prompt recovery of the whole limb. Next, he himself, or an obliging friend ignited the top of the tinder, which was suffered to burn down to the very flesh, wherein a corresponding sore or cavity was inevitably produced. . .25. As parturifacients, three plants are chiefly valued and used to this day among the Carriers. . .the elder *Sambucus racemosus*[*pubens*] hot infusions of which are drunk previous to parturition or before the after-birth is expelled."

1915 Speck-Tantaquidgeon Mohegans 318. "Flowers of the elder are made into a tea to be given to babies for colic. The bark of the elder made into a tea is an excellent purgative; when scraped upward from the branch it acts as an emetic, when scraped off downward it is a physic."

1916 Waugh IROQUOIS 128. Berries of *S. canadensis* eaten.

1928 Parker SENECA 11. Diuretic, late elder.

1923 H. Smith MENOMINI 27. "(*S. canadensis*) The dried flowers are made into a tea which is used as a febrifuge. . .Red elderberry. . .The Menomini recognise that it is a very powerful medicine and only to be used when the instructions for use are very carefully followed, and when other remedies for the same complaint are of no avail. Four joints of the trunk are chosen, the diameter of a man's finger, say three-quarters of an inch. These sticks are of a measured length, from the point of the ulna to the point of the humerus. If these sticks are now peeled downward, the resulting inner bark and rind are steeped and boiled, then thrown away. The liquid is drunk and saves the life of one threatened with serious constipation. This remedy is only used in extreme cases, for there are many other remedies for constipation and this is a dangerous one unless needed, when it becomes a drastic purgative. If these same sticks were peeled upward and the tea drunk, then it would have acted as a powerful emetic. There is probably no doubt of its emetic and purgative properties, but the mechanical difference in preparation is surely pure superstition". . .1932 OJIBWE 360. Same account of use given, Smith adds; "The writer can testify to its strength, but notes that it works both ways at once, no matter how prepared, so that the method of preparation is doubtless superstitious."

1928 H. Smith MESKWAKI 207. "(*S. canadensis*). . .The root bark of the elder is used by them to free the lungs of phlegm. The bark tea is used only in extremely difficult cases of partutition, when the baby is born dead. . .256. While the Meskwaki like to eat these raw [the berries], they also cook them into a conserve. They prefer them without sugar when cooked. . .268. They punch out the pith and make water squirt guns for playing, or else popguns for shooting pith corks."

1933 H. Smith POTAWATOMI 46. "Red-berried elder. The inner bark of the Red-berried elder is accounted the most powerful physic which the Forest Potawatomi have and it is used in the same manner as the Menomini use it."

1934 Stone IROQUOIS 531-2. "The Iroquois recognise the syndrome of a dry hot skin, chills, thirst, prostration and muscular pains. Their management of the case seems quite modern as it included rest, sweating, purgation, diuresis and a restriction of the diet to liquids. Copious infusions of elderberries (*Sambucus canadensis*), either the fruit or the inner bark, were given to cause sweating and diuresis, which properties the medicine actually possesses."

1945 Rousseau Quebec Transl. 99. "The stems with the pith removed were used as spindles in weaving."

1955 Mockle Quebec transl. 84-5. "*Sambucus canadensis*. The internal bark and the fresh root are given as a purgative; the leaves are laxative and the flowers diuretic, diaphoretic and sudorific. The flowers and the leaves contain rutoside. Red-berried elder the same uses as *S. canadensis*. *Sambucus Ebulus* [European sp. introd. s. Que.] a purgative drink from the roots."

Elder flowers are picked and left in heaps for a few hours until the petals fall off. These are dried or mixed with salt to preserve them, this method changes the disagreeable odor of the flowers into a pleasant fragrance. They can be used, fresh or pickled to make elder flower water. They contain rutin. The fresh flowers in melted fat become elder flower ointment. The dried flowers are taken as a tea which promotes urine and perspiration. The fresh ripe fruit contains tyrosin. The leaves contain sambunigrin, readily converted into prulaurasin which is decomposed by an enzyme, prunase into benzaldehyde, hydrocyanic acid and dextrose. (T.E. Wallis 1967:167-8).

1970 Bye IROQUOIS mss "Used elder for ague and inflammation. The berries as a sauce which was a valuable remedy in fevers of patients and convalescense. The blossoms in hot water as a tea. The flowers were sometimes used with cornmeal."

1972 Garrett 7. "The ubiquitous wild elderberry bush has been a source of culinary treasure for generations of cooks. Its froth of creamy white bloom produces delicious fritters and delicate wines and champagnes. Its autumn harvest of tiny purple berries that hang in clusters heavy with juice is as versatile as it is abundant. Elderberry jelly and jam, spiced elderberries and chutney for cold meats, elderberry pie laced with a grating of lemon peel, elderberry syrup for pancakes, and elderberry wine."

The fruits contain vitamin C and reduce fever, help chronic catarrh as well as being antispasmodic, the flowers do the same. They are taken for rheumatism; used as a gargle; in the bath. The fruit juice relieves migraine, neuralgia and pain (Stary & Jirasek 1973:196).

MALECITE and MICMAC Indians of the maritime provinces of Canada use the common elder as a purgative and soporific, emetic and physic. (Chandler, Freeman & Hooper 1979:61).

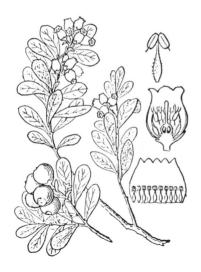

BEARBERRY

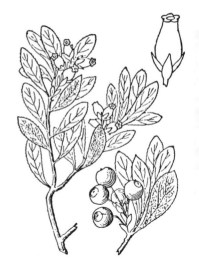

ALPINE BEARBERRY

BEARBERRY   *Arctostaphylos uva-ursi* (L.) Spreng. Ericaceae
A spreading evergreen shrub growing like a mat on rocky, sandy soil. The leaves are leathery, 1-3 cm long, round at the tip and narrow at the hairy stalk. The under side clearly cross veined, without spots. The flowers whitish, bell-shaped, 4-6 mm long. The fruit bright red, mealy, containing 5 nutlets attached to each other.
Range. Circumpolar, in Am. s. to Va., n. Ind., Ill., N.M. and Calif.
Common names. Sagakomi, jackashepuck, kinnikinik, bear's berry, mountain box, mountain tobacco, mountain crawberry, barren myrtle, Yukon holly, universe vine. Kinnikinik is an Algonkian, Cree or Ojibwa word that means 'that which is mixed'. A smoking mixture, varying as to ingredients from tribe to tribe and place to place. (Dict. Canad.1967:406).

ALPINE BEARBERRY   *Arctostaphylos alpina* (L.) Spreng. including *A. rubra*.
The leaves are not evergreen but wither and stay on the prostrate branches. The berries are red to black, juicy, 6-10 mm with separate nutlets.
Range. Circumpolar, in Am. s. to the higher mts. of Me. and N.H. May-June.
1070-1320 A.D. Juntunen site Mich. bearberry seeds found at four locations archeologically and also at the Isle Royale site (Yarnell 1964:61).
1703 Lahontan 11; 53. "They are forc'd to buy up Brasil Tobacco, which they mix with a certain Leaf...called Sagakomi."
Sagakomin an Algonkian word meaning 'smoking leaf berry'; Ojibwa and closely related dialects (Dict. Canad. 1967:652).
1709 Raudot Quebec 345. "The men and women savages smoke very much, or one could better say always. Previously they used an herb called mountain tobacco, but now they smoke black tobacco, or that which is grown here and is very nearly of the same quality as that cultivated in France."
1743 Isham Hudson Bay 132. "Jac'kashepuck, so called by the natives, is a Leaf Like unto a box Leaf, itt Grow's about 2 foot high, and Run's in long branches spreading itt Self upon the Ground, the Stalk's not being of Substance to bear itt up, this Leaf they Dry and pound, mixing itt with their tobacco when they smoak, if they Can not procure this, they take a sort of shrub a black Berry grows on, which they style, (auskemenaw)."
1749 Kalm Quebec Cap aux Oyes September 1st. 489. "The bear berries (*Arbutus uva ursi*) grow in great abundance here. The Indians, French, English and Dutch, in these parts of North America, which I have seen, call them Sagackhomi, and mix the leaves with tobacco for their use. Even the children use only the Indian name for these berries...579. N.Y. State. The bearberry was also found here. The French gathered it and mixed it with the tobacco which they smoked."

1778 Carver 31. "A weed grows near the great lakes, in rocky places, they use in the summer season. It is called by the Indians, Segockimac. . .These leaves, dried and powdered, they likewise mix with their tobacco; and as was said before, smoak it only during the summer. . .as they are great smoakers, they are very careful in properly gathering and preparing them."

1799 Lewis Mate. Med. 263. "*Arctostaphylos uva ursi*. . .It had fallen into disuse till about the middle of the present century, when it first drew the attention of physicians as a useful remedy in calculus and nephritic complaints; and in almost all others to which the urinary organs are subject, such as ulcers of the kidneys and bladder. . .nay even by some it was considered as a solvent of the human calculi [stones]; however from a multiplicity of experiments it has not appeared to possess this dissolving power; yet still may be considered as a valuable remedy, if only it lessens the torture, and thereby renders life more tolerable. Whatever good effects it produces, they seem to be derived from its astringent power."

1817-20 Bigelow 68. "The leaves and stems of the Uva ursi are used in Sweden and Russia for the purpose of tanning leather. According to Linnaeus large quantities are annually collected for this use. When chewed in the mouth, the leaves have an astringent taste, combined with some degree of bitterness. . .Some years ago the Uva ursi was recommended as a remedy in pulmonary consumption. . .to have a very sensible effect in diminishing hectic fever and abating the frequency of the pulse dependent on it. We do not find however that subsequent experience has justified the expectations formed of it in this disease."

1823 Franklin 741. "Jackashey-puck. . .has received the name of sac à Commis, from the trading clerks carrying it in their smoking bags."

1820's Materia Medica Edinburgh-Toronto mss 36. "*Arbutus Uva Ursi* the leaves have a bitter astringent taste without odour; from its astringency it has been employed in menorrhagia & other fluxes more particularly in. . .calculus & ulceration of the urinary organs, has been recommended in Phthisis & some species of cough accompanied with symtoms of hectic fever."

1828 Rafinesque 263. "*Arbutus uva-ursi*, other vulgar names Wortleberry, Foxberry, Checkerberry, &c. The plant often dies the urine black; the berries are sometimes eaten in milk like those of the Vaccinium genus, they are aromatic and diuretic."

1830 Trans. Lit.& Hist. Soc. Quebec 1:91. "Saccacommi is frequently used to smoke in lieu of tobacco, by the traders engaged in the fur countries."

1842 Christison 930. "The period of the introduction of this plant into medical practice is unknown. Geiger says it was used in the south of Europe for the first time about the beginning of the last century, and in Germany not fifty years later. It cannot be traced with confidence to any of the medicinal plants of the Greeks or Romans. . .is apt to be confounded with the leaf of the *Vaccinium Vitis-idaea*, or whortleberry,. . .The uva ursi leaf however is reticulated [cross veined] beneath, while the whortleberry leaf is dotted. Uva-ursi is a powerful astringent; and according to some it is also diuretic. Its astringent virtues led to its being much employed in chronic mucous discharges more especially from the genito-urinary organs. . .It seems to have sometimes a soothing as well as an astringent effect in such disorders."

1859-61 Gunn 874. "The leaves are the part used, and may always be found in drugstores. . .It is serviceable. . .in constant or frequent desire to pass the urine. . .the decoction is made by boiling for a few minutes an ounce of the leaves in a quart of water; dose half a teacupful three or four times a day."

1884 Holmes-Haydon CREE Hudson Bay do not mention any use of bearberry although Holmes does mention that the leaves of the alder have a flavor recalling that of the bearberry.

1892 Millspaugh 100. "The principal substitute leaves for the Uva-ursi of commerce are those of *Vaccinium Vitis Idea* of which Mr. J.H. Sears says: 'This is the plant that the Shakers gather instead of the Uva-Ursi; they go 40 or 50 miles for it when Uva-Ursi is abundant in their own ground. Uva Ursi is an ancient astringent, though used but little until the 13th century by the physicians of Myddfai.'. . .In late years it has been called attention to as a uterine excitant, very useful in prolonged parturition from atony [debility]; it is claimed that it is fully as sure as Secale, while the contractions resulting are more prolonged, while less painful, and dangerous to the child. . .The American Aborigines smoked the dried leaves with tobacco, making a mixture called Sagack-homi in Canada, and Kinikinik among the Western tribes; this is the Larb of the Western hunters. . .Should we prescribe on the palliative principle, and at the same time believe in disinfection by killing germs, I could hardly point to a drug more adapted to diseases of the kidneys, bladder, and urethra than arbutin, which is changed in the renal tract to hydrokinone, a sort of phenol, which is in itself a germicide, the arbutin being more or less innocuous and at the same time a diuretic; it has, however, caused an eruption on the skin."

1908 Henderson & Lusk Materia Medica Toronto. Dried leaves of uva-ursi contain an active principle, the glucoside arbutin.

1910 Morice DENE 128. "Nor should we omit. . .the berry of the kinnikinik. . .which is prepared for eating by roasting in a frying pan and mixed with salmon oil or the grease from any animal."

1923 H. Smith MENOMINI 35. "It is used as a seasoner, to make certain female remedies taste good."

1924 Youngken 500. "The leaves were dried by several aboriginal tribes and ground with tobacco or red willow as a smoking mixture. A decoction of the stems, leaves and berries was drunk by many tribes for pain in the back and sprained back."

1926-27 Densmore CHIPPEWA 318. The red berries of this plant were cooked with meat as a seasoning for broth. . .336. The dried and pulverized leaves were combined with tobacco or red willow, smoked in a pipe and smoke inhaled for a headache. . .376. Smoked in a pipe to attract game.

1928 Reagan CHIPPEWA 239. The leaves are smoked causing intoxication. They are much used in medicine ceremonies, and also as medicine.

1935 Jenness Parry Island Lake Huron OJIBWA 114. "Tobacco: so far as the Parry Islanders are aware, none of their forefathers cultivated tobacco, but obtained it from an Iroquoian tribe in exchange for furs. There was no smoking for mere pleasure in earlier times; it was a strictly religious ceremony, practised, by medicine-men when healing the sick. When tobacco was scarce the Indians substituted willow bark, labrador tea, dried and pounded bearberry roots, or the berry-like tips of the white ash."

1955 Mockle Quebec transl. 69. "The leaves are astringent and diuretic, frequently used for incontinence of urine and as an urinary antiseptic. They contain 6 to 7% of tannins. The Indians used to smoke the leaves as tobacco under the name of Sagakomi."

Collect the leaves in the spring and dry in open. Arbutin in the leaves taken by mouth becomes in the urine arbutin and hydroquinone. The stimulant and antiseptic properties of the leaves is said to be partly due to the latter substance. They are used in diseases of the urino-genital tract (T.E. Wallis 1967:128).

The dried leaves, when smoked, relax the smoker (Assiniwi 1972:129).

Andrometoxin and arbutin in many species of the genus *Pernetya*, Ericaceae, may account for these species narcotic properties. (Emboden 1972:76).

[The use of bearberry leaves should not be undertaken without the advice of a doctor as excessive dosing and long term use can cause chronic impairment of the liver, especially in children].

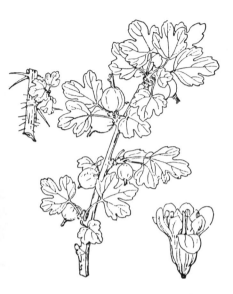

NORTHERN GOOSEBERRY

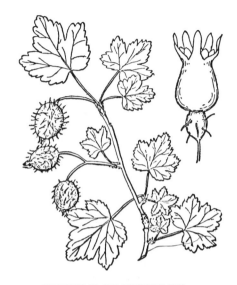

PRICKLY GOOSEBERRY

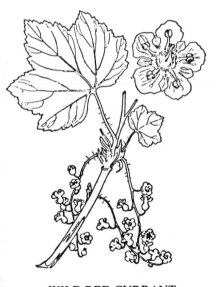

WILD RED CURRANT

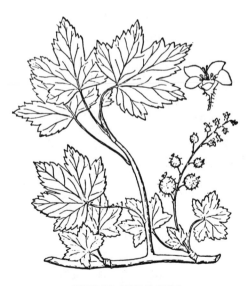

SKUNK CURRANT

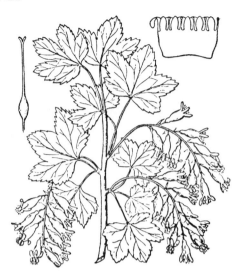

WILD BLACK CURRANT

NORTHERN GOOSEBERRY   *Ribes oxyacanthoides* L. Saxifragaceae (*Grossularia o.*)
Branches rather stout, yellowish, densely bristly when young, the leaves hairy and their stalks
with glands. The gooseberry smooth, reddish-purple when ripe, edible.
Range. Transcontinental, Nfld., N.B., N.S., P.E.I., Que., Hudson Bay to B.C. Yukon, Alaska. in
wet woods and low grounds.

PRICKLY GOOSEBERRY   *Ribes cynosbati* L. (*Grossularia c.*)
Prickles on the branches, few and weak or none. The leaves usually hairy when young. The fruit
covered with prickles, reddish purple to black when ripe.
Range. N.B., Que., Ont. to Minn. s. to N.C. and Okla. in rocky woods.
Common names. Dogberry.
1534 Cartier St. Lawrence transl. 33-4. "There were many gooseberries."
1604 Champlain Tadoussac 181. "There are in these parts great store of Vines,. . .Goose-berries,
red and greene." [The red probably red currants as the gooseberries ripen later.]
1609 Leascarbot-Erondelle Port du Mouton 86. "We saw there, being a sandy
land. . .goose-berries.
1633 Gerarde-Johnson 1324-5. "Goose-berries or Fea-berry bush. . .The fruit. . .greene at the
first, but waxing a little yellow through maturitie. . .The fruit is used in divers sauces for meate,
as those that are skilfull in cookeries can better tel than myselfe. They are used in broths in stead
of Verjuice, which maketh the broth not onely pleasant to the taste, but is greatly profitable to
such as are troubled with a hot burning ague. . .The juice of the greene Gooseberries cooleth all
inflammations, Erysipelas, and Saint Anthonies fire. . .The young and tender leaves eaten raw in
a sallad, provoketh urine, and drive forth the stone and gravel."
1668 Marie de l'Incarnation Quebec 346. "We also make jam from gooseberries."
1743 Isham Hudson Bay 133. "Goose Berries Very plenty but never see any but the black when
ripe, some Grow's as high as in England, other's which grow's at this Barren and Rocky place are
not above 6 inches spreading along the Ground."
1916 Waugh IROQUOIS 126. "Gooseberries were freed from prickles by tying them up in the
skin of an animal and later in an ordinary grain-bag. They were rubbed until the prickles were
broken off. . .127. Various species of wild gooseberries were eaten."
1926-7 Densmore CHIPPEWA 356. "*Grossularia oxyacanthoides*, the root used in decoction for
pain in the back and female weakness."

1923 H. Smith MENOMINI 71. "Prickly gooseberry. . .Gooseberries are one of the staple berries gathered by the Menomini and are preserved and stored for winter use."

1928 H. Smith MESKWAKI 246. "Prickly gooseberry. McIntosh uses the root of this to cure uterine trouble caused from bearing too many children. . .264. The prickly gooseberry is cooked with sugar as a dessert. Mrs. Joe Tesson, the informant did not know of any combination with other fruits."

1932 H. Smith OJIBWE 410. "Prickly gooseberry. The Flambeau Ojibwe relish these berries when ripe and make them into preserves for winter use. . .The smooth gooseberry (*R. oxyacanthoides*). . .The Flambeau gather this berry for fresh food, and also make it into preserves for winter use. It is often cooked with sweet corn."

1933 H. Smith POTAWATOMI 82. "Prickly gooseberry. The Prairie Potawatomi. . .employ the root bark for a uterine remedy. The Forest Potawatomi make a tea of the root for treating sore eyes. . .109. Both. . .use the berries for food and make up jams and jellies with maple sugar for their winter food supply."

WILD RED CURRANT   *Ribes triste* Pallas

Stem often lying on the ground and rooting, without prickles. Leaves sometimes softly hairy beneath, mostly with 5 lobes. The fruit many on a drooping stalk often with hairs that are gland tipped. The fruit red and sour, smooth, edible.

Range. Lab. to Alaska. s. to N.J., Mich., Wis., Minn. and in n. Asia in bogs and wet woods.

SKUNK CURRANT   *Ribes glandulosum* Grauer

Stems lying on the ground without prickles. The leaves like the red currant. The fruit along a stalk that stands upright covered with gland tipped hairs, the fruit also covered with gland tipped hairs, dark red. Whole plant has a disagreeable odor.

Range. Transcontinental, Lab. to Alaska, s. to Me., Vt., Mich., Minn. and in the mts. to N.C. in swamps and wet woods.

WILD BLACK CURRANT   *Ribes americanum* Mill.

Stems erect without prickles. Leaves 3 to 5 lobed, the undersides dotted with glands and some hairs. The fruit along a drooping stalk, black and smooth.

Range. N.B., N.S., s of James Bay to Alta., s. to Del., W. Va., Ind., Io., Nebr. and Colo. in moist woods.

1663 Boucher Quebec transl. 50. "There are currants or red gooseberries."

1743 Isham Hudson Bay 133. "Currans both Red and black the same as in other parts."

1748 Kalm Philadelphia September 20th. 47. "The ladies make wine from some of the fruits of the land. They principally take red and white currants for that purpose. . .An old Sailor who had frequently been in Newfoundland told me that red currants grew wild in that country in great quantity."

1830 Rafinesque 258. "Roots in infusion, bark in gargles used for eruptive fevers, dysentery of cattle, fruits and jelly for sorethroat. Anodyne, diuretic, pellent, depurative, used in angina, exanthems, dysentery, hydrophobia, scabs and ictus. A fine cordial made of black currants. . .Wine made with currants and gooseberries."

1852 Nickle Family book Galt Ont. mss "In all the farm houses here they still follow the old custom of making wine, mostly from the Currants and Raspberry."

1916 Waugh IROQUOIS 128. Wild black and wild red currants eaten.

1926-27 Densmore CHIPPEWA 321. Eaten raw as well as dried for winter use the wild red currant, *R. triste* and *Ribes* species. . .348. The root and stalk of *Ribes triste*; decoction made from 4 plants in 1 quarter of water, 'boiled quite a while', for gravel. . .The leaves and stalks of *Ribes* species mixed with those of *Caltha palustris* (marsh marigold) in decoction drunk for stoppage of urine. . .356. *Ribes glandulosum*, skunk currant; the root in decoction for pain in the back and female weakness. . .358. *Ribes triste*; the stalk mixed with the root of spikenard and wild sarsaparilla in a decoction drunk for stoppage of periods.

1928 H. Smith MESKWAKI 246. "Black currant McIntosh uses the root bark as a medicine to expel intestinal worms. . .264. The Meskwaki make use of the wild black currants as a food."

1932 H. Smith OJIBWE 389. "*R. triste*. . .Wild red currant. The Flambeau Ojibwe use the leaves as some sort of a female remedy. . .410. (*R. americanum*) Wild black currant. The Pillager Ojibwe eat these berries fresh, in jams and preserves and dry them for winter. In the winter, a favorite dish is wild currants cooked with sweet corn. The Flambeau Indians use them in a like manner. . .they gather the wild red currant and use them as they do the wild black currants."

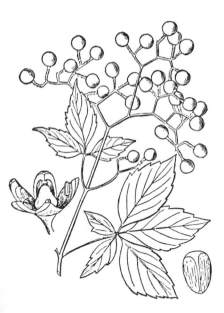
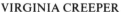

VIRGINIA CREEPER

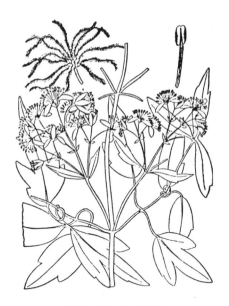

VIRGIN'S BOWER

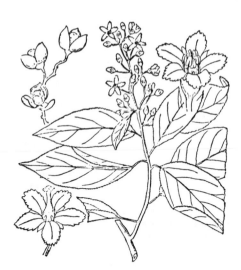

BITTERSWEET

VIRGINIA CREEPER *Parthenocissus quinquefolia* (L.) Planch. Vitaceae (*Ampelopsis q.*)
A climber that has long branched tendrils with adhesive disks at their tips. The leaves consisting
of 5 leaflets or sometimes 3-7, spread like the palm of a hand, dull pale green, decidedly paler
beneath and stalked. The dark blue fruit rarely over 7 mm thick with at most 3 seeds.
Range. s. Me., Que., Ont., s. to Mex. Tex. and Fla. in moist woods and thickets.

WOODBINE   *Parthenocissus inserta* (Kerner) Fritsch
The tendrils do not have any adhesive disks, the plant rests loosely on rocks, fences etc. The leaves are green and glossy above and green beneath. The fruit to about 1 cm thick with 3 or 4 seeds.
Range. New. Engl., Que., Ont., to Man., s. to Calif., N. Mex., Kans., and Pa. in moist woods and thickets.
Common names. American ivy, five leaved ivy, false grape.
1633 Gerarde-Johnson 857. "There is kept for novelties sake in divers gardens a Virginian, by some (though unfitly) termed a Vine, being indeed an Ivy. The stalks of this grow to a great heighth, if they be planted nigh anything that may sustaine or beare them up: and they take hold by certaine small tendrels, upon what body soever they grow, whether stone, boords, bricke, yea glasse, and that so firmely, that oftentimes they will bring pieces with them if you plucke them off. The leaves are large, consisting of foure, five, or more particular leaves, each of them being long, and deeply notched about the edges, so that they somewhat resemble the leaves of the Chestnut tree: the floures grow clustering together after the manner of ivy, but never with us shew themselves open, so that we cannot justly say anything of their colour, or the fruit that succeeds them. . .It may as I said be fitly called *Hedera Virginiana*."
1868 Can. Pharm. J. 6; 83-5. American ivy, *Ampelopsis Quinquefolia*; the bark and twigs included in list of Can. medicinal plants.
1892 Millspaugh 40. "This indigenous vine is being cultivated in Europe much as the European ivy is here, for adorning walls. Ampelopsis is not mentioned in the U.S. P h[arm]; in the Eclectic Materia Medica its preparations are Decoctum. . .and Infusum. . .The fresh young shoots and bark are chopped and pounded to a pulp. . .mixed with alcohol. . .Chemical constituents; Pyrocatechin in the green leaves, Cissotannic acid. . .in the autumnal colored leaves." [with different properties]. The leaves when green contain also free tartaric acid and its salts, with sodium and potassium. Glycollic acid and Calcium glycollate exist in the ripe berries. Little or nothing is known of the action of this drug upon man. . .[In] 1876 reports that two children. . .after chewing the leaves and swallowing the juice were quickly seized with vomiting and purging. . .collapse, sweating and faint pulse. . .four hours after attack before they were normal [again]." [No other reference found in the literature to poisoning from virginia creeper].
1925 Wood & Ruddock. Virginia creeper bark; leaves and twigs a remedy for dropsy, diseases of the skin and bronchitis. Dose of the fluid extract 15-30 drops.
1926-7 Densmore CHIPPEWA 320. "*Parthenocissus quinquefolia*. . .The stalk was cut in short lengths and boiled, then peeled. Between the outer bark and the wood there was a sweetish substance which was eaten somewhat after the manner of eating corn from the cob. The water in which the woodbine had been boiled was then boiled down to a sirup. If sugar were lacking, wild rice was boiled in this sirup to season it."
1923 H. Smith MENOMINI 58. "Virginia creeper. . .This was not used by the Menomini but has been used by the white man for its acidulous foliage. The tartaric acid and its salts in the foliage have been used as a refrigerant and diuretic."
1928 H. Smith MESKWAKI 252. "Specimen 5111 of the Dr. Jones Collection is the root. . .It is boiled and made into a drink to cure diarrhoea."
1932 H. Smith OJIBWE 411. "The Pillager Ojibwe say that the root of this vine was cooked and eaten a long time ago by their people and that it had been given as a special food by Winabojo."
1933 H. Smith POTAWATOMI 88. "The Forest Potawatomi make no use of the plant to our knowledge although they have a name for it."
1960 (1918) Meyer Herbalist 8. "American Ivy. The bark and twigs are the parts usually used. Its taste is acrid and persistent, though not unpleasant, and its decoction is mucilaginous. The bark should be collected after the berries have ripened. . .An old author affirms that there is very great antipathy between wine and ivy, and therefore it is a remedy to preserve against drunkeness, and to relieve or discourage intoxication, by drinking a draught of wine in which a handful of bruised leaves of ivy have been boiled."

VIRGIN'S BOWER   *Clematis virginiana* L. Ranunculaceae
A climbing vine with leaves consisting usually of three leaflets, these may be without teeth but usually have a few deep teeth or may be lobed. The many white flowers are followed by hairy plumes 2-4 cm long, at the ends of the seeds.

Range. N.B., N.S., P.E.I., s. Que., s. Ont., se. Man. to Minn., Nebr. and Mo., s. to Ga. and La. in low grounds, thickets and borders of woods.

Common names. Traveler's-joy. Love vine, devil's hair or darning needle, wild hops, woodbine.

1633 Gerarde-Johnson 885. "Travellers-Joy. The plant which Lobel setteth forth. . .whose long wooddy and viny branches extend themselves very far. . .decking with his clasping tendrels and white starre-like floures (being very sweet) all the hedges, and shrubs that are neere unto it. . .Great tufts of flat seeds, each seed having a fine white plume like a feather fastened to it, which maketh in the winter a goodly shew, covering the hedges white all over with his feather-like tops. The root is long, tough, and thicke, with many strings fastened thereto. . .These plants have no use in physicke as yet found out, but are esteemed only for pleasure, by reason of the goodly shadow which they make with their thicke bushing and clymbing, as also for the beauty of the flours, and the pleasant scent or savor of the same."

1830 Rafinesque 210. "Clematis, Virgin bower. Almost all species medical. . .The bark and blossoms acrid, raising blisters on the skin; a corrosive poison internally, loses the virulence by coction [cooking] and dessication. The extract used for osteocopic pain, dose 1 or 2 grains; frictions of an oily liniment cure the itch. Our *Cl. virginica* and *Cl. viorna* also used as diuretic and sudorific, for chronic rheumatism, palsy, and ulcers in minute doses. All ornamental vines. The flowers hold a peculiar substance, Clematine, similar to gluten. Bruised green leaves used by our empirics as escharotic for foul venereal ulcers, and detergent of other sores."

1868 Can. Pharm. J. 6; 83-5. *Clematis viginiana*, virgin's Bower, bark leaves and blossoms included in list of Can. medicinal plants.

1928 H. Smith MESKWAKI 239. "Leather flower, (*Clematis viorna*) [a southern species with purple leather-like flowers], Indian weed. The root of this species is used to make a drink for any kind of common sickness. McIntosh did not use it."

1950 Rudakov, C.A. 46:2240. Clematis species-Volatile oil containing protoanemonin which is polymerized to anemonin. [see buttercups]

1955 Mockle Quebec transl 42. "*C. virginiana, C. verticillaris*; Leaves when crushed vesicant and detergent." *C. verticillaris*, purple virgin's bower has single, large blue through purple to red flowers, range. Ont. to N.B. on rocks, open woods.

1968 Forsyth London 33. "Traveller's Joy. . .All parts of the plant are poisonous. It is a severe irritant and the juice, if applied to the skin, causes blistering. If eaten it causes enteritis and severe abdominal pain with diarrhoea, which in the end may be fatal. Poisoning by traveller's joy is rare, because of its acrid taste and the severe irritation it causes to the mouth of animals; they may bite but seldom swallow it. . .36. Administer raw eggs and sugar, in skimmed milk, to allay the severe irritation of the mouth and stomach as early as possible. Further treatment should be prescribed only by the medical practitioner or veterinary surgeon."

BITTERSWEET
Celastrus scandens L. Celastraceae

A climber that climbs by twining up trees and fences. The leaves 5-10 cm long, alternate. The flowers around a 3-8 cm long stem are small, greenish. Followed by berries having a pulpy orange outer pod that opens to show a scarlet interior.

Range. Que., Ont., Man., Sask., s. to Okla., La., Ala. and Ga. in thickets, streambanks and woods.

Common names. Staff tree, fever twig, waxwort, staffvine, redroot.

1670's Radisson. See Smith below.

1801 Coues NORTHWEST 1 172. "There is also an abundance of bois tors. . .a short shrub that winds up the stocks of larger trees; the wood is soft and spongy, with a thick bark, which is often eaten by the natives in time of famine."

1830 Rafinesque 206. "Equivalent of Dulcamara and Mezereon, but weaker, Bark used, emetic, antisyphilitic, discutient; externally it expels indurated tumors, and the swelling of cow bags."

1859-61 Gunn 749. "The Bitter Sweet. . .is common throughout the United States. . .The root is creeping, of a bright orange color, about the size of the middle finger or thumb, and several rods in length. . .The bark of the root. . .has a sweetish and rather a sickening taste; it is both a powerful and useful medicine, although like most of the valuable medicinal plants of our country, which nature has so bountifully furnished to our hands, its virtues are but little known or appreciated. . .It increases all the secretions and excretions, particularly perspiration; acts gently as a diuretic, or increases the flow of urine. It is highly valuable in liver complaints, and in all general weakness, in disorders of the skin, and rheumatism; in scrofula or king's evil it is one of the most valuable medicines; also in swellings, ulcers, jaundice, weakness, and obstructions in women. To be taken inwardly, boil half a pound of the bark of the root in a gallon of water down to two quarts, and take a wineglassful two or three times a day. It may be made into a sirup by adding sugar. . .To make Bitter Sweet Ointment, add half a pound of the bark of the root to a pound of lard, simmer slowly over the fire for several hours, then strain for use. It is good for swelled breasts, discuss or drive away tumors or swellings, and also for piles."

1860 Kohl Lake Superior 284. "They [the Indians] have. . .a creeping plant, called by the Canadians 'bois'tors'. . .They smoke the bark."

1868 Can. Pharm. J. 6; 83-5. *Celastrus scandens*; the bark of the root included in list of Can. medicinal plants.

1882 Can. Pharm. J. 224. "Mr. C.H. Bernard made the bark of *Celastrus scandens*. . .subject of an inaugural essay. . .and found the drug to contain sulphuric, hydrochloric, phosphoric, and nitric acids in combination; and potassium, sodium, magnesium, calcium, and iron salts; an acid resin, and a neutral resin, starch, sugar, gum, and a caoutchouc-like body, coloring matter, extractive, and a volatile oil. . .It is more than probable that the activity of the bark depends on the resin and volatile oil."

1892 Millspaugh 42. "The common Bittersweet. . .(*Celastrus scandens*). . .has been largely used in domestic practice, as an alterative, diuretic and cholagogue in various diseases where it seemed necessary to 'cleanse the blood.' It was considered without equal for the removal of hepatic obstruction."

1926-7 Densmore CHIPPEWA 344. A decoction of the root is used especially as a physic for babies. . .348. A decoction of the roots is drunk for stoppage of urine. "This, is one of the Winabojo remedies, the native name being Winabojo onagic, meaning 'Winabojo's intestines.' The legend is that Winabojo was once walking on the ice when he heard something rattling behind him. He looked back and saw that his intestines were dragging behind him and part had become frozen to the ice. He broke off part and threw them over a tree, saying, 'This shall be for the good of my future relatives.'". . .350. A decoction of the stalk was drunk for eruptions.

1923 H. Smith MENOMINI 63. "Bittersweet is abundant on the reservation, and is found in dense woods climbing to the tops of trees thirty feet or more in height. The curled and twisted liane stems curiously resemble the intestines of a man, and doubtless inspired the story. It is recognized by the Menomini that the inner bark is palatable and will sustain life when food is hard to get."

1928 H. Smith MESKWAKI 208. "The Meskwaki do not know what plant this is, nor do they use it. McIntosh did not know the Potawatomi use of it, although he said that he knew that the Menomini use it. Specimen 3656 in the Dr. Jones Collection is the root of *Celastrus scandens*. . .and is used to mix with the root of *Arctium minus* [burdock] and an unidentified Umbellifer for the relief of women in labor."

1932 H. Smith OJIBWE 362. "The Pillager Ojibwe use the red berries of this plant for stomach trouble. . .398. When food is unobtainable in the winter, because the snow is too deep and game is scarce, the Ojibwe gather this bark and separate the inner bark to make a thick soup for a meal. While it is not very palatable, it is sustaining and they may subsist on it for a considerable time."

1933 H. Smith POTAWATOMI 97. "This is one of the real aboriginal foods encountered by the early white voyageurs and often indispensable. . .The inner bark is prepared and cooked. . .The first white man to call attention to it was Radisson. He said, 'The greatest subsistence that we can have is of rind (Vine) tree, which grows like ivie about the trees, but to swallow it we cut the stick some 2 foot long, tying it in faggotts, and boyle it, and when it boyles one houre or two ye rind or skinne comes off with ease, which we take and drie it in the smoake and then reduce it to powder betwixt two grainstoan, and putting the kettle with the same water upon the fire, we make it a kind of broath, which nourished us, but [we] became thirstier and drier than the woods we ate.'

1945 Rousseau MOHAWK 54. "For anemia make an infusion of a fistful of the bark of the roots in a gallon of water. By boiling reduce to a pint. Mix with wine and an infusion of wild grape vines."

1955 Mockle Quebec transl. 57. "The bark has cholagogue, emetic, cathartic, diaphoretic properties. It contains a naphtoquinon, celastrol."

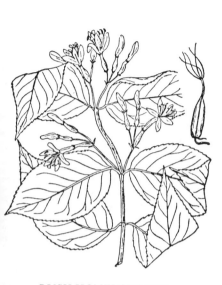

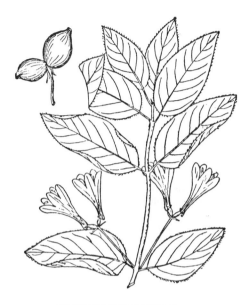

BUSH HONEYSUCKLE

FLY HONEYSUCKLE

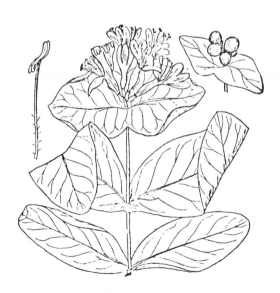

WILD HONEYSUCKLE

BUSH HONEYSUCKLE   *Diervilla lonicera* Mill. Caprifoliaceae
Shrub to 120 cm with leaves 8-15 cm long, pointed, toothed and hairy around their edges, sometimes hairy beneath. The flowers 3-7 on each stalk, yellow turning reddish, hairy within. The fruit is a slender capsule with a beak 10-15 mm long.
Range. Nfld. to Sask., s. to Va., Ga., Ind. and Io. in dry or rocky soil.
1887 Penhallow 48. "In the year 1706, Diéreville visited. . .Port Royal in Acadia. . .He carried a number of plants back to Europe, and submitted them to Tournefort, one of the three great botanists of that day. Among other plants, was a specimen of the bush honeysuckle, a plant entirely new to Tournefort, who dedicated it to its discoverer under the generic name of *Diervilla*."
1830 Rafinesque 216. "Nauseous, pellent, antisyphilitic; has been used for disury, gonorrhea and syphilis, but is not efficient."
1926-7 Densmore CHIPPEWA 304. *Diervilla lonicera* Constituents: Alkaloid believed to be narceine; a glucoside similar to fraxina in *D. lutea*. . .342. The leaves in decoction for a pain in the stomach. Used only in combinations.
1923 H. Smith MENOMINI 27. "The root of this plant is credited with being a cure for senility. It is also a mild diurient. In both cases a tea is brewed from the root."
1928 H. Smith MESKWAKI 206. "Specimen 5117 in Dr. Jones collection. . .is the root of *Diervilla lonicera* and some other unidentified root. It is mixed, boiled and made into a drink for the treatment of gonorrhea. The root is also. . .used as a tea for one who is urinating blood. . .Eclectics among the whites have used the fruit for its cathartic and emetic properties. The plant is also valued by them as a diuretic and as a means to alleviate itching in the urethral tract."
1932 H. Smith OJIBWE 360. "The Flambeau Ojibwe use the root together with other plants such as the Ground Pine, for their most valued urinary remedy."
1933 H. Smith POTAWATOMI 45. "The Bush Honeysuckle is used by many of our Indian tribes of the north and is especially valuable according to them, in urinary troubles. The Prairie Potawatomi make a tea of the root of the Bush Honeysuckle to be used as a diuretic and for the treatment of cases of gonorrhoea. Mrs. Spoon makes a medicine for vertigo in which this. . .is used. Her recipe for the medicine is Red Baneberry root (*Actaea rubra*), the twigs of (*Diervilla lonicera*), the leaves and root of Liverleaf Hepatica (*Hepatica triloba*), and the roots of Sweet Cicely (*Osmorhiza longistylis*). The writer saw her mix this material in her wooden mixing bowl about four inches in diameter with a wooden spoon and afterwards he tasted the infusion which had a sweetish taste. . .The National Dispensatory [1916] says that the whole plant is considered diuretic and has been applied to relieve itching."
1945 Raymond TETE DE BOULE transl. 128. "The leaves of the bush honeysuckle are diuretic; they are mixed with those of bunchberry (*Cornus canadensis*)."
1955 Mockle Quebec transl. 84. "The bark is purgative. The roots are said to be effective against retention of urine."

FLY HONEYSUCKLE   *Lonicera canadensis* Marsh.
Shrub to 2 m with straggling branches. Leaves 3-12 cm long with hairy but not toothed edges. The 2-3 cm long stalk bearing two flowers grows from where the leaf joins the stem. The yellowish flowers 12-22 mm long and smooth. The fruit two red berries.
Range. N.S. and e. Que. to Sask., s. to Pa., O., Ind. and Minn. and in the mts. to N.C. in dry or moist woods. May-June.
Common names. Medaddy-bush.

WILD HONEYSUCKLE   *Lonicera dioica* L.
A climbing shrub with smooth branches. The leaves 5-12 cm long, the upper one or two pairs joined together to make one leaf out of the centre of which the several flowers grow. These are greenish yellow tinged with purple. They are followed by bright red berries.
Range. Mass., Que., n. Ont. to Wisc., Mack., B.C., s. to N.J., N.C., Ind. and Okla. in moist woods, swamps, dunes. May-June.
1830 Rafinesque 240. "All sp. leaves and flowers bitterish, mucilaginous, astringent, detersive, &c. A sirup used for sorethroat, irritation of the lungs."

1915 Speck MONTAGNAIS 315. "The vines of *Lonicera canadensis*. . .are steeped for urinary trouble. As an example of efficiency, a boy at Tadousac whose abdomen was distended with retained water, was relieved in twenty minutes after taking this medicine."

1926-7 Densmore CHIPPEWA 340. "*Lonicera* sp. A decoction of the root with other ingredients not specified drunk for lung trouble.

1923 H. Smith MENOMINI 27. "The bark of this bush (*Lonicera canadensis*) is used in the treatment of urinary diseases. It is used in combination with other plants to cure gonorrhoea. All of the local species of Lonicera have been used by the white men as medicine, though only as non-offical drugs. Many of them have more than a local repute as emetic and cathartic drugs."

1928 H. Smith MESKWAKI 207. "*Lonicera dioca*. The berry and sometimes the root bark is used in a tea to cure worms in pregnant women, who are poor and weakly. It is also used in combination with other roots."

1933 H. Smith POTAWATOMI 46. "*Lonicera canadensis*. . .The Forest Potawatomi combine the bark of this species with Juniper foliage and berries and with the twigs of the Bush honeysuckle to make a 'tea' which is used as a diuretic."

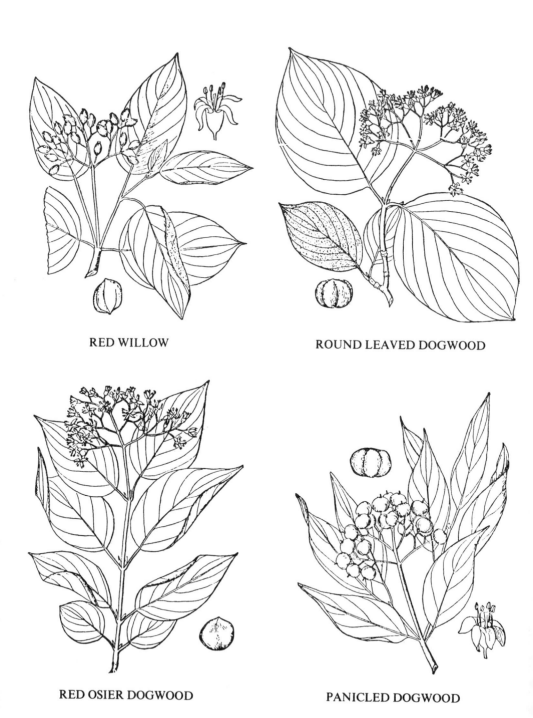

RED WILLOW

ROUND LEAVED DOGWOOD

RED OSIER DOGWOOD

PANICLED DOGWOOD

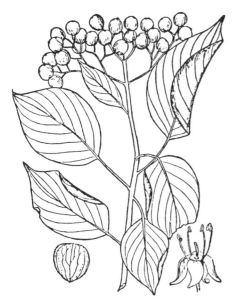

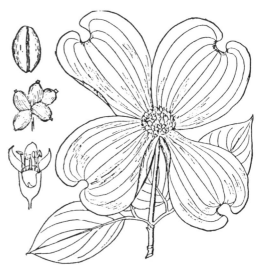

ALTERNATE LEAVED DOGWOOD   FLOWERING DOGWOOD

FLOWERING DOGWOOD   *Cornus florida* L. Cornaceae
Large open shrub or tree to 10 m, Leaves mostly 6-10 cm and half as wide, pale beneath. The large white or sometimes pink flowers are really the four petal-like bracts 3-6 cm long in the middle of which is a cluster of 20-30 yellowish tiny flowers. The fruit is bright red 10-15 mm long.
Range. Me. to s. Ont., Mich., Ill. and Kan., s. to Fla. and ne. Mex. May-June in woods, blooming before the leaves are fully grown.
Common names. Box-wood, arrow-wood, white cornel.
1748 Kalm Philadelphia Nov. 30th. 196. "Several people peeled the roots of the *Cornus florida*, or dogwood, and gave this peel to the patients; and some people, who could not be cured [of ague] by the Jesuits' bark [cinchona], recovered by the help of this."
1779 Zeisberger DELAWARE 51. "Dogwood is also found in these parts. The rind of the root is used in the apothecary shops in place of Jesuit-bark [quinine]. This tree grows to be neither large nor high."
1828 Rafinesque 133. "This tree grows very slow, and the wood is hard, compact, heavy and durable; it is white outside and chocolate color in the centre, taking a very fine polish. . .All kinds of tools and instruments are made with it, also cogs of wheels, teeth of harrows, spoons, &c. most abundant in swampy and moist woods. The bark of the root, stem and branches is bitter, astringent, and slightly aromatic. By analysis it has been found to contain in different proportion the same substances as *Cinchona*. . .The fresh bark frequently disagrees with the stomach, and is improved by keeping at least one year. Tonic, astringent, antiseptic, coroborant and stimulant. It is one of the best native substitutes for Cinchona [quinine], although evidently different in some respects; the powdered bark quickens the pulse, and sometimes produces pains in the bowels. . .Used in intermittent and remittent fevers, typhus and all febrile disorders. . .It is often used in decoction in the country, and even the twigs are chewed as a prophylactic against fevers. Drunkards use the tincture of the berries as a bitter for the same purpose and for indigestion. The flowers have the same properties, and are chiefly used by the Indians, in warm infusion for fever and cholic. . .It is said that the twigs rubbed or chewed, clean and keep sound the gums and teeth. A decoction of the bark is used to cure the distemper of horses called yellow water. Joined with sassafras it is employed in strong warm decoction to clean foul ulcers and cancers. Lastly a kind of black ink can be made with the bark, in the usual way, instead of galls. . . .266. The southern Indians use it in poultice for sores."

1859-61 Gunn 787. "It is the best native tonic and substitute for quinine and the peruvian bark that we have, being very similar in its properties to the Cinchona, and very near as good. The flowers are sometimes used as a mild strengthening bitters, especially for female weakness. The bark of the root is preferable to that of the tree; and the best way to use it, as a tonic, or ague medicine, is in the form of extract, made by boiling water, and evaporating down to a thick stiff extract."

1892 Millspaugh 71. "A peculiar feature in the blossoming of this species is the great regularity in time of appearance of its short lived blossoms; so characteristic is this that the Indians always planted their corn when the blossoms appeared. . .The bark of the roots afforded the aborigines a scarlet pigment. The previous medical use of dogwood bark dates from the discovery of this country, as it was then used by the Indians. . .The fresh bark in doses of from 20-40 grains causes increased action of the heart, heat of the skin, and severe pain in the bowels. The American Indian, true to the principle that seems to have guided him in the use of all medicines, used the bark for fever and colic. . .it increases [the] temperature of the skin and the general perspiration. . .Some experimenters have observed a constant tendency to sleep. . .This does not indicate any specific narcotic properties, but is the result of cerebral fullness. Whether the remote effects. . .are the direct effects of the introduction of the active principles into the blood, is not certainly known; although the latter is most probable, since the cold infusion or the alcoholic extract produces the same effects. . .It is very evident that the bark has properties calculated to invigorate the vital forces, and the organic nervous energy."

1894 Household Guide Toronto 117. "Dogwood is a familar tree, the bark of which is good in fever and ague. It is also used as an appetizer. Make a strong tea by boiling a handful of the bark in a quart of water. Take a wineglassful three times a day."

1915 Speck MICMAC-MONTAGNAIS 317. Bark dried and smoked mixed with tobacco.

1955 Mockle Quebec transl 68. "*Cornus florida*. The bark is astringent and febrifuge. It contains a principal glucoside, cornine that Reichert and later Cheymol identified with verbenaloside, as well as betulic acid."

RED WILLOW   *Cornus amomum* Mill. Cornaceae (*C. sericea*)
A shrub 1-3 m tall, the pith of the young twigs dark brown. The leaves are opposite each other, 6-12 cm long and half as wide or wider. On each side of their centre vein are 4-6 side veins. The fruit is light blue.
Range. New England and Que. to Ont., s. Ind., and s. Ill., s. to S.C. and Ala, May-June in moist woods or along streams.
Common names. Silky cornel, kinnikinik, swamp dogwood, squaw bush, red osier, rose willow, blueberry cornel.

ROUND LEAVED DOGWOOD   *Cornus rugosa* Lam. (*C. circinata*)
Shrub 1-3 m tall, the twigs yellowish-green, often shaded or mottled with red, pith white. Leaves round mostly 7-12 cm with soft white hairs beneath, 7-8 veins on each side of the centre one. Fruit light blue.
Range. Que. to central Ont. and s. Man., s. to N.J., Pa., n. O, n. Ind. and Io., and in the mts. to Va. May-July in moist or dry, sandy or rocky soil.
Common names. Alder leaved dogwood, green osier, bois de calumet.

RED OSIER DOGWOOD   *Cornus stolonifera* Michx. (*C. alba*)
Shrub 1-3 m tall, often forming dense patches by root runners. Young branches bright red, older grey, pith white and large. Leaves opposite, 5-10 cm long and a fourth to two thirds as wide, distinctly whitish beneath. The veins on each side of the centre 5-7. The fruit white to bluish.
Range. Nflfd. to Alaska, s. to Pa., Ind., Ill. and n. Mex. May-June in wet woods and on streambanks.
Common names. Kinnikinik, squaw bush, waxberry cornel, dogberry-tree, gutter-tree, grey willow.

PANICLED DOGWOOD

Cornus racemosa Lam. (*C. paniculata*)

Shrub 1-5 m tall often forming thickets, the twigs reddish soon turning grey. Pith nearly always brown; leaves opposite, 4-8 cm long with 3-4 veins on each side of the centre one, whitish beneath. Fruit white.

Range. Me. to s. Ont. and Man., s. to Fla. and Ark. May-June in moist soil.

ALTERNATE LEAVED DOGWOOD

Cornus alternifolia L.f.

Shrub or small tree to 6 m the twigs with a white pith; the leaves alternate, 5-10 cm long, 4-5 veins on each side, pale green beneath, tending to be found near the tips of the branches. Fruit blue.

Range. Nfld. and N.S. to Minn., s. to Fla., Ala. and Ark. May-June in rich woods.

1380 Crawford Lake site Ontario McAndrews, Byrne and Finlayson 1974. "Three *Cornus* seeds recovered archeologically.

1743 Isham Hudson Bay 135. "Their is a willow they styl, (misqua pemeque,) or red willow, which makes an Excellent Dye upon bone, Ivory, Qhils, or cloth &c.: taking the out side bark of, and boiling the under bark, for a Considerable time, over a moderate fire, and Boyl a Comb for ½ an hour, will come out a fine Deep Red, the Root of which tree makes a finer & Deeper Dye than the Bark, mixing it with the bark, as also Cranberries." [*C. stolonifera.*]

1749 Kalm Fort St. Frederic 22 October 588. "*Bois de calumet* (wood for pipes) is what the French called the *dogwood*, which has green branches and stem and not red like the cornel. It sent forth each year long, narrow, even shoots without branches which had a fairly large pith. Both Indians and French took these shoots or branches, removed the outer bark so that they became smooth, then bored out the soft kernel and used the branches as their pipestems. . .The pith of this tree is so soft that a long narrow stick cut from the same tree will force out the kernel when it is pushed through a branch of it. This is not true of the red dogwood, the core of which is harder. On paring the bark from this branch people loosened it so that it remained attached at one end. Then they put the other end of the cutting in the ground a little distance from the fire and allowed the bark to dry a bit, whereupon they placed it in their tobacco pouch and smoked it mixed with their tobacco. They also used the bark of the red dogwood in the same manner. I inquired why they smoked this bark and what benefit they derived therefrom. They replied that the tobacco was too strong to smoke alone and therefore was mixed. This is one of the customs which the French learned from the natives, and it is remarkable that the Frenchman's whole smoking etiquette here in Canada, namely the preparation of the tobacco, the tobacco pouch, the pipe, pipe-stem, etc. was derived from the natives, with the exception of the fire-steel and flint, which came from Europe, and which the natives did not have before the French or Europeans came here. Red dogwood the French called *bois rouge* and knew of no other use for it than the one mentioned above."

20th. October Fort Nicholson 606. "The wife of Colonel Lydius told me that when she had arrived in Canada she had suffered from pain in her legs as the result of the cold. It became so severe that for a period of three months she could not use one leg and had to go about with a crutch. She tried various remedies without avail. Finally a native woman came to the house who cured her in the following manner. She went into the forest, took twigs and cuttings of the dogwood, removed the bark, boiled them in water and rubbed the legs with this water. The pain disappeared within two or three days and she regained her former health."

1778 Carver CHIPPEWA Lake Michigan 31. "Near this Lake, and indeed about all the great lakes, is found a kind of willow, termed by the French, bois rouge, in English red wood. Its bark, when only of one year's growth, is of a fine scarlet colour, and appears very beautiful; but as it grows older, it changes into a mixture of grey and red. The stalks of this shrub grow many of them together, and rise to the height of six or eight feet, the largest not exceeding an inch diameter. The bark being scraped from the sticks, and dried and powdered, is also mixed by the Indians with their tobacco, and is held by them in the highest estimation for their winter smoking. . .and as they are great smoakers, they are very careful in properly gathering and preparing them."

1791 Long Wisconsin River 149. "We encamped [in 1780] on the banks, and intended setting off at break of day, but one of the Indians was bitten by a rattlesnake. . .which had fourteen rattles. . .This unfortunate accident retarded our journey till the unhappy sufferer relieved himself by cutting out the wounded part from the calf of his leg, and applying salt and gunpowder, and binding it up with the leaves of the red willow tree; he was soon able to proceed, bearing the pain with that fortitude for which the Savages are so eminently distinguished."

1828 Rafinesque 134. "Almost all the species of this genus have more or less the same tonic properties, and may be substituted to the *C. florida*. Three of them best known as most efficient will be mentioned here. *C. sericea* [red willow] or blueberry cornel, vulgarly called swamp dogwood or Rose Willow. The bark is less bitter, more astringent and pleasant to the taste. . .Round leaved cornel. . .an ounce of the bark yields by boiling 150 grains, of an astringent and intensly bitter extract. In use it is found preferable to Columbo and Cinchona, it is much employed in the Northern States, in substance and otherwise, for diarrhoea, dyspepsia; but it is too heating in fevers. . .1830 213. *C. paniculata* has been substituted for *C. florida*."

1857 Daniel Wilson 254. "The Saultaux Indians—as the Chippeqays of the far west are most frequently designated. . .make use of various herbs to mix with and dilute tobacco, such as the leaves of the cranberry and the inner bark of the red willow, to both of which the Indian word kinikinik is generally applied."

1857-61 Gunn 850. "Rose willow (*Cornus sericea*). . .The bark of the root and stalks is the part used and is tonic and somewhat astringent, and very similar in its properties to the common Dogwood. . .It is said to be an excellent remedy to relieve the nausea and vomiting of pregnant females. It is also good as an antiseptic wash for foul and gangrenous ulcers."

1868 Can. Pharm. J. 6; 83-5. Bark of *C. circinata* [*C. rugosa*] included in list of Can. medicinal plants.

1879 H.M. Robinson Hudson Bay 338. "The native carries a fire-bag—a long leather bag, containing pipe, tobacco, knife, flint and steel, and *barouge*, the inner bark of the grey willow." [Barouge = bois rouge = *C. stolonifera*.]

1884 Holmes-Haydon CREE Hudson Bay 303. "Milawapamule. Red willow bark. This bark occurs in two qualities, one being in the form of slender quills, 3-4 inches long. . .the inner surface light orange brown, and the exterior of a deep chesnut brown colour, but when fresh of a bright crimson; the taste is bitter, and the flavour resembles that of tea. The second quality consists of fine scrapings of the young bark. The latter is the form in which the bark is used as an emetic in coughs and fevers. For coughs the bark is boiled in water and the decoction strained and given while still warm in the dose of a wineglassful every few minutes until vomiting supervenes. For colds and fevers a teaspoonful of the decoction is taken occasionally. The scraped wood is also smoked, mixed with tobacco. Boiled with rust of iron, it is used as a black dye."

1892 Millspaugh 71. "The berries of the Red Osier Dogwood. . .are claimed by Murion to yield about one-third their weight of a pure limpid oil, resembling olive and fit for table use or for burning. . .73. [Red Willow] The use of this species in general medicine has mostly been as a substitute for *C. Florida*, than which it is less bitter, while being more astringent. . .This species seems to act stronger on the heart than C. Florida and to cause more cerebral congestion."

1926-7 Densmore CHIPPEWA 360. For sore eyes scrape and steam the root of *C. alternifolia*, using a handful to about a pint and a half of water. Let it cool and strain well. Bathe the eye and let some of the liquid get into the eye, or use it on a compress. Take an equal part of this root and that of *C. stolonifera* and make a decoction, use it as a wash or compress for sore eyes. . .370. Formula for red dye. Take the outer and inner bark of *C. stolonifera* and the inner bark of the white birch and the oak, boil in hot water. Prepare the ashes by burning about an armful of scraps of cedar bark. This should make about 2 cups of ashes, which is the correct quantity for about 2 gallons of dye. Sift the ashes through a piece of cheesecloth. Put them into the dye after it has boiled a while, then let it boil up again, and then put in the material to be colored. Do not let a man or any outsider look at the dye. . .Take equal amounts of the inner bark of *C. stolonifera* and *Alnus incana* or alder and boil in hot water. Colored a white blanket a light red. [See bloodroot for a scarlet dye for quills using this dogwood also]. . .The inner bark mixed with alder and oak and black earth or grindstone dust in hot water let it stand a long time before using, dyes black. . .376. The root of *C. alternifolia* put on muskrat traps as a charm. *C. rugosa* and *stolonifera* used for smoking.

1928 Reagan CHIPPEWA 239. "The Bois Fort Ojibwa of our day smoke tobacco and must have it on all occasions of ceremony. Formerly he used kinnikinnik, which he obtained as the pulverized inner bark (or leaves) of several plants. . .the red dogwood (*Cornus stolonifera*) and a *C. sericea*. [*C. amomum*] The latter was the plant most used and is now still used in certain ceremonies. . .In preparing the kinnikinnik from it, the stems of the plant are gathered green and the red outer bark removed with a sharp knife. The inner fibrous bark is then scraped off of the wood and dried in some container before the fire till it is crisp and brittle and is readily crushed in the hand. It is then 'kinnikinnik' and is ready for smoking. Among the Bois Fort Indians tobacco and kinnikinnik are frequently used as an offering to Manabush and the other manido. They are also sprinkled on the grave boxes to aid the dead on the journey to the spiritland. Tobacco is also used as a peace offering, and so was kinnikinnik in the old times. Its origin is regarded as mystic."

1923 H. Smith MENOMINI 32. "*Cornus amomum* silky cornel and *C. alternifolia* both known as kinnikinik. The bark of this shrub is gathered to yield a liquid pile remedy. The use of the various pile remedies was interestingly given by my informant. The tepid liquid is placed in a special rectal syringe. This is made from the bladder of the deer or bear, into the neck of which is bound a two-inch hollow duck bone. This is tied on with sinew. By compressing the bladder, the liquid is forced into the rectum where it is retained for intervals of half an hour for each application. . .is also used for diarrhoea. . .in the special rectal syringe. . .The bark is also pulverized and put upon a bandage, where a wet application is bound to the anus. The strength of the medicine in this case is supposed to travel upwards. This bark is the species used by a Menomini at Neopit to cure cancer. . .His wife made a poultice of this bark with something else and cured the cancer. But the Menomini would not divulge the exact formula or method of use of this medicine. . .Silky cornel is also used for diarrhoea. In this case an infusion of the bark is used in a rectal injection. . .80. The inner bark of both species was used by the Menomini for smoking tobacco. In these latter days it is mixed with real tobacco, but in olden times it was used alone. It was gathered and toasted to prepare it, the manner of preparation being well told in Dr. Barrett's 'Dream Dance of the Chippewa and Menomini Indians of Northern Wisconsin'. Bull. Pub. Mus. Milwauke Vol. 1 357-368."

1928 H. Smith MESKWAKI 219. "(*C. paniculata*). This is an important medicine. The bark tea was used to cure the flux, in which case it was injected into the bowel as an enema. . .It was often used upon children. When the teeth are sore or one has neuralgia, the same tea is held in the mouth to stop this pain. McIntosh also tells of using the bark in a smudge the same as a reviver. Specimen 5164 of the Dr. Jones collection is the root. . .The root tea was used to cure consumption. . .272. Smoked as ceremonial tobacco."

1932 H. Smith OJIBWE 366. "The Pillager Ojibwe use the inner bark [alternate leaved dogwood] for an emetic. . .The bark [panicled dogwood] is used as a tea for flux. An aggregate of this bark is compressed into a stopper shape and is forced into the anus as a stopper as a treatment for piles. . .399. The twig bark is peeled and toasted over coals on a crude drying form, then further shredded to carry in their tobacco pouches and smoke in their pipes. . .417. Alternate leaved dogwood. . .the twigs are used in thatching and for various purposes by the Pillager Ojibwe. . .430. The root is boiled by the Flambeau Ojibwe to wash a muskrat trap and make it lure the muskrat."

1933 H. Smith POTAWATOMI 54. "Alternate leaved dogwood. The Forest Potawatomi use the bark of the alternate leaved dogwood to make an infusion which is used as an eye-wash. . .Red Osier dogwood, *C. stolonifera*. The Potawatomi say that the root bark is the most efficacious remedy they have for the treatment of diarrhoea and flux. . .118. Bark from the twigs smoked."

1935 Jenness Parry Island Lake Huron OJIBWA 89. "Dysentery; boil the stem of the red osier dogwood, *C. stolonifera* and drink the decoction."

1945 Rousseau MOHAWK transl. 55. "*C. stolonifera*. For dyspepsia, the infusion of the bark of seven branches each one foot long in one pint of water. The very flexible branches are used in drying muskrat skins. . .and in basketry."

1945 Rousseau Quebec transl. 95. "*C. stolonifera*, hart rouge. The flexible branches are used in basketry. There are many baskets made of them on Isles aux Coudres."

1959 Mechling MALECITE maritime provinces of Canada used the red osier dogwood, *C. stolonifera*, for sore eyes, sore throat, catarrh and headache.

1960 Walpole Island CHIPPEWA mss "*Cornus Amomum*, red willow to stop diarrhoea, a handful of the bark from young plants added to a cupful of boiling water, boiled ten minutes, a glass taken in half an hour is effective. . .To treat poison ivy, take only young smooth bark, one cup of bark to a quart of water, boiled, after slightly cooling spread over affected area and allow to dry. Several applications may be necessary. The itching generally stops within a day."

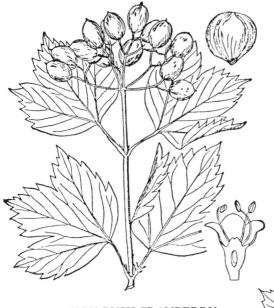

HIGH-BUSH CRANBERRY

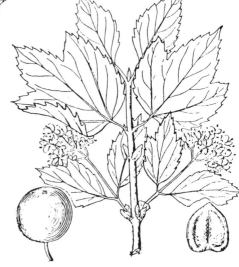

SQUASHBERRY

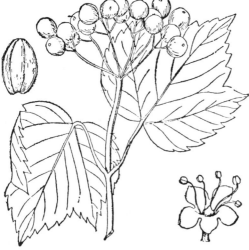

ARROW-WOOD

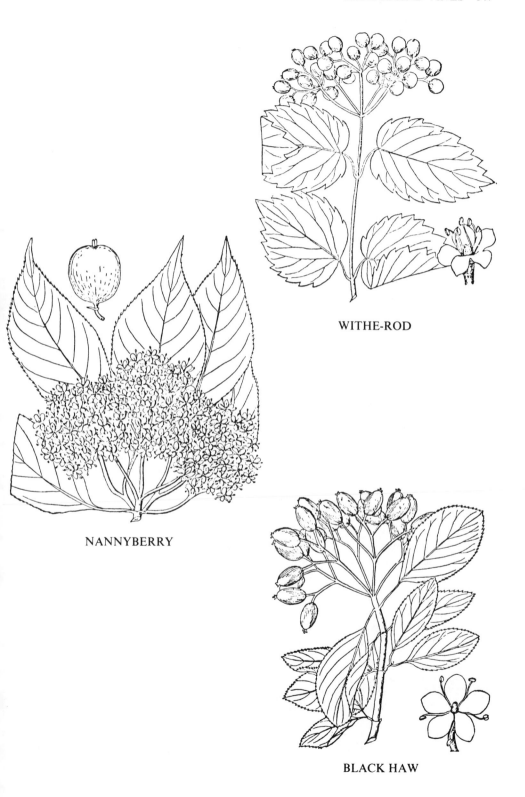

WITHE-ROD

NANNYBERRY

BLACK HAW

HIGH-BUSH CRANBERRY   *Viburnum opulus* L. var. *americanum* Ait. Caprifoliaceae
A shrub 1-5 m tall, stems smooth, leaves like those of the maple 2-5 cm wide, the veins runing
from the stem, the teeth large, hairy beneath. The flowering stem 2-5 cm long, the outer flowers
larger than those in the middle, white. The fruit is a brilliant translucent red, the berries hang on
the shrubs all winter.
Range. Nfld. to B.C., s. to Pa., n.O., Io. and Wash. in moist woods and fields.
Common names. Guelder rose, cranberry tree, cramp-bark, marsh or water elder, dog rowan tree,
gaiter tree or gatten, whitten tree, pembina, pimbina.

SQUASHBERRY   *Viburnum edule* (Michx.) Raf. (*V. pauciflorum*)
Straggling shrub 0.5-2 m the stems often covered with glands. The leaves 5-10 cm often hairy on
the veins beneath. The flowering stem short, usually less than 50 white flowers. The fruit light red
not translucent.
Range. Lab. to Alas. s. to Pa., Mich., Minn., Colo. and Ore. in cold mountain woods.
1668 Marie de l'Incarnation Quebec 346. "We also make jam from gooseberries and from pimi-
nan, a wild fruit that sugar renders very pleasant."
1749 Kalm Fort St. Frederic October 1th. 565. "The cranberry tree, a kind of opulus, flourished
in some places on the shore. We consumed great quantities of the berries which were ripe. They
had a pleasant acid flavor and tasted right well. Even if we had had some other fruit, we should
not have scorned these."
1760 Jefferys New France 41. "The Pemine, another plant peculiar to this country, is a different
shrub, growing along the sides of rivulets, and in meadows, which also bears a clustering fruit of
a very sharp and stringent taste."
1836 Trail Backwds Can. 61. "For richness of flavour, and for beauty of appearance, I admire
the high-bush cranberries; these are little sought after, on account of the large flat seeds, which
prevent them being used as jam: the jelly, however, is delightful, both in colour and
flavour. . .The berries. . .when just touched by the frosts are semi-transparent, and look like pen-
dant bunches of scarlet grapes. . .I was tempted one fine frosty afternoon to take a walk with my
husband on the ice. . .recognised. . .high-bush cranberries. . .stripped the boughs. . .hastened
home, and boiled the fruit with some sugar to eat at tea with our cakes. I never ate anything
more delicious than they proved; the more so perhaps from having been so long without tasting
fruit of any kind."
1853 Reid, 31. "The name, however, by which it is known among the Indians of Red River is
'anepeminan,' from 'nepen,' summer, and 'minan', berry. This has been corrupted by the fur
traders and voyageurs into 'Pembina': hence the name of a river which runs into the Red and
also the name of the celebrated but unsuccessful settlement of 'Pembina' formed by Lord Selkirk
many years ago."
1868 Can. Pharm J. 6; 83-5 The bark of the high-bush cranberry, *V. opulus*, included in list of
Can. medicinal plants.
1870 Briante 39. "Whooping cough, take two ounces of Wild snow ball bark, and steep it in a
quart of water. Dose, one table-spoonful, three times a day. . .95. Sedative, astringent and expectorant."
1892 Millspaugh 74." The High Cranberry (*Viburnum opulus*), now proving valuable in many
forms of uterine affections and puerperal diseases."
1913 Hodge & White 384. "Pembina. A Canadian name for the acid fruit of *Viburnum opulus*,
the high-bush cranberry. . .The word is a corruption of Cree nipiminan, 'watered-berry' i.e. fruit
of a plant growing in, or laved by, water."
1915 Speck PENOBSCOT 310. "High-bush cranberries. . .are steeped and drunk for swollen
glands and mumps. (Also a Malecite remedy)". . .316 MONTAGNAIS. "Plant is boiled and the
mess rubbed in the eyes for sore eyes."
1925 Wood & Ruddock. Cramps in the legs. . .make a strong tea of cranberry bush bark. Drink a
third of a cupful, will stop cramps in 20 minutes. Best to take it night and morning for several
weeks, the trouble seldom returns. Also bark of root of black haw, *V. prunifolium*. [see below]
1926-27 Densmore CHIPPEWA 307. Fruit of *Vibrunum pauciflorum* [*V. edule*] eaten.
1923 H. Smith MENOMINI 63. "These are rather scarce on the Menomini reservation, but are
favored as a fruit whenever they can be found."
1928 H. Smith MESKWAKI 208. "(*Viburnum opulus* L. *americanum*). . .Specimen 3618 of the Dr.

Jones collection is doubtfully identified as the root of this species and. . .'used when in cramps all over'. It is boiled and drunk by one who feels pain over his entire body."
1932 H. Smith OJIBWE 361. "The Pillager Ojibwe used the inner bark as a physic, and also drank the tea to cure cramps in the stomach. Among the white men, *Viburnum opulus* is considered to be the same as *Viburnum prunifolium*, only less potent. It is recommended as an antispasmodic in asthma, hysteria, puerperal convulsions, and dysmenorrhea."
1955 Mockle Quebec transl. 85. "The bark is used in treating functional uterine troubles. It contains viburnin and salicoside."

ARROW-WOOD   *Viburnum acerifolium* L.
Shrub 1-2 m tall, the young stems, leaf stalks and flowering top are covered with fine hairs. Leaves like maple leaves, flowers on a 3-5 cm long stem. The fruit is purple black.
Range. Sw. Que. and N.B. to Minn., s. to Fla. and La. in moist or dry woods.
Common names. Dockmackie, squash-berry.
1830 Rafinesque 274. "Leaves applied to inflamed tumors by the Indians."
1926-27 Densmore CHIPPEWA 344. The inner bark in a decoction drunk from cramps. . .346. The inner bark and that of the alder (*Alnus incana*). In preparing these scrape the stalks carefully, removing only the thin outer covering and using the green part underneath. Put the scrapings of this green bark from both trees in boiling water to make a decoction and drink as an emetic.
1923 H. Smith MENOMINI 28. "The inner bark of this bush yields a tea which is drunk for cramps or colic."

WITHE-ROD   *Viburnum dentatum* L. var. *lucidum* Ait. (*V. pubescens*)
Shrub 1-5 m with close gray-brown or reddish bark. Leaves not lobed, 4-10 cm, sharply toothed, often with hairs on veins beneath. Flowering stem 3-6 cm tall. Fruit blue-black. This is a very variable shrub and can be hairy.
Range. Me. and N.Y. to O., s. in mts. to Ga. the common northern form.

NANNYBERRY   *Viburnum lentago* L.
Tall shrub or small tree to 10 m usually smooth, the leaf stalks 1-2 cm with flatened edges. Leaves 5-8 cm with fine teeth, 6-10 per cm of margin of leaf. The flowering head has no stem. The fruit blue-black with a whitish bloom.
Range. Que. to Man., s. to N.J., Ga. and Mo., Wyo. and Colo. in woods.
Common names. Wild raisin, tea plant, black haw.

BLACK HAW   *Viburnum prunifolium* L.
Like the nannyberry, the leaf stalks nearly always without the flat edges. The fruit blue-black.
Range. Conn. to Mich. and Kan., s. to Ga. and Tex. most common westward in woods.
1830 Rafinesque 274. "Many sp. medical and useful. . .Bark of many smoked like tobacco by Western tribes. Leaves of. . .prunifolium used for tea in the South. *V. dentatum* (Mealy tree, Arrow wood and Tily of Indians.) Bark used by the Indians and Shakers as a diuretic and detergent, bitterish, contains a peculiar fragrant oil; used in decoction daily and freely to prevent and remove cancerous affections, extract, pills and plaster also used."
1859-61 Gunn 761. "The fruit is pleasant and agreeable to the taste and generally liked. In eating it the seeds should be rejected, on account of their powerful tendency to constipate. . .The bark of the root is the part used in medicine. . .used. . .[as a] strong tea. As a tonic astringent it is valuable in chronic diarrhea and dysentery. Its most valuable application however, is in cases of threatened abortion. . .decoction. . .one or two tablespoonfuls (owing to its strength) two or three times a day. . .The decoction is also good to relieve after-pains during confinement: also said to be good to relieve palpitations of the heart."
1881 Can. Pharm. J. 181. "An examination of the bark of *Viburnum prunifolium*, by Mr. A. Van Allen. . .gave as the constituents. . .viburnin of Kramer; a volatile acid answering to all the tests of valerianic acid. . .tannic acid. . .oxalic acid; citric acid; malic acid; sulphates; chlorides of calcium, magnesium, potassium and iron."

1882 Can. Pharm. J. 275. "First introduced to the profession in 1866 by Dr. E.W. Jenks, of Detroit. . .But it is particularly valuable in preventing abortion and miscarriage, whether habitual or otherwise; whether threatened from accidental cause, or criminal drugging. It tones up the system, preventing or removing those harrassing nervous symptoms that so often torment and wear out the pregnant woman. . .It enables the system to resist the deleterious influence of drugs so often used for the purpose of producing abortions. . .Black haw was largely employed in slavery times as a preventative of abortion, and to counteract the effects of cotton root taken with criminal intent by the negresses. . .In dysmenorrhoea [profuse menstrual discharge]. . .by its sedative and anodyne influences, enables the uterus to bear the burden cast on it with much less suffering. In neuralgic dysmenorrhoea, it is a valuable addition to the other antispasmodics indicated, cannabis indica, camphor, conium etc."

1916 Waugh IROQUOIS 128. Berries of *V. Lentago* and *V. opulus* eaten.

1923 H. Smith MENOMINI 63. *V. lentago*, some Menomini eat them.

1932 H. Smith OJIBWE 361. "*V. lentago*. The Pillager Ojibwe collect the inner bark of the trunk, down low next to the ground, to yield a tea which is used as a diuretic. . .Among the white men, Nannyberry is often sold as *Viburnum prunifolium* which is official in our pharmacopoeia. . .398. The berries are eaten when ripe, fresh from the bush, and are also used in jam with wild grapes. . .417. *V. pubescens* [*dentatum*.]. . .The bark of this species furnished one of the ingredients of a Pillager Ojibwe kinnikinnik, which the writer smoked and pronounces good."

1930 Can. Form. 51. Extract of Black Haw with alcohol. . .71. Black haw is the dried bark of *Viburnum prunifolium*. . .It has a slight odour and an astringent taste.

1945 Raymond TETE DE BOULE transl. 134. "For migraine rub the head with the crushed leaves of Hobble bush, *V. alnifolium*."

Black haw bark from the southern states contains 0.2% salicin and isovaleric acid, formerly named viburnin. It is used for asthma, dysmenorrhoea and hemorrhage. It is supposed to prevent threatened abortion (T.E. Wallis 1967:85).

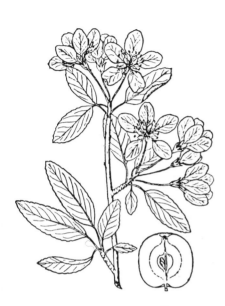

WILD-CRAB APPLE

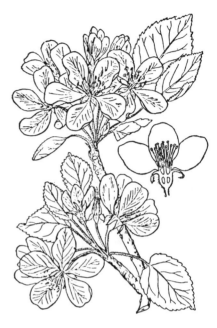

CULTIVATED APPLE

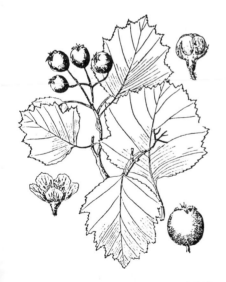

ROUND LEAVED HAWTHORN

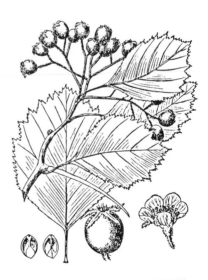

LONG SPINED HAWTHORN

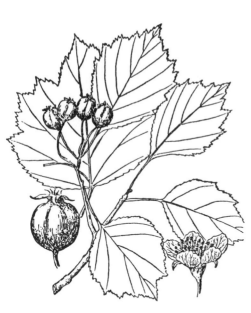

WAXY FRUITED HAWTHORN

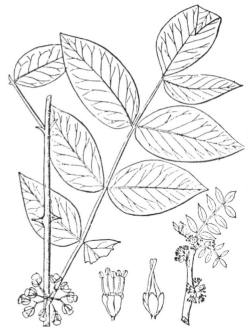

PRICKLY ASH

WILD CRAB-APPLE   *Pyrus coronaria* L. Rosaceae (*Malus c.*)
Tall shrub or low tree, rarely to 10 m. Leaves 4-10 cm often with lobes, toothed, a few hairs beneath when young. Flowers pink or salmon color, fruit greenish, 2.5 cm thick.
Range. N.Y. to s. Ont. to Mich. and Kan., s. to Ga. and Ala. in woods and thickets.
1619 Champlain-Macklem HURON 41. "They also grow grapes and plums, raspberries, strawberries, crab-apples and nuts". . .1632 Bourne transl. 70. Raspberries, strawberries, little wild apples, nuts."
1650 Representation New Neth. 295. "The indigenous fruits consist principally of. . .plums, medlars, wild cherries, black currants, gooseberries, hazel nuts in great quantities, small apples, abundant strawberries throughout the country."
1710 Raudot ILLINOIS 386. "The orchards are full of apple trees whose fruit is acrid and not larger than is the api." footnote. A French variety of small red apple.
1778 Carver 502. "The crab-apple tree bears a fruit that is much larger and better flavoured than those of Europe."
1779 Zeisberger DELAWARE 46. "Crabapples grow in great plenty and the Indians, being very fond of sharp and sour fruit, eat them in abundance."
1830 Rafinesque 254. "*P. coronaria* (wild crab) fragrant blossoms and fruits, austere, good preserve. *P fusea* (Oregon Crabapple) has brown acid pulpy fruits, wood very hard, used for wedges."
1916 Waugh IROQUOIS 129. "Eat the crab-apple." Among the various actions ascribed to the 'The Evil-Minded' is the creation of the crab apple."
1928 Parker SENECA 11. Tonic use. . .wild apple root. . .12 Tuberculosis use. . .wild apple root. . .Malaria use. . .wild apple root.
1928 H. Smith MESKWAKI 242. "Wild crab-apple. The Indians say that fifty years ago this was used to cure smallpox. However, it is not so used now. . .263. Dr. Jones. . .specimen 3717, was dried and prepared for storage by a woman of the Pheasant Clan. These fruits are also reduced to jelly by the Meskwaki women."
1970 Bye IROQUOIS mss. Apples so liked by the Indians that many large orchards existed long before settlers arrived.

CULTIVATED APPLE SPECIES   *Pyrus malus* L. Rosaceae (*Malus sylvestris*)
1609 Lescarbot-Erondelle Quebec 144. "Monsieur Champlain is in another place, to wit in the great river of Canada, near the place where Captain James Cartier did winter, where he hath fortified himself, having brought thither households, with cattle and divers sorts of fruit-trees."
1619 Champlain-Macklem Quebec 102. "By now our gardens were lovely. We had some fine Indian corn and some young trees and grafts that de Monts had given me in Normandy."
1663 Boucher Quebec transl. 53. "Trees from France have not yet been planted here, except for a few apple trees which bear very good apples and in quantity, but there are very few trees."
1668 Marie de l'Incarnation Quebec 346. "We are beginning to have rainette and calville apples, which are very fine and good here, but the species are brought from France. . .1670. 364. There was still ice in our garden in the month of June; our trees and our grafts, which bore exquisite fruit, are dead from it. The whole country suffered the same loss, and particularly the Hospitalière Mothers, who had one of the most beautiful orchards that might be seen even in France. The trees bearing wild fruit are not dead. . .We have become accustomed to this in the thirty-two years we have been in this country and have had time to forget the sweetness and delights of ancient France."
1880 Can. Horticulturist 3; 126. "Mr. J.A. Mackay, Winona, writes. . .'Forty five years ago a road was cut through the old Jesuit orchard at Quebec. The trees were said to be over a hundred years old, and though neglected were said to bear well. Under each tree was a flag of magnesian limestone, which must have been brought from a distance."

LONG SPINED HAWTHORN WHITE THORN   *Crataegus succulenta* Link   (*C. tomentosa*)
Rosaceae
Tree to 8 m or sometimes a shrub, twigs smooth or slightly hairy when young, armed with stout thorns 3-4.5 cm long. The dark green glossy leaves are mostly 3-6 x 2-5 cm, hairy when young, at least along the veins beneath when older, their stalks 1-2 cm long. Flowers 1-1.7 cm wide, white or rose. Fruit bright red, 0.7-1.2 cm thick, flesh succulent when ripe, nutlets mostly 2-3(4), rounded at the ends, deeply pitted on the inner face.
Range. P.E.I., N.S., N.B., N. Engl., Que., Ont., Man. to Pa., w. to Iowa in dry or rocky ground. Fruit ripe September.

ROUND LEAVED HAWTHORN   *Crateagus rotundifolia* Moench
Shrub or small tree to 7 m with smooth or hairy, thorny twigs, thorns curved, 2-7 cm long. The dark yellow-green, hairy or smooth leaves 2-9 x 1.5-6 cm, generally with several pairs of shallow scallops on the edges. The stalks ¼ to 2/3 as long as the leaf. Flowers 1.2-2 cm wide, fruit red with a soft flesh, rarely yellow, tending to become mellow or succulent, 0.8-1.5 cm thick with 3-5 nutlets.
Range. P.E.I., N.B., N.S., Que., Ont., to B.C., s. to N.Y., Mont., N. Mex.

WAXY FRUITED HAWTHORN   *Crataegus pruinosa* (Wendl.) K. Koch
Shrub or small tree to 8 m with intricate thorny branches, thorns 3-6 cm long, curved, chesnut brown. The blue-green leaves 2.5-6 x 2-5 cm and smooth, their stalks 1/3 to nearly as long as the leaf. Flowers 1.2-2 cm wide. The fruit strongly angled, frosted or waxy, apple-green becoming scarlet or purple, with hard thick flesh. Nutlets 3-5.
Range. Nfld., sw. Que., s. Ont., s. to Ark., Ky., and N.C., w. to Wis. and Okla. on rocky ground.
1380 Crawford Lake site Ontario McAndrews, Byrne and Finlayson 1974.3. *Crataegus* seeds; 9 recovered archeologically from four locations.
1535-36 Cartier Quebec transl. 123-4. "Stadacona. . .hawthorns, which bear fruit as big as Damas plums."
1541-42 Cartier Purchas 21. "Moreover there are many white Thornes, which beare leaves as bigge as oken leaves, and fruit like unto Medlars."
1590 Harriot Virginia 18. "Medlars a kind of verie good fruit, so called by us chieflie for these respectes: first in that they are not good untill they be rotten: then in that they open at the head as our medlars, and are about the same bignesse: otherwise in taste and colour they are farre

different: for they are as red as cheries and very sweet, but whereas the cherie is sharpe sweet, they are lushious sweet."

1609 Lescarbot-Erondelle Port Royal 301. "As for the trees of the forest, the most comon in Port Royal be. . .whitethorns. . .302. There is a kind of medlars, the fruit whereof is better and bigger than that of France."

1622 Gerarde-Johnson 1454. "There is a dwarfe kinde of Medlar growing naturally upon the Alpes, and hils of Narbone [France]. . .the fruit is very like the Haw, or fruit of the white Thorne, and of a red colour. . .Medlars do stop the belly, especially when they be greene and hard, for after that they have been kept a while, so that they become soft and tender, they doe not binde or stop so much, but are then more fit to be eaten. . .1327 Of the white Thorne, or Hawthorne Tree. . .It is like to the wild Peare tree,. . .The Hawes or berries of the Hawthorne tree. . .do both stay the laske, the menses, and all other fluxes of bloud; some Authors write, that the stones beaten to pouder, and given to drinke are good against the stone."

1642 De Vries New Neth. 219. "Medlars grow wild and reversely from what they do in our country, as they grow in Holland open and broad above, but here they grow up sharp, the reverse of those in Holland."

1663 Boucher Quebec transl. 49. "White thorn, which bears fruits larger than those of France & of better flavor."

1698 Hennepin Lake Michigan 129. "Our Men found some Hawthorn-Berries and other wild Fruit, which they ate so greedily, that most of them fell sick, and were thought to be poison'd."

1710 Raudot ILLINOIS 384. "These woods are full of. . .medlars, mulberries, chestnuts, and plums. . .The medlars and the mulberry bear fruits as good as those in France."

1830 Rafinesque 213. "Hawthorn, Thorn trees many species, Fruits of several edible, red or yellow, acid or sweetish, making a fine stomachic preserve, useful in diarrhoea and antiemetic; such are *Cr. coccinea, Cr. tomentosa. Cr. crusgalli.* The leaves and flowers of this last, used as pectoral in coughs and whooping cough, as a tea; the shrub makes fine hedges."

1840 Gosse Quebec 139. "The native thorn (*C. Coccinea*); the leaves are shaped almost exactly like those of our English hawthorn, but the berries are much larger. This is not a very common plant here, though I know of several large shrubs within the compass of a mile: but near Quebec [city] it is very common. The Heights of Abraham, and the sloping sides of the cliff, in many places, so thickly clothed with thorn-bushes as to form almost impenetrable thickets. . .I collected about a quart of the haws. . .last autumn, and buried them in the garden a few inches below the surface; they will not, however, sprout until next spring. I also took the pains to collect about a dozen suckers and young plants, which I planted in a line last spring: many of them lived through the summer and are now budding. There are many other plants which might be put to this purpose [live fence or hedge]."

1855 Trail Can. Sett. Guide 75. "The large spurred hawthorn, also, may be found near creeks, and on the banks of rivers, on gravelly soil. This is, if anyting, more beautiful than the common English white thorn. . .The Canadian hawthorn. . .fruit as large as a cherry, and when ripe very agreeable to the taste. The thorns are so large and so strong that it would make a formidable hedge, if any one would plant it, but few will take the time and trouble."

1916 Waugh IROQUOIS 82. "It is likely that other roots, seeds, and fruits were formerly used in bread-making. A suggestion of the former use of haws in this connexion is found in the name djgahedts (On.). Footnote by Waugh; the name is said to signify 'use for bread,' which is applied to such species as *Crataegus pruinosa* and *C. submollis*. . .128 Haws eaten."

1926-27 Densmore CHIPPEWA 321. "Crataegus, species doubtful, Thornapple. These were prepared by squeezing them in the hands, after which they were made into little cakes without cooking, dried on birchbark and stored to be cooked in winter. . .356. Root in decoction for pain in back and female weakness. . .378. The thorns of the thornapple tree were gathered by the women and used as awls in their sewing."

1928 H. Smith MESKWAKI 241. "Pear thorn (*Crataegus tomentosa*). . .The apples are used as medicine for bladder ailments. They are used unripe by the Indians. . .Specimen 5133 of the Dr. Jones collection is the twigs of a species of Crataegus. . .The tea is used for a pain in the side or bladder trouble. . .Specimen 5152 of the Dr. Jones collection is the root bark of a species of *Crataegus*. . .The tea is used for general debility. . .263. Although not of the best, the little apples of the pear thorn are eaten as a food by the Meskwaki and are sometimes cooked."

1932 H. Smith OJIBWE 384. "Hawthorn, *Crataegus* sp. The Flambeau Ojibwe use both the fruit and the bark for medicine, a kind not made now, other than for women. . .409. The Pillager

Ojibwe use the haw apples as a food in the fall of the year. . .423. The Flambeau Ojibwe women use the sharp thorns for sewing awls on finer work such as buckskin sewing with sinew. . .431. The bark of the Hawthorn was used by the Flambeau Ojibwe in making up their deer scent for smoking to attract deer while hunting."

1933 H. Smith POTAWATOMI 76. "Bicknell's thorn (*Crataegus rotundifolia*). The Forest Potawatomi use the apples as a medicine to cure stomach complaints. . .The 1916 Dispensatory of the U.S. says [p. 1403] that the apples have been used for their astringent and heart tonic properties. . .107. The Forest Potawatomi say that the deer and bear are very fond of these apples and they themselves sometimes eat them."

1945 Rousseau MOHAWK transl. 45-6. "Know now four kinds:-1. with large red fruit. . .2. with yellowish fruit. . .3. with medium sized fruit and 4. with little fruit, which are rare. An infusion of the little twigs, without leaves, is drunk when the stomach seems to be getting large, mixed with the roots of elecampane."

1955 Mockle Quebec transl. 58. "English hawthorn (*C. Oxyacantha*). The flowers feebly diuretic and tonic for the heart; they are also used as a neuro-vascular sedative. The chemical composition is complex and not well known. . . .The other Canadian species considered to have more or less the same properties are: *C. rotundifolia*, *C. mollis*, *C. coccinea*, *C. crus-Galli*, *C. succulenta*, and *C. flabellata*." [The names given by Mockle *C. Brunetiana, canadensis, submollis, holmsiana, ferentaria, tomentosa, Victorinii* and *Grayana*, as well as *Crus-galli*].

1970 Bye IROQUOIS mss. Cites Rousseau, in Taylor & Ludwig 1960, where he describes the Iroquois burning the land to clear it. After about 20 years the soil was exhausted and abandoned, the village moved. Hawthorn invaded the fields as the Iroquois were very fond of the haws, the shrubs hybridised. Black locust was associated with the hawthorn.

1973 Garrett 28. "Hawthorn wine. Early settlers to this continent valued hawthorn wine as a heart remedy. . .5 qts. hawthorn berries, 1 gal. water, 2½ lbs sugar, ½ cup lemon juice. 1 pkg yeast. Gather the haws on a sunny day in the fall, after the frost has touched them. Wash them and boil them in water until they are soft. They will become muddy, and you will be quite certain that such an ugly-looking mess could not possibly produce a drinkable wine. Strain off the liquor into a crock and add the sugar, yeast and lemon-juice. The addition of the lemon-juice will turn the liquid to a delicate clear-pink shade. Set the covered crock in a warm place for 2 weeks. Add another cup of sugar, stir well, then strain into the fermentation jar. After three months you may rack and bottle it, if it is clear. But do not fasten the corks in tightly for another month or more. Hawthorn wine is a suprisingly lively brew, and its stillness is sometimes deceptive. We have made a rich, headywine, using the above recipe, substituting 3 lbs of Clover honey, added at one month intervals, for the one cup of sugar."

1973 Stepka & Winters Lloydia 36:4;436. Several species of hawthorn lower the blood pressure. Hawthorn species are hypotonic and have antiarrhymthic activity (Lewis and Elvin-Lewis 1977: 193).

PRICKLY ASH   *Zanthoxylum americanum* Mill. Rutaceae (*Xanthoxylum a.*)
Tall shrub or rarely a small tree up to 8 m with thorns on the stem and branches. The leaves consist of 5-11 leaflets, hairy when young and smooth when old, with resinous dots. They smell of lemon when crushed. This is a member of the same family as the bitter orange. The greenish flowers, in clusters on last years wood, appear before the leaves. They are followed by reddish-brown rough capsules containing black seed or seeds; the taste is spicy.

Range. sw. Que., s. Ont.. to N.Dak., s. to Okla., Mo., Ala. and Ga. in moist woods.

Common names. Toothache tree, angelica-tree, suterberry. There is a southern shrub, *Aralia spinosa*, also called angelica tree but not discussed in this book.

1724 Anon ILLINOIS-MIAMI mss 224. "The bark of the prickly type of ashwood to draw off pus."

1778 Carver 393. "Soon after I set out on my travels, one of the traders whom I accompanied, complained of a violent gonorrhoea with all its alarming symptoms: this increased to such a degree, that by the time we had reached the town of the Winnebagoes, he was unable to travel. Having made his complaint known to one of the chiefs of that tribe, he told him not to be uneasy, for he would engage that by following his advice, he should be able in a few days to pursue his journey, and in a little longer time be entirely free from his disorder. The chief. . .prepared for him a decoction of the bark of the roots of the prickly ash, a tree scarcely known in England. . .by the use of which, in a few days he was greatly recovered, and having received directions how to prepare it, in a fortnight after his departure from this place perceived that he was radically cured."

1817-20 Bigelow 160. "It is not only a popular remedy in the country, but many physicians place great reliance on its powers in rheumatic complaints, so that apothecaries generally give it a place in their shops. It is most frequently given in decoction, an ounce being boiled in about a quart of water. Dr. George Hayward of Boston informs me, that he formerly took this decoction in his own case of chronic rheumatism with evident relief. . .It was warm and grateful to the stomach, produced no nausea nor effect upon the bowels, and excited little, if any, perspiration. . .It produces a powerful effect when applied to secreting surfaces and to ulcerated parts."

1830 Rafinesque 115. "The whole shrub is possessed of active properties; the leaves and fruit smell and taste like the rind of lemons, and afford a similar volatile oil. The smell of the leaves is more like orange leaves. The bark is the officinal part, the smell and taste are acrid, pungent, aromatic. . .Appears to be equivalent to Mezereon and Guayacum in properties. The acrimony is not felt at first when the bark or liquid is taken in the mouth, but unfolds itself gradually by a burning sensation on the tongue and palate. . .This is a great article in the Materia Medica of our Indians; it is called Hantola by the western tribes; they prefer the bark of the root, and use it in decoction for cholics, gonorrhea, syphilis, rheumatism, inward pains, chewed for tooth-ache, and applied externally in poultice, with bear'grease, for ulcers and sores. it is a great topical stimulant, changing the nature of malignant ulcers. In tooth-ache it is only a palliative, as I have ascertained on myself, the burning sensation which it produces on the mouth, merely mitigating the other pain, which returns afterwards. Some herbalists employ the bark and seeds in powder to cure intermittent fevers. A tincture of the berries has been used for violent cholics in Virginia. It is very good in diseases conected with a syphilitic taint."

1851 Schoolcraft 4 502. Prickly ash used by Indians for dropsy.

1859-61 Gunn 838. "A saturated tincture of the berries is found to be an excellent article in cholera, and other diseases of the bowels. . .Bark of the root as well as the berries, is considered a good remedy for rheumatic affections, in a. . .tincture in whisky. . .It warms up and invigorates the stomach, improves and strengthens the digestive organs, opens the pores and promotes general perspiration, and tends to equalize the circulation. For purposes of this kind, and as a strengthening stimulating bitters, there is nothing better grows in our woods. . .Dose of the powder, either of the berries or bark of the root, ten to thirty grains three or four times a day; of the tincture, one to two teaspoonfuls."

1868 Can. Pharm J. 6; 83-5. Prickly ash, the bark and berries included in list of Can. medicinal plants.

1892 Millspaugh 33. "Its speedy relief of rheumatism is said to occur only when it causes free perspiration; for this disease a pint a day is taken of the decoction of one ounce of the bark boiled in a quart of water. It is a powerful stimulant to healing wounds or indolent ulcerations. . .In Asiatic cholera, during 1849 and 1850, it was much employed by our (Eclectic) physicians in Cincinnati, and with great success; it acted like electricity, so sudden and diffusive was its influence over the system. In typhus fever, typhus pneumonia, and typhoid conditions generally, I am compelled to say that I consider a tincture of prickly ash berries superior to any other form of medication."

1915 Harris Algonquin 50. "Prickly Ash was one of the most valuable remedies known to the Algonquins for the cure of rheumatism. They freely chewed the inner bark, and the roots of the tree they boiled, and drank liberal draughts of the water during the day. The inner bark steeped for hours in bear's oil they applied as poultices or embrocations. . .56. Is common around Montreal where I first met it."

1926-7 Densmore CHIPPEWA 342. Root in decoction gargled for a sore throat, also drunk. This was used for quinsy and swelled or ulcerated throat. . .364. The root in decoction was used as a bath to strengthen legs and feet of a weakly child, especially if the limbs were partially paralyzed. . .305. *Zanthoxylum americanum*, constituents, Zanthoxylin and an alkaloid resembling berberine.

1928 Parker SENECA 10. "It is certain that many remedies once common among the Indians were passed on to the settlers and found to be potent. Among these we may mention. . .prickly ash. . .used as a tonic."

1923 H. Smith MENOMINI 51. "The bark, root bark and fruit of this tree are all medicines with the Menomini. The ripe berries thrown into hot water make a medicine which is used in the mouth to spray on the chest and throat in bronchial diseases or on sores. It is also used as a seasoner in mixtures. The root bark is used in poultices. This, along with other medicines, is often put upon swellings in a special method by the Menomini medicine man. The teeth of the gar fish are moistened with the medicine. The medicine man makes three striking motions with this in his hand, saying with each motion 'wehe'. the fourth time, saying 'we ho ho', he strikes the swelling and makes it bleed so that the pulverized or liquid medicine may enter the flesh. He strikes the swelling three or four times. Then a poultice of the medicines is kept on for four days, when it should be healed. The berries. . .the liquid in which they are soaked is often drunk for minor maladies."

1928 H. Smith MESKWAKI 244. "Four distinct parts of this plant are used; the bark of the trunk, the bark of the root, the berries and the leaves. The bark and berries are a strong expectorant and are used in making cough syrup and medicine. It is also used for stopping hemorrhages and tuberculosis. Specimen 3653 of the Dr. Jones collection is a mixture [of the]. . .inner bark of pickly ash, the root of *Aralia nudicaulis*, and another undetermined root. It is drunk to give strength to one who is ill. . .A tea used to cure kidney trouble."

1932 H. Smith OJIBWE 387. "Both the Flambeau and Pillager Ojibwe make trips further south to get this bark. . .they want it for treating quinsy and sore throat. They say that even the berries are good for a hot tea to treat sore throat, and also to use as a spray on the chest to cool and relieve congestion in bronchitis."

1933 H. Smith POTAWATOMI 80. "We found none of the. . .Forest Potawatomi using this medicine. . .undoubtedly they do use the prickly ash as all of other Wisconsin Indians do.

1955 Mockle Quebec transl. 53. "The bitter aromatic bark is used in chronic rheumatism and as a stimulant in gastro-intestinal flatulence and diarrhea; it is used for chewing and for toothache."

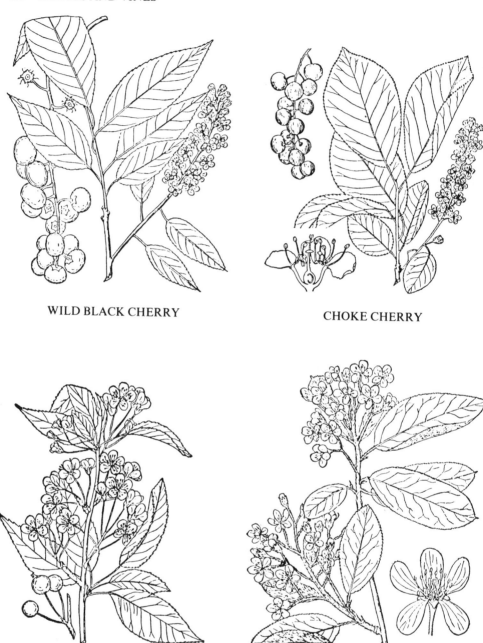

WILD BLACK CHERRY

CHOKE CHERRY

PIN CHERRY

CHOKE BERRY

WILD BLACK CHERRY

Prunus serotina Ehrh. Rosaceae

Tree to 25 m with reddish brown branches, the inner bark aromatic. The leaves 6-12 cm pointed at ends, edges incurved with short stubby teeth. The 20 or more white flowers have petals 4 mm on 3-6 mm stalks. The fruit purplish black with a slightly bitter and vinous flavor.

Range. N. B., N.S., s. Que., s. Ont., Minn., N.D., s. to Fla. and Guatemala. Woods and roadsides.
Common names. Rum cherry, whiskey, cabinet cherry.

CHOKE CHERRY
Prunus virginiana L.

Tall shrub to small tree to 10 m with grayish bark, the inner layers with a disagreeable odor. The leaves 5-12 cm abruptly pointed with sharp teeth. The roundish white petals on a spike of over 20 flowers with stalks of 5-8 mm. The fruit from red to deep black when ripe. Puckers the mouth on eating.
Range. Nfld., N.S., James Bay, to B.C., s. to Va. and Ark. in many habitats.

PIN CHERRY
Prunus pensylvanica L.f.

A small tree to 10 m or a straggling shrub, the tree bark a shining reddish brown with darker flecks. The leaves bright green on both sides with fine teeth 6-12 cm commonly less than half as wide. Flowers not more than 12, on 1-1.5 cm long stalks. The fruit bright red the size of a pin head with little sour flesh covering the seed.
Range. Lab., Nfld., James Bay to B.C., s. to N.J., w. Va., n. Ind., S.D. and Colo. Rocks, woods, fence rows.
Common names. Pigeon, fire, birdcherry.

1070-1320 Juntunen site *p. pensylvanica*, pin cherry, found archeologically at fourteen locations. Seed of some cherry sp. found archeologically at Alway site Ont. Jury 1937:2.
1624 Wassenaer New Neth. 71. "In the woods are found all sorts of fruits: plums, wild cherries. . ."
1634 Journey into MOHAWK country 146. "We bought some [corn] bread, that we wanted to take on our march. Some of the loaves were baked with nuts and cherries and dry blueberries and the grains of sunflowers."
1637 Le Mercier HURON Jes. Rel. 13;261. When smallpox was rampant in the village of Ossa-sane the Huron medicine man ordered the chief to take: "the bark of the ash, the spruce, the hemlock and the wild cherry, boiling them together well in a great kettle and washing the whole body therewith, and that care should be taken not to go out of their cabins barefooted, in the evening. He added that his remedies were not for women in their courses."
1653 Bressani HURON Jes. Rel. 38;243. "And the cherries are no larger than a pea,—being little else than stone and skin and very sour."
1663 Boucher Quebec transl. 45. "The tree called Cherry-tree (Merisier), grows large and tall, very straight. Its wood is used for furniture, & the stocks [the butts] of muskets. It is red inside & the best for the work done here. . .50. There are little trees which are called cherry trees, which bear two or three kinds of fruit; the taste isn't disagreeable but they are small; the trees never grow very large."
1724 Anon ILLINOIS MIAMI 222. "The bark of the root of the cherry tree chewed and held a long time on the gum cures the mal du Terre [scurvy]."
1748 Kalm Delaware 12th. Dec. 220. "The wood of the wild cherry tree [black cherry]. . .is very good and looks exceedingly well; it has a yellow colour, and the older the furniture is, which is made of it, the better it looks. But it is already scarce, for people cut it everywhere without replanting. . .340. We lodged with a gunsmith. . .The best and most expensive stocks for his muskets were made of wild cherry, and next to these he valued most those of the red maple. They scarcely use any other wood for this purpose."
1764 William Wood New England. 16. "The cherrie trees yeeld great store of cherries which grow in clusters like grapes; they be much smaller than our English Cherrie, nothing neere so good; if they be not very ripe, they so furre the mouth that the tongue will cleave to the roofe, and the throate wax horse with swallowing those red Bullies (as I may call them) being little better in taste. English ordering may bring them to be an English cherrie but yet they are as wilde as the Indians." [*P. virginiana*]
1785 Cutler. Black cherry, an infusion or tincture of the inner bark is given with success in the Jaundice. Fruit infused in rum and brandy for the sake of giving them an agreeable flavour.
1779 Zeisberger DELAWARE 45. "Of the wild cherry, there are three kinds, not found in Europe at all, and having a very good taste. The one sort grows on high thick trees, which are found in large numbers and yield a very fine red wood that is well suited for cabinet work."

1830 Rafinesque 253. "Few wild cherries are esculent. . .*P. virginiana* chokecherry, *P. canadensis* [cf. *P. pumila* and sand cherry] and *P. serotina*, are active medical, berries in racemes, called Black Cherries. The bark is bitter astringent, contains Prussic acid, tannin, gum and mucus. Tonic, febrifuge, sedative. Very useful in fevers, agues, hectic fever, dyspepsia, lumbar abscess, chronic asthma and hysteria, cardialgy, &c. . .heat drives off the Prussic acid. Bark of the root stronger. Reduces pulse from 75 to 50. In large doses narcotic and vermifuge. Leaves poison cattle, berries intoxicate birds, used for cherry bounce, baneful: kernels equal to bitter almonds."

1855 Trail Can. Sett. Guide 77. "Of wild cherries there are many different species, but they are more medicinal than palatable: steeped in whiskey, with syrup added, the black cherry is used as a flavour for cordials and the inner bark made into an extract, is given for agues, and intermittents, and also in chest diseases. . .The red choke-berry. . .the bark is tonic and bitter: when steeped in whiskey it is given for ague. No doubt it is from this that the common term of 'taking his bitters', as applied to dram drinking, has been derived. Bitter indeed are the effects of such habits upon the emigrant."

1895-61 Gunn 880. 'Wild cherry [black]. The bark is the part used. . .An infusion may be made by adding a pint of water to an ounce of powdered bark, and let it stand overnight, when it will be ready for use. . .Dose of the infusion, half a wineglassful, three times a day."

1868 Can. Pharm J. 6; 83-5. *P. Virginiana*; bark included in list Can. medicinal plants. . .Black cherry. The bark is used to make a very pleasant syrup, which is coming into General use as an ingredient in cough mixtures. . .Advertisement: To Chemists & Druggists—The undersigned desires to bring before the Notice of the Trade, his CHERRY TOOTH PASTE. It is the most agreeable and at the same time the cheapest article in the Canadian market, and will fully justify any recommendation it may receive. For price, address A Havard, manufacturer, 290 Queen Street. . .Toronto. . ."

1879 Can. Pharm J. 322. "Yellow poplar bark used with wild cherry bark, prickly ash, dogwood bark, and wahoo [*Euonymus atropurpurea*] is good for consumption."

1884 Holmes-Haydon CREE Hudson Bay 303." *Prunus virginian*—The bark is used fresh, as a rule. It is used as a cure for diarrhoea. For this purpose a handful of the bark is scraped off a young bough and boiled in about a pint of water and a wineglassful used as a dose."

1885 Hoffman OJIBWA 199. "Choke cherry. . .The branches are used for making an ordinary drink; used also during gestation. The fruit is eaten. Wild black cherry. . .The inner bark is applied to external sores, either by first boiling, bruising, or chewing it. An infusion of the inner bark is sometimes given to relieve pains and soreness of the chest. . . .Wild red cherry, *P. pensylvanica*. . .A decoction of the crushed root is given for pains and other stomach disorders. Fruit is eaten and highly prized. This is believed to be synonymous with the June cherry of Minnesota, is referred to in the myths and ceremonies of the 'Ghost Society.'"

1894 Household Guide Toronto 123. "Wild Cherry. This is good for general weakness, poor digestion, lack of appetite, nervousness and coughs. It is also considered an excellent remedy for the first stages of consumption or palpitation of the heart. The parts used in medicine, are the berries and inner bark of the roots and branches. Dose. A heaping teaspoonful of the dried and powdered bark, soaked twenty-four hours in one quart of cold water. Take a wineglassful four or five times a day."

1915 Speck PENOBSCOT 310. "Black cherry. . .bark is steeped and drunk for a cough, and the berries, steeped, make a fine bitter tonic. . .Chokeberry. . .bark steeped and drunk for diarrhea."

1915 Speck-Tantaquidgeon MOHEGAN 318. "Ripe wild cherries (*P. serotina*) are put into a bottle and allowed to ferment as they are, in their own juice, for about a year, when they are thought to become an excellent remedy for dysentery. Wild cherry leaves and boneset steeped together make a tea beneficial for colds, 'to be drunk hot at night, cold at morn.'"

1916 Waugh IROQUOIS 128. "All three kinds of cherries eaten. . .153. "A salt remedy, obtained among the Cayugas of Brant county, was claimed to be effective for 'inflammation of the bowels.' Salt is placed in the patient's hands and on the feet. A decoction of black cherry bark is administered internally, and a poultice of the boiled bark is applied to the abdomen."

1926-7 Densmore CHIPPEWA 317. "The twigs of the chokecherry and wild cherry were tied in a little bundle by a strip of bark long enough to permit the lifting of the bundle and dropping it into hot water without burning the hand. The bundle of twigs for one infusion was about 4 inches long and each packet was perhaps 1 inch in diameter. . .Chokecherries were pounded, stones and all, between two stones, and dried on birchbark and stored to be cooked in winter. . .Black cherries were eaten raw as well as dried for winter use. . .334. Inner bark of the white pine, the wild plum, and the wild cherry used for gangrenous wounds. [See description in full of preparation and treatment under pine.]. . .340. The inner bark of the chokecherry, the root of hazel and white oak and the heart of the wood of ironwood were steeped together and the decoction drunk for hemmorhages from lungs. . .342. The inner bark of the chokecherry was made into a decoction and used as a gargle for sore throat. This was said to be very astringent. . .344. The decoction was also drunk for cramps in the stomach. . .346. A decoction made with root of wild plum and the black cherry drunk for worms. The root of the black cherry, boil a handful of the prepared roots in about a pint of water and drink for cholera infantum. . .350. The bark of the chokecherry in decoction used as a wash to strengthen the hair and make it grow. . .354. The root of the black cherry and that of labrador tea, dried, powdered and mixed, but not cooked. After this powder had been on the flesh for a time it becomes damp. It is then removed, the sore washed, and a fresh application made. Applied to a severe burn or ulcer or any condition in which the flesh is exposed. . .The root or inner bark of the black cherry for scrofulous sores. Use the fresh roots mashed as a poultice; or scrape the inner bark, boil and use water as a wash. This remedy is especially useful for scrofulus neck. . .Drunk at the same time is a decoction made from 4 roots of Culver's-root and a large handful of the inner bark of the chokecherry, in a pint of water. Dose, one swallow taken before breakfast and at frequent intervals, usually before eating. The action of this remedy is a mild cathartic intended to cleanse the blood. . .366. A decoction of the inner barks of the choke cherry, black cherry, wild plum and the shadbush used as a disinfectant wash. . .333. "The use of a knife in amputation was mentioned by Maingans, whose limbs were amputated below the knee, the only instrument used being a common knife. When he was a boy his feet and limbs were badly frozen and in a hopeless condition. The pain was so intense that he begged a man to amputate them in this manner, and he did so. This was followed by a dressing of pounded bark (*Prunus serotina* Ehrh.) applied dry and renewed as often as it became damp—usually twice a day. Nothing else was used and the healing was perfect."

1923 H. Smith MENOMINI 50. "The Chokecherry inner bark is pounded to make a poultice and Manapus, the culture hero, pointed it out as a medicine to heal a wound or gall on man or beast. The inner bark is also dried, then steeped in water, the tea being drunk for diarrhoea. When administered to children it is sweetened. In aboriginal times, it was also a kind of beverage or tea to drink with meals. The liquid made by boiling the dried berries is also used to cure diarrhoea. . .71. The writer has observed women and children working on baskets and keeping a continual stream of choke cherry seeds dropping from their lips as they stripped small branches of cherries to eat. . .Black cherry, if eaten when they have been picked and allowed to stand for some time, are said to make the Indian drunk. They are also eaten fresh."

1928 H. Smith MESKWAKI 242. "Chokecherry. The root bark tea is sedative and is used for stomach troubles. Specimen 5077 of the Dr. Jones collection is the root bark of *P. virginiana*. . .The bark is boiled and made into a drink and it is also used as a rectal douche fluid for curing piles. The fluid is astringent and is spoken of by the Indians as 'a puckering'. . .264. These cherries are eaten avidly when fresh and ripe and the women and children gather whole branches to carry to their working places, stripping the fruit at their leisure while they work."

1932 H. Smith OJIBWE 385. "Pin cherry. The inner bark is a valued remedy for coughs. . .409. The Pin cherry is abundant around the Flambeau Reservation and the Ojibwe are fond of it. It is an education in itself to see a group of Ojibwe women working on mats with a supply of fruit laden branches beside them. With one hand they start a stream of berries into the mouth and the stream of cherry stones ejected from the other corner of the mouth seems ceaseless. The Pillager. . .use it in the same manner. . .385. The chokecherry. The Pillager make a tea for lung trouble from the inner bark. . .409. The Pillager like it, especially after the fruit has been frosted. . .385. Black cherry. The Flambeau Ojibwe value the bark of this species to make a tea as a remedy for coughs and colds. . .409. They prefer this cherry to all other wild cherries and dry it for winter use. Some of them also make whiskey from the ripe cherries."

1933 H. Smith POTAWATOMI 77. "Black Cherry. The Forest Potawatomi used the inner bark. . .as a seasoner for other combinations of medicines. . .108. While [they] use this cherry for food, they esteem it mostly for using in wine or whisky. The first thing that occurs to the Forest Potawatomi when this cherry is mentioned is. . .(whisky). . .77. *P. pensylvanica*. . .[they] use the inner bark. . .to make a tea to cure a cough and alleviate internal pain. . .Chokecherry [they] use the bark for an eye-wash and make a tonic drink from the berries. . .108. Use the choke cherry for food and also for seasoning or flavoring wine."

1945 Rousseau MOHAWK transl. 46. *P. serotina.* "Used when 'the blood seems thick'."

1945 Rousseau Quebec transl. 91. "*P. pensylvanica.* The bark with that of the white plum is used in making a syrup for coughs."

1945 Raymond TETE DE BOULE transl. 130. "*P. pensylvanica.* The inner bark is grated, the scrapings are boiled and applied to an umbilical cord which bleeds or is placed on at the time it is cut."

1955 Mockle Quebec transl. 60. "*P. serotina.* The bark is used as a sedative and expectorant in bronchial affections. . .The leaves contain a flavonic glucoside, serotin."

1956 Leechman Native Tribes 109. "An especially nice kind, called berry pemmican, was made by adding crushed choke cherries or berries. The ripe cherries were pounded, just as the meat had been, and the cherry paste, stones and all, was stirred in with the meat and fat. Now and then, as a very special touch, a few crushed leaves of peppermint were added."

1959 Mechling MALECITE of maritime provinces of Canada used the pin cherry wood for chafed skin, the bark for erysipelas. The black cherry bark for consumption, coughs and colds and berries for a tonic.

The bark of the wild black cherry is collected in the autumn. The thin green bark contains most hydrocyanic acid, between 0.12 to 0.16%. The bark of the root is said to be more active. The bark when dried is odorless but when moistened smells of bitter almonds and has a bitter astringent taste. It contains prunasin which yields when moistened with water hydrocyanic acid and benzaldehyde. It has mild tonic and sedative properties useful for coughs and chest complaints. The bark of the other cherries is occasionally substituted for that of the black cherry (T.E. Wallis 1967:85-6).

[Fresh wild cherry leaves are toxic to animals, particularly when wilting for it is then that they contain the largest amount of cyanide. The berries are not poisonous but eating large amounts at one time can be dangerous.]

1970 Bye IROQUOIS mss *P. virginiana,* chokecherry. The Iroquois used the fruit fresh or dried to make a drink. The Seneca used the branches in a drink to aid digestion, the inner bark for diarrhoea, also for a tea like drink. *P. pensylvanica,* pin cherry, was not commonly eaten by the Iroquois, but was used to make a drink. Several Indian tribes used the crushed root in treating stomach troubles. It was sometimes used as stock for grafting. Black cherry, *P. serotina,* the Iroquois tapped the bark for a drink and also used the bark to make medicine.

CHOKE BERRY   *Aronia arbutifolia* (L.) Ell. Rosaceae (*Pyrus melanocarp*)

Shrub 1-2 m (3) with hairy branches when young. Leaves 3-7 cm long, the centre vein of the leaf with a row of glands. This is the easiest way to identify the aronia in the field. The fruit is red in this variety and purple to black in var.*melanocarpa,* which has smooth stems.

Range. Nfld, N.S., N.B., P.E.I., Que. and Ont., s. to S.C., n. Ga. and Tenn., Fla. and Tex. in swamps, bogs, acid soil, woods, on rocks.

Common names. Choke-pear, dog-berry.

1830 Rafinesque 196. "The chokeberries are produced in 4 or 5 species of shrubby aronia: they are astringent and unpalatable."

1933 H. Smith POTAWATOMI 76. "Black chokeberry (*Pyrus melanocarpa*). . .The Forest Potawatomi steep the berry to make a tea to cure a cold. Among the whites [Nickell] the berries are used for their astringent properties. The 1916 Dispensatory says that the bark has been used among eclectic practioners for its astringent properties. . .107. The Forest Potawatomi say that they eat the berries from this plant but they are entirely too bitter to suit the white man."

1936 Yanofsky. The fruit used in the preparation of pemmican in north eastern U.S.

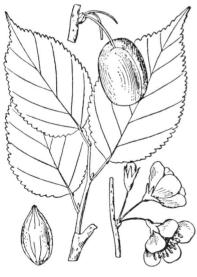
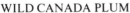

WILD CANADA PLUM

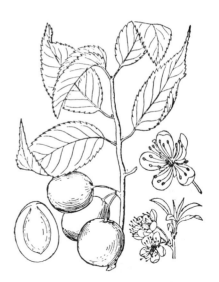

AMERICAN WILD PLUM

WILD CANADA PLUM
Prunus nigra Ait. Rosaceae

Small tree to 10 m with thorns. The leaves 7-12 cm, half as wide as long, with rounded teeth that have glands at their tips, fine hairs underneath. The flower stalk 1-2 cm bearing a cluster of 3 or 4 white or roseate petalled flowers, the petals 10-15 mm. Fruit red to yellow, 2-3 cm. stones flattened.

Range. N.B., N.S., Que., n.w. shore Lake Superior., to s.e. Man., s. to Io., Va., Ga., N.Y. in moist woods and thickets, or fence rows.

Common names. Pomegranate, horse plum, guignier.

AMERICAN WILD PLUM
Prunus americana Marsh.

Shrub or small tree to 8 m spreading from roots and forming thickets. Leaves 6-10 cm with sharp coarse teeth without glands at their tips. The 2-4 flowers in a cluster have white petals 10-15 mm long. The fruit is red and shining, 2 cm thick.

Range. sw. Que. to Sask., s. to Ariz., Ark. and n. Fla. in moist woods roadsides and fence rows.

200 A.D. ± Hopewell culture *P. nigra* found archeologically in Serpent Mound Ontario, Canada; *P. americana* in McGraw site Ohio. Yarnell 1964.

1070-1320 A.D. *P. nigra* found archeologically at Ripley, Westfield N.Y.; Moccasin Bluff, Verchave 11 sites Mich.; Juntunen Lake Huron Mich. and Alway site Ont. Jury 1937. Middleport, Sidney-MacKay, and Lawson 15th and 16th cent. sites Ont. Wintemberg 1939-46. *P. americana* found archeologically Verchave 11, Mich.; Baum, Gartner, Feurt, Baldwin, Cramer, Merion and Franks sites in Ohio; and Dutton's Ash Pit Ont. Yarnell 1964:62.

1400 Draper Site Ont. Finlayson 1975:225. Plum pits, 214 found archeologically.

1534 Cartier Gaspe transl. 62-3. The Indians [St. Lawrence Iroquois] come to the sea only at the time of fishing, "had with them. . .as well prunes, which they dry as we do, for winter, which they call honnesta". . .1535-36 Stadacona [Quebec] transl. 123-24. "full of many beautiful trees, of the same kind as those in France, such as. . .plum trees."

1609 Lescarbot-Erondelle Port Royal 297. "The most part of the woods of this lands be. . .likewise plum-trees which bring forth very good plums."

1612 Capt. Smith Virginia Indians 91-2. Plums, they preserve them as Pruines.

1619 Champlain-Macklem HURON 40-41. "Cahiague [near Orillia, Ont.] itself is the largest of all the villages. . .The soil is good and the savages grow a great deal of Indian corn. . .They also grow grapes and plums, raspberries, strawberries, crab-apples and nuts."

1632 Champlain-Bourne 70. "There are a great many vines and plums, which are very good."

1624 Sagard HURON 329. "As for the plums, named Tonestes, which are found in the country of our Hurons, they resemble our violet or red damsons, except they are not so good by far. The color deceives, and they are sour and acrid to taste, if they have not felt the frost; that is why the Indian women, after having carefully gathered them, bury them several weeks in the ground to soften them, then take them out, dry them, and eat them. But I believe that if these plums were grafted, they would lose this acridity and roughness, which renders them disagreeable to the taste before the frost."

1624 Wassenaer New Neth. 71. "In the woods are found all sorts of fruits; plums. . ."

1636 Brebeuf HURON Jes. Rel. 10;187. For the bowl game, six wild plum stones. . .were put into a large wooden bowl. These dice were painted black on one side and white or yellow on the other. The players, squatting on the ground in a circle, took the bowl in turn in both hands and, lifting it a little from the ground, struck it sharply so that the dice sometimes fell on one side and sometimes on the other. A side scored when the stones fell either all white or all black.

1639 Lalement HURON Jes. Rel. 17;159. The use of this bowl game to cure is described. . .The man who was selected to play either previously had had a dream that he would win or had a charm. One man who had such a charm rubbed the plum stones with an ointment and rarely failed to win.

1663 Boucher Quebec transl. 50. "Plum trees which bear red plums of the size of the Damascene, & which have a good taste; but not always as good as those of France."

1668 Marie de l'Incarnation Quebec 346. "As for trees, we have plum-trees which, when well manured and cultivated, give us fruit in abundance for three weeks. We do not cook the plums in the oven, for then only a pit covered with skin remains, but make marmalade out of them with sugar, which is excellent. We make ours with honey, and this is quite sweet enough for us and our children."

1698 Hennepin north end Lake Erie 109. "The Forests are chiefly made up of Walnut-trees, Chestnut trees, Plum-trees and Pear trees [Service berry?], loaded with their own Fruit. . .641-42. MIAMIS. Their Village is situated on an Hill, from whence one may discover the largest Meadows in the World, adorn'd at certain distance with Groves and Woods. The soil is very fertile, and produces a great quantity of Indian Corn. They preserve also Plums and Grapes."

1710 Raudot MIAMI 385. "The plums are as beautiful as those of France. There are several kinds, but they have very thick skins and do not come loose from the seed, nor do they have the agreeable taste that plums should have."

1778 Carver 503. "The Plum-tree. There are two sorts of plums in this country, one a large sort of a purple cast on one side and red on the reverse, the second totally green and much smaller. Both these are of good flavour, and are greatly esteemed by the Indians, whose taste is not refined, but who are satisfied with the productions of nature in their unimproved state."

1830 Rafinesque 253. "Plums esculent, some cult. by Indians, make good pies, preserves, &c."

1885 Hoffman OJIBWA 200. "*Prunus Americana*. . .The small rootlets, and the bark of the larger ones, are crushed and boiled together with the roots of the following named plants, as a remedy for diarrhea. The remaining plants were not in bloom at the time during which the investigations were made, and therefore were not identified by the preceptors."

1916 Waugh IROQUOIS 145. "A so-called coffee was also stated to be sometimes made from the wild plum. The plums are cut along one side, the stones removed, and the fruit dried on boards or in evaporating baskets in the sun. The beverage is made by adding boiling water to the dried fruit. . .128. Fresh plums eaten and dried for winter use."

1926-27 Densmore CHIPPEWA 346. A decoction made of the roots of *P. americana* and the wild cherry, *P. serotina* drunk for worms. . .352. Trunk of young white pine, the inner bark of the wild cherry and the inner bark of a young tree of the wild plum: "'Cut the first named into sections and boil with the barks until soft, strain, keeping the decoction, pound the woody material into a mash and dry; when needed, soak the mash thoroughly in the decoction and apply; care should be taken that the barks after boiling do not come in contact with rust or dirt.' The informant stated that he used this successfully on a gunshot wound after gangrene had set in. This could be applied to any form of 'rotten flesh', after which a knife was used to cleanse the wound". . .360. The dried roots were used in decoction or fresh roots were scraped and mashed, and the decoction applied externally to broken breast. . .366. The bark was used in decoction as a disinfectant wash. Also mixed with the inner bark of the three wild cherries and the shadbush. . .371. Formulae for red dyes. . .Third formula. This formula was used by Mrs. Razer in dyeing porcupine quills for the writer, the result being a brilliant scarlet which closely resembled analine dye. The quills were seen in the dye. Bloodroot, 2 handfuls of the root; wild plum 1 handful of the inner bark; red-osier dogwood 1 handful of the inner bark; alder one handful of the inner bark; hot water 1 quart. All boiled before the quills were put in the dye. Fourth formula (dark red), 1 handful of root of bloodroot and 1 handful of inner bark of wild plum in 1 quart of hot water. . .374. Dark yellow, Double handful of shredded root of bloodroot and single handful of shredded root of wild plum in hot water boiled together. . .Sixth formula inner bark of sumac and wild plum with the root of the bloodroot in hot water. The inner bark of the plum was scraped, and it was said that this was used 'to set the color'.

1928 H. Smith MESKWAKI 242. "Wild plum (*P. americana*). . .The bark of the root is an astringent medicine used to cure canker in the mouth. There is no recorded use of this as a medicine by the white man. Canada plum. . .The bark tea of this species is used to settle the stomach when it will not retain food. It has no medicinal use among the whites. . .263. The Meskwaki gather the wild plum in quantities and make it into a plum butter to use in the winter time. They are also fond of it fresh. The Canada plum is esteemed as highly as the wild plum, and is preserved and eaten in the same manner."

1932 H. Smith OJIBWE 409. "The Pillager Ojibwe find quantities of the wild plum (*P. nigra*, Canada plum) in thickets and gather it for food and for preserves. . .426. The Flambeau Ojibwe use the inner bark as an astringent color fixative in dyeing with other plant materials."

1970 Bye IROQUOIS mss. The Iroquois used the plum fresh or dried to make a drink, possibly making a coffee-like drink from the dried fruit. They planted it around their villages and along their trails, by dropping the stones.

Phloretin in the bark and root of plum trees is an active agent against gram positive and negative bacteria. Essence of prune added to flavor cigarettes (Lewis and Elvin-Lewis 1977 362, 95).

The first Europeans to land in America carried dried plums—(prunes), with them. They became an important article of trade with the Indians who relished their sweetness. Used by the Jesuits as medicine in Huronia and in the hospitals in Quebec. No European plum trees planted in Quebec in 1663 (Boucher 1663).

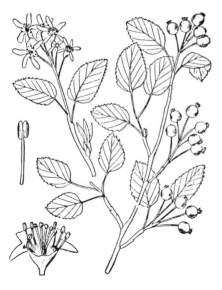

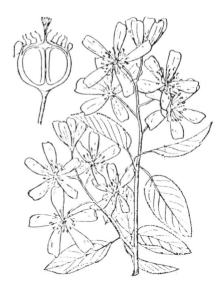

LOW JUNEBERRY   SERVICE BERRY

Service Berry, shadbush, little pear, juneberry are some of the names of this confusing genus, the Amelanchiers. A name according to Gray that is said to be barbaric and not satisfactorily explained. They are often called medlars.—The European medlar is not a native tree in north America. The distinguishing feature is a small fruit a few centimeters in size that contains 10 cells each with one seed. It is in most varieties sweet and edible. The Indians are very fond of it and have spread the different varieties. Weigand noticed that hybrids were abundant in areas where recent disturbances such as fires or clearings had occured. There is no agreement on the number of species, their names etc. as they tend to blend into one another. The fruit either has wool on its top or it does not. This is one clear way to tell the *A. canadensis, arborea* and *laevis* from the low juneberry, *A. spicata* or as it is also called, *A. stolonifera*, whose fruit is densely wooly on top.

SERVICE BERRY   *Amelanchier canadensis* (L.) Medic. Rosaceae
A tree to 8 m or a bushy shrub usually in clumps. The alternate leaves have fine teeth around their edges, they are half grown and white wooly when the flowers open. Later they become almost smooth and green when full grown. The 5-15 mm stalk bearing the flowers is erect. This is an early flowering variety with conspicuous flowers. The fruit is smooth, dark purple to black and sweet.
Range. N.S., P.E.I., N.B., Que., Ont., s. to Ga. and Miss. in low ground, swamps and thickets.
A. arborea and *A. laevis* also have fruit that is smooth on top but the stem bearing the flowers droops. The half opened leaves of *A. laevis*, the smooth juneberry, are smooth and purplish bronze. It has smooth topped sweet and juicy fruit. It is found in the same kinds of places and in the same range as the service berry.

LOW JUNEBERRY   *Amelanchier spicata* (Lam.) K. Koch *A. stolonifera* Weig.
Single or clumped shrub 2-3 m tall or less frequently a shrubby tree 3-6 m tall. The leaves with coarse teeth along upper 2/3 of their margins, densely wooly when half open at flowering time, which is late in this species. The leaves are smooth when mature. The flowers in a compact spray on a wooly flowering stem less than 4 cm long. The fruit wooly on top, dark purple.
Range. Nfld., N.B., P.E.I., N.S., Que., James Bay, Ont. to Minn., s. to Mich, Io.,' in mts. of N.C., Ga. and N.Y. in rocky, sandy open ground or woods, either wet or dry.
1534 Cartier Voyages Gaspe transl. The Indians have pears.
1604 Champlain-Purchas Tadoussac 181. "There are in these parts great store of Vines, Peares."

1609 Lescarbot-Erondelle Port Royal 301. "In the woods. . .I have seen there small pears very delicate."

1620 Mason Newfoundland A;iv. "The Countrie fruites wild, are cherries small, whole groaves of them, Filberds good, a small pleasant fruite, called a Peare."

1624 Sagard HURON 329. "There are pears, certain small fruits a little larger than peas, of a blackish color and soft, very good to eat by the spoonful like blueberries, which grow on small trees, which have leaves similar to the wild pear trees here, [probably *Crataegus punctata*, hawthorn] but their fruit is entirely different."

1663 Boucher Quebec transl. 52. "There are a quantity of little fruits whose names I know not, and which are not very special, but they are eaten when others are lacking."

1698 Hennepin Lake St. Clair 109. "The Forests are chiefly made up of Walnut-trees, Chesnut-trees, Plum-trees and Pear-trees, loaded with their own Fruit."

1789 Mackenzie Voyages 107. "There are plenty of berries, which my people called poires; they are of a purple hue, somewhat bigger than a pea, and of a luscious taste."

1804 Grant SAUTEUX 309. "There is a fine fruit not larger than a currant, tasting much like a pear and growing on a small tree about the size of a willow."

1818 Description P.E.I. "A fruit in this Island, called the Indian pear, is very delicious."

1820 Harmon Journal 81. "Different kinds of berries are now ripe, such as strawberries, raspberries, and what the Canadians call paires, which the Natives denominate Misasquito-minuck."

1820 Franklin Journey 88. "Under the name of meesasscootoomeena it is the favorite dish at most Indian feasts, and mixed with pemmican, it renders that greasy food actually palatable."

1830 Trans. Lit. & Hist. Soc. Quebec 111 126. "In the country parts this small fruit is dignified with the name of poire, more from its fine flavor, it is presumed, than from any resemblance to pears."

1840 Gosse Quebec 148. "The wild Service Tree. . .its profuse corymbs of white blossoms give it the appearance of a large snowball. Its fruit is about the size of a cherry, but more resembling a medlar in form: it ripens in August. The tree is not common with us."

1843 Lefroy 62. "The poire is mixed up in large quantities with a fine pemmican for the use of the officers and this makes what is called berry pemmican."

1852 Richardson Arctic Exped. 428. "*Amelanchier canadensis*. . .is La Poire of the voyageurs. . .Its wood being tough, is used by the natives for making arrows and pipestems, and has obtained on that account the name of bois de fleche from the voyagers."

1871 Palmer. *Amelanchier canadensis*; berries eaten fresh and dried, boiled in broth of fat meat for feasts. "In preparing the fruit for future use a favorite plan is to take a tub holding 20 or 30 gallons, in the bottom of which bark of spruce is placed; upon this bark a quantity of berries is laid; stones nearly red hot are next laid on; then berries then stones until the tub is filled. It is allowed to remain untouched for 6 hours when the fruit will be thoroughly cooked. It is then taken out, crushed between the hands, spread on splinters of wood tied together, over a slow fire, while drying the juice which was pressed out in cooking in the tub is rubbed over berries. After 2 or 3 days drying the berries will keep a long time. Very palatable, more so when a few huckleberries mixed with them."

1913 Hodge & White 410. "Saskatoon. A name in use in w. and s.w. of Canada for the service berry. . .probably a corruption of misaskwatomin which is the name applied to the fruit in the Cree dialect of Algonquian, signifying 'fruit of the misaskwa, the tree of much wood'." [*A. alnifolia*].

1916 Waugh IROQUOIS 128. Fruit of Juneberry eaten. . .144 "Loskiel. . .observed that they 'prepare a kind of liquor of dried bilberries, sugar and water, the taste of which is very agreeable to them.' These were probably some or one of several species of Vaccinium or blueberry, although the name is sometimes popularly applied to the juneberry, *Amelanchier canadensis*, and related species."

1926-7 Densmore CHIPPEWA 321. "*Amelanchier canadensis*, Shadbush. These are called 'Juneberries' by the Chippewa and are found abundantly in their country. They are considered the simplest form of refreshment. 'Take some Juneberries with you,' is a common saying among the Chippewa. A certain song contains the words 'Juneberries I would take to eat on my journey if I were a son-in-law.'" 344. A decoction made of the root of this combined with roots of cherry and young oak, drunk for dysentery. . .356. Bark in combination with pin cherry, choke cherry and wild cherry made into a decoction and drunk for female weakness. . .385. Root steeped and drunk for excessive flowing. This was given to a pregnant woman who had been injured, to prevent miscarriage.

1923 H. Smith MENOMINI 71. "The Juneberry or service-berry is a favorite food of the Menomini, seemingly as important as blueberries. It is gathered and dried for winter use the same as blueberries."

1932 H. Smith OJIBWE 384. "Smooth Juneberry (*Amelanchier laevis*) according to Charley Burns. . .the bark was used for medicine, but he did not know what it was to treat. The Pillager Ojibwe. . .say that the bark is to make a tea for the expectant mother. . .408. According to John Whitefeather, Flambeau Ojibwe. . .knew it only as food, although some tribes use the bark as a medicine. Juneberries were also dried for winter use, the Indians often preferring them to blueberries."

1933 H. Smith POTAWATOMI 77. "*A spicata*, low juneberry. The Forest Potawatomi use the root bark to make a tonic. . .The Ojibwe of Lac du Flambeau use the bark for medicine but we do not know for what ailment. The Pillager Ojibwe. . .say that the bark is used to make a tea for the expectant mother. . .107. The Forest Potawatomi relish the berries as a fresh food and also dry and can them for winter use. Other Wisconsin tribes are also fond of them."

1945 Rousseau Quebec transl. 90. "The fruits of the Amelanchier were already called poires in the writings of Champlain and Lescarbot, and this name used by Cartier probably designates this fruit. Sagard writes on the subject. . .This means that it is surely a very ancient french meaning."

1970 Bye IROQUOIS mss *Amelanchier canadensis*. The fruit is used as a blood remedy to treat after pains and hemorrhages of childbirth. The branches were used to make a tea.

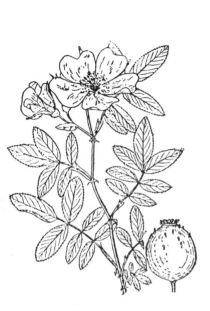

SWAMP ROSE

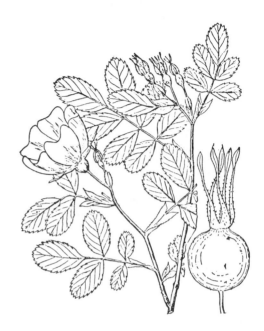

SMOOTH ROSE

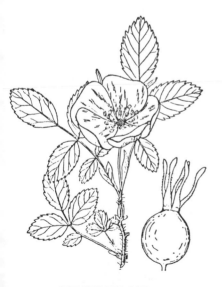

PRICKLY ROSE

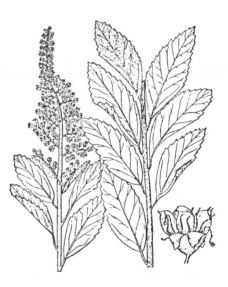

HARDHACK

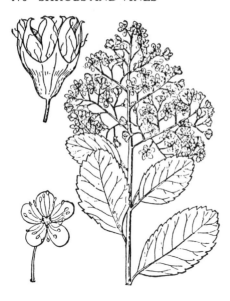

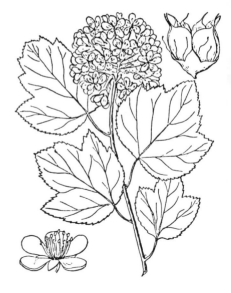

MEADOW SWEET   NINEBARK

SWAMP ROSE   *Rosa palustris* Marsh. Rosaceae
A small shrub to 2 m, the leaves consisting mostly of 7 leaflets, a few spines on the stems with
their tip turning down, about 3-6 mm long. Their base at least half as long, flattened. The flowers
solitary or a few together, the cup that holds each one covered with gland tipped hairs. The hip is
covered with glandular hairs.
Range. N.S., N.B., Que., s. Ont. to Minn., s. to Gulf of Mexico. In swamps, shores, stream banks.

SMOOTH ROSE   *Rosa blanda* Ait.
Stems to 1.5 m without thorns or very few slender prickles, towards their base but not on the
flowering branches. Leaflets five to seven, flowers solitary or a few together, petals pink, 2-3 cm,
cup and stalk smooth. Hips smooth, leaflets around the top of the hip hairy.
Range. N.S., N.B., Que., Ont., District of Mackenzie, Man., s. to N.Y., Pa., Ind. and Mo. in dry
woods, dunes, prairies.

PRICKLY ROSE   *Rosa acicularis* Lindl.
Stems to 1 m usually covered with straight slender prickles. Leaflets 3-7 with coarse teeth. The
flowers usually single with pink petals 2-3 cm long. The hips are smooth, with erect smooth
leaflets around the top.
Range. N.B., Que., northernmost Ont. to Alaska and Yukon, s. to Ida., n. N.M., S.Dak., Minn.,
and Vt. and in Siberia, in woods, rocky banks.

CATTLE ROSE   *Rosa arkansana* Porter
Stems usually die back in the winter, bristly, to about 50 cm. Leaves of mostly 9-11 leaflets.
Flowers large, pink fading to white.
Range. Man. to B.C.s to Mont., N.Mex., Tex. and Mo. in dry prairies and open woods. Used by
the Chippewa see Densmore below.
1475 Bjornsson Icelandic mss transl. Larsen 117. "Rosa is rose, dry and cold in the first degree. If
one crushes rose and applies to erysipelas, it helps. It is good for too much heat of the stomach or
the heart. Roses crushed and drunk with wine are good for diarrhoea. All eye-ointments should

have the juice of roses. If one dries roses and crushes them fine, that is good to put in the mouth with honey for sores of the mouth. If one drinks fresh roses crushed with honey, it is good for great heat. If one wets the bee-hive with rose juice and milk, the bees will not go away. Roses are also good for the sting of the spider. If one crushes roses with salt it is good for a tumor, though it be old. A woman, too, may be purged with rose juice boiled in salt. The same, too, is good to drink for pustules which come internally. It is also good for dysentery. Salt and roses crushed together is good for dog's bite. If one holds rose juice in his mouth, it is good for the teeth. If one crushes roses with honey and rubs upon the eyes, that lets him see well. . .32. Electuary of rose juice, which is made of juice of roses and many other spices. . .Cleanses too, those who are convalescing from tertian and quotidian fever without any danger or harm."

1534 Cartier St. Lawrence transl. 33-4. "There are lots of gooseberries, raspberries, and rose of Provins."

1609 Lescarbot-Erondelle Acadia 86. "We saw there, being a sandy land. . .musk-roses."

1613 Champlain fac. ed. transl and original 313. "Arrived at Quebec. . .[at] the habitation then I had some repairs made & planted some roses, & took some oak (de sente) to try out in France. (laditte habitation, puis y fis faire quelque reparations & planter des rosiers, & fis charger du chesne de sente pour fair l'epreuvé en France)."

1653 Marie de l'Incarnation Quebec 210. "You ask me for seeds and bulbs of the flowers of this country. We have those for our garden brought from France, there being none here that are very rare or very beautiful. Everything is savage here, the flowers as well as the men."

1663 Boucher Quebec transl. 84. "For the flowers, there have not yet been many brought from France, except roses. . .86 Wild roses are not double flowered."

1693 Memoir of the medicines necessary for the King's troops in Canada transl. 3 L rose honey. . .15 L pure rose oil; 5 L simple rose oil [this was the largest amount of any of the oils ordered]. . .2 L conserve of rose of Provins, liquid. . .6 L Syrop of roses. . .2 L Roses of Provins mundified (Vallee 1927:273-5 where he reproduces the list of over 123 items ordered on the 5th. Oct.1693)

1741 Farrier's Dispensatory London 17. "Red roses, petals effectual astringent. Honey of Roses, take a good handful of red rose petals, the whites being picked off [the white heel of the red petal], infuse upon them a Pint of boiling water when they have stood for some Hours, pour off the Infusion; warm it over a gentle Fire in a cover'd Vessel and pour in another handful of fresh Leaves [petals]; let this be repeated till the Infusion is very strong, then add twelve ounces of Honey and boil it to the consistence of a Syrup. This is a very useful Medicine in many external applications, where the Bones or Sinews are wounded and laid bare, in which case it is always better, when mixed with Brandy or Spirit of Wine, Aqua Vitae or Tincture of Myrrh. Conserve of Roses, take any quantity of Red Rose Leaves [petals] beat them in a marble or stone mortar, with treble their quantity of loaf Sugar, till they are thoroughly incorporated with it. This is of good use inwardly to the human body, in Pectoral Disorders; but to Horses, it is chiefly beneficial to be apply'd as a Cataplasm to the eyes when they are hot and inflamed."

1785 Cutler. Wild rose, blossoms red, berry pale red, common in moist land. The blossoms gathered before they expand and dried, are astringent, but when full blown are purgative. This species is generally preferred for conserves. A perfumed water may be distilled from the blossoms. The pulp of the berries, beat up with sugar, makes the Conserve of Hips of the London Dispensatory. The dried leaves of every species of rose have been recommended as a substitute for Indian tea, giving out a fine colour, a sub-astringent taste, and a grateful smell."

1812 Clarke Disp. 43. "Confection of red rose. . .astringent in hemorrhages &c. It is very rarely employed unless combined with nitrate of potassium, alum, opium, sulphuric acid and similar medicines. Externally as a cataplasm in chronic inflammation."

1820's Materia Medica mss Edinburgh-Toronto 36. "Rosa Gallica. The petals have a slight degree of astringency, the infusion in water forms a pleasant astringent gargle."

1830 Rafinesque 258. "Roots, galls, buds, and fruits all astringent, sweetish, corroborant, used in dysentery and diarrhea; contains tannin, sugar, myricine, resin, fat oil, volatile oil, acids, salts. Blossoms of red roses similar, styptic, have gallic acid, fine conserves; while pale or white roses. . .are laxative, a fine syrup for children. Rose water fine perfume, useful for sore eyes."

1833 Howard Quebec 29. "To cure a Bruise in the Eye apply a plaister of the conserve of roses. . .62. To cure the Itch beat together the juice of 2 or 3 lemons with the same quantity of the oil of roses. Anoint the parts affected. It cures in 2 or 3 times applying. . .92. To cure a Quincy in the Throat. Swallow slowly white rose water mixed with syrup of mulberries."

1842 Christison 798-9. "The petals. . .are used fresh for making a conserve, and are dried for other pharmaceutical purposes. . .The honey. . .a very old remedy, is still used by some in sore throat and ulcerations of the lining membrane of the mouth. . .The conserve is one of the best, if not the very best, of all materials for making pill-masses. . .which may be kept long without becoming hard. The infusion. . .as a tonic, refrigerant and astringent, especially for compounding gargles. . .But the active properties it possesses depend mainly on the sulphuric acid it contains."

1885 Hoffman OJIBWA 200. "*Rosa blanda*. . .A piece of root placed in lukewarm water, after which the liquid is applied to inflamed eyes."

1894 Toronto Household Guide 258. "Lait Virginal. . .Many skins will not stand constant washing, but need to be cleansed after a dusty ride or walk by other means than soap and water. Lait Virginal is a delicious preparation and can be made as follows: One pint of rose, orange flower, or elder flower water, half an ounce of simple tincture of benzoin and ten drops of tincture of myrrh."

1926-7 Densmore CHIPPEWA 292. Hips used as food. . .R. *arkansana*, cattle rose. . .336. Decoction of the roots of the wild rose, prairie sage, seneca snakeroot and the ground plum taken for convulsions. . .356. Root in decoction applied externally to wounds. . .356. Inner bark of the root of the rose and red raspberry for cataract. "These two remedies are used successively, the first for removing inflammation, and the second for healing the eye. They are prepared in the same way, the second layer of the root being scraped and put in a bit of cloth. This is soaked in warm water and squeezed over the eye, letting some of the liquid run into the eye. This is done 3 times a day. It was said that these would cure cataract unless too far advanced, and that improvement would be shown quickly if the case could be materially helped". . .364. The roots of the seneca snakeroot, prairie sage, ground plum and wild rose made into a tonic. They were dried; "the first name is pounded and kept seperately. Equal parts of the last three are pounded together until powdered. . .A quart of water is heated and about 1/3 of a teaspoon of the mixed ingredients is placed on the surface of the water at the 4 sides of the pail. A very little of the first [seneca snakeroot]. . .is placed on top of each. The ingredients soon dissolve. A stronger decoction was secured by boiling. The medicine was taken 4 times a day, the dose being small at first, and gradually increased to about a tablespoonful. A measure made from birchbark was used for this remedy."

1933 Can. Formulary 41. "Aqua Roasae. Rose water of commerce is prepared by the distillation of the flowers of *Rosa Damascena*, . . .*centifolia*. . .or *moschata*, diluted immediately before use with twice its volume of distilled water. . .is a saturated solution of the volatile oil of the fresh rose flowers."

1923 H. Smith MENOMINI 50. "Pasture rose (*R. humilis*) [R. *carolina*]. The Menomini believe that eating the rose hips of this species will cause a healthy person to get an itching like the piles. The medicinal part is the skin of the fruit. This is eaten to cure stomach troubles."

1928 H. Smith MESKWAKI 242. "Smooth rose, (*R. blanda*). The skin of the rose hip is used for stomach trouble. . .McIntosh and the Meskwaki use it for itching piles or for an itch anywhere on the body. The whole fruit is boiled down to a syrup."

1932 H. Smith OJIBWE 385. "The smooth rose. The Pillager Ojibwe use the skin of the fruit for stomach trouble. The Flambeau Ojibwe. . .dry and powder the flowers for use in relieveing heartburn. The skin of the rose hips is a medicine for indigestion."

1933 H. Smith POTAWATOMI 78. "Smooth rose. The Forest Potawatomi use the root of the smooth rose for medicine whereas the Prairie Potawatomi use the skin of the rose hips. The Forest Potawatomi make a tea for the treatment of lumbago and headaches."

1945 Rousseau MOHAWK transl. 47. "*R. Eglanteria*. An astringent intestinal used by the coureurs des bois. An introduced species, but other native species may be used by the Indians in the same way."

The petals are gathered by picking the buds before they expand and cutting off the white heels, then dried at about 35 C. to kill any insect eggs, then stored in a tightly closed jar away from the light. The fresh petals are used for the conserve. The hips, rich in vitamin C, running from 75 to 1303 mg of Vitamin C for each 100 grams of hips depending on variety and habitat. They should be simmered with just enough water to cover, mashed and put through a jelly bag to remove the skins and trichomes [hairs] inside. These hairs are very irritating to the bowel and must be carefully removed in making a conserve or syrup. (T.E. Wallis 1967). [When making the tea of rose hips, soak over night and simmer next day, do not boil or simmer for long. Drink the liquid. It contains sugar from the hips].

HARDHACK
Spiraea tomentosa L. Rosaceae

A shrub with a few stems to 1 m tall. The leaves 3-5 cm long are silvery white or reddish beneath, the veins easy to see. Leaves are dark green above, toothed. The flowers grow like a steeple up the top of the stem, and are a beautiful bright pink, or occasionally white.

Range. N.B., P.E.I., N.S. to Man., Minn., s. to N.C., Tenn. and Ark. in swamps and wet meadows.

Common names. Silver-leaf, poor-man's-soap, spice hardhack, steeple bush.

1830 Rafinesque 92. "The whole plant is inodorous, but the taste is pleasantly bitter and powerfully astringent. It contains tannin, gallic acid, bitter extractive &c. all soluble in water. Formerly used by the Mohegan tribe of Indians and the herbalists; brought to notice only towards 1810, by Dr. Cogswell of Hartford. Schoepf and Cutler have omitted it. Drs. Mead, Ives, and Tully have since recommended it as a very good astringent and tonic. The whole plant may be used, but the root is the least valuable part. The extract of it, prepared by the Shakers and others, is the best form; dose 4 to 6 grains, every two or three hours, in dysentery and chronic diarrhoea, cholera infantum, debility of the bowels and the system, hemorrhage of the bowels, and other diseases where astringents are required. It appears to be equal if not superior to Kino [*Pterocarpus*] and Catechu [*Acacia*], because it never disagrees with the stomach, all its virtues are soluble in water, is a bitter tonic, and can be had pure and genuine. It is peculiarly useful in the secondary stages of bowel complaints, when the inflammation has been partly subdued, either alone or combined with ipecac, opium, &c. It has been used abroad by seamen, with great benefit, in the cholera morbus and chronic diarrhoea of the tropical climate, even in the first stage. United to milk and sugar, it forms a very pleasant drink for the protracted stage of cholera. It is said to be equivalent to *Geranium maculatum* and *Cornus circinata* [*C. rugosa*] in most cases, but the first is less tonic, and the last a better tonic. The Honskokaogacha of the Osage Indians is probably this shrub; they use the dry root and stem as a powerful styptic and astringent, to stop blood and hemoptysis, by chewing them, or drinking the cold infusion; the women use it in tea and as a wash for female complaints, as a restringent, &c."

1870 Briante 91. "Hardhack-Tonic and astringent, good for weak state of the Stomach."

1915 Speck-Tantaquidgeon MOHEGAN 319. "Leaves of hardhack are steeped to make medicine for dysentery."

1932 H. Smith OJIBWE 386. "The Flambeau Ojibwe make a tea from the leaves and flowers of the Steeple bush to drink for the sickness of pregnancy and to act as an easy parturient. The whites have used the root and the leaves as an astringent and tonic, in diarrhea, hemorrhages, gonorrhea, ulcers etc."

1955 Mockle Quebec transl. 61. "A decoction of the flowers is used as a diuretic, and the roots for diarrhea."

MEADOW SWEET
Spiraea alba DuRoi (*S. salicifolia* of some reports; *S. latifolia*)

A shrub to 2 m. with dull brown or yellowish brown twigs, smooth or sometimes hairy. The northern variety has red or purple brown twigs. The leaves are long and narrow with fine teeth, not white underneath. The flowers crowd the summit of the stem like a pyramid and are white with a flush of red or lavender, and nearly always covered with fine hairs.

Range. Nfld. to Alta., s. to Va., N.C., Ind., n. Mo. and S.D. in wet meadows and swamps or on rocky soil.

1830 Rafinesque 265. "*Spiraea salicifolia* used as an agreeable subtonic and subastringent tea near Albany, &c."

1888 Delamare Island of Miquelon transl. 17. "The infusion of the leaves of this plant is so like that of china tea, that it is considered on Miquelon as a substitute for that tea. It tastes better and is better for the health than the tea of James [Labrador tea], the red tea [wintergreen tea], and other teas used by the inhabitants."

1928 H. Smith MESKWAKI 243. "Specimen 3628 of the Dr. Jones collection is the immature seeds of *Spiraea salicifolia*. . .It is made into a medicine to stop blood flux."

1932 H. Smith OJIBWE 386. "The Flambeau Ojibwe use the root as a trapping medicine."

1933 H. Smith POTAWATOMI 80. "Among the Forest Potawatomi, the bark is considered medicinal but the use of this medicine was not stated. Among the whites [Nickell 1911: 130] the root of this plant is valued for its tonic and esculent properties, while the herbage is used for its astringent and diuretic properties."

1945 Rousseau MOHAWK transl. 47. "*Spiraea latifolia*, the Indian name translates as Indian tea. To prevent nausea and vomiting, drink a decoction of the spiraea and the leaves and branches of yarrow after they have been mashed and left in cold water for two days. The plant is used in Quebec as a substitute for tea."

1955 Mockle Quebec transl. 62. "Tonic and astringent. The plant is used as a substitute for tea, which it tastes like, in certain places."

NINEBARK   *Physocarpus opulifolius* (L.) Maxim.
Shrub with many stems up to 3 m, the bark comes off in strips which has given it the name of nine bark and in french, seven bark (à sept ecorce). The maple-like leaves have teeth around their edges. The balls of white or purplish flowers are at the ends of 1-2 cm long stems. The brownish capsules contain the seeds, these can be either shining or scurfy.
Range. James Bay, Que. to Minn., S.D., and Colo., s. to N.C., Tenn. and Ark. in moist, sandy or rocky soils and shores. May-July.

1812 Peter Smith. Weavers quills are made of the pith. The root is said to be a great cathartic, but I have never proved it. The Indians use a decoction of these roots for fomenting and poulticing. . .It removes the anguish and cures a burn beyond credibility; cases verging on mortification, fellons, swellings, rising of a woman's breast etc. yield to its application beyond anything else. To apply it boil the roots and make a strong decoction, then take of the liquor and thicken up a poultice with bran or Indian meal, this may be put into a little bag made of thin cloth, and apply it as warm and as moist as will be agreeable; this may be repeated as often as you will, until the pain or inflammation is quite gone. Linen or cotton cloths dipt in the liquor, hot, and applied as warm as can be born and then kept close while the case remains and so repeated, will be a good way to apply it."

1830 Rafinesque 93. "Ninebark has nearly the same properties as hardhack, and is an equivalent. I have used the extract with equal success. It is chiefly used by herbalists in external applications for fomentations, poultices, burns, mortification, swelling."

1901 Morice CARRIER Arctic 22. "When a wound or sore manifested a tendency towards decomposition, a sort of blister of the inner bark of the willow and of the outer bark of the bear berry bush was applied, generally with good results. . .The plant I refer to is a shrub four or five feet high, whose name seems to be unknown to all the English-speaking people I have met, though the plant is very abundant all through my district. French Canadians in the service of the Hudson's Bay Company call it, it would seem, l'arbre aux sept ecorces, though it is no tree at all. The medical properties of its leaves, bark, and root are highly valued by the Indians. The word I call it by is merely a translation of its Carrier name—soes mai teon, bear-berry-stick or bush. . .26-7. Cataract is easily discerned by the natives who treat it in this wise. . .In stead of birch bark, others use for the same purpose a piece of calcined bone which, coming in contact with the waste tissue formed on the eye, seems to have the same drawing properties as a magnet on a bit of iron. In either case, the eye is left sore and bloody. It is now carefully washed and as a final treatment, it is bathed with a cooled infusion of the inner bark of the bear berry bush to which a little woman's milk has been added. The former especially is reputed to be quite a specific against any soreness of the eyes, though its mordant properties render its application very trying at first. With this last preparation the patient is made to retire, and when he wakes up on the morrow, he generally feels quite well. Such operations are even now quite common and as uniformly successful. But I am inclined to believe that, considering the primitive way they are performed, at least as much credit is due to the endurance of the patient as to the skill of the oculist.

1923 H. Smith MENOMINI 49. "The bark of this shrub yields a valuable drink for female maladies. It cleans out the system, and if the patient is barren, the drinking of this renders them again fertile, according to the Menomini."

1955 Mockle Quebec transl. 59. "Astringent and diuretic."

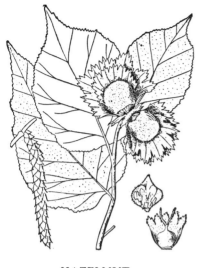

HAZELNUT

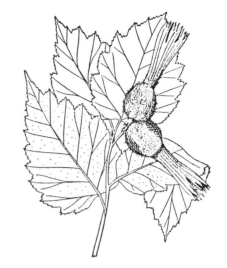

BEAKED HAZEL

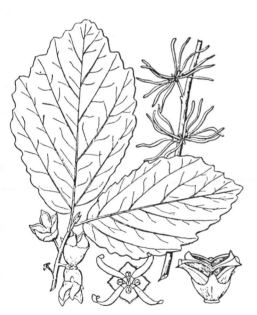

WITCH HAZEL

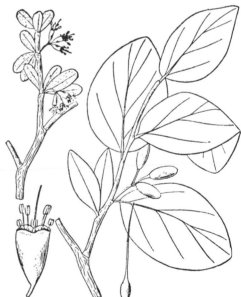

LEATHERWOOD

HAZELNUT   *Corylus americana* Walt. Betulaceae

Shrub 1-3 m tall with young twigs and leaf stalks hairy, these red when young, also usually with glands. The leaves with two sets of fine teeth, paler and often hairy beneath. Two hairy lacey leaflets around the nut.

Range. Me. to s. Ont and s. Man., s. to Ga., and Okla. in dry or moist woods. Nuts ripe July-Aug.

Common names. American filbert.

BEAKED HAZEL *Corylus cornuta* Marsh. (*C. rostrata*)
Shrub 1-3 m tall young twigs hairy at first but without glands. The leaves with wide spaced deep teeth, hairy on the veins beneath and paler. The nuts with a long slender beak prolonged beyond the end of the nut, bristly hairy.
Range. Nfld. to Lake Superior to B.C., s. to N.J., Pa., O., Mo. and Oreg. and in the mts. to n. Ga. in moist woods and thickets. Fruit ripe Aug-Sept.
800-1400 A.D. *C. americana* found archeologically by Wintemberg (1936:12) at the Roebuck, Iroquoian site in Grenville county Ontario: at Boyer's Run Rock shelter in Penn. and at 3 sites and 3 caves in Ohio. Yarnell 1964:63). *C. cornuta* found archeologically at 25 locations at the Juntunen site, Michilimackinac and at Indian Point, Isle Royale (Yarnell 1964:63).
1535-6 Cartier Isle aux Coudres, St. Lawrence transl. 118-9. "This island. . .there are several wild hazel bushes which we found covered with nuts as big and of better taste than ours but a little harder; and for this reason we call it Island of Hazel bushes."
1642 De Vries New Netherlands 219. "The Indians dry the nuts of trees and use them for food. . .There also grow here hazel-nuts, large nuts in great quantities."
1830 Rafinesque 213. "Hazelnut, Filberts. Good fruit, giving relief in nephritis: afford much oil of a bad smell, anodyne, odontalgic."
1888 Delamare Island of Miquelon transl. 28. "The bark slightly febrifuge, not used."
1915 Harris HURON 50. "For ulcers and tumors the Hurons applied to the affected parts poultices made from the bark of the hazel-nut tree. . .56. The species 'rostrata' more common northward is also common throughout the western states. It is very common in Ontario. The bark is astringent and a febrifuge."
1916 Waugh IROQUOIS 122. "A considerable variety of edible nuts are met with throughout the Iroquois country and were not only eaten raw, but were also incorporated into other foods. . .123. Hazelnut, common and beaked were used. . .124. Nut meat oil was often added to the mush used by the Falseface Societies. The oil was also formerly used (like sunflower oil) for the hair, either alone or mixed with bear's grease. Lafitau remarks that the mixture was used as a preventitive of mosquitoes." [See walnut].
1926-7 Densmore CHIPPEWA 338. Stalk burned and the charcoal combined with bear's gall and pricked into the temples with needles for convulsions. . .[see cedar]. . .340. The root of the hazel and that of the white oak steeped together with the inner bark of the chokecherry and the heart of the wood of the ironwood and the decoction drunk for hemorrhages from the lungs. . .372. The black rushes were colored with the inner barks of the hazelnut. *C. americana* and that of the butternut boiled together. "It was necessary to dip the rushes every day for about two weeks, boiling them a short time and then hanging them up to dry. These rushes are a clear heavy black. When the process was completed and the black rushes were dry they were rubbed thoroughly with a little lard 'to make them shiny and limber'". . .Fourth formula for a black dye the green-burs of the hazelnut and the inner bark of the white oak in hot water and boiled; then the inner bark of the butternut and some black earth was added. Let it stand a long time before using. . .Seventh formula was used in dyeing a piece of white blanket for the writer. The result was not a heavy black, but this was said to be due to the insufficient quantity of the dye. The inner bark of oak, green hazel burrs, grindstone dust, iron and a little ochre dust in hot water was the formula. . .377. Drumming sticks were made from the hazel. . .307. The nuts were eaten.
1923 H. Smith MENOMINI 26. "The inner bark of the hazel bush is used with other herbs as a binder to cement the virtues of all together. . .63. The Menomini are very fond of these nuts when they are in the milk stage, and also gather and dry them for winter use."
1928 H. Smith MESKWAKI 267. "Hazel twigs used to be employed in making home-made brushes for cleaning the earthen floors of wigwams. They were also used in making twig baskets. . .256. Used for food."
1932 H. Smith OJIBWE 359. "Bearskin said that the bark of the hazelnut bush is medicine. It is boiled and used as a poultice on cuts to close and heal them. . .The Pillager Ojibwe used only the hairs of the hazelnut husk as a medicine to expel worms. . .398. Especially fond of the newly gathered nuts before the kernel has hardened. . .417. A crooked stick with an enlarged base such as can often be obtained in a hazel bush makes the favorite drum stick for the Flambeau Ojibwe. The finest twigs are bound into a bundle, with the tips sheared to serve as a primitive broom. . .The finer twigs may also be used as ribs in making woven baskets for collecting or storing acorns or hard fruits. . .425. The Flambeau Ojibwe make use of the seed hulls of the Hazelnut

in setting the black color of butternut dye. They are boiled together and the tannic acid of the hulls sets the color."

1933 H. Smith POTAWATOMI 44. "Use the inner bark in medicinal combinations very much the same as they use the inner bark of the willow. It is used as an astringent. . .97. Gather and eat as Ojibwe do."

1945 Rousseau MOHAWK transl. 38. "The stalk cut into pieces is used to make a collar to alleviate the pain babies suffer when teething. An infusion of one-year-old stalks of hazel with the root of field horsetail is used for the same purpose."

1945 Rousseau Quebec transl. 85. "The nuts are eaten after being lightly cooked in the oven. The twigs are used for rheumatism."

1945 Raymond TETE DE BOULE transl. 128. "A tea made of the tips of the branches is used to cure heart troubles."

1955 Mockle Quebec transl. 34. "*C. americana* the bark astringent and febrifuge. . . *C. rostrata*, the bark astringent and febrifuge. The oil from the nuts is used for toothache."

WITCH HAZEL   *Hamamelis virginiana* L. Hamamelidaceae
Shrub to 5 m tall, leaves 5-15 cm long with rounded teeth and slight lobes, often hairy beneath. The bright yellow flowers open in the fall when the leaves are falling. They consist of 4 long, thin, wavy petals. The capsules contain usually two hard shiny seeds which ripen a year later.
Range. N.B., N.S., s. Que., s. Ont. to n. Mich. and se. Minn., s. to Fla. and Tex. in moist woods.
Common names. Spotted-alder, snapping hazel, tobacco wood, pistachio, winter bloom. The wood is hard, weighing 43 lbs per cu. foot.

1590 Harriot Virginia Indians 24. "They are a people clothed with loose mantles of Deere skins. . .those weapons that they have, are onlie bowes made of Witch hazel, & arrows of reeds."

1633 Gerarde-Johnson 1481. "Witch Hasell or the broadest leaved Elme [Ulmus montana]. . .This prospereth and naturally groweth. . .in good plenty in moist places in Hampshire where it is commonly called Witch Hasell. Old men affirme, that when long boughes [bows] were in great use, there were very many made of the wood of this tree, for which purpose it is mentioned in the statutes of England by the name of Witch Hasell."

1931 Grieve England 283. "Branches of Wych Elm were formerly used for making bows and when forked were employed as divining rods. [*Ulmus montana*, Wych elm]." [This common elm of northern England grows up as several branches like a shrub. It is possible that the name witch hazel was given to *Hamamelis* by the first English settlers because its leaves looked so like those of the witch hazel elm and the hazel of England. They used it for divining rods as they did the elm. The shrub has no association with witches or their works other than the name given it in English. It was the hazel that was associated with witches in England].

1744 Colden Letter 3;89 to Gronovius in Leyden. "I shall tell you what I learn'd of the use of the Hamamelis from a Minister of the Church of England who officiates among the Mohawk Indians. He saw an allmost total blindness occasioned by a blow cur'd by receiving the Warm Stream of a Decoction of the Bark of this Shrub through a Funnel upon the place. This was don by direction of a Mohawk Indian after other means had for a considerable time prov'd ineffectual. I have since experienc'd the benefit of it used in the same manner in an Inflammation of the eye from a blow."

1778 Carver 508. "The Witch Hazel grows very bushy, about ten feet high, and is covered early in May with numerous white blossoms. When this shrub is in bloom, the Indians esteem it a further indication that the frost is entirely gone, and that they might sow their corn. It has been said, that it is possessed of the power of attracting gold or silver, and that twigs of it are made use of to discover where the veins of these metals lie hid; but I am apprehensive that it is only a fallacious story, and not to be depended on; however the supposition has given it the name of witch hazel." [Here Carver is referring to a different shrub, the *Fothergilla* or witch-alder of the southern States, which seems to have been given the attributes of the witch-hazel.]

1785 Cutler 412. "The Indians considered this tree as a valuable article in their materia medica. . .They applied the bark, which is sedative and discutient, to painful tumors and external inflammations. A cataplasm of the inner rind of the bark, is found to be very efficacious in removing painful inflammations of the eyes. The bark chewed in the mouth is, at first, somewhat bitter, very sensibly astringent, and then leaves a pungent, sweetish, taste, which will remain for a considerable time."

1828 Rafinesque 229-30. "[Seeds] in the South where they are called erroneously Pistachoe nuts, although quite unlike the *Pistacia vera*. . .They are similar in shape to the esculent Pine seeds of *Pinus picea*, cylindrical, shining black outside, white and farinaceous inside, rather oily and palatable. The shrub resembles very much in the appearance of the leaves and nuts, the common hazelnut. . .but the blossoms are totally different. It has become in the United States the Witch hazel, affording divining rods, employed by the adepts of the occult arts, to find or pretend to find Water, Ores, Salt, &c. under ground. The *Alnus* [alder] and *Corylus* [hazel] are often substituted, a forked branch is used, the two branches held in both hands; when and where the point drops, the springs or metals sought for, are said to be! A belief in this vain practice is as yet widely spread. . .The Indians value this shrub highly, and it is much used in the North by [white] herbalists. The bark affords an excellent topical application for painful tumors and piles, external inflammations, sore and inflamed eyes, &c. in cataplasm or poultice or wash. A tea is made of the leaves, and employed for many purposes, in amennorrhea, bowel complaints, pains in the sides, menstrual effusions, bleeding of the stomach, &c. In this last case, the chewed leaves, decoction of the bark or tea of the leaves, are all employed with great advantage. A strong infusion is given in injection for bowel complaints. . .268. Called Shemba by the Osage Indians, and used for ulcers, tumors, sores, &c. in poultice."

1959-61 Gunn 883. "Both leaves and bark are used in medicine. . .mostly in decoction, which is good as an astringent in diarrhea, dysentery, and in bleedings from the lungs, stomach, and urinary organs, taken freely internally; and also good as a wash to old and foul ulcers, and as an injection in leucorrhea, flooding, and falling of the womb, and as a gargle and wash in sore mouth and throat. Dose of the decoction, from half to a teacupful, three or four times a day. The Witch Hazel may generally be had in drug stores."

1868 Can. Pharm. J. 6;83-5. Bark and leaves of Witch Hazel, *Hamamelis Virginiana* included in list of Can. medicinal plants.

1892 Millspaugh 58. "This plant, about which was formerly draped, by those versed in the occult arts, a veil of deep mystery, and whose forked branches were used as a divining-rod while searching for water and ores, grows profusely in the damp woods of Canada and the United States. . .The many varied uses of a watery infusion of Witch-hazel bark were fully known to the aborigines, whose knowledge of our medicinal flora has been strangely correct as since proven."

1905 Muldrew Muskoka Ont. 50. "A rather tall branching shrub, often growing in clumps in moist soil. The yellow flowers appear in October while the fruit of the previous year yet remains, which fact, with its fame as a divining rod, may account for the popular name. It is reported as rare east of Toronto, but I have found it rather common in parts of Durham county, and frequent in Muskoka. An extract of the bark has medicinal properties."

1915 Speck PENOBSCOT 312. A concoction of seven herbs is taken as a sudorific before entering the sudatory [sweat bath]. It comprises [among the seven] witch-hazel twigs.

1916 Waugh IROQUOIS 148. "Witch-hazel. . .was stated by Chief David Jack to be made into a decoction of suitable strength, sweetened with maple sugar and used as a tea at meals."

1923 H. Smith MENOMINI 37. "A decoction of witch hazel was used by the participants in games, to rub on their legs to keep them limbered up. The twigs of witch hazel are steeped and the decoction is used to cure a lame back. The seeds were also used as the sacred bead in the medicine ceremony. These black beads were called 'megise'."

1933 H. Smith POTAWATOMI 59. "This was one of the remedies that the Forest Potawatomi use in their sweat baths. They place the twigs in water and with hot rocks create steam which bathes sore muscles."

1928 Parker SENECA 11. Sedative: use witch hazel.

1955 Mockle Quebec transl. 63. "A powerful astringent when used as distilled water of the leaves or an extract of the bark for the care of the skin and against varicose veins, hemorrhoids, phlebitis, varicose ulcers and also as a hemostatic. There has been found a crystallised tannin, hamamelitannin, a combination of gallic acid and a hexose, hamamelose, and also quercetol and choline."

The seeds suddenly are driven out of their dry capsules with a loud snap, heard clearly if a branch is brought into the house in the autumn. The dried powdered leaves will stop bleeding from small cuts (Harlow 1957:194).

The bark should be collected in the spring, it contains 6% tannin and is used for hemorrhage from nose, lungs, rectum or uterus. The leaves are collected in the fall and dried in the shade to keep their green color. The fruit is a small woody capsule breaking open at the top into two halves, each containing a seed which is edible. Distilled witch hazel is prepared from the fresh twigs that bear flowers in the fall. It is used for piles, bruises, and as an astringent lotion (T.E. Wallis 1967:99,142).

An extract made from the leaves of witch hazel is used in suppositories (Lewis and Elvin-Lewis 1977:293).

Witch hazel is used commercially in after shave lotions and mouth washes.

LEATHERWOOD   *Dirca palustris* L. Thymelaeaceae

Shrub growing 1-2 m tall with yellowish green, smooth, jointed twigs and tough, fibrous, light grey bark. The 5-8 cm long leaves on 2-5 mm stalks are hairy when young and smooth or nearly so when older. The clusters of 2-4 small yellow flowers appear before the leaves. They are protected from cold winds by dark hairy scales, 'which look like folds of fur around the silky yellow calyces'. The berries are long, narrow, to 8 mm, reddish and poisonous.

Range. s. Que. and s. Ont. to Minn., s. to Fla., Ala., Ark, and Okla. in rich moist woods.

Common names. Rope wood, poison berry, wicopy, wickup, swamp wood, American mezereon, bois de plomb.

400 B.C.-250 A.D. Identified in Ohio Adena and rock shelter textiles by Whitford 1941:10. Yarnell 1964:190.

1708 Sarrazin-Vaillant, Quebec-Paris, Boivin 1978 transl. 198. "I do not know why it is called bois de plomb, [lead wood] for it is very light. . .The bark is very thick, supple, very strong; and it separates easily from the wood. It is pounded and applied to malign ulcers. It is said the abbé Gendron used it for cancer and that he learnt this use of it from our savages. . .Here the cooked bark is used as a cataplasm to alleviate the pains of hemorroids and old ulcers. It is said that this is the remedy of abbé Gendron for cancer, but I know well that it is powerless in these cases."

1724 Anon ILLINOIS-MIAMI mss 224. "The bark of leatherwood boiled for all sorts of wounds, I have seen a cancer cured by it; it serves to stop the bloody flux. We must carry some of this wood to France."

1749 Kalm Albany April the 17th. 284. "Leatherwood. The *Dirca palustris*, or moose-wood, is a little shrub which grows on hills, near swamps and marshes, and is now in full blossom. The English in Albany call it leatherwood, because its bark is tough as leather. The French in Canada call it bois de plomb, or lead wood, because the wood itself is as soft and as tough as lead. The bark of this shrub was used for ropes, baskets, etc. by the Indians, while they lived among the Swedes. And it is really very fit for that purpose on account of its remarkable strength and toughness, which is equal to the lime tree bark [basswood]. The English and Dutch in many parts of North America, and the French in Canada, employ this bark in all cases where we in Europe use the lime tree bark, especially for binding purposes. The tree itself is very tough, and one cannot easily seperate a branch from the trunk without the help of a knife. Some people use switches of this tree for whipping their children."

1778 Carver 507. "The moose wood. . .makes equally as good cordage as hemp."

1817-20 Bigelow 158. "The fruit of the Dirca has been suspected of narcotic properties. . .A child which had eaten these berries [suffered] effects like those produced by Stramonium, such as stupor, insensibility, and dilation of the pupils. An emetic brought up the berries and the child gradually recovered. . .Dr. Locke (my assistant) gave the freshly dried root to various patients in doses of from 5 to 10 grains which quantity in most instances proved powerfully emetic and sometimes cathartic. . .Applied portions of the bark moistened with vinegar to the skin of his arm. In twelve hours no effect was produced, in twenty four some redness and itching took place and in thirty a complete vesication followed. . .I have introduced the Dirca in this place, not so much because it has been yet applied to any medical purpose of great importance; but because it would be improper, in a work like the present, to pass over unnoticed a shrub of such decided activity. . .The Indians used it for cordage."

1828 Rafinesque 159. "The bark is very tough, can hardly be broken, and tearing in long strips is used yet in many parts for ropes, a practice borrowed from the Indian tribes; the wood is also flexible. The berries are poisonous, children must avoid them, if eaten by mistake an emetic must be resorted to. The bark and root have a peculiar nauseous smell and unpleasant acrimonius taste. . .They are active and dangerous medicines to which less acrimonius substances ought to be preferred."

1829 MacTaggart 1307. "The timbers of the bark canoe. . .are sewed with strips of the leatherwood-tree."

1830 Trans. Lit. & Hist. Soc. Que. 3; 88. "Leatherwood, the whole plant is remarkably pliable, and the bark so strong and flexible as to be frequently used for ligatures, and for straps to carry burdens; it is easily stripped off the plant its whole length when required for use; whence probably the name of Bois de pelon, usually pronounced Bois de plomb."

1836 Trail Backw. Can. 113. "Leather-wood, called American mezereon, or moose wood; this is a very pretty, and at the same time useful shrub, the bark being used by farmers as a substitute for cord in tying sacks, etc.; the Indians sew their birch-bark baskets with it occasionally."

1840 Gosse Quebec 125. "I found a shrub very numerous in the woods, covered with yellow flowers, very small, with thick downy envolopes. I have a twig of it; I was obliged to cut it off; for, small as it is, the bark was so tough that I could not tear it. That is the Leather plant. . .extreme toughness of the inner bark, which is so strong that the stoutest man could not break, by pulling a strip of an inch in width, taken from the main stem. The bark is used for strings for many purposes, especially by millers, who collect great quantities for the purpose of tying their flour bags. The wood, when stripped of the bark, is remarkably soft and brittle, snapping with the slightest effort, almost like the pith of elder. It is here commonly known by the name of Wickaby."

1868 Can. Pharm. 6;83-5. Leatherwood, *Dirca palustris*, the bark included in list of Can. medicinal plants.

1892 Millspaugh 146. "The fibrous bark afforded material for ropes, thongs, cordage and baskets to the American aborigines. The medical history of the drug is slight, the only reference to its use is that of the Indians as a masticatory for aching, carious teeth. . .Dirca acts as an irritant to the mucous membranes of the gastro-intestinal tract and bladder, as well as to the nerves."

1920 Fyles 65. "This plant, so useful to the North American Indians. . .The bark contains poisonous properties similar to its relative mezereon and, when fresh, causes severe irritation to the skin, followed by blisters. All parts of the plant have a burning, nauseous taste. The poison is most powerful during the flowering and fruiting. . .All parts of mezereon are acrid and poisonous, especially the bark and berries. They contain an extremely acrid resin mezerin, a bitter poisonous glucoside daphnin, as well as a vesicating fatty oil. . .In case of human poisoning an emetic may be given, followed by a soothing drink such as rice water, barley water, iced milk, or white of an egg beaten up in cold water while waiting for medical advice, which should be promptly summoned."

1926-7 Densmore CHIPPEWA 346. Cut up the stalk and dry it, pulverize, put about a tablespoon in warm water, steep but do not let it boil. Do not eat after taking it. Green stalks may be chewed. This is taken as a physic. . .350. Make a decoction of the roots of Dirca and mugwort (*Artemisia dracunculoides*), use it as a wash to strengthen the hair and make it grow.

1923 H. Smith MENOMINI 54. "Name in Menomini means 'variegated urine'. The roots are steeped to make a tea, which heals kidney troubles. It is diuretic. It has been used by the white man in chronic skin diseases. . .76. The tough bark or even twigs of the leatherwood was used for cordage by the aboriginal Menomini. Even now emergency cordage is made from the leatherwood."

1932 H. Smith OJIBWE 390. "The Potawatomi name 'djibe gub' means a dead person, or ghost or spirit. The bark is very soft, strong and elastic, so that twigs can be tied in knots. The Pillager Ojibwe say that all their people use it as a tea for a diuretic.

1933 H. Smith POTAWATOMI 85. "The Forest Potawatomi use the inner bark. . .to make a tea for its diuretic properties. . .114. 'Dead man's bark.' This is one of the ready cordages that are to be found in the woods. The bark is tough and stringy and makes a good substitute for twine."

1945 Rousseau MOHAWK transl. 50. "The bark, twisted, is used to make rope. With the bark one can pull a considerable load. The wood and the bark is used as an energetic purgative. The infusion mixed with the wood and bark of the black walnut is used as a vomitive to drive 'the yellow' from the stomach. The 'yellow' is a sickness of the whites that they brought along with tea, butter and tobacco. The 'yellow' accumulates in the stomach and cannot 'pass'. . .Like the Indians, the whites use the bark to make twine. The drastic character of this plant is well known in modern medicine."

1955 Mockle Quebec transl. 66. "The bark is vesicant; it is given in infusion as a drastic purgative and mixed with black walnut as a vomitive. According to Choquette the rubefacient and drastic action is due to a resin and the emetic action to a saponiside."

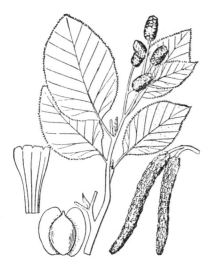

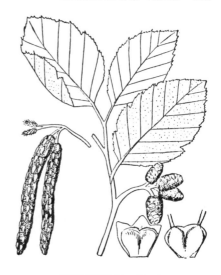

GREEN ALDER   SPECKLED ALDER

GREEN ALDER   *Alnus crispa* (Ait.) Pursh Betulaceae (*A. viridis*)
A shrub to 3 m high, the younger leaves more or less glutinous and hairy, the buds without stalks. The leaves with sharp, fine teeth, when mature dark green above. The fruit only 1-2.1 mm wide and surrounded by pale membranous wings.
Range. Lab. to Alaska, s. to Mass., N.Y., Mich. to N. Calif.; higher mts of N.C. and Tenn. in bogs, shores and cold woods.
Common names. Mountain alder

SPECKLED ALDER   *Alnus rugosa* (DuRoi) Spreng. (*A. incana, A. serrulata*)
Tall shrub or tree with leaves that have double teeth or even small lobes, pale green beneath, usually hairy on the veins. The fruit 2-3.5 mm with very narrow wings.
Range. Nfld. to Mack. and B.C., s. to Md., Va., Iowa, Calif.; also in Eurasia, in wet soil.
Common names. Common-tag- hazel alder.
1633 Gerarde-Johnson 1477-78. "The European alder. . .the wood or timber is not hard, and yet it will last and indure verie long under the water, yea longer than any other timber whatsoever: wherefor in the fenny and soft marish grounds they do use to make piles and posts thereof, for the strengthening of the walls and such like. This timber doth also serve very well to make troughs to convey water instead of pipes of Lead. . .The leaves of Alder are much used against hot swellings, ulcers, and all inward inflammations, especially of the Almonds and kernels of the throat. The barke is much used of poor country Diers, for the dying of course cloth, cappes, hose, and such like into a blacke colour, whereunto it serveth very well."
1748 Kalm Philadelphia October the 14th. 104. "I found afterwards, myself, that the alders in some places of Canada were but little inferior to the Swedish ones. Their bark is employed here in dyeing red and brown. A Swedish inhabitant of America told me that he had once cut his leg to the very bone, and that some blood had already congested within; that he had been advised to boil the alder bark, and to wash the wound often with the water; that he had followed this advice, and had soon got his leg healed, though it had been very dangerous at first."
1799 Lewis Mat. Med. 83. "Leaves and bark of European alder a bitter styptic of disagreeable taste. Used in intermittent fevers. A decoction of the bark for inflammation of tonsils. Leaves chopped and heated efficacious for dispersing milk in the breast as a cataplasm."
1830 Rafinesque 188. "*Alnus serrulata*. Near streams from Canada to Florida. Leaves vulnerary and astringent, repel the milk when bruised and applied to the breast. Bark styptic, dies brown, and with vitriol black. The cones also die black. The inner bark of the root is emetic and dies yel-

low. The wood produces a light charcoal, the very best for gunpowder. . .called Sulling by the Canada tribes, who use the bark in poultice for swellings and strains."

1833 Howard Quebec 44. "To Kill Fleas and Bugs. Cover the floor with leaves of alder gathered while the dew hangs upon them.—Adhereing to these, they are killed."

1884 Holmes-Haydon Hudson Bay CREE 303. "Nepatihe or Green Alder. This is the bark of *Alnus viridis*. It consists of thin shreds which have evidently been scraped off the young branches. The inner surface is of a pale dull brown and the exterior greenish brown. It has a very astringent taste with a slight bitterness and a flavour recalling that of the leaves of *Arbutus Uva-Ursi* [bearberry, *Arctostaphylos*]. It is used in dropsy."

1915 Speck PENOBSCOT 309. "Alder (*Alnus* sp.) bark boiled in water stops cramps and retching. . .312. A concoction of seven herbs is taken as a sudorific before entering the sudatory [sweat bath]; alder bark, witch hazel twigs, fir twigs, cedar boughs, sweet-flag, prince's pine, lambkill and a kind of brake". . .MONTAGNAIS 315. "Twigs of alder are boiled and drunk for impure blood. . .Alder bark is used as a brew in small quantities for fever."

1915 Speck-Tantaquidgeon MOHEGAN 319. "Twigs of speckled alder are steeped and used for bathing purposes, for sprains, bruises, headache, and backache."

1916 Waugh IROQUOIS 68. "Decoctions of hemlock bark and roots, also the bark of the alder, are used in colouring spoons and other wooden articles a deep red. These become further darkened and polished by usage."

1922 W.D. Wallis MICMAC used the bark for bleeding, hemorrhage of lungs, diptheria.

1926-7 Densmore CHIPPEWA 328. "An informant said that the only regulation concerning the scraping was that the root of alder must be scraped toward the plant". . .346. The inner bark of the alder and arrow wood (*Viburnum acerifolium*). "In preparing these, scrape the stalks carefully, removing only the thin outer covering and using the green part underneath. Put the scrapings of this bark from both trees in boiling water to make decoction to be drunk as an emetic. . .359. The root of the alder. In preparing this remedy the root must be scraped upward. A weak decoction is made from a few inches of the root and a pint of water. The following ingredients are added to this: 4 bumblebees are caught and put in a box to die of themselves. In catching the bees they must be stunned but not injured. It destroys the efficacy if the bees are treated otherwise. The bees are dried, ground to a powder, and put in a leather packet until needed. When the medicine is to be used, a pinch of this powder is put in a small teacup of the above decoction. The dose is about a tablespoonful. Two doses are usually sufficient for difficult labor [in childbirth]. A specimen of the bee was obtained and identified as a common bumblebee.". . .360. A decoction of equal parts of the roots of alder, red-osier dogwood and alternate-leaved dogwood as a wash or compress for sore eyes. . .373. Yellow dye, light yellow. Use only the inner bark of the alder, though both inner and outer bark can be used. Either green or dried bark can be used. Pound the bark until it is in shreds and steep it, putting in the material while the dye is hot and letting it boil up. Nothing is needed to set the color. [See under wild plum for crimson, and dogwood for red and black dye formulas using alder bark by Densmore,]

1928 Parker SENECA 11. "Tag alder used as a diuretic."

1923 H. Smith MENOMINI 26. "The bitter inner bark of this alder is used for poultices to reduce swellings. For more power from the alder, the Menomini employ the root bark. . .When the mucus is too loose in a cold, then it will be congested somewhat by drinking an infusion of the root bark. This infusion may also be used as a wash for sores, being astringent and healing. . .As a wash to cure saddle gall in horses. . .The inner bark is made into an infusion which is used as an alternative. [This last is given under *A. rugosa* and the first part under *A. incana*, which are now considered one species]. . .78. Alder bark is boiled to yield a reddish brown dyestuff. The cloth or other material to be colored is immersed in the boiling liquid."

1928 H. Smith MESKWAKI 206. "Specimen 5137 of the Dr. Jones collection is the root of *Alnus incana*. This is boiled and drunk by children who pass blood in their stools."

1932 H. Smith OJIBWE 358. "The Flambeau Ojibwe use the root for its hemostatic qualities. When one passes blood in his stools, the root tea will act as an astringent and coagulant. . .The eclectic [white] practitioner in the United States and Canada employ it in a powdered condition for dusting upon chafed body surfaces. . .425. The Flambeau Ojibwe use the inner bark for dyeing a light yellow, or with other ingredients to get a red, red brown or black. In occasional cases where sweet grass is dyed yellow, the woman chews the inner bark and draws a wisp of sweet grass through her mouth weaving it in for color."

1933 H. Smith POTAWATOMI 43. "The Potawatomi scrape the inner bark. . .and use the juice obtained to rub on the body to cure the itch. A bark tea is made for flushing the vagina and to make a rectal application with their home-made form of syringe as described previously, [see under white birch], to shrivel the anal muscles and thus cure cases of piles. Potions of the bark tea are also drunk to cure the flux. The powdered inner bark of the speckled alder is used to sprinkle upon the galled spots of their ponies to cure them. Nickell [white] says that the bark has alterative, emetic and astringent properties. The Herbalist says that the bark has been used in the treatment of scrofula and has been considered as alterative and emetic."

1935 Jenness Parry Island OJIBWA Lake Huron 114. "Red dye from boiled alder bark."

1945 Rousseau MOHAWK transl. 38. "To calm the pain resulting from blows, drink every two hours an infusion of fragments of one year old plants. While it is boiling add water three times. When the urine is thick drink a decoction of the twigs of the alder and the roots of *Agropyron repens* [twitch grass]."

1945 Rousseau Quebec transl. 84. "The alder was used formerly to make a brown dye for wool, more intense than that obtained with labrador tea."

1945 Raymond TETE DE BOULE transl. 119. "The alder was the only dye plant known to Neweiacitic. The inner bark gives a clear yellow.

1955 Mockle Quebec transl. 34. "*Alnus crispa* green alder, the bark is astringent and febrifuge, containing 9 to 10% of tannin. The inner bark of the root is emetic. The fresh leaves are used to apply to tumors and inflamed tissues. . .*Alnus incana* the bark astringent."

A tea of the leaves has been used for pimples. The Eskimo boiled the inner bark to produce on orange dye on reindeer skins. Bees use the pollen of alders for spring-brood rearing; the sharp-tailed and ruffled grouse eat the leaves and buds and to some extent the seeds and rabbit and beaver chew the bark. (Harlow 1957:130).

1959 Mechling MALECITE of maritime provinces of Canada used the bark of the black alder, *A. incana* for ulcerated mouths.

1978 Riley personal communication from G. Fireman of Attawapiskat, James Bay. His Cree mother still uses the inner bark of alder as a moist poultice to stop heavy bleeding from wounds.

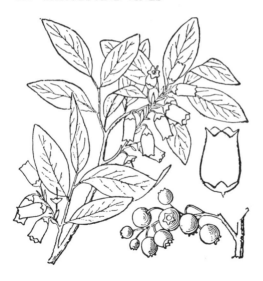

HIGH BUSH BLUEBERRY

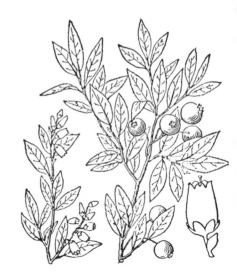

LOW BUSH BLUEBERRY

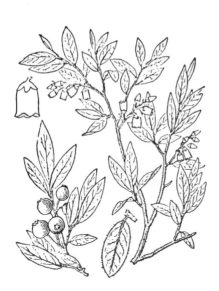

DOWNY BLUEBERRY

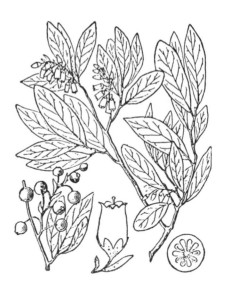

BLACK HUCKLEBERRY

HIGH BUSH BLUEBERRY   *Vaccinium corymbosum* L. Ericaceae

In the middle of bogs grows the high bush blueberry, one of the tallest of the blueberries. Its stems are minutely warty, greenish-brown and round, 1-4 m tall. The leaves, on short stalks, are greeny blue with tiny hairs around their edges, 4-8 x 2-3 cm; the underside may be hairy on the veins or hairy all over, but smooth above. The white, or faintly pink 6-10 mm bell-shaped flowers appear with the leaves. The berry is blue with a whitish bloom on it.

Range. N.S. to Mich., s. to N.J., Pa., O. and Ind.

EARLY OR LOW BUSH BLUEBERRY   *Vaccinium angustifolium* Ait.
The common low blueberry bush in dry rocky places. 5-20 cm tall with green warty branches
and smooth leaves that are only 1-3 cm x 4-10 mm wide with sharp teeth. There are few white or
pinkish 3-5 mm long flowers followed by 7-12 mm thick bright blue berries, sometimes nearly
black, very sweet.
Range. Lab. and Nfld. to Man., s. to N.J., Pa., Mich., Minn. and in the mts. to Va. and W. Va.

DOWNY BLUEBERRY   *Vaccinium myrtilloides* Michx. (*V. canadense*)
In moist or dry soil and in bogs, this 20-40 cm tall shrub has branches densely covered with hair.
Its leaves are thin and soft 1.5-3 cm long and half as wide, softly hairy on both sides. The 4-5 mm
white or pinkish flowers are followed by berries, blue or bluish black, covered with a whitish
bloom.
Range. Lab. to B.C., s. to Pa., Ind. and Minn., and in the mts to Va. and W.Va. These are our
three main blueberries. Other species vary as to sweetness but their medicinal qualities vary not
at all.
1070-1320 Juntunen site Michilimackinac Lake Huron Yarnell 1964:35. Blueberry seeds found
archeologically.
1380 Crawford Lake site Ontario McAndrews, Byrne and Finlayson 1974: Four blueberry seeds
found archeologically.
1500 Draper site Ontario Finalayson 1975:225. 71 blueberry seeds found archeologically.
1619 Champlain-Macklem Ottawa river 1616 34. "We also found—it was almost as if God had
wished to bestow a gift of some sort on this barren and unfriendly country for the succour and
support of its people—that in season the riverbanks were thick with berries of all sorts, including
raspberries and blueberries (a small berry but very good to eat). The savages dry the berries for
use during the winter, much as we in France dry prunes for use during Lent. . .36. Lake
Huron. . .The savages had eaten so much in the early stages of the journey that by this time we
had little left, though for some time we had been eating only one meal a day. Luckily, there was
also plenty of blueberries and raspberries. Without them we might have starved to death. It was
on the French River that we met some three hundred men from a tribe we called the cheveux
relevés or long hairs. . .I made friends. . .their headman. . .explained that when we came upon
them they had been drying blueberries, so they would have something to eat that winter when
their other supplies had been used up. . .78. To make bread they boil the dough, as if they were
making corn soup. This makes it easier to whip. After it is thoroughly boiled they sometimes add
blueberries or dried raspberries, or occasionally (for it is very scarce) pieces of suet. After mois-
tening the batter with warm water they make it up into loaves or biscuits which they bake under
hot coals."
1634-5 Journey into country of the MOHAWK 146. "This day we were invited to buy bear
meat, and we also got half a bushel of beans and a quantity of dried strawberries, and we bought
some bread, that we wanted to take on our march. Some of the loaves were baked with nuts and
cherries and dry blueberries and the grains of the sunflower."
1663 Boucher Quebec transl. 51. "There is another sort of little fruit as large as big peas, they are
called Bluets. & have an excellent taste."
1749 Kalm Philadelphia March 17th. 262. "Huckleberries. The Indians formerly plucked them in
abundance every year, dried them either in the sunshine or by the fireside, and afterwards prepared them for eating in different manners. These huckleberries are still a dainty dish among the
Indians. On my travels through the country of the Iroquois, they offered me, whenever they
designed to treat me well, fresh corn bread, baked in an oblong shape, mixed with dried huckleberries, which lay as close in it as raisins in a plum pudding. . .The Europeans also used to collect
a quantity of these berries. . .Some preserve them with treacle."
1812 Peter Smith 38. "A tea made of the blue berry root, when it comes to be known and proved,
will probably be esteemed as the best antispasmodic in the compass of medicine. That is, it will
prevent and do away spasms of every description in a safe and superior manner. . .such as
cramp, hiccup, cholic, cholera morbus, epilepsy, hysterics, and I suppose every other species of
fits, even the ague. . .The blue berry root is said to be the great medicine that the squaws use at
the birth of their children. Experience has however proved, among white women, that its assistance is very special. It is to be made use of in the following manner—Take a good handful of
green or dry roots, make it into a tea (say half a pint) give half of it, and fill up with hot water;

repeat the drinking every 10 minutes, or oftener until it has effect. . .When a woman finds that she is taken in labor, let her drink as above. . .The delivery will be facilitated with much safety. It is to be noticed that if the anguish attending the delivery is not moderated, the doses have not been strong enough; for they act on the same stimulant principles that opium does. . .The squaws, I have heard, drink a little of a tea of this root for two or three weeks before their expected time. I have given this tea in a case of inflammation of the uterus, and found it a speedy cure. The tea of this root is neither a purge nor a vomit, but acts as a stimulus to the nervous system. . .I believe that it is always safe."

1830 Rafinesque 50. "The Indians made a kind of wine of them, and dried them in cakes. . .Useful in scurvy, diarrhea, dropsy, bilious fevers,&c. . .They stain and dye purplish. Leaves astringent, can tan leather, a tea used for sore mouth."

1859-61 Gunn 884. "There are several varieties. . .they all possess the same properties however. The root is the part generally used as a medicine, and is both diuretic and astringent. A decoction of the root is a good astringent remedy in diarrhea and bowel diseases. . .also good as a gargle and for sore throat and mouth, and for old indolent ulcers. The root and berries, bruised and tinctured in Gin are a good diuretic, and seldom fail to relieve gravelly and dropsical affections; to be drank freely, or as much as the stomach and head will bear."

1892 Millspaugh 100. "Said to be narcotic—a property also ascribed to the wine of Whortleberries (*V. uliginosum*) which is very intoxicating."

1916 Waugh IROQOUIS 126. "Berries not required for immediate consumption are dried. This may be done in several ways. The fruit may be spread out just as it is upon boards, in flat evaporating baskets and dried in the sun or by the fire; or it may be mashed and afterwards placed in small cakes upon large basswood leaves to dry. It may also be cooked and afterwards preserved in the manner just described. It is finally stored away in elm bark boxes or covered baskets. . .When wanted for use, the cakes of dried berries are soaked in warm water and cooked as a sauce, or mixed with corn bread. The dried berries were often taken along as a hunting food."

1926-27 Densmore CHIPPEWA 322. "A Canadian Chippewa said that his people combined dried blueberries with moose fat and deer tallow. . .338. The flowers of *V angustifolium*, low bush blueberry, dried and placed on hot stones and the fumes inhaled for 'craziness'. This was said to be one of the remedies given by Winabojo. These remedies are most highly regarded."

1923 H. Smith MENOMINI 66. "Blueberries are a favorite food with the Menomini. They gather them in large quantities and dry them in the sun as raisins or currants are dried for winter use. They are dried on a scaffold thatched with rushes. Dried blueberries and dried sweet corn are eaten together, sweetened with maple sugar, as a special dish."

1932 H. Smith OJIBWE 369. "The Flambeau use the leaves of this common blueberry for a medicinal tea as a blood purifier. . .401. They cook the berries with wild rice, and venison and make a sweet bread with them."

1933 H. Smith POTAWATOMI 57. "The root bark of the downy blueberry has been used by the Forest Potawatomi for a medicine, but we were not able to discover for what ailment. . .99. It is also the basis of a very considerable industry during the late summer months when the berries are gathered and sold to white traders. . .Make a practice of lining their berry pails with the leaves of Sweet Fern which they claim keeps the berries from spoiling."

1945 Raymond TETE DE BOULE transl. 133. "One part of the harvest is eaten immediately; the other is cooked for ten hours or longer in the course of which the blueberries decompose and solidify into a paste. It is a sort of vegetal pemmican that can be kept for two years and which is eaten during the winter to vary the menu which is too exclusively meat. 'Mother' Dube. . .calls this preparation, savage cheese. . .This is an old Indian recipe."

1971 Jolicoeur Quebec 3. "*V. canadense* (*myrtilloides*) downy blueberry for diabetes."

1972 Pailaiseul transl. 212. "Downy blueberry. A decoction of the leaves, 20 or 30 gr. in a litre of water; boil five minutes, drink 2 or 3 cups a day for inflammation of the genito-urinary tract, notably cystitus, incontinence of urine (children in bed), skin diseases, pruritis, excema. It lowers the blood sugar count. . .Modern work has shown that the berries. . .in decoction sterilise in 24 hours cultures of colibacilla and Eberth's bacilla, responsible for typhoid. They constitute the natural remedy for enteritis, dysentery and intestinal fermentations. With the fresh berries you can make a tincture of myrtille which Abbe Kneipp says 'is the first and most indispensable of all the tinctures in our household pharmacy.' In a litre jar put 100 to 150 gr of fresh berries and fill with alcohol or brandy. It is ready in 15 days but stronger and better if left longer. It is taken for the same illnesses as the decoction, 10-30 drops on a cube of sugar. A second dose after 8 to 10 hours, a third is rarely necessary."

1973 Stary & Jirasek 210. "*Vaccinium myrtillus*. 1. The berries. . .exert an astringent and costive action on the intestines. The leaves also contain tannins and other little known substances reducing the sugar level in the blood. They have a mild disinfectant effect in infections of the kidney and bladder. The fruits are popularly used in the form of a decoction for diarrhea, and also as a gargle for stomatitis. The decoction from the leaves and seedcoats of the berries is an efficient subsidiary medicine in the treatment of diabetes. . .The drug is collected only in the wild. The berries were listed as a medicinal drug by Abbess Hildegarde of Germany in the 12th. century."

BLACK OR HIGH BUSH HUCKLEBERRY   *Gaylussacia baccata* (Wang.) K. Koch Ericacea
Often confused with the blueberry and called highbush blueberry. The name Huckleberry also applied to blueberry. An upright shrub to 1 m tall with stiff greyish branches, the young growth reddish with fine hairs. The best way to identify it is by the leaves which are covered with tiny glands full of resin. Easily seen if a leaf is held up to the light. The leaves are 2-5 cm long, short stalked, green on both sides and usually smooth but with a very fine fringe of hairs around the edges. The flowering stalk has bell-shaped white flowers 4-6 mm long from hairy cups and stalks. The flowers turn reddish with age. The black berries are 6-8 mm, containing ten seed-like nutlets.
Range. Nfld. and Que. to Ont. and Man., s. to Ga., Ala. and Mo. May to June in dry sandy and rocky soil, often around the edges of swamps.
Common names. Black-snap, crackers.
1868 Can. Pharm. J. 6;83-5. Whortleberry, *Vaccinium Frondosum*, the fruit included in list of Can. medicinal plants. This is *Gaylussacia frondosa*, dangleberry, a plant of the Atlantic coast and sometimes inland.
1885 Hoffman OJIBWA 199. "Forms one of the chief articles of trade during the summer. The berry occupies a conspicuous place in the myth of the 'Road of the Dead' referred to in connection with the 'Ghost Society'."
1916 Waugh IROQUOIS 128. *Gaylussacia baccata* eaten.
1970 Bye IROQUOIS mss An important food, dried the berries for winter use, ate fresh, made into drinks, used as a medicine for the liver and blood, smoked the leaves.

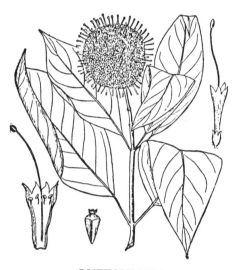

BUTTONBUSH

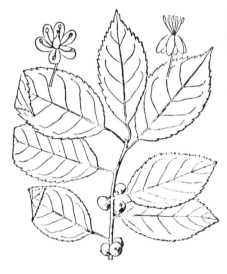

WINTERBERRY

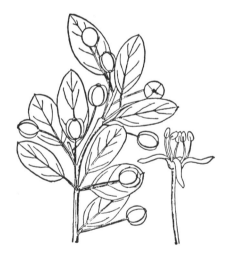

MOUNTAIN HOLLY

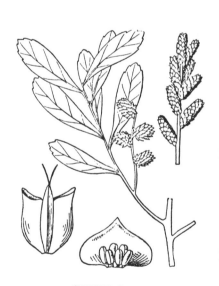

SWEET GALE

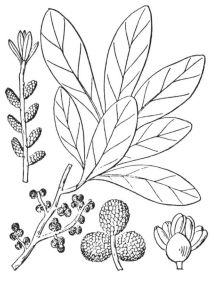

BAYBERRY

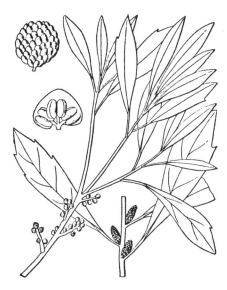

WAX MYRTLE

BUTTONBUSH   *Cephalanthus occidentalis* L. Rubiaceae
Shrub 1-3 m tall or even a small tree in the south. Leaves opposite or in whorls of threes, 8-15 cm long, mostly smooth or inconspicuously hairy in the north, lower leaf surfaces and twigs evidently hairy in the south. The many fragrant flowers are white on a long stem, growing in the form of a round button 3 cm thick, followed by hard seeds.
Range. N.B. and Que. to Minn., s. to Mex. and the W.I. in swamps and streamsides.
Common names. Pond dogwood, pin-ball, little snowball, crane-willow, crouper. (Buttonwood is a common name of the sycamore, *Plantanus occidentalis* L.)
1828 Rafinesque 102. "Buttonbush. . .it is peculiar to North America. . .The whole shrub active, and bitterish, the bitterness is most enfolded in the bark of the roots; this bark and the inner bark of the stem are brittle, somewhat resembling Cascarila and Dogwood in appearance and qualities. Tonic, febrifuge, cathartic, diaphoretic. The flowers, leaves, bark of stems and root are used by the Southern Indians and the French settlers of Louisiana. It has not yet been noticed in our Materia medica and is even omited by Schoepf but it deserves further attention. A fine fragrant syrup may be made with the flowers and leaves, which is a mild tonic and laxative. The most efficient part is the bark of the root. A decoction of it cures intermittent fevers acting on the bowels, at the same time is useful in relaxed bowel. . .1830 206. Inner bark agreeable bitter, much used for coughs, and in a wash for palsy in Carolina; also diuretic, taken in pills for gravel."
1892 Millspaugh 76. "Rubiaceae.—This large and important order has but few representatives in North America but yields many valuable drugs in the hotter climates. . .The cinchonas or Peruvian barks. . .Gambier or pallid catechu (*Uncaria Gambier*), coffee, ipecacuanha (*Cephaelis Ipecacuanha*). . .madder, cleavers. . .The medical history of Cephalanthus is not important; it has been used with accredited success in intermittent and remittent fevers, obstinate coughs (Elliot), palsy, various venereal disorders (Merat), and in general as a tonic, laxative and diuretic. Part used. . .The fresh bark of the stem, branches and root. The root apparently contains the greatest proportion of the bitter principle of the plant."
1925 Wood & Ruddock. "*Cephalanthus occidentalis*, the bark very useful in coughs and colds and diseases of the throat and lungs generally."
1928 H. Smith MESKWAKI 243. "The inner bark of this species was a very important medicine with McIntosh and was used as an emetic. With the white man, *Cephalanthus* bark has been gathered as a sort of substitute for quinine [cinchona], and indeed belongs to the same family."

1955 Mockle Quebec transl. 83. "The leaves and the bark of the stems and root are febrifuge, diaphoretic and cathartic."

1960 Walpole Island CHIPPEWA mss. "Buttonbush used to stop menstrual flow. About a cupful of the stems and leaves boiled 5 minutes and 3 cups a day drunk during flow. The result varies with individual. Plants gathered in July and August and stored. Also the root, 6" or so 1" in diameter added to quart of boiling water and boiled ½ hour. Several cupfuls a day effective in 24 hours for pains and cramps of unusually long menstrual flow."

WINTERBERRY   *Ilex verticillata* (L.) Gray Aquifoliaceae (*Prinos v.*)

Shrub to 5 m, leaves deciduous, dull green above, smooth or hairy beneath, with fine teeth, generally broadest above the middle. Flowers white, a few together on the stem where the leaves join it. Berries bright red lasting all winter.

Range. Nfld. N.B., N.S., P.E.I., Que. Ont. to Mich., s. to Md., Va. and Ind. in swamps and wet woods.

Common names. Fever bush, black alder, striped, white or false alder, inkberry.

MOUNTAIN HOLLY   *Nemopanthus mucronatus* (L.) Trel.

Branching shrub to 3 m, the stalks of the leaves usually red, 5-15 mm long. Leaves 2-5 cm, without teeth or only very fine and sparse ones. Flowers yellowish, on 1-2 cm stalks growing from the stem where the leaves join it. Followed by red berries 6 mm thick.

Range. Nfld., N.B., N.S., P.E.I., Que., Ont. James Bay, to Minn., s. to W. Va and Ind. in damp woods, swamps, bogs.

Common names. Catberry, false holly, brick-timber.

1749 Kalm Quebec October the 14th. 563. "The inkberry grew as a rule here in the woods in level and somewhat low-lying places. The branches are now full of red berries which I tasted and found rather bitter. A man who accompanied me told me the same; he called the shrub bois de marque, but did not know any use for it." [In France, wood used to tally purchases in a store was called a 'marque'.]

1778 Carver 510. "The Fever Bush grows about five or six feet high; its leaf is like that of the lilac, and it bears a reddish berry of spicy flavour. The stalks of it are exceedingly brittle. A decoction of the buds or wood is an excellent febrifuge, and from this valuable property it received its name. It is an ancient Indian remedy for all inflammatory complaints, and likewise much esteemed on the same account by the inhabitants of the interior parts of the colonies."

1817-20 Bigelow 144-5. "The Black alder has had a considerable reputation as a tonic medicine, perhaps more than it deserves. The late Professor Barton tells us, that the bark has long been a popular remedy in different parts of the United States, being used in intermittents fevers and some other diseases as a substitute for the Peruvian bark [quinine]; and on some occasions, he thinks it more useful than that article. . .'It is supposed to be especially useful in cases of great debility accompanied by fever. . .and as a tonic in cases of incipient gangrene. In the last case. . .it is unquestionably a medicine of great efficacy. It is given both internally and employed externally as a wash.' Dr. Thatcher recommends a decoction or infusion of the bark taken internally in doses of a teacupful, and employed also as a wash, for the cure of cutaneous eruptions, particularly of the herpetic kind. . .the *Prinos* is not entitled to hold a very exalted rank in the list of tonics. As a bitter it is at best but of the second rate, and in astringency it falls below a multitude of the common forest trees. The berries are recommended by the writers above cited, as possessing the same tonic properties with the bark. . .I have known sickness and vomiting produced in a person by eating a number of these berries found in the woods in autumn."

1830 Rafinesque 253. "*Prinos*, black alder, Fever bush, winterberry. . .Inner bark emetic, cathartic, tonic, antiseptic. Used in agues, fevers. . .herpatic eruptions, gangrene, jaundice, foul ulcers &c. in powder, decoction and tincture, a wash or poultice. Berries purgative and vermifuge. . .Bitters made with them. Popular remedies. . .8. *Nemopanthus*. . .the bark is also employed for bird lime, and the wood by turners, &c."

1859-61 Gunn 746. "Black Alder (*Prinos Verticillatus*). Known also as the Winterberry. . .The bark, both of the stalk and root, is the part used as medicine. . .by some Botanic physicians has been highly recommended in liver complaint, jaundice, diarrhea, intermittent fevers, and a debilitated state of the system. . .A strong decoction of the Black Alder bark is an excellent application to foul and gangrenous ulcers, and when thickened with a little powdered elm bark, is a good poultice in such cases. . .The dose of the decoction. . .is about a wineglassful three or four times a day."

1869 Porcher 428. Leaves are substituted for tea. [Sturtevant 1919: *I. verticillata.*]

1892 Millspaugh 106. "Our only other proven species in this order is the South American Mate or (*Ilex Paraquayensis*) the leaves of which are used like Chinese tea and are considered slightly nervine, diaphoretic, and diuretic. . .The Black Alder. . .is another of the growing list of plants handed down to us by the aborigines, who used the bark internally and externally as a tonic, astringent, and antiseptic, and is probably as well-known to domestic practice as any indigenous shrub. The berries are purgative and vermifuge, forming one of the pleasantest adjuvants in children's remedies, for the expulsion of lumbrici [worms]. Schoepf first noted the plant as having the above field of utility and also mentioned its usefulness in anascarca. The bark is officinal in the U.S. Ph. [arm.]"

1905 Muldrew Muskoka Ont. 42. "The birds avail themselves of the berries when better fare is denied them by the snow, and it is credited with giving its peculiarly unpleasant flavour to the flesh of grouse in December."

1925 Wood & Ruddock. "*I. verticillata*. A decoction of the bark of the root and stalk sucessfully used in jaundice, liver and intermittent fever."

1923 H. Smith MENOMINI 22. "Winterberry, *Nemopanthus*. . .So far as my informant knew these berries were considered poisonous to human beings, though he said that bears eat them. He thought if they were used by the Menomini, it was for some evil purpose."

1932 H. Smith OJIBWE 355. "*Nemopanthus*. . .the berries are used as medicine, but the writer was unable to discover for what disease or how used. . .*Ilex verticillata*. The bark of this native holly is medicine among the Flambeau Ojibwe, but the use could not be discovered, other than that it might be used for diarrhea."

1933 H. Smith POTAWATOMI 39. "*Nemopanthus* is the species the Forest Potawatomi use. Small branches of the Mountain Holly are cooked. The resulting liquid is again boiled until it resembles a syrup and this syrup is used as a tonic. Mrs. Spoon named this species as one of the fifty she used to combine and boil down as a syrup which became a sort of 'shot-gun prescription' for many different kinds of diseases. She did not enumerate all of the fifty kinds that went into the medicine but they must have been varied enough to cure almost any ill to which the human flesh is heir. Among the whites, the uses of Mountain Holly are divided into two classes; the bark of the shrub is tonic, bitter, alterative, febrifuge and astringent. The fruit is used as a cathartic and a vermifuge. . .95. While these berries are edible, they are quite bitter and not relished by the white man, but the Forest Potawatomi claim that they keep the berries for a food."

1955 Mockle Quebec transl. 56. "*Ilex verticillata* bark and leaves astringent and febrifuge; fruits emetic, purgative and vermifuge.".

1970 Bye IROQUOIS mss. *Ilex verticillata* bark used as an astringent, tonic, and antiseptic. The leaves as a tea substutute.

SWEET GALE   *Myrica gale* L. Myricaceae

A deciduous shrub to 1.5 m in height with many branches. The resin dotted, fragrant, stalkless leaves are 3-6 cm long, smooth or finely hairy on both sides, their blunt ends sometimes with a few teeth. Some shrubs bear fruiting catkins, others only male catkins which are 1-2 cm long, appearing before the leaves, looking at a distance of an orange-red color. The female fruiting catkins are 10-12 mm long, the fruit is a series of nutlets in the shape of an elongated cone that is sticky and aromatic to touch or taste.

Range. Circumboreal, in Am., s. to L.I., Pa., N.C., Mich., Minn. and Wash. along the shores of lakes and streams, swamps, April-May.

Common names. Dutch or Burton myrtle or gale, scotch gale, bay-bush, sweet willow.

BAYBERRY   *Myrica pensylvanica* Loisel.

A deciduous shrub 0.5-2 m high with 4-8 x 1.5-3 cm leaves that are smooth above, often finely hairy beneath with a few teeth at their blunt ends. The male catkins 6-15 mm, the female 5-10 mm, their fruits few or only one nutlet thickly covered with wax, giving them a bluish-white color.

Range. e. Que. to La., also on the shores of Lake Erie and at a few isolated places inland. April-May on dry hills and shores.

1475 Bjornsson Icelandic mss Larsen transl. 92. "Myrtus is called sweet gale, cold in the first degree, dry in the second. Its fragrance counteracts shooting-pains in the head. Sweet gale crushed dries boils. The juice of sweet gale dries matter in the ears and kills their worms. Small sweet gale is good for flux of blood and other purgation. Green sweet gale crushed with vinegar stops nosebleed if applied to the flesh; (better the head) oil of sweet gale gives the hair strength to grow more. . .S17. Item for headache, take sweet gale green, crushed well and mixed with sour wine, and wash the head therein."

1748 Kalm Philadelphia Oct. 13th. 101-3. "Bayberries. There is a plant here from whose berries the settlers make a kind of wax. . .From the wax. . .they likewise make a soap here, which has an agreeable scent, and is the best for shaving. This wax is also used by doctors and surgeons who reckon it exceedingly good for plaster upon wounds. . .An old Swede mentioned that the root. . .was formerly used by the Indian as a remedy against toothache. . .Another Swede assured me that he had been cured of the toothache by applying the peel of the root to it.

1749 Cape aux Oyes 1st. Sept. Gale or sweet willow (*Myrica gale* L.) is likewise abundant here. The French call it *laurier*, and some *poivrier* [pepper]. They put the leaves into their broth to give it a pleasant taste. . . .Quebec Sept. 7th. 496. The women dye their woolen yarn yellow with seeds of gale. . .26th. Sept. 549-50 The Hereditary Princess. . .gave me instructions. . .[to bring to Sweden]. . .'The seeds that we wish you to bring in great quantities are seed of. . .myrtle from which candles are made, bayberry'."[*Myrica cerifera* southern shrub]

1791 Lewis ed. Aitkin Mat. Med. 123. "The leaves are said to be used by the common people [in England] for destroying moths, and cutaneous insects, being accounted an enemy to insects of every kind; internally in infusions, as stomachic and vermifuge, and as a substitute for hops for preserving malt liquors, which they render more inebriating and of consequence less salubrious." [*M. gale*].

1778 Carver 509. "The Myrtle [*M. pensylvanica*] is a shrub about four or five feet high. . .It bears small berries, which are generally called Bay Berries and these are full of a gluey substance, which being boiled in water, swims on the surface of it, and becomes a kind of green-wax, this is not so valuable as bees-wax being of a more brittle nature, but mixed with it [it] makes a good candle, which as it burns sends forth an agreeable scent."

1830 Rafinesque 244. "Myrica. . .All the sp. equiv. Valuable evergreen shrubs. Leaves fragrant, balsamic, containing like the bark tannin, resin, gallic acid and mucilage. Useful in uterine hemorrhages, hysterical complaints, palsies, cholics and scrofula in powders, decoction and tea. The tea of *M. gale* milder, formerly drank in Europe as tea, and leaves put in soups, used in Russia for gout, fevers, itch and insects. The bark chewed is a good sialagogue, made into a snuff it is a powerful errhine: taste acrid, stimulant, in large doses of a drachm it produces a burning sensation and vomiting, sometimes diuresis. Bark of the root used for the tooth ache. The inner bark pounded soft dispels scrofulous swellings and sores, a strong tea of the leaves being drank also. A tincture of the berries with *Heracleum* [Cow parsnip] is used for violent flatulent cholics and cramps. The buds dye yellow. The berries [*Myrica cerifera*] are covered with a peculiar wax, easily extracted by boiling, cooling and purifying, they give 32 per cent of wax, fragrant, greenish, and brittle, used for beautiful fragrant candles, soap, blacking balls, plasters. It contains cerine, Myricine, insoluble in alcohol, and a peculiar oil. It is actively medical, astringent, vulnerary, anodyne, subnarcotic. Dr. Fahnestock announced in 1822, that it is a specific for typhoid dysentery; this valuable property has been confirmed, I have verified it myself in diarrhoea, others in cholera morbus. . .It is used in powder, pills, or lozenges, made with sugar and mucilage."

1859-61 Gunn 739. "Bayberry (*Myrica cerifera*) This shrub is frequently called Candleberry, and Wax Myrtle. It grows from New England to Louisiana. . .[Here *M. pensylvanica* is obviously included]. . .in Massachusets, where it is very abundant. . .I consider this plant to be one of the most valuable of this, or any other country. . .The root should be collected early in the Spring, or late in the Fall, freed from dirt, then beat with a mallet or club to separate the bark. This bark should be perfectly dried without exposure to the wet or damp. . .generally found in drug-stores in the form of a fine powder. . .a sovereign remedy for scrofula, applied in the form of a poultice, by bruising the bark, simmering it in rain-water, and applying the poultice to the ulcers, and injecting a strong decoction into the ulcer or little crevice. . .The tea is useful as a wash in all old sores. In the Eastern States it is used as a remedy in scarlet fever with great success, also as a gargle in putrid or ulcerated sore throat. . .When taken in very large doses, it produces a narcotic effect. . .When the stomach is very foul, it may act as an emetic. It is valuable as a remedy in diarrhoea, dysentery, etc. on account of its astringent properties. A decoction administered in the dose of a teacupful about three times a day, generally effects a cure. The dose is a table-spoonful of the powdered bark steeped in a teacupful of boiling water, and sweetened to taste. The Bay Berry is one of the principal ingredients in the celebrated Thomsonian Composition Powders."

1892 Millspaugh 160. "Sweet gale, whose berries in infusion are said to be an efficient remedy for itch, and a vermifuge; the leaves are said to be substituted for hops in Sweden in the manufacture of beer."

1932 H. Smith OJIBWE 425. "Sweet Gale, in the fall of the year, the tips of the branches grow into an abortive scale or gall-like structure that is plucked and boiled to yield a brown dye stuff. The Flambeau Ojibwe seem to be the only Ojibwe that know this."

1933 H. Smith POTAWATOMI 65. "Sweet Gale. The Forest Potawatomi have no medicinal use for this plant to our knowledge. . . .121. Used to line the blueberry pail. . .It was also thrown on the fire to make a smudge to keep the mosquitoes away."

1935 Jenness Parry Island OJIBWA Lake Huron 114. "Yellow dye from the boiled seeds of *Myrica gale*."

1955 Mockle Quebec transl. 33. "Piment royal, bois-sent-tous-bon. Astringent, balsamic and expectorant. The fresh leaves contain 0.50% of a stupifying essence, a drastic resin and myricitrin."

1974 Lawrence & Weaver 385. "The fresh leaves of *Myrica gale*. . .were obtained from a wet bog near Barry's Bay, Ontario, Canada. . .In each case the oil was obtained by steam distillation of the dried leaves. . .Found to contain 41 compounds. . .Showed some marked differences to the previously published results, particularly the presence of selin-11-en-4-ol(14.6%) and alpha bisabolol (5%)."

1977 Evans & Barber Science 197; 338. "There is a need to develop rhizobial strains with capabilities to colonize and infect legume roots and to fix nitrogen in soils with appreciable contents of fixed nitrogen. . .Enormous areas in the country are used for the production of forest trees. . .In these areas nitrogen is fixed by blue-green algae associated with lichens, liverworts, and mosses and by symbiotic associations between endophytes and woody species such as *Alnus*. . .*Myrica*. . .If the biology of some of these systems were better understood, the endophytes of the non-leguminous symbionts could be cultured and inocula prepared and used to increase nodulation and nitrogen fixation."

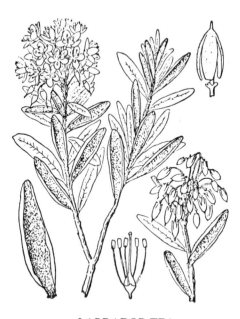

LABRADOR TEA

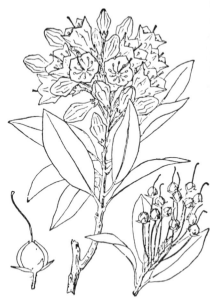

MOUNTAIN LAUREL

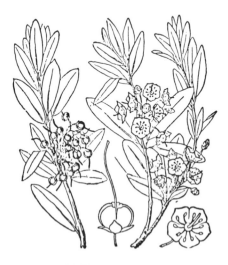

SHEEP LAUREL

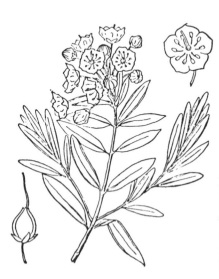

SWAMP LAUREL

LABRADOR TEA   *Ledum groenlandicum* Oeder Ericaceae (*L. latifolium*)
A shrub to 1 m tall with woody stems covered with reddish hairs. Alternate, stalkless, evergreen, leathery leaves 2-5 cm long, dark green on the upper side whose edges roll over the underside. This is covered with browny reddish wool like a thick felt. The newest shoots may not have this fur yet. The white flowers are at the end of the stems and are 1 cm wide. The fruit is slender and egg shaped, 5-7 mm and hairy.
Range. Greenl. to Alas., s. to n. N.J. and Pa., Mich., Wis. and Minn. June-July in acid bogs and wet shores. *L. Palustre* an arctic plant with shorter leaves.
1743 Isham Hudson Bay 134. "Plants of Physicky Herb's. Several are growing in these parts one of Which they styl (wishakapucka) which is us'd as a perge or fomentation, but the English in these parts makes a Drink of itt, going by the Name of wishakapucka tea, being of a fine flavour, and Reckon'd Very wholesome,—I was troubled Very much my Self with a Nervious Disorder, but by Constant Drinking 1 pint made strong for three months Entirely cur'd me. . .217. [1749] And here I can but Observe that the plant Wizzakapuckka, intirely cur'd me, being Very much Efflicted with a Nervious Disorder, when I went into that country Last, and have Known a person since my arrival in England, Which was troubled with a giddiness in his head, and Subject to fainting fitts by using this plant made strong, twice a Day, has found a Great Deal of Benefitt by itt. But as to the Indians using itt I must conterdict the Author [Henry Ellis], for to my certain Knowledge, their is none of the Indians usd. it in any shape; so fair from using itt I have offer'd some to them when have Refus'd itt with a Great Dislike;Shaggamittee also they do not use when they are indispose'd, any more then at another time, being as common a Drink to them as small Beer is to us &c." [Isham seems to imply that the Indians used labrador tea as a purge, so they would not want to drink it with him, or used it as a fomentation.]
1812 Rush Diary Dec. 15th. 303. Records that Francois André Michaux, who had just returned from a trip to northern parts of Quebec told him that labrador tea was a popular beverage among the Indians of that region, but not the French, who from their diet of salt meat, suffered from scorbutic complaints. (Vogel 1963; 65.)
1821 Franklin Journey 43. "Not being able to find any tripe de roche, we drank an infusion of the Labrador tea plant (*Ledum palustre*) and ate a few morsels of burnt leather for supper. . .363. Since our departure from Point Lake we had boiled the Indian tea plant. . .which produced a beverage in smell much resembling rhubarb."
1828 McGregor Maritime Colonies 23. "The Indian tea or Labrador shrub, is grateful to the taste and considered an effectual antiscorbutic."
1830 Rafinesque 236. "Contains 20 chemical substances, even wax and osmazome, very near to Chinese tea, but stronger, owing to fragrant resin. Leaves bitterish nidorose [reeking] cephalic, pectoral, exanthemic, &c. Useful in coughs, exanthema, itch, scabies, leprosy &c. In strong decoction kills lice and insects. Said to be narcotic and phantastic by Schoepf."
1857 Report from the Select Committee. . .Westminster, England 373. "It was formerly imported into this country by the Hudson's Bay Company under the name of Weesukapuka."
1874 Can. Pharm. J. 68. "A new insecticide to replace pyrethrum '*Ledum palustre*' said to destroy fleas, bed bugs, lice, beetles and their larvae and many other insects. An alchoholic tincture of the plant to which a little glycerine is added is said to drive away mosquitoes from any surface to which it has been applied. It is also said to be a remedy for mosquitoe bites. The fresh plant is best for all these purposes but the dry is also effective. Try the powder of the plants for the potato beetle."
1884 Holmes-Haydon 'CREE Hudson Bay 303. "Karkar-pukwa or Country Tea (*Ledum latifolium* L.). The fresh leaves are chewed and applied to wounds. The flowering tops are used as tea and should be gathered when in full bloom. The dried flowers have an odour between that of tansy and chamomile. . .By homoeopaths it is used as a remedy for tender feet, especially when associated with rheumatism, and the tincture is highly esteemed for relieving the pain of the sting of insects."
1887 Journal of the Senate of Canada 166. "The Labrador or country tea. . .was used very extensively in the country before our entrance into Confederation. In the hay and harvest fields it was considered by many of the old settlers of the Red River colony to be superior to any other beverage in allaying thirst. I know of homes in this country where this tea is still used."
1888 Delamare Island of Miquelon transl. 25. "An infusion of the leaves is used in Saint-Pierre and Miquelon to replace tea and in Canada it is used to put a head on small beers."

1892 Millspaugh 100. "Marsh Tea used in dysentery, diarrhoea, tertian ague, and in some places to render beer heady, though it is said to bring on delerium."

1915 Speck MONTAGNAIS 313. "The leaves and twigs of Labrador Tea are steeped and drunk to purify the blood and taken in case of chills."

1915 Speck MICMAC-MONTAGNAIS Newfoundland 316. "The leaves are steeped to make a tea which has a beneficial effect on the system. It is the common native beverage. . .317. The leaves in a decoction drunk as a tea as a diuretic."

1926-27 Densmore CHIPPEWA 317. "It is interesting to note that the Chippewa did not commonly drink water encountered in travelling but boiled it, making some of the following beverages from vegetable substances that were easily available. Fresh leaves were tied in a packet with a thin strip of basswood bark before being put in the water. Dried leaves could be used if fresh leaves were not available. The quantity was usually about a heaping handful to a quart of water. Beverages were usually sweetened with maple sugar and drunk while hot. . .Leaves of Labrador tea. . .354. The roots of Labrador tea and wild cherry dried, powdered and mixed but not cooked. Applied to a severe burn or ulcer or any condition in which the flesh is exposed. After this powder has been on the flesh for a time it becomes damp. It is then removed, the sore washed, and a fresh application made."

1930 Grieve England 460. "Of infusion, 2 to 4 fluid ounces three to four times a day. Overdoses may cause violent headache and symptoms of intoxication."

1932 H. Smith OJIBWE 401. "The Flambeau Ojibwe used the tender leaves of this plant as a beverage tea, and will even eat the leaves in the tea. It is well known tea to many northern and Canadian Indians."

1933 H. Smith POTAWATOMI 57. "Wesawabaguk meaning yellow leaf. Mrs. Spoon used the leaves in one of her medicinal combinations, but did not say what ailment it was intended to correct [see Mockle below]. . .The U.S. Nat. Dispensatory [1916] records that the leaves in full doses cause headache, vertigo, restlessness and a peculiar delirium. The infusion of the leaves augments a secretion of saliva, of perspiration, urine, and dilates the pupil of the eye. It is a remedy rarely employed now except in cases of chronic bronchitis. A decoction of the leaves has been used as a vermin exterminator, while fresh twigs have been placed among woollen clothes to keep moths from them. . .99. The Forest Potatwatomi use the leaves of Labrador tea to make a beverage. . .120. Also as a brown dye material."

1935 Jenness Parry Island OJIBWA Lake Huron 114. "When tobaco was scarce the Indians substituted labrador tea."

1945 Rousseau Quebec transl. 96. "Used to dye wool brown, known generally throughout the Province as Labrador tea, rarely as wooly tea."

1955 Mockle Quebec transl. 71. "The tea of the leaves is digestive and pectoral. The pulverised leaves are taken for a headache. The Indian women make a decoction which they take three times a day when delivery is near. The leaves contain 3% tannins, arbutoside and ursolic acid."

MOUNTAIN LAUREL   *Kalmia latifolia* L. Ericaceae
Shrub or small tree often 2-3 m forming dense thickets on sandy or rocky acid soil. The evergreen, alternate 5-10 cm leaves are on stalks 1-2 cm long, smooth and green on both sides. The flowers in clusters at the ends of the stems, white to rose with purple markings, 2-2.5 cm wide.
Range. N.B. to s. Ont. and s. Ind., s. on the coastal plain and in the mts. to Fla. and La. May-July. The wood very hard and brown with a weight of 44 lbs per cu. ft.
Common names. Clamoun, ivy bush, wood or small laurel, spoon wood.

SHEEP LAUREL   *Kalmia angustifolia* L.
This shrub has a woody stem up to 1 m tall. The leaves are mostly opposite, evergreen, leathery, stalked, dark green on top, light green beneath, 3-5 cm long, half as wide. The flowers, on hairy 2 cm long stalks, grow from the stem below the top. There will be leaves on the stem above the flowers. These are purple or crimson, see illustration for their shape and the seed pod that follows them. These are divided into five segments with a fine thread sticking out from their tops.
Range. Nfld. and Lab. to Hudson's Bay, s. to Va., Pa., and Mich. In dry acid soils.
Common names. Lambkill, wicky, spoon wood, dwarf laurel, sheep poison.

SWAMP LAUREL   *Kalmia polifolia* Wang.

A sparingly branched shrub to 1 m tall with sharply two edged twigs. The evergreen leaves are opposite, practically stalkless, 1-3.5 cm long, dark green and leathery above, whitened beneath with very fine hairs. The rose purple, 10-16 mm wide flowers are at the end of the stem.

Range. Lab. to Alas., s. sparingly to Conn., Pa., Mich., Minn. and Calif. May to June in sphagnum bogs.

1748 Kalm 335. "The leaves are poison to some animals and food for others. . .Form the winter food for stags, and if killed during the time of feeding and the entrails given to dogs to eat, they become quite stupid, and, as it were intoxicated, and often fall so sick that they seem to be at the point of death, but the people who have eaten the venison have not felt the least inconvenience."

1778 Carver 507. "The spoon wood is a species of the laurel, and the wood when sawed resembles box wood."

1779 Zeisberger DELAWARE 153. "Laurel, also called wild box, grows along river banks, or in swamps in cool places or on the north side of mountains. It grows so thickly that it is impossible to get through it. In swamps of laurel, bears like to make their winter quarters. The wood is fine and hard. The Indians make spoons of it. The main stem does not become thicker than a leg. The leaves are green summer and winter." [*K. latifolia*]

1810 Barton "Nearly allied to the Rhododendron is the genus *Kalmia*. Of this we have several species and all of them are poisons. The *Kalmia Latifolia*, or broad leaved laurel is best known to us. It kills sheep and other animals. Our Indians sometimes use a decoction of it to destroy themselves."

1830 Rafinesque 17. "A beautiful genus of evergreen shrubs peculiar to north America, dedicated to Kalm, a Swedish traveller and botanist. . .It has been by many deemed poisonous to men and cattle. It is certainly deleterious to horses, calves, and sheep feeding on it in the winter. . .Sheep if not soon relieved by oil, will swell and die. Yet deer and goats feed on the leaves, and can digest them. . .The wood is soft when fresh, but becomes hard and dense, nearly similar to box, much used for tools, instruments, and spoons. The Kalmias grow very slowly, and live a century or more. All the species of this genus having equal properties. . .Narcotic, errhine, antisyphilitic, antiherpetic. &c. Rather dangerous internally, if it be true that the Indians kill themselves by a strong decoction of it. More useful externally; powdered leaves employed in tinea capitis, and in some fevers; with lard, they form a good ointment for herpes. . .Thomas asserts its narcotic qualities, and that the decoction even in small doses produced vertigo. . .Elliot states that the negroes of Carolina use it. . .in a strong wash to cure the itch of men and dogs; it smarts but it cures effectually. It has been used in psora and other cutaneous affections. It is stated to have been used in syphilis, but how is not told, probably in sores and ulcers. The brown powder of the leaves and seeds are errhine. Their tincture is powerful and dangerous; a few drops killed a rattlesnake."

1840 Gosse Quebec 300. "Resembling the small woods of Newfoundland, on the borders of the large marshes, I found also the same plants that inhabit such situations in that country. . .Sheep laurel (*Kalmia Angustifolia*), Swamp Laurel (*Kalmia glauca*) there called Gould."

1859-61 Gunn 816. "*Kalmia latifolia*. . .known as Poison Laurel, being indeed a narcotic poison. . .When used for medicine, must of course be used with caution. . .The leaves are the part used. In large doses or overdoses, like most of the vegetable narcotics; it produces headache, vertigo, loss of sight, depressed action of the heart, general weakness, cold extremities and the like. In medicinal doses, it is a powerful sedative, and a valuable alterative, used mainly as an alterative in syphilis, and as a sedative in enlargement and over-action of the heart, and in inflammatory diseases. It has also been found very useful in hemorrhages, and in dysentery. As a remedy for that wretched disease, syphilis, it is regarded by some as among the best and most efficient. It must however, in all cases be used with prudence and caution, and should any of its dangerous symptoms appear, must be at once discontinued, or the dose lessened. It is generally used in the form of a strong or saturated tincture, which may be made by bruising the leaves if fresh, or if dry, crumbling them up, and covering them with dilute alcohol or good spirits and let stand one or two weeks. The dose will then be ten to twenty drops three or four times a day, beginning with ten, and increasing a drop or two a day, up to twenty; and carefully watching all the symptoms. This in the case of syphilis, diseases of the heart, and where it is necessary to continue the medicine for some days. . .The leaves stewed in lard make an excellent ointment for scald head, and that tormenting complaint the itch."

1868 Can. Pharm. J. 6;83-5. Sheep Laurel, *Kalmia Latifolia*; Leaves included in list of Can. medicinal plants.

1884 Holmes-Haydon CREE Hudson Bay 303. "We-suk-a-pup (*Kalmia angustifolia*) Bitter Tea.—The twigs with leaves and flowers are used in bowel complaints and as a tonic. A small handful is boiled in two pints of water, and a teaspoonful taken occasionally. A nearly allied species, *K. latifolia* is said to have cured an obstinate case of diarrhoea. In this instance an ounce of the leaves was boiled in eight ounces of water down to four ounces, and thirty drops of the decoction were given four times a day. When given six times a day this quantity caused vertigo. A case of poisoning from the use of *Kalmia latifolia* is on record, in which glowing heat in the head, loss of sight, coldness of extremities, were followed by nausea and vomiting (Edinburgh Med. Journ, 1856, 1014). . .Great prostration of the circulation. . .It is pointed out in the United States Dispensatory (p. 1678) that *K. angustifolia* most likely possesses similar properties. It is remarkable. . .that it should be used as a tonic by the Cree Indians. The coldness of the climate may. . .modify the development of the poisonous principle and species closely allied to a poisonous one are not always poisonous."

1888 Delamare Island of Miquelon transl. 24. "This plant is toxic for ruminants; it will be toxic for man according to Dr. Gras, who during his stay on Miquelon observed a case of poisoning due to the drinking an infusion of this plant." [*Kalmia angustifolia*]

1892 Millspaugh 103. "The previous uses of this plant *K. latifolia*, in medicine were of a very limited character. A decoction was used in domestic practice for. . .secondary syphilis. It has been recommended in inflammatory fevers as a cardiac depressor; its astringency was ultilized also by the application of the drug in diarrhoeas and hemorrhages of the bowels. Kalmia is not official in the U.S. Ph. [arm]. . .Laurel leaves have always been deemed poisonous, especially by the Indians and the laity. Dr. Bigelow states. . .that it is common belief that the flesh of the Partridge, after feeding upon the leaves and fruits, becomes itself poisonous. . .The flesh of the bird impairs the functions of the brain and acts directly as a sedative poison. . .The symptoms. . .are: Vertigo and headache; almost complete loss of sight. . .thirst, nausea and vomiting. . .great palpitation and fluttering of the heart. . .great prostration. . .*K. angustifolia* seems. . .to be the most poisonous species."

1915 Speck PENOBSCOT 311. "Several more elaborate cures are as follows: Lambkill (*Kalmia angustifolia*), cedar bark, and salt used to be pounded together and made into a poultice. A specimen poultice obtained was put up in a small birch-bark cup. By means of a scratching instrument scars were cut into the skin directly over the part affected with pain and the poultice smeared over and rubbed in. This was a nostrum used in olden times for all kinds of trouble." [See Potentilla]

1915 Speck MONTAGNAIS 314. "The leaves of sheep laurel (*Kalmia angustifolia*), bitter flower powder, are known for their poisonous properties. A very small quantity is steeped and drunk for colds and backache. This was so strong that they say 'it runs through the whole body.'"

1915 Speck MICMAC-MONTAGNAIS Nfld. 316. "Sheep laurel is known to be very poisonous. A poultice is made of the crushed leaves and bound to the head to cure headache over night. As a non-specific remedy a small dose, not more than a spoonful, of tea made with a few leaves is considered valuable." Cartwright, in the early part of the last century obtained a list from the same people. . .*Kalmia angustifolia*, the leaves in a hot water infusion drank for stomach complaints. . .very poisonous if strong."

1920 Fyles 78. "*Kalmia latifolia* L. all parts of the plant except the wood contain the very poisonous constituent andromedotoxin. . .Cases of human poisoning have been known from eating the honey from the flowers, or chewing the leaves in mistake for wintergreen. . .*Kalmia angustifolia*. . .Of an intensive poisonous nature similar to the mountain laurel. No doubt other species of Kalmia, including the pale or swamp laurel (*Kalmia polifolia* Wang) are equally injurious."

1955 Mockle Quebec transl. 71. "*Kalmia angustifolia*. The plant is given in decoction or lotion for ulceration. There is found in the leaves a glucoside, arbutoside and a toxine andromedotoxin. *Kalmia latifolia*. The leaves are used for falling hair and mange and as well for syphilis. They also contain arbutoside and andromedotoxin and as well asebotoside, identical, according to some authors with phloridzoside."

WET OPEN PLACES

seasonally wet meadows, lake and stream banks, swamps and acid bogs, or all moist open places. This section starts with plants that float in the water, moves to those that like water on their roots and then to those at the water's edge. Also found in wet open places but discussed under other sections are St. John's wort, raspberries, cleavers, violets, may apples, pepper grass, goldenrods and stinging nettles

WET OPEN PLACES

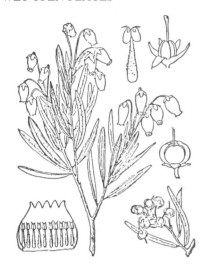

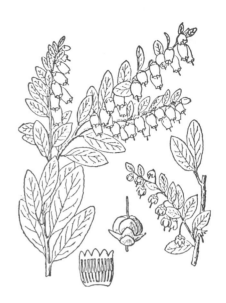

BOG ROSEMARY   LEATHERLEAF

BOG ROSEMARY   *Andromeda glaucophylla* Link. Ericacea (*A. polifolia*)
A shrub up to 50 cm tall with leathery, narrow, blue green leaves, 3-5 cm long, their edges rolled in over their undersides which are covered with a fine white wool, consisting of erect hairs. The flowers are lilac bells that hang down. Their fruit is 5-6 mm thick and has a tip sticking straight up that is as long as it is thick.
Range. Nfld. Lab., to Sask., s. to N.J., W.Va., n. Ind., and Minn. in acid bogs, floating sphagnum. May-June.
1888 Delamare Island of Miquelon transl. 24. "A narcotic-acrid plant poisonous to sheep according to Provencher (?)."
1892 Millspaugh 100. "The leaves of the European and North American *Andromeda polifolia* are an acrid and dangerous narcotic and are said to kill sheep if browsed upon."
1923 H. Smith MENOMINI 35. "Not used."
1932 H. Smith OJIBWE 400. "Bog Rosemary (*Andromeda glaucophylla*). Young tender leaves and tips of this plant are used by the Flambeau Ojibwe to boil for a beverage tea. While they often pick and use it fresh on the hunting trail, they also gather and dry it for later use. It is not a bad substitute for 'store tea'."
1955 Mockle Quebec transl. 69. "The plant is narcotic-acrid and poisonous with the toxicity due to andromedotoxin."

LEATHERLEAF   *Chamaedaphne calyculata* (L.) Moench Ericaceae
A stiff erect shrub to 1.5 m with many branches. The stiff, evergreen, leathery leaves are 1.5-5 cm long with stalks 1-3 mm long, and with barely visible teeth. The spray of tiny white bells at the end of the twigs is beautiful. Their buds form the year before and should be looked for. Brown seed capsule, no berries.
Range. Circumboreal, s. to N.J., O., n. Ind., n. Ill. and in the mts. to N.C. April and June in bogs and around the edges of swamps, often in masses.
Common name. Cassandra.
1923 H. Smith MENOMINI 35. "This is not used so far as is known by the Menomini."
1923 H. Smith OJIBWE 400. "This is another beverage tea highly prized by the Flambeau Ojibwe. The Pillager Ojibwe also use it in the same manner."

1933 H. Smith POTAWATOMI 56. "Gather the leaves to make an infusion to be used in the treatment of fevers. The leaves themselves as a poultice are used to treat inflammation. We have no record of use by Whites."

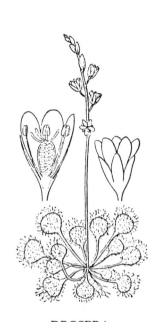

DROSERA

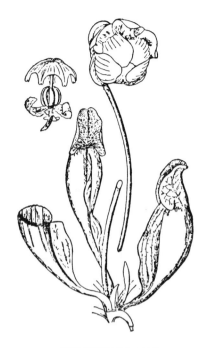

PITCHER PLANT

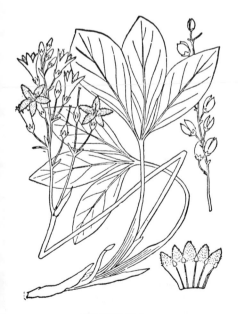

BOGBEAN

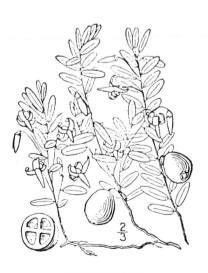

CRANBERRY

ROUND LEAVED SUNDEW   *Drosera rotundifolia* L. Droseraceae
This tiny plant grows in acid bogs and in sand by the edge of serpentines. The round leaves form a rosette spread out on 1-1.5 cm long stems, they are only 4-10 mm long, shorter than their stems. They are covered with red erect hairs. These have globs of sticky 'dew' on their ends. The flowering stem appears later, 7-35 cm tall with 3-15 white flowers. The seeds are like chaff. The plants stain paper purple.
Range. Circumboreal, in America s. to S.C., Ga., Tenn. and Calif.
Common names. Rosa solis, eyebright, youth wort, lustwort, red rot, moor grass.
All plants need nitrogen and usually obtain this through their roots in the form of soluble nitrates. Decayed plants, as a result of the work of nitrifying bacteria in the soil, supply these nitrates. These bacteria need oxygen to do their work. In sphagnum bogs where the sphagnum is floating on water, oxygen is rare. So plants growing there have to find some other method. Insectivorous plants have found a way around this problem. Drosera have glandular reddish hairs with a glob of sticky glistening fluid at their ends, all over the upper side of their leaves. The sparkle of this 'dew' in the sun attracts insects. The lightest touch on a hair is felt by the other hairs, these, aware of their prey, bend over the insect, gumming it fast and suffocating it by blocking its breathing pores. The glands in the hairs eject then an acid peptonizing ferment, which acting upon the proteins, dissolves all the soft parts of the insect's body. This fly broth is absorbed by the leaves and so nourishes the plant. Afterwards the tentacles expand, the indigestible parts blow away and the leaves manufacture and secrete more sticky fluid. (Perry 1972:102)
1633 Gerarde-Johnson 1557. "The leaves stamped with salt do raise blisters, to what part of the body soever they be applied. The later Physitions have thought this herbe to be a rare and singular remedie for all those that be in a consumption of the lungs, and especially the distilled water thereof. . .but the use thereof doth otherwise teach. . .bin observed, that they have sooner perished that used the distilled water hereof, than those that abated from it, and have followed the right and ordinarie course of diet. Cattell of the female kind are stirred up to lust by eating even a small quantity. . .because through his sharp and biting qualitie it stirrith up a desire to lust, which before was dulled, and as it were asleepe. It strengthens and nourisheth the body, especially if it be distilled with wine, and that liquour made thereof which the common people call Rosa Solis. If any be desirous to have the said drinke. . .let them lay the leaves of Rosa Solis in the spirit of wine, adding thereto Cinnamon, Cloves, Maces, Ginger, Nutmeg, Sugar, and a few grains of Muske, suffering it to stand in a glasse close stopt from the aire and set in the Sun by the space of ten daies, then straine the same and keep it for your use."
1830 Rafinesque 217. "Juice used to destroy warts and corns, with milk for freckles and sunburns; it makes milk solid, but sour like bonyclabber, liked in Sweden. Deemed pectoral in South America, a sirup used for asthma."
1888 Delamare Island of Miquelon transl. 15. "These are astringent, bitter, acidulous and even slightly caustic plants. The use in persistent cough is not known to the inhabitants [of the Island]."
1892 Millspaugh 29. "A fit summary of all this practice may be found in Hahnemann's observations. 'Drosera is one of the most powerful medicinal agents in our country. It was formerly used externally, but without success, in cutaneous affections, and it seems to have been taken with greater advantage internally'. . .Chemical constituents Alizarin. . .Drosera asserts altogether a peculiar action upon the lungs and, in fact, the whole respiratory tract, thus leading us to value it deservedly in pertussis, bronchial irritation and even phthisis, where in fact it gives many a patient a restful night, and more peaceful day when the disease is too far advanced for still greater benefit."
1894 Toronto House. Guide. 180. "How to use all kinds of Homeopathic remedies. . .For consumption or for whooping cough give drosera."
1930 Grieve England 782. "In America it has been advocated as a cure for old age; a vegetable extract is used together with colloidal silicates in cases of arterio sclerosis."
1955 Mockle Quebec transl. 50. "This plant is used in infusion or as a tincture for asthma, pulmonary catarrh, whooping cough and coughs. The juice of the leaves is used for pimples and corns. . .Other species used in the same way are *D. anglica, D. linearis,* and *D. longifolia.*"
The leaves and flowers are collected in the wild just as they begin to flower. Pinched off at ground level and spread to dry in a shady spot with good air circulation. In many places in the world it is a protected plant and very difficult to collect. The active principles are not precisely known. It is a diuretic and lowers the blood sugar level. It is used in herbal tea mixtures for stub-

born coughs, asthma and bronchitis and popular with older people with hardening of the arteries and hypertension (Stary & Jirasek 1973:122).

Drosera are endangered in Wisconsin and rare in Minnesota and Ontario. They should never be collected as there are many better remedies more easily available. Sphagnum bogs are damaged by being walked upon.

PITCHER PLANT *Sarracenia purpurea* L. Sarraceniaceae

This very odd plant grows in floating sphagnum bogs. The 10-20 cm tall, round, hollow leaves have a 1-5 cm wide thin wing down one side. The perfect hollow tube, which is the inside of the leaf, has downward pointing hairs all over it. Insects that fall in cannot climb out and decay at the bottom of the tube. The plant feeds on this decayed matter, see sundew. The top of this tubular leaf bends over to form a hood. The flowering stem is 30-50 cm tall with a 5-6 cm wide deep purple red, nodding, leather like flower. The whole plant is red in the fall.

Range. Lab., Nfld., N.B., P.E.I., N.S., Que., James Bay, Ont., Man., Athabaska, s. to Sask., Minn., n. Ill., Ohio and Del.

1633 Gerarde-Johnson 412. "Clusius in the end of his fourth book of Historia Plantarum, sets forth this, and saith, hee received this figure with one dryed leafe of the plant sent him from Paris from Claude Gonier an Apothecarie of that citie, who received it (as you see it here exprest) from Lisbone. Now Clusius describes the leafe that it was hard, and, as if it had been a piece of leather, open at the upper side, and distinguished with many large purple veines on the inside, &c. for the rest of his description was only taken from the figure (as he himselfe saith) which I hold impertinent to set downe, seeing I here give you that same figure, which by no means I could omit, for the strangenesse thereof, but hope that some or other that travell into forraine parts may finde this elegant plant, and know it by this small expression, and bring it home with them, that so we may come to a perfecter knowledge thereof."

[The statement by Gerarde that Clusius had received the dried leaf from Claude Gonier an apothecary in Paris, who had received it from Lisbon, is one piece of a jig saw puzzle that has intrigued historians of plant movements at the beginning of the seventeenth century. Bauhinus wrote in 1620 of some of the plants in Burser's Herbarium, now in Upsala, that they had been sent him by an apothecary in Paris, who had them from Peru, a Portuguese colony. Juel in 1931 considered this unlikely, as several were north American plants, he thought they probably came from Canada. Rousseau in 1964 considered them sent by Louis Hebert from Port Royal. Here is the name of a Paris apothecary receiving plants from Lisbon and sending them on to botanists in Europe. Perhaps this piece of pitcher plant came from Canada too].

1640 Curtis Botanical Magazine 849. John Tradescant found a pitcher plant in Virginia and brought a live specimen to England.

1700's Sarrazin, Quebec, where he was a physician used the pitcher plant in the treatment of smallpox. He gave a large wineglassful of the infusion of the root to bring out the spots. A second or third dose was given at intervals of four to six hours and caused the pustules to subside with an immediate improvement in the patient. Sarrazin said he had received this remedy from the Indians. Linnaeus named the pitcher plant after him.

Smallpox was unknown in America before the arrival of the white man and so the Indians had no immunity to it. When the germs arrived in a camp, most of the inhabitants died. Densmore tells of an old Sioux who said: "A medicine man usually treated one special disease, and treated it successfully. He did this in accordance with his dream. A medicine man would not try to dream of all the herbs and treat all diseases, for then he could not expect to succeed in all nor to fulfill properly the dream of any one herb or animal. He would depend on too many and fail in all. That is one reason why our medicine men lost their power when so many diseases came among us with the advent of the white man." [See a similar description under sweet flag.]

1640 Lalemont HURON Jes. Rel. 20; 27-31. "A spirit appeared to a man while fishing and said. . .I come to teach you both the reasons and remedies for your misfortune. It is the strangers who alone are the cause of it; they now travel two by two throughout the country, with the design of spreading the disease everywhere. . .this smallpox which now depopulates your houses. . .As for those who are now attacked by the smallpox, I wish you to serve me in curing them; prepare a quantity of such a water, run as fast as possible to the village, and tell the elders to carry and distribute this potion the whole night. . .Six of the elders then bore in silence a great kettle full of that water and made all the sick people drink it. . .the ceremony was repeated the next night." [An infusion of the root of the pitcher plant?]

1768 James Latham in Quebec introduced inoculation for smallpox to Canada.

1800 Dr. Macurdy St. John's Newfoundland received some of Jenner's vaccine from the Rev. John Clinch and vaccinated many people. Clinch by 1802 had vaccinated 700.

1812 Gazette, Kingston Ont. Letter which refers to a bill sent in by a doctor, with a deduction of £6 for 'killing your son'. This was because the doctor had carried the small pox to the son who died of it.

1861 Herbert Miles Quebec. Assistant Surgeon to the Royal Artillery, sent a plant to Dr. Hooker in London who identified it as *Sarracenia purpurea* [pitcher plant]. Mr. Miles wrote that an epidemic of smallpox had broken out among the Indians, the disease had proved virulent in the extreme among the unprotected, because unvaccinated, natives. However the alarm had greatly diminished on an old squaw going amongst them, and treating the cases with the infusion. This treatment it is said was so successful as to cure every case. . .The remedy is given in the form of a strong infusion of the root, which was why, after very considerable difficulty, having obtained a small supply of the plant, he had sent it to Dr. Hooker for identification." (Millspaugh)

1868 Can. Pharm. J. 6; 83-5. The root of the pitcher plant, *Sarracenia purpurea*, included in list of Can. medicinal plants.

1888 Delamare Island of Miquelon transl. 14. "Louvet, pharmacist to the French Navy made a study of *Sarracenia*. . .For our part [Dr. Delamare] the antivariolic [antismallpox] properties of the plant are somewhat less than demonstrated. As to the anti-rheumatic virtues attributed to it, we contest them until we have more ample information, our trials have not been happy and we have had to abandon this plant for salicylate acid or at least only use it as an adjunct."

1892 Millspaugh 19. [After quoting the account given above by Mr. Miles he mentions] "A resolution passed at a meeting of the Medical Society of Nova Scotia held at Halifax. . .the use of Sarracenia in Variola that there was not, any reliable data upon which to ground any opinion in favor of its value as a remedial agent. . .Millspaugh notes that:- "The previous use of this plant by the Indians in smallpox, for which it has been held by them as specific, is corroborated by homeopathic practice, but has in almost all instances been an absolute failure in the hands of the 'old school'. They [the Indians] judged that the use of the root not only greatly shortened the run of the disease and checked maturation, but prevented deep pitting in convalescence."

1915 Speck PENOBSCOT 310. "Pitcher plant is steeped and drunk for spitting up blood, and supposedly for kidney trouble. (Also a Malecite remedy.)". . .MONTAGNAIS 314. The leaves of pitcher plant (Virgin Mary's socks) are steeped for medicine for smallpox. . .MICMAC 316. A strong docoction of the root was drunk, a tablespoonful or tea spoonful frequently during the day with abstinence for several days, for spitting blood and other pulmonary complaints. . .The roots of the pitcher plant, which is very common in the barrens of Newfoundland, are steeped and the liquid is drunk for sore throat. The plant is locally called 'pipe' because the hollow leaf bowl is occasionally used as a makeshift pipe by the Indians."

1926-27 Densmore CHIPPEWA 379. "The leaves of the pitcher plant were called 'frog-leggings' and used as toys, or filled with ripe berries."

1923 H. Smith MENOMINI 52. "This plant is used in Menomini medicine, but data concerning its use was not available. My informant thought it was used by sorcerers."

1932 H. Smith OJIBWE 389. "Bearskin, Flambeau Ojibwe medicine man. . .said that the root is used to make a tea to help a woman accomplish parturition."

1933 H. Smith POTAWATOMI 82. "Mrs. Spoon uses the foliage of the Pitcher Plant to make a 'squaw' remedy, though she could not explain its particular use. . .123. The Forest Potawatomi say that the old time Indians used the leaves of this plant for a drinking cup when they were out in the woods or swamp."

1945 Rousseau MOHAWK transl. 43. "An infusion of the leaves of the pitcher plant and fragments of the entire plant of *Sparganium eurycarpum* (Bur reed) used for a chill."

1945 Raymond TETE DE BOULE transl. 131. "The root is diuretic; mixed with beaver castoreum it cures sickness of the urinary passages. . .At Manouan the dried leaves are found in every house and it is unquestionable that the plant contains an abundance of tannin. . .All the Indian tribes consider the pitcher plant as a stimulant and diuretic. They make a drink from it to hasten birth during delivery. The Indians also use the leaves as goblets when in the woods or swamps. The stylised plant is often seen on baskets."

1955 Mockle Quebec transl. 49. "This plant is considered a stimulant and diuretic and is utilised

in dysentery and smallpox. The Indians make a drink from it to hasten deliverance in child-birth."
1978 The World Health Organisation announced that smallpox had been almost eliminated in the world by the use of vaccination.

BOGBEAN
Menyanthes trifoliata L Gentianaceae

Found in floating sphagnum bogs with the pitcher plant and sundew, often growing in clumps as the roots run along just under the sphagnum. These roots are thick, scaly, sometimes very long, marked by scars of former leaf stalks. The stalks are 10-30 cm tall with three leaflets at the end, each 3-6 cm long or longer. The flowering stalk also 10-30 cm tall is crowded with flowers at its end. These are white or pinkish, 10-14 mm.

Range. Boreal N. Am. and Eurasia, s. to N.J., Va., O., and Mo. May-June.

Common names. Marsh or bean trefoil, buckbean, water shamrock, bitter worm, bog nut, moon flower, marsh clover.

1633 Gerarde-Johnson 1194. "The seed. . .saith Diorcorides, if it be taken with meade or honied water, is good against the cough and paine in the chest. It is also a remedy for those that have weak livers and spit bloud, for as Galen saith it cleanseth and cutteth tough humours, having also adjoined with it an astringent or binding quality."

1724 Anon ILLINOIS-MIAMI mss 224. "The root of bean trefoil, for looseness of the bowels or bloody flux. It is necessary to boil it and not drink anything else until there is a complete cure."

1791 Lewis ed. Aitkins. "They are sometimes, among the common people, fermented with malt liquors for an antiscorbutic diet drink. Their sensible operation is by promoting urine and some-what loosening the belly."

1799 Lewis Mat. Med. 256. "Inveterate cutaneous diseases have been removed by an infusion of the leaves, drunk to the quantity of a pint a day, at proper intervals, and continued some weeks. Dr. Cullen has had frequent experience of their good effects in some of these herpatic and seem-ingly cancerous kinds. Boerhaave relates that he was relieved of the gout by drinking the juice mixed with whey."

1817-20 Bigelow 58. "The root is undoubtedly entitled to a high place in the list of tonics. . .in small doses. . .it imparts vigour to the stomach and strengthens digestion. . . .Large doses. . .produce vomiting and purging and frequently powerful diaphoresis. . .has been employed with benefit in intermittent and remittent fevers. . .Its reputation in the north of Europe, particuarly in Germany, was at one time so high, that it was consumed in large quanti-ties, and deemed a sort of panacea. Its true character, however, is simply that of a powerful bitter tonic, like Gentian and Centaury."

1830 Rafinesque 35. "The whole plant is bitter, like gentian but the root is more intensly so."

1820's Mat. Med. Edinburgh-Toronto mss 24. "The following plants possessing bitterness in a greater or less degree were formerly used but are now discarded from Practice. . .*Menyanthes trifoliata*. . ."

1842 Christison 634. "The Bog-bean. . .has long been used in European medicine, but is now lit-tle employed in this country [England] except in domestic medicine. . .is tonic, stomachic and febrifuge. On account of these actions it is still given for dyspepsia in domestic practice; and when agues were frequent in Scotland, it was in common use as a febrifuge. . .Some physicians believe it is unjustly neglected at present."

1868 Can. Pharm. J. 6; 83-5. Leaves and root of the buckbean, *Menyanthes trifoliata* included in list of Can. medicinal plants.

1888 Delamare Island of Miquelon transl. 27. "This plant, tonic, febrifuge, emmenagogue, is not used [on the Island.]

1892 Millspaugh 129. "A peculiar property pervades the whole of this natural order (*Gentianaceae*). The species when fresh are all emetic and cathartic, and, when dry, tonic, stom-achic in varying degrees. . .As early as 1613 a Swedish writer, Johannes Franckenius, states that a decoction of the herb removes all visceral obstructions, acts as an emmenagogue and diuretic, kills intestinal worms, and is an efficacious remedy in scrofula. . .In Sweden the leaves are often used in brewing; two ounces of which are said to equal a pound of hops, for which they are substituted. . .neither dryness nor heat removes the bitterness of the roots."

1923 H. Smith MENOMINI 36. "This was given a name, though only one shared in common

with other water plants. The Buckbean is a medicinal plant of the Menomini, though my informant did not know its use". [was it as an emmenagogue?]
1955 Mockle Quebec transl. 75. "The leaves are used as a bitter tonic, febrifuge and laxative and also for rheumatism. They contain a glucoside, meliatoside."
An alkaloid strychnicine identical with maliatoside (meliatin) was isolated in 1910 by Bridel from *Menyanthes trifoliata* (T.E. Wallis 1967:207).
The leaves are collected in the wild during the time the plant is flowering and dried. The drug increases the flow of gastric secretions. It is used in herbal teas for the liver and gall bladder and to increase appetite. (Stary & Jirasek 1973:160).

CRANBERRY   *Vaccinium oxycoccos* L. Ericaceae

Lying flat on the edge of the sphagnum or in the middle of it are the slender, creeping stems of the small cranberry, rooting every now and then. The leaves are only 2-10 mm long, evergreen, dark green above, whitish beneath. The hairy flowering stalk 1-4 cm long, grows from among the leaves near the end of the branch. The flowers are pink and the 7-13 mm berry is round and pink.
Range. Circumboreal, s. to N.J., Pa., n. O., n. Ind. and Minn. May-July in bogs.

LARGE CRANBERRY   *Vaccinium macrocarpon* Ait. (*Oxycoccus m.*)

Very like the small cranberry except that the berries are red, oval and 1-2 cm.
Range. Nfld. to Man., s. to Va., O. and n. Ill., and locally in the mts. to N.C. and Tenn. June-Aug. in bogs.
1624 Sagard HURON 238. "Cranberries (toca) were put into little cakes or eaten raw."
1708 Sarrazin-Vaillant, Quebec-Paris, Boivin 1978 transl. 127. "Our savages call them *Atoca*. They make a conserve of them and esteem them for medicine for stomach problems." Note in hand of J.-F. Gaultier, "in Canada *atoca* or good fruit."
1743 Isham Hudson Bay CREE 155. "The Leg's and thigh's [of a caribou] they cure otherways, they cutting all the flesh of the bones and Cutt itt in slices, which to be dryd. . . .when dry'd they take and pound, or beat between two Stones, till some of itt is as small as Dust, which they styl (Ruhiggan) being Dryd. so much that their is Little moisture in itt;—when pounded they putt itt into a bag and will Keep for several Years, the Bones they also pound small and Boil them over a moderate fire to Reserve the fatt, which fatt is fine and as sweet as any Butter or fatt that is made,. . .Pimmegan as the Natives styles itt, is some of the Ruhiggan, fatt and Cranberries mixd. up togeather, and Reckon'd by some Very good food by the English as well as Natives."
1791 Long, Lake Superior 106. "The wind proving favourable, we proceeded to Cranberry Lake, so called from the great quantities of cranberries growing in the swamps. We stopped here two days to refresh ourselves after the great fatigue we had undergone in struggling against the rapids. . .arrived at Lake Schabeechevan. . .the swamps are full of wild rice and cranberries. . .On this lake there are about one hundred and fifty good hunters. . .this was one inducement for settling here which was increased by the prospect of a plentiful supply of fish, rice and cranberries, which are winter comforts of too great consequence to be slighted."
1830 Trans. Lit. & Hist. Soc. Que. 111; 99. "This pleasant fruit is yearly collected in the autumn, and brought to market under the Indian name of atoca, the proper French name of canneberge not being in use here."
1830 Rafinesque 49. "All the cranberries are very acid and somewhat acerb. yet become very palatable with sugar in the form of tarts, preserves, &c. They are cooling, slightly laxative, and form an excellent diet both in health and disease. The large cranberries, peculiar to America are the ones most usually gathered for our markets, and are even exported to Europe and the West Indies; keeping pretty well in barrels, and still better in bottles. . .Useful in fevers, diarrhoea, scurvy, dropsy, and many other diseases. Their acid is said to be the oxalic and malic. Cranberry tarts are one of the American table luxuries. Their juice mixed with sugar or alcohol keeps a long while, and forms a fine acidulous drink with water allaying thirst, and lessening the heat of the body. The berries last throughout the winter on the bushes."
1833 Howard Quebec 12. "Cancer to cure. Take cranberries, crush them well and apply them to the sore and it will soon be well."
1855 Trail. 81-2. "The Indians are the cranberry gatherers: they will trade them away for old clothes, pork or flour. The fruit is sometimes met with in stores; but it is of rare occurrence now:

formerly we used to procure them without difficulty. . .The cranberry will keep a long time just spread out upon the dry floor of a room, and can be used as required, or put into jars or barrels in cold water. . .The Indians attribute great medicinal virtues to the cranberry, either cooked or raw: in the uncooked state the berry is harsh and very astringent: they use it in dysentery, and also in applications as a poultice to wounds and inflammatory tumours, with great effect."

1857 Daniel Wilson 254. "The Indians accordingly make use of various herbs to mix with and dilute the tobacco, such as the leaf of the cranberry." [See bearberry]

1860 Kohl Lake Superior 321. "These ottakas do not require drying or preserving, for they keep through the whole winter in the Indian lodges."

1888 Delamare Island of Miquelon transl. 23. "The inhabitants make an excellent conserve with the berries which when raw are acidulous and antiscorbutic."

1892 Millsapugh 100. "Cranberries. . .refrigerant and a fine pallitative dressing for acute erysipelas."

1915 Speck MONTAGNAIS 316. "Cranberry branches are steeped as a medicine for pleurisy."

1916 Waugh IROQUOIS 128. Cranberries eaten.

1925 Wood & Ruddock, Japanese remedy; cranberries will end a case of piles, cook and eat a fruit dish full two or three times a day. . .cranberries are the best cure for recent erysipelas ever known if applied early. This dangerous malady yields at once. Pound berries and spread on old cotton and apply over entire diseased area and inflammation speedily subsides.

1926-27 Densmore CHIPPEWA 321. "Cranberry, cooked, probably eaten with sugar."

1923 H. Smith MENOMINI 65. "This is Menomini food that is sweetened with maple sugar and eaten the same way as the blueberry."

1932 H. Smith OJIBWE 369. "A tea for a person who is slightly ill with nausea. . .401. This is an important wild food. . .cranberry pie."

1933 H. Smith POTAWATOMI 58. "The Forest Potawatomi do not use the cranberry as a medicine, except insofar as they claim that all of their native foods are also at the same time medicines and will maintain health. . ."

1945 Raymond TETE DE BOULE transl. 134. "The atocas are eaten by the Indians fresh or boiled with sugar."

1955 Mockle Quebec transl. 72. "The berries are acidulous, refreshing, antiscorbutic, antibilious, diuretic and laxative. They are made into a conserve that is very appreciated. They contain an anthrocyanoside, oxycoccriyanine."

1975 Trevor Robinson 90. The complexity of these chemical compounds [in plants]. . .finding 41 component fragments [of a compound] in the cutin of cranberries. . .

1977 Globe & Mail Toronto Nov. 17th. F5. "Women can help protect themselves against UTIs, [Urinary tract infection]. . .find it helpful to drink cranberry juice daily (and several times a day when an infection is present or threatening)."

The cranberry shows experimental hypoglycemic activity. (Lewis and Elvin-Lewis 1977).

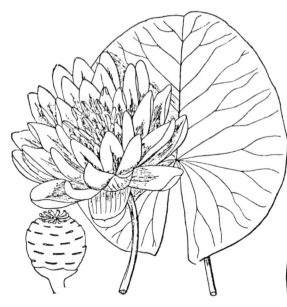

FRAGRANT WHITE WATER LILY

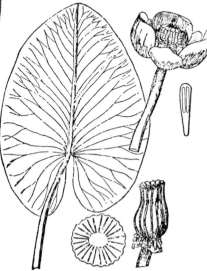

YELLOW WATER LILY

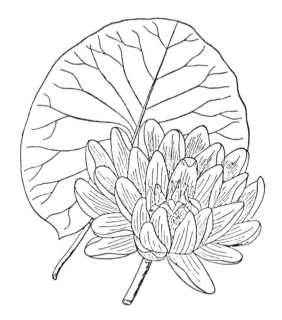

TUBEROUS WATER LILY

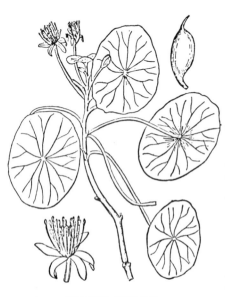

WATER SHIELD

YELLOW WATER LILY *Nuphar variegatum* Durand Nymphaeaceae (*N. advena, Nymphaea a.*)
Floating leaves 10-25 cm, two thirds as wide, submersed leaves few or none. The leaf stalks are
flattened on top and widen into wings. The yellow petals (sepals) are few and thick usually with a
reddish base. There is a 1 cm wide green disk in the centre.
Range. Lab. Nfld., P.E.I., N.S., N.B., Que. Hudson Bay, Ont., Man., Dist. Mackenzie, Yukon
B.C. s. to Del., n. O., Io., Kans. and Ida. in ponds in summer, inlets, lakes.
Common names. Beaver root, spatter-dock, bullhead-lily. *Nuphar luteum* of Europe is a closely
related plant.

FRAGRANT WHITE WATER LILY *Nymphaea odorata* Ait. Cas.
The leaves are 10-20 cm long and mostly not over 20 cm wide, commonly purple beneath, with a
plain stem without stripes. The fragrant white flowers open in the morning and close by 4 oclock.
Range.. Nfld., N.B., N.S., P.E.I., Que., Ont., n. shore Lake Superior, Man., s. to Fla. and Tex. in
quiet waters.

TUBEROUS WATER LILY *Nymphaea tuberosa* Paine
The leaf stems are usually striped, the leaves 20-30 cm broad, usually green beneath. The white
flowers scarcely fragrant, close much later than the fragrant lily.
Range. sw. Que., Ont. to English river, Minn. to Nebr., s. to Ark., Ill., Ohio and Md. *Nymphaea
alba* L the European white water lily, is a similar species.
1633 Gerarde-Johnson 820. "Water Lillie with yellow floures [*Nuphar luteum* of Europe] stoppeth
laskes, the over overflowing of seed which commeth away by dreames or otherwise, and is good
for them that have the bloudie flix. But water Lillie which hath the white floures [*Nymphaea alba*
of Europe] is of greater force, insomuch, as it staieth the whites. . .being stamped and laid upon a
wound, it is reported to stay the bleeding. The Physitions of our age do commend the floures of
white Nymphaea against the infirmities of the head which come of a hot cause: and do certainly
affirme, that the root of the yellow water lily cureth hot diseases of the kidneys and bladder, and
is singular good against the running of the reines. The root and seed of the great water lilie is
very good against venery of fleshly desire, if one do drinke the decoction therof, or use the seed
or root in powder in his meates, for it dryeth up the seed of generation, and so causeth a man to
be chaste, especially used in broth with flesh. The conserve of the floures is good for the diseases
aforesaid, and is good also against hot burning fevers. The floures being made into oile, as yee
do make oil of roses, doth coole and refrigerate, causing sweete and quiet sleepe and putteth
away all venerous dreames: the temple of the head and palmes of the hands and feet, and the
brest being annointed for the one, and the genitors upon and about them for the other. The
greene leaves of the great water Lillie, either the white or the yellow laid upon the region of the
backe in the small, mightily cease the involuntary flowing away of the seed called Gonorhea, or
running of the reines, being two or three times removed, and fresh applied thereto."
1672 Josselyn New. Engl. 72. "Roots of yellow water lily after long boiling, eaten by the Indians,
tasted like sheep liver. . .stamped between two stones made into a plaister to eat proud flesh."
1785 Cutler. "The white flowers open about seven in the morning and close about four in the
afternoon. A conserve is made of the leaves of the blossoms. The roots of [the white and yellow]
both species are much used, in the form of poultices, for producing suppuration in boils and
painful tumors, and are very efficacious. The root of the yellow water lily is generally preferred.
Dr. Withering says the roots are used in Ireland. . .to dye dark brown."
1799 Lewis Mat. Med. 191. "Alvine fluxes, gleets. The roots are supposed by some to be in an
eminent degree narcotic, but on no very good foundation. . .in some parts of Sweden in times of
scarcity, used as food, and did not prove unwholesome. [referring to the European water lily]
1817-20 Bigelow 138. "The roots of this plant (*N. odorata*) are among the strongest astringents,
and we have scarcely any native vegetable which affords more decided evidence of this property.
When fresh, if chewed in the mouth, they are extremely styptic and bitter. Their decoction
instantly strikes a jet black colour with sulphate of iron. . .The roots of the water lily are kept by
most of our apothecaries, and are much used by the common people in the composition of poultices. They are no doubt injudiciously applied to suppurating tumours. . .They are occasionally
used by physicians in cases where astringent applications are called for. . .The Nymphaea of
Europe which appears perfectly similar in its qualities to the American plant, was celebrated by

the ancients as an antaphrodisiac and as a remedy in dysentery and some other morbid discharges."

1830 Rafinesque 45. "White water lily the properties similar to those of *N. alba* of Europe, but much more efficient and decided. The roots are chiefly used, and are kept in shops in New England. . . .Externally, the roots and leaves are used for poultices in piles, tumors, scrofulous sores, lockjaw, and inflamed skin. Internally the roots are useful in diarrhoea, dysentery, gonorrhea, leucorrhea, scrofula, and many fevers. . .The fresh leaves are excellent for cooling and emollient cataplasms; they are eaten by cows and cattle, and in Canada they are eaten in the spring, boiled for greens. The fresh root is used sometimes like soap. A conserve of the flowers is said to be very cooling and even anti-erotic. . .The fresh juice of the roots, mixed with lemon juice, is said to be a good cosmetic, and to remove pimples and freckles of the skin. . .Upon the whole, this plant has important properties, and deserves the attention of the medical practitioners, although many writers totally omit it. The yellow water lilies belonging to the genus *Nuphar* have the same properties, although less efficient."

1859-61 Gunn 881. "White pond lily. The root is astringent, demulcent, and somewhat anodyne; and said to be antiscrofulous. Used internally in. . .affections of the lungs; externally in the form of poultices, as an application to sores, tumors, swellings, scrofulous ulcers and the like. The infusion is also good as a wash and gargles for sore and ulcerated mouth and throat."

1868 Can. Pharm. J. 6; 83-5. The white water lily, *Nymphaea odorata*, the root included in list of Can. medicinal plants.

1892 Millspaugh 18. "The roots [of the white water lily] in decoction, were much esteemed by Indian squaws as an internal remedy, and injection or wash for the worst forms of leucorrhoea, its properties in this direction being due to its great astringency. The macerated root was also used as an application in the form of a poultice to suppurating glands; its styptic properties were also fully known and utilized."

1915 Speck PENOBSCOT 310. "A mash made of the leaves is used for swellings of the limbs. (*N. odorata*)"

1915 Speck-Cartwright MICMAC-MONTAGNAIS Newfoundland. "The expressed juice of the root of the white water lily drunk for coughs. The root, boiled, used as a poultice for swellings. The root of the yellow water lily bruised with flour or meal and used as a poultice for swellings and bruises."

1916 Waugh IROQUOIS 82. "Bread was sometimes made of other materials than corn such as. . .of roots. . .of the yellow pond lily and others. . .119. The roots of the yellow pond lily. . .are referred to as having been used in the Iroquois area, but have been practically forgotten by present day Iroquois."

1926-7 Densmore CHIPPEWA 342. White water lily, the root dried and finely powdered put in the mouth for a sore mouth.

1923 H. Smith MENOMINI 42. "Yellow water lily. This plant is described by the Menomini as belonging to the 'Underneath Spirits' and is accounted a great medicine. The large fibrous. . .underwater stems are pulled and the so-called root is dried and then powdered. This powder is used for poultices to heal cuts and swellings. The Menomini say that this plant makes the fogs that hover over the lakes. . .69. The large fleshy rhizomes are starchy and firm. They are cooked in the same manner as rutabaga."

1932 H. Smith OJIBWE 376. "White water lily, the Ojibwe use the root as a cough medicine for those who have tuberculosis. The root of the yellow water lily is the only medicinal part and is grated to make a poultice for sores. Other ingredients such as skunk cabbage root are added to this poultice. The Ojibwe gather a goodly quantity of the large underwater stems; which we are prone to call roots, dry them, and reduce them to powder. The powder alone is supposed to heal cuts and swellings. . .407. The Flambeau Ojibwe eat the buds of the white water lily before they open."

1933 H. Smith POTAWATOMI 65. "According to Pokagon, the root of the sweet scented water lily was used as a poulticing material when it was pounded, but our informant did not tell us what ailments it was supposed to cure. The Forest Potawatomi gather large quantities of the root of the yellow pond lily and give it the name of pine snake, because of the appearance of the roots where the water has dried away exposing them. The writer made a trip with Mrs. Spoon to obtain a supply of this root and gathered perhaps a two-bushel sack of it. The roots were cut in quarters to dry better. The root is pounded into a pulp, either fresh or dried to use as a poulticing material for many inflammatory diseases."

1945 Rousseau MOHAWK transl. 43. "An infusion of the root of the yellow water lily with that of sweet flag and the entire plants of *Myriophyllum*, drunk hot by adolescents (16-17 years) whose blood 'does not circulate quickly enough' Also when 'the blood goes to the head'"

1945 Raymond TETE DE BOULE transl. 129. "The seeds of the yellow water lily are eaten and the stem sucked to quench thirst."

1955 Mockle Quebec transl. 43. "White water lily, the root is astringent, the leaves as poultices are emolient, the juice of the roots mixed with lemon juice is supposed to be efficacious for pimples and freckles."

1962 Montgomery 41. "After pollination the flowers are drawn beneath the water by the shortening of the flower stalk and the seeds mature under water". . .(White water lily, *Nymphaea ordorata*).

The large rounded rootstock about as thick as a banana stem, floating on the water in late summer is the root of the yellow water lily. Use it boiled or scrape it, and remove any black spots, leave it in the hot ashes of the camp fire all day and by night it will be ready to eat. It can also be boiled, or dried and ground to make flour, or kept for use later. The seeds removed from their green outer shells make a good gruel when boiled. Or they can be fried in fat to make a kind of popcorn. Use the large leaves to wrap other vegetables for cooking (Assiniwi 1972:89).

WATER SHIELD
Brasenia Schreberi Gmel. Nymphaeaceae

The smaller leaves floating on the water near the lilies could be those of the water shield. Its leaves are attached to their stem at the centre of the underside of the leaf. The stems are up to 2 m long, and round leaves 4-12 cm long and half as wide. The flowers are purplish red on stems up to 15 cm long that grow from the main stem.

Range. N.S. and e. Que. to Minn., s. to Fla. and Tex.; also on the Pacific slope and in Tropical America and the old world.

Common names. Water target, deer-food, little water lily, frog leaf.

1828 Rafinesque 90. "The underside of the leaf is covered with a coat of pale jelly, sometimes purplish, first described by Schreber. . .the leaves afford one of the few instances of pure homogenous vegetable jelly, being spontaneously produced, and covering the whole under surface of the leaves and the stem. Deer and cattle are very fond of eating these leaves; even swim in the water in search of them. They are mucilaginous, astringent, demulcent, tonic and nutritious. The fresh leaves may be used like lichen in pulmonary complaints and dysentery. When dry the gelatinous matter almost disappears yet they impart mucilage to water. . .unnoticed as yet by all medical writers but well known to the Indians."

1923 H. Smith MENOMINI 42. "Not used. The rhizomes of Brasenia have been used by white men in the treatment of phthisis, also in dysentery."

1928 H. Smith MESKWAKI 197. A remedy for the menses; stomach trouble; the best for flux. The flowers of water target, the root of bloodroot, the inner bark of choke cherry and of Maindenhair and ginseng, mixed.

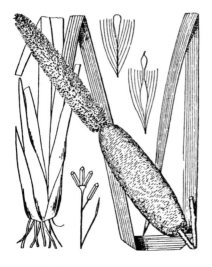

BROAD LEAVED CAT-TAIL

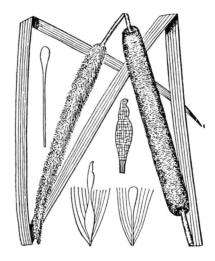

NARROW LEAVED CAT-TAIL

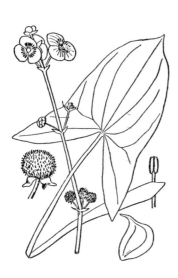

ARROWHEAD

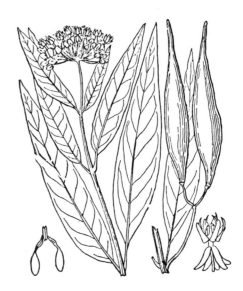

SWAMP MILKWEED

BROAD LEAVED CAT-TAIL   *Typha latifolia* L. Typhaceae
Stems 1-3 m tall with flat leaves that are 1-2 cm wide. The flowering stalk is surrounded by two
different brown cylinders, the one at the end with fuzzy, loose, pollen-bearing tips, and immedi-
ately below it, the 2.5 cm thick and 10-15 cm long fruiting cylinder that looks hard and dense.
Range. Nearly cosmopolitan throughout our range in marshes, commonest inland.
Common names. Cat-o'nine tails, marsh beetle, bulrush, great reed mace, candlewick.

NARROW LEAVED CAT-TAIL   *Typha angustifolia* L.
Stem 1-1.5 m tall with leaves 4-8 mm wide. There is a gap on the stem between the pollen bearing top and seed bearing lower cylinder.

Range. Nearly cosmopolitan throughout our range commonest near the coast in marshes.

800-1400 A.D. Found archeologically at Kettle Hill and Ash Caves in Ohio. Yarnell 1964:186.

1616 Champlain HURON 85. "During the day they bind the child to a piece of wood and wrap him in furs or skins. . .under the child they spread the silk of a special kind of reed—the one we call hare's foot—which is soft for it to lie on and helps to keep it clean."

1624 Sagard HURON 129. "Babies are put on beautifully soft down of a kind of reed. . .and they clean it with the same down."

1633 Gerarde-Johnson 46. "Cats Taile. The Soft Downe stamped with swines grease well washed, healeth burnings or scaldings with fire or water. . .This Downe in some places of the Isle of Elie, and the low countries adjoining thereto, is gathered and well sold to make mattresses of, for plowmen and poore people. It hath beene also often proved to heale kibed or humbled heeles (as they are termed) being applied to them, either before or after the skinne be broken."

1698 Hennepin 528. "The Indians. . .make mats of bulrushes to lie upon."

1749 Kalm Philadelphia April 9th. 278. "Cat-tail. Flax or cat-tail are names given to a grass which grows in bays, rivers, and in deep whirlpools, and which is known to botanists by the name of *Typha latifolia.* Its leaves are twisted together, and formed into great oblong rings, which are put upon the horse's neck, between the mane and the collar, in order to prevent the horses neck from being hurt by the collar. The bottoms of chairs (now called rush bottom chairs) were frequently made of these leaves, twisted together. Formerly, the Swedes employed the down which surrounds its seeds and put it into their beds instead of feathers; but as it coalesces into lumps after the beds have been used for some time, they have left off making use of them. I omit the uses of this plant in medicine, that being the peculiar province of the physicians."

1830 Rafinesque 270. "Roots subastringent, febrifuge, esculent, yield one tenth of a fine fecula similar to salep, eaten by Indians of Oregon, useful in fevers. Leaves used by cooper and to make mats, chair bottoms. Pollen equal to *Lycopodium* (ground pine) for medical use and pyrotechny. Burs or hairs of seeds used to fill cushions, united to ashes and lime make a cement as hard as marble. Seeds kill mice. Ought to be cult[ivated] in swamps."

1840 Gosse Quebec 317. "Have you ever examined any of that large patch of bulrushes (*Typha Latifolia*) which grow in the bottom of this field?. . .The thick cylindrical head appears like a fine, but very closely set brush, radiating from the axis or stalk, which it covers for about six inches. On picking out a lump of what we may call the bristles of this brush, we are surprised to see we have a handful of the softest down, that which before was not bigger than one's thumb, now on being freed from the stalk, filling one's hand. . .the whole head is composed of this very expansive down; and I am told that poor persons sometimes collect quantities of it to make beds, which are said to be soft and elastic."

1868 Can. Pharm. J. 6; 83-5. "Cat-tail Flag *Typha Latifolia*, the root included in list of Can. medicinal plants."

1885 Hoffman OJIBWA 200. "The roots are crushed by pounding or chewing, and applied as a poultice to sores."

1916 Waugh ABENAKI 149. "It is probable that infusions of many other materials, including various edible roots, and forming broths or soups, with more or less food value, were used from time to time. A suggestion of this is found in the use by the Abenaki of the juice from the bruised roots of the cat-tail and other plants."

1924 Youngken 499. "Every part of this plant was used by various Indian tribes for some ailment. . .The Omaha tribe used the roots and ripe blossoms for scalds. For this purpose the root was powdered, wetted and spread as a paste over the scald. The ripe blossoms were then applied as a covering and the injured part bound, so as to hold the dressing in place. The Cheyenne used an infusion of the powdered roots and white bases of the leaves for the relief of abdominal cramps."

1923 H. Smith MENOMINI 77. "The root is used as a natural oakum for caulking leaks in boats. The leaves are used to make mats to cover the winter lodges, much as the bulrush mats are made. Because of the heavy flat layers, they keep out the rain and snow and are well adapted to winter thatching. In summer they are stored away for the next year's use."

1928 H. Smith MESKWAKI 248. "Children born in the winter are wrapped in a quilt of this fuzz to keep them warm. Old sores on the neck are padded with this fuzz to help them get well. . .269.

Several parts of the cat-tail are useful to the Meskwaki. The root is used as a natural oakum to caulk his canoe. The leaves furnish him with rainproof and windproof side wall for the wigwam. . .The fuzz of the fruit makes good pillow and comfort material. The mats made of cat-tail leaves are produced in an entirely different way from those made of rushes. They are sewed and their edges are woven and sewed also. Nettle fiber is the strongest cord, and is used for sewing and binding the edge. A curved bone of a calf is shaped into a needle with an eye to carry the nettle cord which is about the size of a carpenter's line and the leaves are sewed with an invisible stitch. . .They are made several layers thick and the mats are quite large. . .flag-reed lodge. . .the walls were made from the mats of *Typha latifolia*. The covering or support for the roofing mats were woven from the twigs of pussy willow. The overlapping of the leaves. . .renders the shelter waterproof and keeps the wind out."

1932 H. Smith OJIBWE 390. "The Flambeau Ojibwe used the fuzz of the fruit for a war medicine. They claim that the fuzz thrown into an enemy's face will blind him. . .423. The Flambeau Ojibwe women use the cat-tail leaves to make. . .mats to be placed on the sides of the medicine lodge or any temporary wigwam or sweat lodge. . .They are not quite rain-proof as a roofing material, so birchbark rolls are used for that purpose. The fuzz or seed. . .is used to make mattresses and sleeping bags. . .They gather the heads and boil them first, which causes all the bugs to come out of them. Then they dry them and strip the fuzz, to make a mattress, which they claim is as soft as feathers, but very prone to mat together, so it must be shaken often and thoroughly. They also make a quilt of it, and from the quilt, a sleeping bag. This is declared to be soft and warm in the coldest weather. . .they used to throw the fuzz. . .into the eyes of their enemies."

1933 H. Smith POTAWATOMI 85. "The Forest Potawatomi used the root to make poultices for various inflammations. The fresh roots are pounded and reduced to poulticing material. . .114. Names translate 'shelter weed' and 'fruit for babies bed'. Make mats for sides of wigwam, use fuzz for quilt upon which to place the infant."

1926-27 Densmore CHIPPEWA 378. "Bulrush mats for the floor were woven on frames, the basswood twine being passed 'over and under' the rushes. . .380. The outer covering of cat-tail rushes was formed into toys representing human beings and ducks. The latter were usually made in groups of five. They were placed on the surface of smooth water, and the child agitated the water by blowing across it, which caused the ducks to move in a lifelike manner."

1945 Rousseau QUEBEC transl. 107. "The fuzz used to fill puffs to sit upon."

1945 Raymond TETE DE BOULE transl. 132. "The Indians gather the fuzz to make mattresses."

It has been claimed that competent chemists find the cat-tails's food value nearly equal to that of corn or rice. . .cat-tail roots are said to contain as high as thirty percent sugar and starch. . .when macerated and boiled a syrup of excellent flavor is produced. Cat-tails could be grown commercially for the flour and cornstarch from the roots. The flour can be fermented to produce ethyl alcohol, the fibers used to make burlap, an adhesive can be made from the stems, the fuzz compressed to make insulation, the seeds produce oil and the waste makes chicken feed (Cat-tail Research centre, Syracuse Univ, Leland Marsh, Ernest Reed cited Charles Ben Harris 1961:102).

ARROWHEAD   *Saggitaria latifolia* Willd. Alismataceae

Growing in shallow water from short fibrous roots, the leaves are on long stems. The many shapes of the leaf are confusing but most are from 5-40 x 2-25 cm and shaped like a large arrow with points on either side of the stem. The flowering stem, 10-120 cm tall has heads of 2-15 flowers. They have three 1-2 cm long, white petals followed by a ball of beaked seeds. The beak on this variety of arrowhead is horizontal and 1.-2.5 mm long.

Range. N.S., N.B., P.E.I., Que. James Bay, Ont., Man., Sask., Alta., B.C., s. to Calif., and Tex.

1749 Kalm Philadelphia March 17th. 259. "*Sagittaria, Katniss* is another Indian name of a plant, the root of which they were also accustomed to eat, when they lived here. . .The Indians either boiled this root or roasted it in hot ashes. Some of the Swedes ate it with much relish at the time when the Indians were so near the coast; but at present none of them make any use of the roots. Nils Gustafson told me. . .the Indians, especially the women, travelled to some islands, at about Whitsuntide, dug out the roots, and brought them home; and while they had them they desired no other food. They were said to have been destroyed by the hogs [brought over by the Europeans] which were exceedingly greedy for them. The cattle are fond of their leaves. I afterwards got some of these roots roasted, and in my opinion they tasted good, though they were rather dry. The taste was nearly the same as that of potatoes. . .The katniss is an arrow-head or Sagittaria, and is only a variety of the Swedish arrow-head or *Sagittaria sagittifolia*, for the plant above the ground is entirely the same, while the root underground is much greater in the American than in the European variety. . .Further north in this part of America I met with the other species of Saggitaria which we have in Sweden."

1830 Rafinesque 259. "Arrowleaf, Katnip of Lenaps, Wapatu of Oregon tribes, twelve species equally valuable esculent roots of Indians (Cult. in China and Japan) trade with it, make bread, soups, dishes &c. Refrigerant, subastringent; useful applied to feet or yaws and dropsical legs; leaves applied to breast to dispel milk of nurses."

1926-27 Densmore CHIPPEWA 342. "The root steeped and drunk if a 'person's food did not agree with them'. . .319. This is commonly called the 'wild potato' and grows in deep mud. At the end of the tubular roots are the 'potatoes' which are gathered in the fall, strung, and hung overhead in the wigwams to dry. Later they are boiled for use."

1923 H. Smith MENOMINI 61. "This is one of the Menomini valued wild potatoes and hard to get on their reservation. . .The Indians usually see them in the water, washed out by the current, or see them near the burrow of a muskrat or home of a beaver."

1928 H. Smith MESKWAKI 254. "This is one of their valued wild potatoes."

1932 H. Smith OJIBWE 353. "While they are chiefly prized for food, they are also taken as a remedy for indigestion among the Pillager Ojibwe. . .396. Use it as a medicine for man and horse. . .The corms are a most valued food source to the Ojibwe. They will dig them if they cannot get them more easily. Muskrat and beaver store them in large caches, which the Indians learn to recognize and appropriate. It is difficult to dig them out still attached to the plant, because the connection between the roots and the corm is so fragile and small. The round corms are attached by a tiny rootlet to the main mass of fibrous roots, and are capable of reproducing the plant. . .They are. . .pure white inside, sweet and quite starchy. . .For winter use, the potato is boiled, then sliced and strung on a piece of basswood bark fibre and hung up overhead for storage. They also use the fresh corms, cooking them with deer meat and maple sugar. Some of the potatoes are kept over after the cooking and the maple sugar is thickened until they might almost be called candied sweet potatoes."

1933 H. Smith POTAWATOMI 94. "Similar use to that of the Ojibwe."

1945 Rousseau MOHAWK transl. 65. "For children who cry suddenly in the night give an infusion of the roots of sweet flag and the entire plant of arrowhead. I do not know whether the Iroquois eat the tubercules. Waugh and Parker do not say, but most of the Indians of North America used to eat them."

SWAMP MILKWEED   *Asclepias incarnata* L. Asclepiadaceae

An almost smooth stem or if hairy, then in lines up the stem, which is up to 1½ m tall. The leaves are opposite, abruptly narrowed to a rounded base, 7.5-15 mm long, 1-4 cm wide. The flowers are pink to red, 5-7 mm. The pods stand upright in pairs, are smooth and sparingly hairy. The juice of the plant is milky and contains caoutchouc as does the juice of the common milkweed.

Range. N.B. to Ont., Sask., S.D., Ariz., Mex. and Fla. June-Aug. in swamps.

Common names. Rose milkweed, white Indian hemp, water nerve root.

300 B.C.-500 A.D. *A. incarnata* fiber found archeologically in Ohio Hopewell sites by Whitford 1941:10. Yarnell 1964:191.

1828 Rafinesque 76. "*A. incarnata* has been noticed by Tully and Anderson in a thesis as a useful emetic and cathartic. . .1830 196. Indians of Louisiana use *A. serpentaria*, for the bite of rattle snakes. The *A. debilis* makes a kind of flax. The *A. phytolacoides* dies yellow green, the milk appears similar to opium; silk gloves have been made with the silk of the pods. The Oregan and Western tribes call many species Nepesha, they use the roots in dropsy, asthma, dysentery, and as emetics, chiefly the *A. syriaca A. incarnata* and *A. obtusifolia*."

1868 Can. Pharm. J. 6;83-5. The root of the rose-colored silkweed, *A. incarnata* included in list of Can. medicinal plants.

1926-27 Densmore CHIPPEWA 364. Put 1 root in 1 quart of water, steep, strain, and when cool bathe the child in it. Also good for grown people when sick or tired. Soak feet in it and lie down. . .304. Constituents a volatile oil, resins, and the glucoside asclepiadin. . .300. The root is alterative, anthelmintic, cathartic and emetic.

1923 H. Smith MENOMINI 62. "When these milkweeds are in bloom, or even better, in bud, the heads are highly esteemed as food, much like the asparagus tips of the white man. They are made into soup with deer broth or fat of some sort. They are also cut and dried and stored for winter use."

1928 H. Smith MESKWAKI 205. "The root of this species is used as a taenifuge. McIntosh related to the writer how he recovered four long tape worms from a woman by its use. The root tea is said to drive the worms from a person in one hour's time. The roots are extensively used in the same manner as the officinal drug *Asclepias tuberosa* [see Dry open places] as a diuretic and carminative, and in large doses as a cathartic and emetic."

1970 Bye IROQUOIS mss. Fibers used for wampum belts, fine cords, fish nets, burden straps, the root cathartic.

See under Dry Open Places for the other milkweeds.

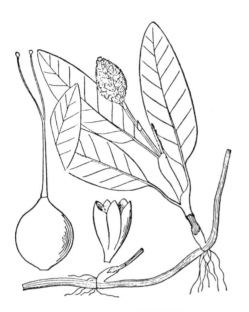

WATER SMARTWEED

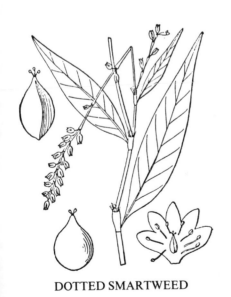

DOTTED SMARTWEED

SMARTWEED

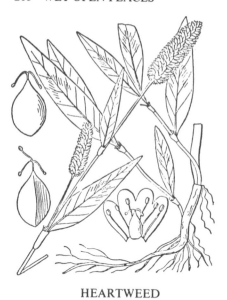

HEARTWEED

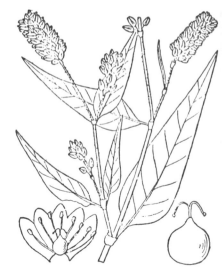

PENSYLVANIA PERSICARIA

The name smartweed derives from an old English word, smeorten, bite. The botanical name is *Polygonum* or many knees, because these plants have stems with a succession of swollen joints covered with sheaths, as if they had many knees. Most of them when tasted, leave the tongue smarting. Another common name for them is Knotweed. There are many different species and they are difficult to identify.

WATER SMARTWEED   *Polygonum amphibium* L. Polygonaceae (*P. natans*)
This grows both in the shallow water and on land nearby. Plants on land will be hairy all over, the upper sheaths have a flaring, scalloped, green edge, very easy to see. Those growing in the water will have tight tops to their sheaths. Their leaves will be smooth or nearly so. The leaves of the land plants can be up to 20 cm. long. Both plants have a conspicuous flowering stalk shaped like a cone, covered with shocking pink flowers. This cone is rarely over 3 cm. long.
Range. Iceland, Lab.?, Nfld., N.B., P.E.I., N.S., Que., James Bay, Ont., to Alaska and Yukon, s. to Utah, Colo., Nebr., Pa., and N.J. There is a form without the flaring edge to the sheath. A very closely related species, *P. coccineum* (*P. muhlenbergii*) does not have a flaring edged sheath either and its flowering stalk is only 14-15 cm. long and 1 cm. thick, the flowers ranging fron scarlet to pink or rarely white. It is not known from N.B. or Nfld. nor Alaska and the Yukon but grows s. to Calif., Mex. Both these species have several subspecies.
Common names. Water persicaria, willow-weed, ground willow, heartsease, red shanks.
1785 Cutler. "Blossoms red in wet meadows. The root is said to be one of the strongest vegetable astringents."
1928 H. Smith MESKWAKI 197. "An emetic for poisons. Antidote for peyote poisoning. Root of Water smartweed (*P. muhlenbergii*) and the leaves of Indian tobacco (*Nicotiana tabacum*). . . .236. Meskwaki name translates 'white or water potato'. The root is used for treating sores in the mouth. The Meskwaki use it for a tea when it is 'young or soft', as they express it. The leaves and stems furnish a tea for the treatment of flux in children. The Indians soak the drug without heat, as they claim the active principle is destroyed by heating. Specimen 5092 of the Dr. Jones collection is a mixture incorporating the root of this water smartweed with five other ingredients. . .The mixture is boiled and made into a drink to cure women with an injured womb."
1932 H. Smith OJIBWE 381. "The Flambeau Ojibwe use this plant for a tea to cure a pain in the

stomach." 431. They dry the flower and then include it in their hunting medicine, which is smoked to attract deer to the hunter."

1933 H. Smith POTAWATOMI "*P. amphibium* The Forest Potawatomi used the root of this as a medicine but the particular use was not stated. Among the whites the root of this plant has been used as a blood purifier."

1966 Campbell, Best & Budd. 74. "Persicarias (*P. coccineum*) that grow in water and can be harvested as sloughs dry up make excellent aromatic hay, but those which have developed entirely on dry land are harsh and unpalatable. Leafy and green hay will contain 15 per cent or more protein with corresponding levels of crude fibre. . .Persicarias that are pastured are credited with causing 'yellows' in livestock with white skins; this condition is seldom, if ever, produced when fed in well-cured hay."

DOTTED SMARTWEED.   *Polygonum punctatum* Ell. (*P. acre*) Polygonaceae
A slender stem to 1 m. tall, with sheaths that are long and tight, sometimes with bristles at their tops. The leaves are smooth and narrow, to 20 x 2 cm. The flowers are only 2 mm long and greenish. They are far apart at the bottom of the erect flowering spike, closer together at the tip, which may droop a little. The leaves and the outer petals (sepals) of these flowers are covered with tiny bumps filled with oil which burns the mouth when tasted.
Range. N.B., P.E.I., N.S., Que., Ont., Man., to B.C., s. to Calif., Mex., Tex. and Fla. in wet places and swampy ground.

SMARTWEED   *Polygonum hydropiper* L. Polygonaceae
The stems smooth, green or reddish, up to 2 m. tall. Some of the sheaths will be swollen at the base by the development of several tiny flowers within these sheaths. The narrow leaves are rough on the vein beneath. The visible flowers are continuous on their stem which usually droops at the end. The flowers are greenish, the leaflets (sepals) surrounding them are dotted with glands and usually have a white edge. The seeds are often three sided. 2.2-3.3 mm.
Range. Both native and introd. Nfld., N.B., P.E.I., N.S., Que., Ont., s. to Ala. and Tex. in damp soils and ditches. The plant may be entirely introd. in N. America.
Common names. Pepperplant, biting persicaria, knotweed, snake or sickle weed.
1687 Clayton Virginia Indians 6. "The great success they have in curing wounds and sores, I apprehend mostly to proceed from their manner of dressing them: For they first cleanse them by sucking, which though a very nasty, is no doubt the most effecheal and best way imaginable; then they take the biting Persicary, and chaw it in their mouths, and thence squirt the juice therof into the wound, which they will do as if out of a syringe. Then they apply their salve-herbs, either bruised or beaten into a salve with grease, binding it on with bark and silk grass."
1791 Lewis Materia Medica ed. Aitkin 199. *P. hydropiper* bitter arsmart, water pepper, the leaves in phlegmatic habits, it promotes urinary discharge. . .good success in scorbutic complaints. The fresh leaves are sometimes applied externally for cleansing old fistulas, ulcers and consuming fungus flesh, for these purposes they are said to be employed by farriers, among whom they have principally been made use of.
1785 Cutler. Arsmart, water pepper, *P. punctatum*. It occasions severe smarting when rubbed on flesh. The taste is acrid and burning. It dyes wool yellow. Dr. Withering says it cures little apthous ulcers in the mouth. That the ashes mixed with soft soap is a nostrum in a few hands, for dissolving the stone in the bladder; but perhaps not preferable to other caustic preparations of the vegetable alkali."
1859-61 Gunn 858. "Smartweed (*Polygonum punctatum*). It has an intensely hot, acrid, and peppery taste. Smartweed is stimulant, diaphoretic, diuretic, emmenagogue and antiseptic, and is a valuable medicine. A strong tincture of the herb is highly recommended in amenorrhea, or suppressed menses, in doses of one or two teaspoonfuls three times a day. . .A cold infusion of the herb has been used with success in gravel, and affections of the kidneys and bladder; and a cold infusion of the herb and wheat bran is said to be an excellent remedy for bowel complaints, drank freely. Smartweed makes an excellent fomentation, along with hops and other bitter herbs, to be applied warm to the abdomen in inflammation of the bowels; and a strong decoction is good to wash foul and gangrenous ulcers, and parts tending to mortification. . .The tincture and extract of Smartweed should be made of the fresh herb, as it loses some of its strength by age; it

is also injured by heat or boiling. To make an infusion, hot water should be poured on it, and allowed to macerate till cold."

1868 Can. Pharm. J. 6; 83-5. The root of *P. hydropiper* included in list Can. medicinal plants.

1892 Millspaugh 141. "The use of Smartweed (*P. punctatum*) among the laity, who include *P. hydropiper* is very general and extended, especially as a fomentation in amenorrhoea. . .enteritis and mastitis, and internally in the same troubles and in coryza. . .A cold infusion has been found very serviceable in nursing sore-mouth, mercurial ptyalism, gout and dysentery, and externally as a wash for indolent ulcers and painful hemorrhoids. In Mexico. . .put into the baths of persons afflicted with rheumatism."

1926-27 Densmore CHIPPEWA 344. Flowers and leaves of *P. punctatum* drunk as a decoction for pains in the stomach, used only in combination with other herbs.

1928 Parker SENECA 11-12. Smartweed used as a tonic, smartweed tea with salt in copious quantities for coryza.

1945 Rousseau MOHAWK transl. 40. "*P. hydropiper*. In ancient times the whole plant except the roots, was used instead of pepper. For pains in the head, cut it into bits, wet it and apply to the head. It is easy to understand the culinary use of this plant."

1955 Mockle Quebec transl. 37. Hemostatic. The plant contains an essence which gives it a piquant and peppery taste.

HEARTWEED   *Polygonum persicaria* L.

The smooth erect stem is much branched and up to 80 cm tall. The sheaths are tight, nearly smooth and fringed with short bristles. The leaves are long and narrow with a dark blotch near the centre and oil glands all over. The tight cylinder of the pink to rose purple flowers is erect. The seeds are shining black, 1.8-2.5 mm averaging four-fifths as wide.

Range. Native of Europe now common in our range, s. to Fla. and Tex. and w. to Alaska and Calif. June-Oct. in waste places.

Common names. Peachwort, blackheart, common persicary, spotted knotweed, Lady's thumb, lover's pride, arsemart, smartweed.

1633 Gerarde-Johnson 447. "It is reported that the Dead Arsemart is good against inflammations and hot swellings, being applied at the beginning: and for greene wounds, if it be stamped and boyled with oyle Olive, waxe and Turpentine."

1791 Lewis ed. Aitkin. "This plant is said to be a good vulnerary and antiseptic; decoctions of it in wine restrain the progress of gangrene (according to Tournefort, Paris 1703)."

1830 Rafinesque 66. "It has. . .very strong properties, is an acrid diuretic, burning the tongue and even the skin. . .it has been much used in gravel, commonly infused in wine; is said to have cured odontalgy, sores of the ear, and apthous sore mouth. . . .All cattle avoid them; they kill fish in ponds, and even snakes fear them. They die wool a fine yellow, with alum; called *Curage* in Louisiana, and much esteemed. Schoepf says they cure the ulcers and sores of horses. The *P. persicaria* grows near water all over the United States, and is easily known by its lanceolate leaves, with a black spot above, and oblong spikes of red flowers. The *P. hydropiper*, *P. amphibium*, *P. pensylvanicum*, & c. are equally medical and equivalent to *P. persicaria*."

1854 Trail 180. "The common yellow dye used by the settlers, is either a decoction of the golden-rod; or of a weed known as Smart-weed (a wild persicaria it is)."

1926-27 Densmore CHIPPEWA 344. The decoction of the flowers and leaves a strong medicine, drunk internally alone or in combinations, for pains in the stomach, yet one sprig not enough for a treatment.

1955 Mockle Quebec transl. 38. "The plant is astringent and vulnerary. It is also used to ease stomach pain and is said to have the power to kill worms."

1968 Forsyth England 79. "Several species of Polygonum have been recorded as having caused gastro-enteritis in animals that have eaten large quantities of them. They include water pepper, (*P. hydropiper*), knotgrass (*P. aviculare*) [see dry open places] and *P. persicaria*. . .All these plants are known to contain a sharp acrid juice which is extremely irritant if applied to the skin. . .poisoning by them is not very likely to occur."

1968 Adrosko 34. "During the 18th and early 19th centuries it was recommended by professional dyers because of the durable yellow color it imparted to woolens, cottons, and linens. . .Plants were cut while in bloom, then dried, and soaked for several days to induce fermentation. The dye liquid was then heated and alum mordanted cloth immersed in it. One 19th century dyer suggested its use in compound colors such as black, smoke, snuff and green."

PENSYLVANIA PERSICARIA   *Polygonum pensylvanicum* L.
The smooth erect stem grows up to 1 m. tall. The sheaths are plain, papery, smooth and without hairs. The leaves are long and narrow with an edging of fine hairs. The flowering stalk is 1.5-3 cm long with a blunt end. There are tiny glands at the end of minute hairs on this stalk. The flowers are rose to white, the seed is concave on both sides, mostly broader than high, 2.6-3.4 mm.
Range. N.S. and Que. to Minn. and S.D., s. to Fla. and Tex. in moist rich soils, July-Sept. highly variable.
1923 H. Smith MENOMINI 47. "This is a bitter leaf which is dried by the Menomini for tea. When one has a hemorrhage of blood from the mouth, this is drunk to stop it. Mixed with other herbs, it is drunk by women after childbirth, and heals them internally."
1928 H. Smith MESKWAKI 236. "This is used to cure the bloody flux by wiping the anus with it. It is also a cure for piles."
1933 H. Smith POTAWATONI 72. "The Forest Potawatomi use the entire plant [*of P. Careyi*] to make a tea to cure a cold that is accompanied by fever. They also use *P. lapathifolium* to make a tea for curing fevers."
1963 USSR C.A. 61-8609e Irradiating the seeds of species of smartweed increased the protein content in the fruit of the plant. It was better to irradiate before sowing. The nitrogen content rose also.
There is a very long history of the use of *Polygonum amphibium, aviculare, hydropiper, persicaria* and other species to treat various forms of cancer. The roots, juice, and plant all seem to have been used in folk medicine. (Hartwell 1970:373)
1972 USSR C.A. 99083x Extracts of smartweed can be used together with syntans for tanning hides. The leather was found to be of uniform color with satisfactory water absorption and mechanical strength for shoe soles.

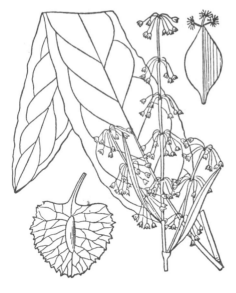

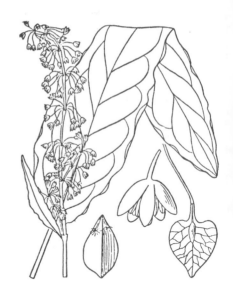

GREAT WATER DOCK   YELLOW DOCK

1962 Compt. Rendu Lille France 254;1492-4. By periodic examination of the leaves of ascorbic acid and oxalate rich plants of the Polygonum and Rumex families it was determined that during growth the ascorbic acid and oxalate content increased or decreased in parallel. This was especially true of the Polygonaceae whose high oxalate content, between 2500 and 3500 mg per 100 grms of fresh leaves, coincided with a high ascorbic acid or Vitamin C content.

Other members of this family are the sorrels and docks, *Rumex*. They too have joints on their stems covered with sheaths, that are brittle and disappear with age. Their stems are grooved. See under dry open places for the sheep sorrel.

The flowers of all the docks, (*Rumex*) to be described create beautiful triangular wings by the three inner petals (sepals) joining together, back to back at their centre veins, their edges curving out. There is usually a grain attached to the centre vein of each wing. The seed is inside this grain. The identification of the different docks is based to a large degree on where this grain is attached, how many grains there are in each flower, and the shape and size of the wings, which are called valves. The illustrations show these differences.

GREAT WATER DOCK   *Rumex orbiculatus* Gray (*R. britannica*) Polygoneceae
Stout erect stem to 2.5 m with long flat leaves, smooth and dark green. The flowers are on several branches up to 50 cm tall. The wings (valves) are each 5-8 mm both ways with crisped edges. The grain is above the stalk of the wing and half as long.

Range. Nfld. and Que. to N.D., s. to N.J., Ind., and Nebr. in swamps and shallow water July-Aug.

Common names. Sorrel, Horse-sorrel.

1070-1320 Juntunen site Mich. Seed of Rumex found archeologically in one location Yarnell 1964:35.

1785 Cutler. The Indians use this root with great success in cleansing foul ulcers. It is said they endeavoured to keep it a secret from the Europeans.

1830 Rafinesque 259. "*R. britannica, sanguineus* and *aquaticus*, chiefly used. Roots astringent, deobstruant, tonic, diaphoretic: useful in scurvy, cutaneous eruptions, syphilis, ulcers of the mouth, foul ulcers, itch, cancerous tumours, &c. in decoction, wine, lotion. They dye yellow. Contain sulphur, starch, oxalate of lime, &c. Syrup with Prunus. . .used for dysentery. Leaves edible equal to spinach."

1904 Henkel 18. "Yellow rooted water-dock. *Rumex britannica* L. The root, which is the part to be collected for medicinal purposes. . .in late summer or autumn after the fruiting tops have ripened, then washed, split lengthwise into halves or quarters and carefully dried. The docks are largely employed for purifying the blood and as a remedy in skin disease. Rumex or dock roots are imported into this country (U.S.) to the extent of about 125,000 pounds annually. The price ranges from 2 to 8 cents a lb. Also collected are the roots of the bitter dock and the yellow dock."
1928 H. Smith MESKWAKI 237. "Specimen 5124 of the Dr. Jones collection is the root of *R. britannica*. . .It is boiled and made into a drink that is an antidote for poison."
1932 H. Smith OJIBWE 381. "The Flambeau Ojibwe use the root, which contains considerable tannin, for closing and healing cuts. . .431. The dried seeds of this dock are smoked by the Flambeau as a favorable lure to game when mixed with kinnikinnik."
1933 H. Smith POTAWATOMI 73. "While there is no Potawatomi name given for this plant. . .as far as we know, still they use the root as a blood purifier."
1950 Wintemberg German-Canadians 12. "A tea of the leaves for dysentery."

YELLOW DOCK

Rumex crispus L. Polygonaceae

A slender, erect, grooved green stem up to 1 m tall bears long stalked, long leaves, rounded at their base and with wavy or curly edges. There are many erect, flowering branches. The tiny dark green flowers hang down on their 5-10 mm stalks. The three wings each have a grain that is half as long as they are, it is also two thirds as long as it is wide.
Range. Native of Europe found as a weed of roadsides, fields and moist ground.
Common names. Sorrel, curled or narrow dock.
1749 Kalm Albany April 18th. 285. "Sorrel. Both the Swedish and English settlers are in the spring accustomed to prepare greens from various plants of which the following are the most important; *Rumex crispus* L. is a kind of sorrel which grows at the edge of cultivated fields and elsewhere in rather low land. Farmers choose a variety which has green leaves instead of pale colored ones. All sorrel is not suitable for greens, for the leaves of some are very bitter. These green leaves are gathered at this time everywhere, and used by some people in the same way that Swedes prepare spinach. But they generally boil the leaves in the water in which they had cooked meat. Then they eat it alone or with meat. It is served on a platter and eaten with a knife, which is different from the Swedish custom. Here also vinegar is placed in a special container on the table to be used on the kale. I must confess that the dish tastes very good."
1785 Cutler. "The roots are cathartic. The seeds are said to have been given with great advantage in the dysentery. The fresh root bruised and made into an ointment or decoction to cure the itch."
1830 Rafinesque 259. "*R. patienta, obtusus, acutus* and *crispus*, similar but root less astringent, laxative or purgative, diuretic, seeds used in dysentery."
1859-61 Gunn 885. 'The fresh leaves bruised and simmered in sweet cream, fresh butter, or lard, make a good ointment for scrofulous ulcers, scrofulous sore eyes, glandular swellings, and it is said, will cure the itch."
1868 Can. Pharm. J. 6; 83-5. The root of yellow dock, *R. crispus* included in list of Can. medicinal plants.
1885 Hoffman OJIBWA 200. "The roots are bruised or crushed and applied to abrasions, sores, etc."
1892 Millspaugh 143. "The root has been used in medicine from ancient times, as a mild astringent tonic, laxative and depurent, its use being similar to that of rhubarb and sarsaparilla [Mexican *smilax*]. A decoction of the root has been found useful in dyspepsia, gouty tendencies, hepatic congestion, scrofula, syphilis, leprosy. . .An ointment of the powdered root with lard, or a cataplasm with cream, has been considered a specific for the cure of itch, and a useful application to cancers, as well as a discutient for indolent glandular tumors. Whatever use the root may have in these latter troubles must reside in the peculiar acid contained in it. Rumex is also considered an excellent dentifrice, especially where the gums are spongy. As a pot-herb the young root leaves are well known in all country localities. . .The acid. . .acts as a rubefacient and discutient and is a valuable agent for destroying parasites of the skin."
1916 Waugh IROQUOIS 117. "The young leaves, before the stem appears are eaten cooked like spinach. . .118. A number of plants such as. . .yellow dock. . .are considered to be European

introductions, a further illustration of the readiness of the Iroquois in the adoption of new materials."

1924 Youngken 497. "The root and green leaves of the Yellow Dock were used by many tribes as a medicine and a dye. The Cheyenne drank an infusion of the powdered root for hemorrhage of the lungs. They also moistened the powdered root and applied it as a poultice to wounds and sores."

1926-27 Densmore CHIPPEWA 350. The root, dried and powdered, is moistened, spread on a cloth and applied as a poultice in cases of great itching of the skin and eruptions. The root of bitter dock, *R. obtusifolius*, is steeped and applied externally for eruptions. It is used especially for children. . .*R. crispus*, yellow dock, the root dried and pounded was used externally for a clean cut. . .354. The dried and pounded root was applied externally to ulcers. . .366. A poultice of the root would cure a swelling in one day if there were no suppuration.

1945 Rousseau MOHAWK transl. 41. "Rumex sp. notably *R. mexicanus, R. crispus* and *R. verticillatus*, an infusion of the grains of dock and fragments of yarrow for diarrhea."

The MALECITE of the Maritime provinces of Canada used the root of the yellow dock as a purgative and for cold in the bladder. Mechling 1959.

Man has always considered it a kind act of providence that docks grow near the stinging nettles because rubbing dock leaves on the sting relieves it instantly.

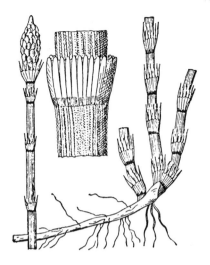

GREAT SCOURING RUSH

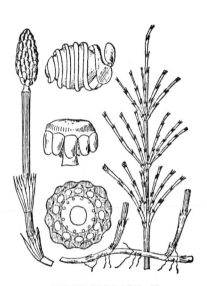

FIELD HORSETAIL

GREAT SCOURING RUSH   *Equisetum hyemale* L. Equisetaceae (*E. praealtum*)
Stems all alike, 5-7 mm thick, evergreen, without any branches, erect, 20-150 cm tall with mostly 18-40 broad, rounded, roughened ridges. The hollow centre is about 3/4 the diameter of the stem. The sheaths about as long as broad with a dark band at the top and bottom. The teeth fall off as the plant matures. Spore bearing cones at the top of the stem.
Range. Circumboreal, in Am. s. to Fla. and Calif. in sandy banks and moist slopes.
Common names. Horse-pipe, scouring rush, dutch rush, shave grass, prèle, gunbright.
1633 Gerarde-Johnson 1116. "Dioscorides saith, that Horse-taile being stamped and laied to, doth perfectly cure wounds, yea though the sinews be cut in sunder, as Galen addeth. It is of so great and so singular a vertue in healing of wounds, as that it is thought and reported for truth, to cure wounds of the bladder, and other bowels, and helpeth ruptures or burstings. The herbe

drunk either with water or wine, is an excellent remedy against bleeding at the nose and other fluxes of bloud. It staieth overmuch flowing of womens floures, the bloudy flix, and the other fluxes of the belly. The juice of the herbe taken in the same manner can do the like, and more effectually. Horsetail with his roots boiled in wine, is very profitable for the ulcers of the kidnies & bladder, the cough and difficultie of breathing. . .Is not unknown to women, who scoure their pewter and woodden things of the kitchen therewith."

1830 Rafinesque 217-8. "Polish wood, metals and utensils, good food for cattle in winter. All the rough species used to scour and clean. Used in Italy for a cattle diuretic, given to oxen voiding blood. . .Some tall species called Nebratah by the Missouri tribes, are used for brooms, mats, wicks, thatch. Their roots produce great thirst; they are powerfully stimulant and diuretic, used in dropsies, menstrual and syphilitic diseases."

1859-61 Gunn 851. "It is diuretic and astringent; and said to be good in dropsies, suppressed urine, gravel, and affections of the kidneys-to be used freely in decoction or infusion made of the tops or stems. The ashes of the rush are said to be an excellent article for sour stomach and dyspepsia, better than ordinary alkalies."

1868 Can. Pharm. J. 6; 83-5. The plant of the scouring rush, *Equisetum hyemale* included in list of Can. medicinal plants.

1892 Millspaugh 179. "It is gathered into bundles by many housewives and used to brighten tins, floors, and woodenware, and in the arts of polishing woods and metals. This plant is not mentioned in the U.S. Ph. and is not officinal in the Eclectic Materia Medica . . .It is said that where cattle have been given too large quantities of an infusion as a diuretic, it has caused the voidance of blood."

1901 Morice Arctic DENE 25. "As parturifacients, three plants are chiefly valued and used to this day among the Carriers. They are the horse-tail (*Equisetum hyemale*) which is taken in strong decoctions. . ."

1922 Thomson & Sifton 27. "In ancient times the Horsetail family was one of the most important. The fossil record shows that its members formed a striking part of the coal forest swamps, their jointed stems, two feet or more in thickness, rising to heights of fifty to one hundred feet. To-day there are only a few isolated species of a single genus."

1915 W. R. Harris HURON 43. "When hard on the trail of a deer or when pursued by his enemy over poorly watered lands the Indian suffered severly from blood-spitting. When this happened and to stop the hemorrhage he chewed and swallowed, while on the run, the Hon-kos-koa-ga-sha, an astringent root which he carried with him when leaving his tent." [May refer to horsetail]

1925 Anderson 149. "Horse-tail, or, as it is called by the French Canadians, 'prèle', used to be considered excellent horse feed, and when possible the Hudson's Bay Company's brigades were halted where it was abundant."

1926-7 Densmore CHIPPEWA 379. "Rushes were tied in small bundles and used for scouring utensils, the two varieties thus being used being *Equisetum hyemale* and *E. praealtum*. . .366. Burned as a disinfectant."

1923 H. Smith MENOMINI 34. "The water in which these are boiled is used to cure kidney troubles, and is drunk by women after childbirth to clear up the system."

1928 H. Smith MESKWAKI 220. "The Meskwaki drink an infusion of the whole plant as a cure for men or women of gonorrhea. . .273. This plant is fed to the Meskwaki ponies to make them fat. It is said that they will fatten on this food in about a week."

1933 H. Smith OJIBWE 418. "The Pillager Ojibwe, besides using this for a medicine, employ a handful of the stems to scour their kettles and pans."

1945 Rousseau MOHAWK transl. 33. "An infusion of the roots is used by the old men 'when the urine is too red.'"

1955 Mockle Quebec transl. 20. "Even though this species is not used in popular medicine, it is interesting to note that the stems, strongly incrusted with silica, used to be used to clean copper vases and to polish metal."

FIELD HORSETAIL   *Equisetum arvense* L.

This horsetail has two kinds of stems. In the early spring a single hollow stem with 10-12 smooth ridges and sheaths that are 5-10 mm long and have twelve brown teeth, is found. At its tip is a cone that is covered with cases containing spores. This stem dies and a new stem appears that has fine, jointed, branches. The distance between the main stem and the first joint on a branch is longer than the length of the sheath it is growing from. The central cavity of this main stem is 1/4 the diameter of the stem.

Range. Cosmopolitan in moist or dry sandy soil. The roots can go down as far as one meter and run for long distances.

Common Names. Bottle brush, horse-pipes, snake-pipes, mare's tail, joint grass.

1830 Rafinesque 217. "Astringent and diuretic, good in hematuria, gonorrhea, phthisis.&c."

1920 Fyles 11. "The harmfulness of field horsetail has for many years been the subject of much discussion and difference of opinion, but in Canada it was found to be the cause of much loss. The toxic principle has not been determined. . .Horses suffer most from eating this weed in hay, particularly young horses. It is also known to be injurious to sheep, but there is a difference of opinion as to its effect on cattle. The weed does not appear to be as poisonous when eaten in the fresh green state."

1928 H. Smith MESKWAKI 272. "This plant is gathered and fed to captive wild geese. It is said it will make them fat in a week's time."

1932 H. Smith OJIBWE 368. "The Pillager Ojibwe use the whole plant to make a tea to cure the dropsy. . .400. Gather this for their domesticated ducks to eat and also to feed their ponies, to make their coats glossy."

1933 H. Smith POTAWATOMI 55. "The whole plant was used by the Forest Potawatomi to make a tea for the treatment of kidney and bladder trouble. They claim that it is very good to cure lumbago. . .one local name is 'squeaky noiseweed'. . .among the whites the infusion of the plant has been used as a wash for putrid wounds and ulcers."

1945 Rousseau MOHAWK transl. 33. "An infusion of the roots is given to teething infants mixed with the tips of year old hazel. Field horsetail is a remedy one shouldn't abuse. One knows that the dry hay of this plant mixed with oats causes horses that eat it a sickness (equitosis) known in Quebec as 'chambranle.'"

1955 Mockle, Quebec, transl. 20. "The plant is used in decoction as a diuretic, hemostatic and remineraliser. It is particularly rich in silica and salts of potassium and contains traces of a toxic alkaloid, palustrine (or equisetine), a saponoside only slightly toxic, equisetonoside. . .Manske and Marion have found traces of l-nicotine."

1968 Forsyth England 25. "It has been shown that an enzyme, thiaminase, which is capable of destroying Vitamin B_1 is present in horsetail as well as in braken. . .horses poisoned by either plant respond favourably to treatment with aneurin (Vitamin B_1)"

1970 Bye IROQUOIS mss. Growth said to indicate where to find water.

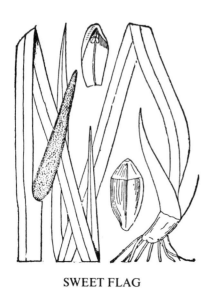

SWEET FLAG

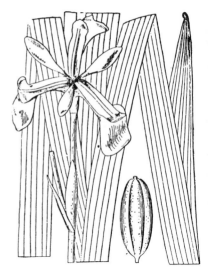

BLUE FLAG

BLUE FLAG   *Iris versicolor* L. Iridaceae
Thick creeping rhizomes, from which leaves grow 20-80 cm tall, straight and stiff, over 1 cm
wide, purplish at the base. The 6-8 cm wide flowers are on short stems, their petals violet blue,
variegated with yellow, green and white. The seed capsule is three sided, its inside shining, 3.5-5
cm long.
Range. s. Lab., Nfld., N.B., N.S., P.E.I., Que., to James Bay, Ont., Man., s. to Va. and Minn. in
wet places, marshes, meadows, shores, pools on rocks.
Common names. Wild iris, poison or water flag, snake-liver or flag lily, flower de luce.
1475 Bjornnson Icelandic mss. Larsen transl. 142. "Iris has blue color and is hot and dry in the
second degree. Its power is all in the root. One shall cut it in round sections and draw on a
thread each piece separately so that they do not touch, and hang them in the shade; and that will
scarcely dry in a twelfth-month. With wine it is good to drink for a cough and it makes one
sleep. If this herb is crushed fine and drunk with wine, it is good for pussy boils in the heart
roots. If one drink it with a little water and a little wine, that is good for a bad humor. But drunk
with vinegar, it helps cramps in the stomach. So also it helps against poison. If crushed fine and
drunk with wine, it is good for cramps. If its root is crushed and drunk, it softens a hard member.
If this herb is put in a man's anus, it is good for pain of the thighs. If the root is crushed and
applied below on a woman, it purges the afterbirth from her. If crushed with honey and applied
to a bone which is without flesh, then flesh grows fully over that bone. If one mixes a third of
white hellebore and two parts of this herb with honey and puts it upon his face, that cleanses it of
freckles and all blotches."
1749 Kalm Fort Nicholson October the 30th. 606. "Colonel Lydius related how the Indians
make use of the iris root as a remedy for sores on the legs. This cure is prepared as follows. They
take the root, wash it clean, boil it a little, then crush it between a couple of stones. They spread
this crushed root as a poultice over the sores and at the same time rub the leg with the water in
which the root is boiled. Mr. Lydius said that he had seen great cures brought about by the use
of this remedy. It is the blue iris, which is extremely common here in Canada, that is used for this
purpose."
1785 Cutler. "A decoction of fresh roots is a powerful cathartic and will sometimes produce
evacuations when other means fail; but it is too drastic for common use. The juice of the fresh
roots may be given in doses of 60-80 drops every two hours. The root loses most of its acrimony
by drying."
1791 W. Bartram 361. [Writing of the Creek Indian town of Attasse] "The town was
fasting. . .taking medicine to avert a grievous calamity of sickness. [They had] laid in the grave an

abundance of their citizens. They fast seven or eight days during which time they eat and drink nothing but a meagre gruel, made of a little corn flour and water, taking at the same time by way of medicine or physic, a strong decoction of the roots of *Iris versicolor*, which is a powerful cathartic. They hold this root in high estimation, every town cultivates a little plantation of it, having a large artificial pond just without the town planted and almost overgrown with it."

1817-20 Bigelow 158. "The root has a nauseous taste and when swallowed or held in the mouth even in small quantities, it leaves behind a powerful sense of heat and acrimony. . .Having myself formerly made use of this root in dispensary practice, I can bear testimony to its efficacy as a medicine, though not altogether to its convenience. A small quantity of the recent roots. . .are generally certain and active in their operation on the bowels. They are apt to occasion a distressing nausea like sea sickness. . .The activity of this article is diminished by age."

1830 Rafinesque 232. "Flower de luce. . .Roots of all more or less medical. *I versicolor* or common blue flag, chiefly used: roots sweetish, mucilaginous, taste nauseous subacrid, it contains white resin and fecula. Cathartic, diuretic and astringent. Much esteemed by the Southern tribes, and kept in ponds for use, as a purgative; very active, a few grains of the fresh root operates on the bowels with much nausea, 60 drops of the juice are drastic, milder when dry. In large doses drastic and emetic; formerly used in syphilis and hydrophobia. The decoction in sore mouth, ulcers and wounds as a wash. . .The leaves used for many diseases of children, being milder, purgative and vermifuge. The sweet blossoms still better, their syrup similar and equal to that of violets, pectoral, laxative, & c. The seeds may be used like coffee, eq. of Okra seeds."

1859-61 Gunn 751. "The root is the part used. It is a powerful and valuable alterative as an antimercurial and anti-venereal remedy. It is generally used in combination with other alteratives, to form a sirop or tincture. . .It is also cathartic and diuretic, and by some regarded as an antidote for worms. It is good in dropsy. . .is also good in scrofula, syphilis, in chronic rheumatism, chronic affections of the liver, spleen and kidneys, to be given in smaller doses. . .Like mercury, it seems to act more specifically on the glands throughout the system, exciting them to a healthy and increased action, yet without any of the bad effects of mercury. . .There is also a concentrated article made from this root, called Iridin, in the form of a soft extract."

1868 Can. Pharm. J. 6; 83-5. *Iris versicolor*, the rhizome included in list Can. medicinal plants.

1884 Holmes-Haydon CREE Hudson Bay 303. "The use of . . .*Iris versicolor* as a cholagogue and purgative approaches closely to present medical practice."

1892 Millspaugh 173. "Iris was highly esteemed by the Aborigines of this country, as a remedy for gastric disturbances, and also by laymen as a domestic remedy, when pytalism [mercury] was considered necessary. The fresh root pounded to a pulp is considered and justly, one of the best poultices that can be applied to a felon, often quickly relieving the pain, even when suppuration is far advanced. It will generally, discuss the affection, if applied early in its development. . .Irisin or Iridin, an acrid resinoid body, results as a constant factor in all the analyses so far made. Iris acts powerfully upon the gastro-intestinal tract, the liver, and especially the pancreas; causing burning sensations and a high state of congestion. . .Upon the nervous system, its action is marked. . .by the severe toxic neuralgia of the head, face and limbs."

1915 Speck MONTAGNAIS 315. "The blue flag is crushed and mixed with flour to be made into a poultice to be placed on any sort of pain." [See Sweet flag, there is a confusion of use reported.].

1920 Fyles 26. "The rootstock is poisonous. It contains the acrid resinous substance Irisin or Iridin. . .It is often mistaken for the sweet flag (*Acorus calamus*) which is not poisonous. . .When in flower the two plants are so dissimilar that they could never be taken for one another, but in the autumn when the roots are gathered, nothing remains but the upper portion of the plants. Even then, however, they may be distinguished by their odour, the sweet flag being pleasant, aromatic, while the blue flag is unpleasant and nauseous."

1926-7 Densmore CHIPPEWA 366. A poultice of the root is applied externally to a swelling. It is said to be very strong medicine.

1928 Parker SENECA 11. Sedative use Iris. . .12. Bruises use iris wash.

1928 H. Smith MESKWAKI 224. "The root is used for colds and lung trouble. The freshly macerated root is used as a poultice for burns and sores. . .195. Mixed with the seeds of the yellow water lily and the berries of wild sarsaparilla it makes a medicine for a sore throat."

1932 H. Smith OJIBWE 371. "The Flambeau use a half inch of the root boiled in water as a quick physic. Under the name 'milk root' the Pillager use a little piece of the root in boiling water, drinking a tablespoonful and a half as an emetic and physic. . .430. Both Flambeau and

Pillager Ojibwe use this as a charm against snakes and claim that Indians all over the country use it the same way. When the Ojibwe go out blueberrying all day, every one carries a piece of it in his clothes and will handle it every little while to perpetuate the scent. They believe that snakes will shun them while so protected. They say that the Arizona Indians use it when they hold their snake dances and are never struck as long as their clothes are fumigated with it. They also chew it to get the odor into their mouths, preparatory to taking rattlesnakes into their teeth. The rattlesnake never offers to bite them so long as the scent of the Blue Flag persists."

1933 H. Smith POTAWATOMI 60. "Use the root to make poultices to allay inflammation...121. The leaves are used to weave mats and baskets."

1945 Rousseau MOHAWK transl. 67. "Two sorts are distinguished by the Mohawks, a small one and a large one. Their rhizomes are macerated and mixed with a little hot water to make a cataplasm which is used for blood poisoning provoked by contusions."

1945 Raymond TETE DE BOULE transl. 129. "The crushed roots are applied to burns and sores."

1955 Mockle Quebec transl. 30. "The rhizome is used in small doses as a cathartic, vermifuge and diuretic. For external use it is put on as a cataplasm for blood poisoning provoked by contusions."

1964 Rousseau transl. 302. "Among the other dye-plants used by the Indians of Quebec are...the leaves of the blue flag (*Iris versicolor*)...for various shades of green."

Iris versicolor yields the drug named Blue Flag. It is the source of the "iridin" of commerce. It is purgative, diuretic and emetic. (T. E. Wallis 1967:396).

Iris versicolor apparently possesses the ability to increase the rate of fat catabolism. It was used in India in the treatment of obesity (Lewis and Elvin-Lewis 1977:212).

SWEET FLAG   *Acorus calamus* L. Araceae

This arum has a thickened end and a long rootstock which has numerous thin rootlets growing from it into the wet mud. The root stock when cut is pinkish or pale red inside and has an aromatic smell. When eaten it has a strong biting and pleasant taste. The glossy, yellow-green leaves are 8-25 mm wide and up to 2 m tall, erect, sharp pointed and sharp edged with a rigid mid-vein running up their whole length. The spathe resembles the leaves, is up to 80 cm long. The cylinder bearing the mass of yellowish brown flowers is up to 9 cm long and 2 thick. It grows about halfway up the three angled stem. In our range the fruit is usually abortive.

Range. N.B., N.S., P.E.I., Que., Ont., to James Bay, to B.C., s. to Wash., Ida., Mont. and Tex. Also in Europe and Asia in moist open places.

Common names. Calamus, flag-root, myrtle flag, beewort, muskrat root.

1609 Lescarbot-Erondelle Acadia 86. "We saw there, [Port du Mouton], being a sandy land...*calamus odoratus*, angelica, and other simples."

1633 Gerarde-Johnson 64. "The decoction of the root of Calamus drunke provoketh urine, helpeth the paine in the side, liver, spleen, and brest; convulsions, gripings, and burstings; it easeth and helpeth the pissing by drops. It is of great effect, being put in broth, or taken in fumes through a close stoole, to provoke womens naturall accidents. The juice strained with a little honey, taketh away the dimnes of the eyes, and helpeth much against poyson, the hardnesse of the spleene, and all infirmities of the bloud. The root boyled in wine, stamped and applied plaisterwise unto the cods, doth wonderfully abate the swelling of the same, and helpeth all hardnesse and collections of humors. The quantitie of two scruples and an halfe of the root drunke in four ounces of Muskadel, helpeth them that be bruised with grievous beating, or falls. The root is with good success mixed with counterpoysons. In our age it is put into Eclegma's, that is, medicines for the lungs, and especially when the lungs and chest are apprest with raw and cold humors. The root of this preserved is very plesant to the taste and comfortable to the stomacke and heart; so that the Turks at Constantinople take it fasting in the morning, against the contagion of the corrupt aire."

1650 Representation New. Neth. 298. "The medicinal plants found in New Netherlands up to the present time, by little search, as far as they have come to our knowledge, consist principally of...sweet flag...[among over 35 others named]."

1820's Materia Medica Edinburgh-Toronto mss. 27. *Acorus calamus*, grows in marshy situations in this [Great Britain] & other countries of Europe. Has a faint aromatic smell & warm bitterish taste. Its flavour resides in its essential oil. It has been used as a Tonic in Intermittent Fever & enters into the combinations of Bitter infusions and tinctures.

1828 Rafinesque 28. "The roots are the most essential part. They form an article of trade in China, Malabar, Turkey. In the early stage of the North American Colonies, it was exported to England; and it is even now occasionally sent abroad. . .Cattle will not eat this plant, and it is noxious to insects; the leaves, therefore, may be used to advantage against moths and worms. This is owing to their strong smell. Leather can be tanned by the whole plant. . .The roots are warm, aromatic, pungent and bitter. . .The infusion in wine or spirits becomes bitter, but acquires a nauseous flavour. The infusion in water preserves the fine smell, and becomes pleasantly warm and bitter. It is useful in disorders of the stomach, flatulency, vertigo, cholics, dyspepsia, &c. candied roots and the extract or chewing the roots and swallowing the juice are efficient in those cases. The warm infusion. . .cures the wind colic of infants, sailors, &c. . .When the root is masticated, a copious salivation is produced, which has cured the toothache. Children are fond of this root in many places, and may be indulged with it; the taste is spicy and pleasant. . .This root enters into many compound preparations, theriaca, mithradate, &c. . .262. It contains also fecula and extractive; decoction destroys its activity."

1859-61 Gunn 765. "Called also sweet Flag. . .It is generally cultivated. . .It is a stimulating, aromatic tonic. It it most useful, perhaps, in cases of flatulent colic, especially for children, and should be used in the form of a tea. A sirup made of Calamus is an excellent substitute for such injurious articles as Bateman's Drops, and Godfrey's Cordial."

1868 Can. Pharm. J. 6; 83-5. *Acorus calamus*, sweet flag the rhizome, included in list of Can. medicinal plants.

1884 Holmes-Haydon CREE Hudson Bay 302. "Pow-e-men-arctic (Fire or Bitter Pepper Root). This is the rhizome of *Acorus calamus* L., or a nearly allied species, and is used for coughs. The rhizome is rather more slender than met with in this country [England], being only about one third of an inch in diameter, but seems to be quite as aromatic and pungent. It is not a little singular that there is hardly a country where this plant grows that the rhizome is not used in medicine."

1894 Household Guide Toronto 123. "Sweet Flag is recommended for pain in the stomach or bowels. It can be taken in the form of a tea, sweetened with a little sugar, or the root may be eaten without any preparation."

1915 Speck PENOBSCOT 305. "The root of sweet flag (*Acorus calamus*), 'muskrat root' (Penobscot and Nanticoke), as a cure for cholera is based on the belief that, serving as the diet of the muskrat and causing its excrements to be meager, the root will have the same effect on man. . .This is perhaps the most important herb in Penobscot pharmocology, and knowledge was imparted to a man by the muskrat spirit in a dream. A plague of sickness was sweeping the Indians away. There was no one to cure the people. One night a man was visited by a Muskrat in a dream. The Muskrat told him that he was a root and where to find him. The man awoke, sought the muskrat root, made a medicine of it, and cured the people of the plague. Sections of the dried root are cut up strung together, and hung up for preservation in nearly every house. . .311. One of the numerous functions of the Penobscot panacea, sweet flag or muskrat root, is to keep away disease in general by being steamed through the house. It is thought to 'kill' sickness. Also while travelling, when disease is likely to attack a person he may keep it away by chewing a piece of the root. . .312. Sweet flag is one of the seven herbs used before the sweat bath. . .316. Sweet flag is employed as a panacea by the Micmac-Montagnais as among the Penobscot. . .320. It is one of the ingredients of a Mohegan spring tonic."

1919 Sturtevant 23. "*Acorus calamus*. The rhizomes are used by confectioners as a candy, by perfumers in the preparation of aromatic vinegar, by rectifiers to improve the flavor of gin and to give a peculiar taste to certain varieties of beer. In Europe and America, the rhizomes are sometimes cut into slices and candied or otherwise made into a sweetmeat. These rhizomes are to be seen on sale on the Street corners of Boston and are frequently chewed to sweeten the breath."

1924 Youngken 488. "In early days the Indians mixed the powdered rhizome and roots with powdered red willow bark and used the mixture for smoking. All of the Indians employed the rhizomes as a carminative. . .Among the Teton-Dakota, warriors chewed the rhizome to a paste which they rubbed on their faces to prevent excitement and fear when confronted with an enemy. The Cheyenne tribe believed the rhizome when chewed and rubbed on the skin to be good for any malady. They tied portions of the rhizome to the dress, blanket or necklet of their children to keep away the night spirits. The leaves were worn by various tribes as garlands."

1926-7 Densmore CHIPPEWA 344. "The measure for preparing this root was according to the age of the patient, the measure being the length of the index finger, whether an infant or an adult. This quantity of the root was scalded (not boiled), and taken warm. Dose about a half cupful. Same dosage for all physics. . .340. For a cold snuff up nostril the pulverized root or drink a decoction of it. . .342. For a sore throat children gargled with the decoction; adults chewed the root. . .For a toothache the dried root was chewed or the decoction drunk."

1928 Parker SENECA 11. Calamus taken as a carminative.

1923 H. Smith MENOMINI 22. "The root of this plant is used to cure cramps in the stomach. It is considered a very powerful remedy and is used only in very minute quantities. The measure of a dose is the length of the finger joint. It is also called. . .'a simple penetrator.' It is a good physic for the whole system, clearing the bile and all, but if too much is taken, the Menomini say that it will kill the patient. The blade of the plant was also used in constructing the wigwam."

1928 H. Smith MESKWAKI 201. "McIntosh said the Menomini call it 'Kaswe'ka', but we remember it under the simple name of 'we'ke'. The Meskwaki use it as a physic, and in combination with other medicines it is a cure for burns. . .Specimen 3612 of the Dr. Jones collection is calamus. . .the root is boiled and then drunk by one afflicted with tuberculosis or with a cough. It appears again in his specimen 5149. . .in which the root is boiled and made into a drink for a cramp expected in the stomach."

1932 H. Smith OJIBWE 355. "The root of Sweet Flag is a quick acting physic, supposed to act in half a day. Bearskin cautioned the writer that no more than one and a half inches was to be used, as more would make one ill, and even this much is quite harsh. The Pillager Ojibwe recognize the Sweet Flag under the name 'we'ke', which is the same word used by another tribe for the Yellow Water lily, and by another for the Blue Flag. John Peper said that the root was used for curing a cold in the throat or for curing a cramp in the stomach. . .428. The root tea of this is used by Big George, Flambeau Ojibwe, on his gill net to bring him a fine catch of white fish. The net still smelled of the calamus root after being in the water more than twelve hours, and he caught 121 white fish in one pull of the net. . .It is combined with the root of Sarsaparilla."

1933 H. Smith POTAWATOMI 39. "Sweet Flag is a valued medicine and used for various ailments. The dried root is powdered and snuffed up the nose to cure catarrh. It is also one of the ingredients of a remedy to stop a hemorrhage. The formula for this remedy is-chips of the heartwood from a four-inch piece of ironwood, and arbor-vitae, root of sweet flag and a handful of the root bark of the common shining willow (*Salix lucida*). These materials are placed in a vessel covered with two quarts of water, which is boiled down to a pint. One tablespoonful of this mixture is taken every hour until the hemorrhage stops. This is one of the bitterest medicines that the Forest Potawatomi have and is described as being bitter as gall. Many of the Indians in speaking of this remedy are inclined to be cautious in the amount used and say that only a very small piece of the root is necessary."

1942 Fenton IROQUOIS 523. "Of the more important medicinal plants used among the Iroquois. . .sweet flag (*Acorus calamus*) in singing."

1945 Rousseau MOHAWK transl. 71. "The Indians distinguish three kinds. First the muskrat root, a plant with knotted rootlets that are very divided. Secondly a plant with very long brown rootlets. Thirdly a cultivated plant with white rootlets. The root of the second variety, reduced to powder, and mixed into a large quantity of hot water, it used for the grippe and chills. Go to bed immediately after having drunk the hot infusion. The root of the third variety, reduced to powder, is taken mixed in a little cold water in half tablespoonful doses when one feels ill after having eaten a meal. For adolescents, whose blood does not circulate very fast, an infusion of *Acorus calamus* (I don't know of which variety) and some *Myriophyllum*, [a water weed]. An infusion of plantain and the roots of the second variety of *Acorus* for painful respiration caused by pains in the bottom of the chest. For children who cry suddenly in the night, give an infusion of *Acorus calamus* (I do not know of which variety) and the entire plant of *Sagittaria latifolia* [arrowhead]. I was not able to see these three varieties of sweet flag. The first two may represent phases of the same plant. On the other hand they could perhaps be species of different families. The third form certainly seems doubtful; there is no sweet flag cultivated in Quebec. One knows that the Indians often base their taxonomy on utilitarian or ecological characteristics, and do not hesitate to place together species of different families. Sweet flag is one of the plants that is most used in the popular medicine of French Canada, above all for neuralgia and digestive troubles. In the district of Montmagny, an infusion of the root of sweet flag cured the great fever, on the condition it was caught in time. Many of the tribes of northeastern America, above all the Missouri and the Ojibwa, use the plant in the treatment of the grippe. For the Penobscot, the Micmac and the Montagnais of Newfoundland, and the Caughnawaga and almost all the Indians of North America, it is a panacea. When it does not grow in a region, they do not hesitate to import it. Thus the Cheyenne, an Algonquin tribe, obtained it from the Sioux."

1931 Grieve England 728. "In powder, Calamus root, on account of its spicy flavour serves as a substitute for cinnamon, nutmeg and ginger. It is also said to be used by snuff manufacturers and to scent hair powder and in tooth powders. . .The highly aromatic volatile oil is largely used in perfumery. . .In the United States, Calamus was also formerly used by country people as an ingredient in making wine bitters."

1955 Mockle Quebec transl. 26. "The rhizome possesses aromatic, tonic and emetic properties. It is used mostly as an aromatic, stomachic, and carminative. For this purpose an infusion of the fresh root, or the dried root mashed, is used. It has been held that chewing the root lessens the pain of the toothache."

To candy the rootstock it is cut in very thin slices and boiled, drained and boiled again in a thick syrup. It can be very strong. The bottom of the stem is like candied ginger when properly prepared (Medsgar 1966:175).

The rhizome contains an aromatic, volatile oil whose chief constituent is asaryl aldehyde and acorin. It is stimulant and tonic and has been used for ague and atonic dyspepsia (T. E. Wallis 1964:396).

1971 Willaman & Li 740. *Acorus* sp. the whole plant above ground contains choline.

The Indians of Montana are reported to have boiled the root of sweet flag in water and drunk the water to bring about abortion (Weiner 1972:11).

Asarone and beta-asarone in the root oils of sweet flag seem to be responsible for the strong visual hallucinations that can result from chewing the root. The Cree of Canada are reputed to have used it for this purpose (Emboden 1972:53).

The root should be collected in the autumn and not peeled as this lowers its essential oil content.

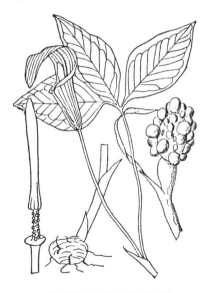

JACK IN THE PULPIT

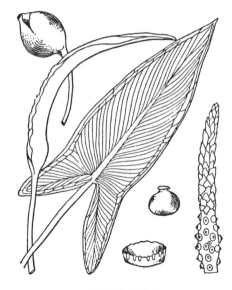

TUCKAHOE

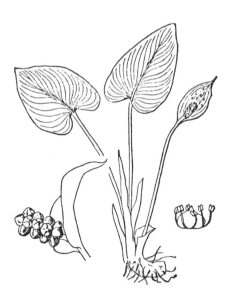

WATER ARUM

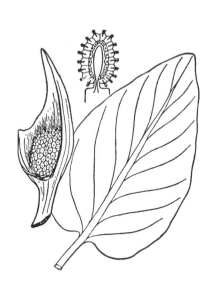

SKUNK CABBAGE

JACK IN THE PULPIT *Arisaema atrorubens* (Ait.) Blume Araceae (*A. triphyllum Arum t.*)
From a sheath at its base grow two leaf stems and a flowering stem. The leaves have three leaflets
at the end of their 30-60 (150) cm stems. The flowering stem is 3-20 cm tall ending in a tube covered at the bottom end with tiny yellow flowers. A leaf, the spathe, green with purple stripes in
some varieties, curls around the flowering part of the tube and bends its end over the open top of
the tube, (the preacher in the pulpit). The flowers are followed by berries, green becoming bright
red and poisonous. The spathe can be all green or all purple in other varieties, the underground
stem of the plant ends in a corm, potatoe like, which should never be eaten raw.

Range. N.B., N.S., Que., Ont., to n. Lake Superior, se. Man., s. to e. Kan., Mo., and S.C. in moist woods and thickets.
Common names. Indian turnip, wild turnip, marsh pepper, bog onion, brown dragon, starchwort, wake-robin, dragon root, cuckoo pint.

TUCKAHOE *Peltandra virginica* (L.) Schott & Endl. (*Arum v.*)

From a fibrous or subtuberous root, a long-stemmed leaf, shaped like an arrow head, grows up to 20 cm long, bright green, strongly veined. The tube bearing the flowers is nearly as long as the leaf. The spathe, tightly furled around the tube, leathery, green with white or pale margins, up to 20 cm long, just longer than the tube. The berries green.
Range. sw. Que., s. Ont., to N.Y., and N.H., s. to Tex. and Fla. in swamps or shallow water.
Common names. Poison arum, virginia wake robin.

WATER ARUM *Calla palustris* L.

This plant creeps over the bogs often making large mats with its green leaves. The leaf stems are 10-20 cm bearing one 5-10 cm long leaf. The flowering stem ends in a cylinder surrounded by a pure white leaf (spathe) which turns away from the flowering and fruiting tube. The berries are bright red at the end of the tube.
Range. Lab., Nfld., P.E.I., N.B., N.S., Que., to James Bay, Ont., Man., Mackenzie dist., Sask., Yukon and Alaska, s. to Colo., Tex. and Fla. and in Eurasia.
Common names. Wild calla, swamp-robin, female or water dragon.

1590 Harriot Virginia Indians 17. "Coscushaw, some of our company took to bee that kinde of roote which the Spaniards in the West Indies call Cassauy, whereupon also many called it by that name: it groweth in very muddie pooles and moist groundes. Being dressed according to the countrey maner, it maketh good bread, and also a good sponemeate, and is used very much by the inhabitants: The juice of this root is poison, and therefore heede must be taken before anything be made therewithal: Either the root must bee first sliced and dried in the Sunne, or by the fire, and then being pounded into floure wil make good bread: or els while they are green they are to bee pared, cut into pieces and stampt: loves of the same to be laid neere or over the fire until it be soure, and then being well pounded again, bread or spone meate very good in taste, and holsome may be made thereof."

1612 Capt. John Smith Virginia Indians 92. "The chief roote they have for foode is called Tockawhough. It groweth like a flagge in low muddy freshes. In one day a Savage will gather sufficient for a weeke. These rootes are much of the greatness and taste of Potatoes. They use to cover a great many of them with oke leaves and ferne, and then cover all with earth in the manner of a colepit; over it, on each side they continue a great fire 24 hours before they dare eat it. Raw it is no better than poison, and being roasted, except it be tender and the heat abated, or sliced and dried in the sun, mixed with sorrell and meale or such like, it will prickle and grate the throat extreamely, and yet in sommer they use it ordinarily for bread."

1624 Sagard HURON 264. "Some little Indians had some roots called *Ooxrat*, like a small turnip or bald chestnut, which they had just pulled up to take to their cabins. A young French boy, living with us, had asked them for some and had eaten one or two. At first he found the taste rather agreeable, but shortly afterwards he felt great pain in his mouth, like a burning pricking flame, and a great quantity of secretions and phlegm continually dropped from his mouth so that he thought he was about to die. In fact we did not know what to do about it, being ignorant of the cause of this symptom and fearing lest he had eaten some poisonous root. But when we spoke to the Indians about it, and asked for their advice they had the rest of the roots brought to see what they were and when they had seen and recognised them, they began to laugh, saying that there was no danger nor any evil result to be feared, but rather good, if it were not for the stinging and burning pains in the mouth. They use these roots to purge the phlegm and moisture in the head of old people and to clear the complexion; in order to avoid the stinging pain they first cook them in hot ashes and then eat them without feeling any pain afterwards; these do them all the good in the world. I am sorry that I did not bring some of them here to France on account of the use which I think would have been made of them."

1633 Gerarde-Johnson 834-5. "Cuckow pint or wake robin [*Arum maculatum* of Europe]. The faculties of cuckow pint doth differ according to the varietie of countries: for the root hereof, as

Galen doth affirm, is sharper and more biting in some countries than in others. If any man would have thicke and tough humours which are gathered in the chest and lungs to be clensed and voided out by coughing, then that Cuckow pint is best that biteth most. . .Dioscorides sheweth, that the leaves also are preserved to be eaten after they be dried and boyled. . .The most pure and white starch is made of the roots of Cuckowpint; but most hurtful to the hands of the Laundresse that hath the handling of it, for it choppeth, blistereth, and maketh the hands rough and rugged, and withal smarting."

1708 Sarrazin-Vaillant, Quebec-Paris, Boivin 1978 transl. 68. *Arisaema triphyllum.* "This plant grows in the shade in the woods. . .The corm is used in this country for stomach troubles, but it must be dried first for green it is dangerous."

1749 Kalm Philadelphia March the 17th. 260. "*Arum Virginicum.* Taw-ho and Taw-him was the Indian name of another plant, the root of which Indians eat. . .It grows in moist ground and swamps. Hogs are very fond of the roots. . .must have been extirpated in places which are frequented by hogs. The roots often grow to the thickness of a man's thigh. When they are fresh, they have a pungent taste, and are reckoned a poison in that fresh state. Nor did Indians ever venture to eat them raw, but prepared them in the following manner: they gathered a great heap of these roots, dug a great long hole; they made a great fire above it, which burnt till they thought proper to remove it; and then they dug up the roots and consumed them with great avidity. These roots, when prepared in this manner, I am told, taste like potatoes. The Indians never dry or preserve them, but always dig them fresh out of the marshes, when they want them. . .It is remarkable that the arums. . .are eaten by men in different parts of the world, though their roots, when raw, have a fiery pungent taste, and are almost poisonous in that state. How can men have learned that plants so extremely opposite to our nature were eatable, and that their poison, which burns on the tongue, can be conquered by fire? Thus the root of the *Calla palustris*, which grows in the north of Europe, is sometimes used instead of bread in an emergency. The North American Indians eat this species of arum. . .67. Mr. Bartram told me that the savages boiled the spadix and the berries of this flower [tuckahoe] and devoured them as a great delicacy. When the berries are fresh they have a harsh, pungent taste, which they lose in great measure upon boiling."

1778 Carver 519. "Wake robin is an herb that grows in swampy lands; its root resembles a small turnip, and if tasted will greatly inflame the tongue, and immediately convert it from its natural shape, into a round hard substance; in which state it will continue for some time, and during this no other part of the mouth will be affected. But when dried, it loses its astringent quality, and becomes beneficial to mankind; for if grated into cold water, and taken internally, it is very good for all complaints of the bowels."

1785 Cutler. 487. "The roots dried and powdered a medicine for asthma, can safely be given to children, 4-6 grains, adults 20 grs. It is given in a fit and repeated as case requires. The Indians told the white men of its antispasmodic use. . .The shredded roots and berries were said to have been boiled by the Indians with their venison."

1796 Simcoe 'Toronto' Diary 328. "I gathered a great many plants (including) dewberries; wild turnip, which cures a cough-it is like arum."

1817-20 Bigelow 59. [*Arisaema atrorubens*] "An acrid stimulant. . .The root contains pure white faecula, resembling the finest arrowroot or starch. To procure this, the fresh root should be reduced to a pulp and placed in a strainer. Repeated portions of cold water should then be poured on it. . .leaving the fibrous portion behind. The faecula thus obtained, loses its acrimony on being thoroughly dried, and forms a very white, delicate and nutritive substance. . .The Laplanders prepare a wholesome bread from the acrid root of *Calla palustris*."

1820's Materia Medica Edinburgh-Toronto mss. *Arum maculatum* [of Europe] resembles pellitory & may be used for the same purposes but its pungency is unpleasant. Internally it has been used as a remedy in paralysis & rheumatism.

1828 Rafinesque 68. "*Arum triphyllum* The whole plant, and particularly the root, is violently acrid, and even caustic to the tongue, but not to the skin. It burns worse than capiscum or Cayenne pepper. The active principle is a peculiar substance, Aroine, highly volatile, having no affinity with water, alcohol, oil or acids, and becoming an inflammable gas by heat or distillation. The roots yield one fourth of their weight of a pure amylaceous matter, like starch or arrow-root, or a fine white delicate nutritive fecula, by the same process as Cassava or *Jatropha manihot*. . .The fresh roots are too caustic to be used internally, unless much diluted, and when dry they are often inert, unless they have been dried very quickly, or kept buried in sand or earth. It must be used in substance mixed with milk or molasses, since it does not impart its pungency to any liquor; or the fresh roots must be grated, or reduced to a pulp, with three times their weight of sugar, thus forming a conserve, the dose of which is a teaspoonful twice a day. In these forms it is useful for flatulence, cramp in the stomach, asthmatic and consumptive affections. It quickens circulation, and promises to be a useful topical stimulant when the acrid principle may be rendered available. It has been found beneficial in lingering atrophy, debilitated habits, great prostration in typhoid fevers, deep seated rheumatic pains, or pains in the breast, chronic catarrh, &c. . .263. The root is not inert when dry, and even the powder is used by Empirics with honey for coughs &c. . .It is said to kill snakes. The Indians use it for coughs with spikenard or *Aralia*, and for fevers with Snakeroots and *Prunus*. . .An ointment is made for external use in rheumatism, tinea, &c. The seeds appear to have all the properties of the root with double the strength, being less liable to lose their activity, ought to become the officinal substitute in half doses. . .126. It is asserted that the Indians can handle Rattlesnakes with impunity, after wetting their hands with the milky juice of the root of this plant *Convolvulus panduratus* or of *Arum triphyllum*."

1859-61 Gunn 810. "[The root] makes an excellent poultice in scrofulous swellings; when dried and pulverized, and mixed with honey or sirup, is a good remedy in coughs, canker, pain in the breast; and given in teaspoonful doses, of the powder, is a valuable remedy in colic. It is said to be very valuable in cases of low typhus fever. An ointment made of the fresh root and lard, is useful, I have been informed, in scald head. The ordinary dose of the powder is ten to twenty grains, two or three times a day; but I have generally found the powder or dry root to be nearly or quite inert and good for nothing! It should be made into sirup, for colds, coughs, and the like while fresh by macerating in a little vinegar, and then mixed with honey or molasses."

1868 Can. Pharm. J. 6; 83-5. *Arisaema triphyllum*, Indian turnip, the corms included in list of Can. medicinal plants.

1915 Speck PENOBSCOT 310. "Jack in the pulpit (*Arisaema triphyllum*). . .is steeped to make a liniment for general external use. The liquid is also a poison."

1915 W. R. Harris ALGONQUIN 50. "Combined with snake-root and the bark of the wild cherry tree, the Chippewa and other Algonquin tribes made use of the Indian turnip for coughs and fevers. The turnip was called by them E-haw-sho-ga (Bite the mouth). . .56. The bulb-like root of this plant has an intensely acrid taste. It was used by the Indians against colic. The whole plant is a powerful poison. I have often found it growing in the ravines and bogs around Toronto."

1916 Waugh IROQUOIS 119. "The roots of. . .Indian turnip. . .are referred to as having been used in the Iroquois area, [for food] but have been practically forgotten by present-day Iroquois."

1920 Fyles 18. "The Jack-in-the pulpit contains acrid properties. The corm is very poisonous. . .a decoction made from it has been used to kill insects."

1926-7 Densmore CHIPPEWA 360. *Arisaema triphyllum*, decoction of the root externally for sore eyes.

1923 H. Smith MENOMINI 23. "The fiery root of this plant [*A. triphyllum*] used as a poultice for sore eyes. The writer. . .was unable to discover how such a poultice felt, as the informant had never tried it himself."

1928 H. Smith MESKWAKI 202. "This [Indian turnip] is one of the diagnostic medicines. The central part of the seed, divested of pulp, is dropped into a cup of water. If it goes around four times clockwise, before dropping to the bottom, the patient will recover. But if it goes down the fourth time, or fails to float at all, the patient will die. Charles Keosatok told us that the Meskwaki used to chop this root fine and put it in the meat they fed to their Sioux enemies and others. A few hours after eating, this would cause them much pain and they would die. The root is not used now by the Meskwaki, since they gave up their medicine lodge, but it was formerly used by them to reduce the swelling from a rattlesnake bite. . .When mixed with a portion of a plant gall found on *Solidago canadensis* (Canada goldenrod) and sweet flag it is used in very small doses to cure insomnia. . .272. This root was one reserved largely for use in war. When the Meskwaki were at war with the Sioux, they would often abandon vessels of meat cooked with this root. The meat was appetizing but some time after the Sioux had partaken of it they would have great stomach pains and would shortly die."

1932 H. Smith OJIBWE 356. "The root was said by John Peper. . .to be used in treating sore eyes."

1933 H. Smith POTAWATOMI 95. "Nicolas Perrot found them using this root *A. triphyllum* for food. . .*Calla palustris.* 40. The Forest Potawatomi find that the root of the Water arum when pounded and applied as a poultice to swellings is very efficacious in reducing them."

1945 Rousseau MOHAWK transl. 69. "To render women sterile, infusion of the roots *A. triphyllum* reduced to powder and mixed with that of *Asclepias syriaca*." [see milkweed for details].

1955 Mockle Quebec transl. 26. "*A triphyllum*, the corm used for anemea, stomach troubles and colics; crushed it is applied externally to produce vesication. The juice of the crushed corms is used to cure skin diseases. The corms contain sitosterol in the proportion of 0.5 g/kg of material dried. . .*calla palustris* astringent."

1968 Forsyth England 109. "*Arum maculatum* [European species]. Children are attracted to the berries which are very poisonous. . .root contains an acrid juice which is an acute irritant when applied to the skin. . .death can result from eating it raw. First aid treatment an emetic and demulcents. . .Food preparations from the baked and powdered root were known as Portland arrowroot and Portland sago."

SKUNK CABBAGE   *Symplocarpus foetidus* (L.) Nutt. Araceae

The spathe (leaf that covers the cylinder that bears the flowers and seeds) appears very early in the spring and can grow 8-15 cm tall. It is thick, swollen, leathery, pale-green, closely streaked and spotted with purple or reddish brown. It envelopes the cylinder which is covered with small purple flowers, and may be underground. Later the leaves grow, as do cabbage leaves, on short stalks from the root. They are up to 60 cm long, bright green and clustered on the root stalk. The plant smells like a skunk when in flower.

Range. N.B., N.S., s. Que., Ont., se. Man., s. to Iowa, Tenn., and Ga. and in e. Asia. Feb.-April in swamps and muddy ground.

Common names. Meadow cabbage, foetid hellebore.

1708 Sarrazin-Vaillant, Quebec-Paris, Boivin 1978 transl. 24. "It smells like garlic, but more foetid. I believe it is suppurative. . .Its root is useful for the suppuration of tumors." A note in the hand of J.-F. Gaultier in the margin reads:- "The inhabitants of Canada use the root of this *arum* for the flux in cows and all livestock. It is also used for the flux in children. It is put in their 'bouillies'. The cooked root is good to eat.'

1749 Kalm Philadelphia March 13th. 257. "Skunk cabbage. . .Dr. Colden told me that he had employed the root in all cases where the root of the arum is used, especially against scurvy etc."

1778 Carver 518. "Skunk cabbage or Poke is an herb that grows in moist and swampy places. The leaves of it are about a foot long, and six inches broad, nearly oval, but rather pointed. The roots are composed of great numbers of fibers, a lotion of which is made use of by the people in the colonies for the cure of the itch. There issues a strong musky smell from this herb, something like the animal of the same name described, and on that account it is so termed."

1785 Cutler. Indians taught white man the uses of this plant.

1817-20 Bigelow 47-8. "An acrid principle exists in the root even when perfectly dry, producing an effect like that of Arum and Ranunculi. . .The seeds when dry are reduced to half their former size, and in this state they have a tough waxy consistence and an animal odour. They contain fixed oil in abundance, which is easily forced out of them by expression. . .They burn with an oily smoke, leaving behind a large coal. . .Cutler was the first who recommended its use in asthmatic cases. . .since the recommendation. . .many country physicians have employed the root in asthma, catarrh, and chronic coughs, with evident benefit. . .Some caution. . .is requisite in its management. . .not only vomiting but headache, vertigo, and temporary blindness [may result]."

1830 Rafinesque 231-2. "The syrup is a mild one, used in senile catarrh. . .The leaves are less powerful, but the seeds most active, requiring smaller doses. . .Leaves externally used for wounds and ulcers, herpes and cutaneous affections, bruised and applied; also used to dress blisters, promoting the discharge. It is said that bears are fond of this plant and feed on it. The lotion of the root cures the itch."

1851 Schoolcraft 4; 502. Skunk cabbage used as a palliative by Indians for asthma.

1859-61 Gunn 857. "The root is the part used, and is a valuable expectorant and antispasmodic."

1868 Can. Pharm. J. 6; 83-5. *Symplocarpus Foetidus*, skunk cabbage, the root and seeds included in list of Can. medicinal plants.

1892 Millspaugh 169. "The skunk cabbage is not official in the U.S. Ph. having been dismissed.

In the Eclectic Materia Medica the use of this drug, especially compounded with others is considerable. The fresh or dried fleshy fruits divested of the seeds, and mashed with an equal portion of Indian meal, have been used in this neighbourhood [Central New York] to a great extent, and with excellent success, as a poultice for caking mammae, promptly, in many instances coming under my notice, dissipating the hardness and restoring the glands to health."

1915 Speck DELAWARE 320. "Skunk cabbage for colds."

1922 Wallis MICMAC Used the plant for headache.

1916 Waugh IROQUOIS 118. "Young leaves and shoots cooked like spinach and eaten. . .119. The roots. . . are referred to as having been used in the Iroquois area for food, but have been practically forgotten by present-day Iroquois."

1923 H. Smith MENOMINI 23. "This is the root that the bear likes to dig and eat. It is employed as a poultice. The root is first dried, then powdered and then sprayed over the surface of the wound. It is also used as a seasoner with other medicines. . .They give the use as a remedy for cramps. The root hairs alone are used for stopping hemorrhages. Skunk root is one of the ingredients of the tatooing set. Tattooing was not employed by the Menomini so much for the design as for the treatment of diseases, being a talisman against their return. The medicines were tattooed in over the seat of the pain. Not all the herbs used were identified for the writer did not see them growing. Among them were powdered birchbark, charcoal pigment, skunk root, deer's ear root (*Menyanthes trifoliata*), red top root (*Lobelia cardinalis*) black root (unknown), and yellow root, probably *Oxalis acetosella*. The medicines were moistened and tatooed into the flesh with the teeth of the gar pike, dipped in the medicines. The various colors stay and form a guard against the disease. After the tatooing is done, the surface is poulticed and painted with medicines. [see also under white cedar, tattooing]. Under the drug name of Dracontium, the white man has employed skunk root as a medicine. . .narcotic. . .It is probably of little value and rarely employed."

1928 H. Smith MESKWAKI 203. "Charles Keosatok accompanied the writer on a long auto trip to a springy place along the Iowa river to get this important remedy. He dug one for us and one for himself to send to his relatives in Oklahoma. The older roots, where the ends had exfoliated or perhaps been eaten off by crayfish, he explained had been eaten by the snake spirit "monito". If one were to have more than four roots of this in his possession at any one time, the snake spirit would cause the rattlesnakes to come into his house and bite the inhabitants. For this reason, he would not take more than one root, because he had three at home. The fine rootlets or root hairs were to be used in curing toothache. The leaf bases furnished a poultice to reduce swellings. The seeds themselves were medicine, but he did not know their use."

1936 Medsger 137. "My friend carefully collected the young leaves with their thick, almost white leafstalks and prepared them for cooking. In the boiling process, he changed the water two or three times. I pronounced them good. All the offensiveness had disappeared and the taste was pleasing."

1955 Mockle Quebec transl. 26. "A powerful antispasmodic. The leaves are used externally in skin diseases."

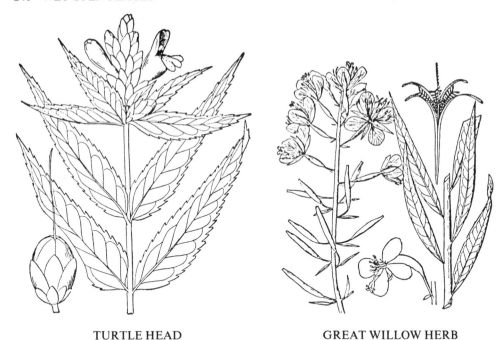

TURTLE HEAD   GREAT WILLOW HERB

TURTLEHEAD   *Chelone glabra* L. Scrophulariaceae
The stout, smooth stem is slightly foursided, 50-80 cm tall. The leaves are stalkless or almost so, opposite, up to 15 cm long with sharp, low teeth. The flowers are tubes 2.5-3.5 cm long with a mouth at one end, somewhat resembling that of a snake or turtle. They are white or faintly reddish or even purple, arranged close together on a spike 3-8 cm long.
Range. Nfld. to Minn., s. to Ga., and Ala. July-Sept. in wet woods, often with their roots in water.
Common names. Balmony, snake head, cod mouth, shell flower, fish mouth, salt-rheum weed, bitter herb.
1830 Rafinesque 118. "I have the pleasure to introduce these active plants into the Materia Medica. . .I am indebted to Dr. Lawrence of New Lebanon, for the first knowledge of their properties, and he to the Indians and Shakers. They are powerful, tonic, cathartic, hepatic, and antiherpetic. The whole plant is used, but strictly the leaves; they are extensively bitter, one of the strongest of our bitters, without any aromatic smell and very little astringency.. . .Their tincture becomes black, and the use of it dyes the urine the same color. It contains gallic acid, a peculiar resinous substance soluable in water and alcohol, similar to picrine and aloes, of a black color and very bitter taste, lignine &c. . .It is useful in many diseases, fevers, jaundice, hepatitis, eruptions of the skin &c. In small doses it is laxative, but in full doses it purges the bile and cleans the system of the morbid or superfluous bile, removing the yellowness of the skin in jaundice and liver diseases. The dose is a drachm of the powdered leaves 3 times daily. . .The Indians use a strong decoction of the whole plant in eruptive diseases, biles, hemorrhoids, sores, &c. Few plants promise to become more useful in skileful hands; it ought to be tried in yellow fever and bilious fever, the tropical liver complaint &c."
1845 Mattson 213. Plant used in composition of rheumatic drops and as a cataplasm for cancerous tumors (Hartwell 1971:213)
1854 King. Ointment of plant for inflamed tumors. (Hartwell 1971:213).
1859-61 Gunn 740. "This herb is exceedingly bitter, and has long been known in New England, as a tonic and laxative. It is employed in costiveness, dyspepsia, loss of appetite, and general languor, or debility. Given to children afflicted with worms, it will generally afford relief. It is a

valuable medicine in diseases of the liver, and in jaundice tends to remove the yellow tinge from the skin and eyes. An even teaspoonful is a dose."

1868 Can. Pharm. J. 6; 83-5. The leaves of *Chelone glabra* included in list of Can. medicinal plants.

1878 Jackson, Can. Pharm. J. 155. "In a recent list of 'Pure Medicinal Preparations prepared *in vacuo*' at New Lebanon [Shakers] occurs a preparation from *Chelone glabra* L. The plant is known as snake head or balmony and grows in damp soils. Its action is described in the catalogue above referred to: Tonic, cathartic, and anthelmintic, valuable in jaundice and hepatic diseases, likewise for the removal of worms."

1892 Millspaugh 113. "Balmony has for years been a favorite tonic, laxative and purgative, among the aborigines of North America and Thomsonian physicians; without sufficient reason however as a tonic, in the doses usually employed."

1933 H. Smith POTAWATOMI 82. "The Forest Potawatomi have no name or use for this plant to our knowledge and consider that it is a more recent plant to their region."

1971 Hartwell 213. "The leaf used in an ointment for tumors by the Potawatomi Indians. (H. Smith, Ethnobotany of Potawatomi)." [Smith said the use for tumors was by the white population. Smith gives no use of *Chelone glabra* by any Indian tribe.].

1955 Mockle Quebec Transl. 78. "The leaves are prescribed as a laxative, purgative and cathartic."

1959 Mechling MALECITE of maritime provinces of Canada used *Chelone glabra* for prevention of pregnancy.

GREAT WILLOW HERB   *Epilobium angustifolium* L. Onagraceae

A straight, smooth stem, 1-3 m tall. The leaves alternate, long and narrow to 20 cm. The many flowered spike, hairy, the flowers pink to purple with petals 1-2 cm long. The pods 3-8 cm long, finely hairy when young. The seeds with white silk attached float away when the pods split in four.

Range. Circumboreal, s. to N.J., O., n. Ill., Kans., and N.M. June-Sept. in dry and wet places often at borders of lakes. Abundant after fires.

Common names. Fire weed, rosebay, purple rocket, Indian wickup, herb wickopy, pigweed, blooming sally, french willow herb, firetop. The common name fireweed leads to confusion as *Erichtites* is also very abundant after fires and is the plant usually meant by fireweed. Also some Indians call the basswood 'wickup' as well as the great willow herb. The botanical name *Epilobium* means a flower upon a pod.

1832 Green Universal Herbal England. The young shoots are said to be eatable, although an infusion of the plant produces a stupifying effect. The pith when dried is boiled and becoming sweet, is by a proper process made into ale. . .As fodder, goats are said to be extremely fond of it. . .The down of the seeds, mixed with cotton or fur, has been manufactured into stockings, etc. (Grieve 1931:848).

1840 Sir John Richardson. The young leaves, under the name of l'herbe fret, are used by the Canadian voyagers as a potherb (Sturtevant 1919:255).

1870 Briante 36. "Take the root of the 'Indian Wickery' and make a poultice of it. It will be found to be one of the best things for old sores or inflammation."

1888 Delamare Island of Miquelon transl. 19. "The inhabitants do not use this plant even though its roots and young shoots are edible in salads and the leaves are used in Canada for making beer."

1925 Youngken 167. "An infusion of the leaves and roots was used for hemorrhage of the bowels by the Cheyenne."

1925 James Anderson 145. "The root or running stock, grated and made into a poultice was considered very healing by my late father. L'herbe froide of the Canadian French, the roots are thoroughly dessicated and pounded so as to separate the filaments from the mealy portions, then a little mixed with water. It forms a tenacious mucilage that is very efficacious as an application to ulcerous sores. In conjunction with the roots of *Smilacina racemosa*, false solomon's seal, it is used in scrofulous cases."

1926-27 Densmore CHIPPEWA 352. Fresh or dried leaves were moistened and made into a poultice and applied to bruises. The same poultice might be used to remove a sliver.

1923 H. Smith MENOMINI 43. "The root of this plant is used to make a wash for swellings."

1932 H. Smith OJIBWE 376. "Flambeau name 'slippery or soap root' The Flambeau Ojibwe say that the outer rind of this root lathers in water and they pound it to make a poultice. This is used to draw out inflammation from a boil or carbuncle. With white men, it is demulcent, tonic and astringent. It has been used internally for its tonic effects on mucous surfaces and its value in intestinal disorders."

1933 H. Smith POTAWATOMI 66. "While the Forest Potawatomi use this for medicine, its use was not explained. The Prairie Potawatomi use the root of *E. ciliatum* to make a tea to check diarrhea."

1945 Raymond TETE DE BOULE transl. 128. "The roots are boiled and applied to sore skins."

1955 Mockle Quebec transl. 65. "The mashed roots are used in cataplasms for tumors."

1966 Campbell, Best, Budd 88. "Reports vary considerably regarding the grazing value of fireweed. Sheep make good use of it, but apparently require other fodder to balance their rations. Cattle will browse it occasionally, while horses and game seldom eat it. Fireweed is excellent bee pasture."

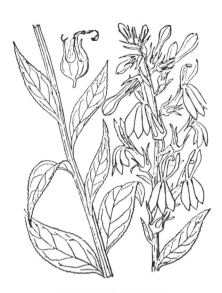

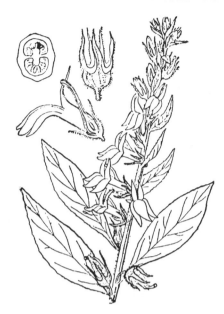

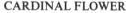

CARDINAL FLOWER   GREAT BLUE LOBELIA

GREAT BLUE LOBELIA   *Lobelia siphilitica L.* Lobeliaceae
A stout, straight, somewhat hairy stem 50-150 cm tall, the upper third with flowers. The leaves alternate, 8-12 cm long, stalkless, sometimes with hairs, finely toothed around their margins. The lowest leaves may be stalked. The flowers are blue with white markings or all blue, or white, 2.5 cm long on hairy stalks in a ridged hairy cup that has five long points.
Range. Maine to Man. and Colo., s. to N.C. and Tex. Aug.-Sept. in wet ground and swamps.
Common names. High-belia, Blue cardinal flower.
1749 Kalm July 17th. 389-90. "Venereal disease is common. The Indians are likewise infected with it; many of them had it, and some still have it; but they are possessed of an infallible art of curing it. There are examples of Frenchmen and Indians who had been 'radically' and perfectly cured by the Indians within five or six months. The French have not been able to find out this remedy, though they know that the Indians employ no mercury, but that their chief remedies are roots which are unknown to the French. I afterwards heard what these plants were, and gave an account of them to the Royal Academy of Sciences". . .1750 Kalm wrote of Lobelia as a specific for Syphilis (in Swedish) published in Kong. Vet. Acad. Hanl. Five species of this herb were described as a cure for veneral disease.
1751 Bartram wrote Description, virtues and uses of sundry plants of these northern parts of America; and particularly of the newly discovered Indian cure for Venereal Diseases, *Lobelia syphilitica* L.
1791 Lewis ed. Aitkin 74. "Edinburgh College seems to give credit to the efficacy of Lobelia by receiving it into their latest catalogue of simples."
1799 Lewis Mat. Med. 176. "The whole plant has a milky juice. It grows in moist places in Virginia and bears the winters of our climate. . .It was long a famous secret among North American Indians for the cure of venereal diseases. The secret was purchased by Sir William Johnson, and has been made public in the writings of Bartram, Kalm and others. . .Notwithstanding the character this plant bears, it has never been confirmed in Britain, nor even in Virginia; for in both countries recourse is almost universally had to mercury in the lues [Syphilis]"
1814 Clarke Consp. 97. "Blue cardinal flower, Diuretic, cathartic. It generally disagrees with the stomach, and possesses no power of curing syphilis, from which supposed virtue it took its name. It is employed in the form of a decoction, made by boiling the dried roots in water."
1830 Rafinesque 25. "It is a lactecent, acrid, and nauseaous plant, which has been deemed long

ago to be diuretic, repellent, cathartic, emetic, and anti-syphilitic; but its properties are rather similar to *L. inflata*, although less active; it is chiefly sudorific and diuretic, and its properties are not so easily destroyed by heat, since it is used in decoction and extract. The root has been chiefly used instead of the plant; dose five to twenty grains of the extract in dropsy. The Northern Indians used it for the cure of syphilis, in conjunction with *Prunus* [wild cherry] and *Podophyllum*, [mayapple] and in strong decoction, washing also the ulcers with it, and sprinkling them with the powder of *Ceonothus* [New Jersey tea]; but it has failed in the hands of physicians, and only availed in cases of gonorrhea, acting then as a diuretic. Henry recommends to unite to it *Geranium maculatum* and willow bark as astringents. It disagrees with the stomach, and often causes griping, purging, and vomiting."

1859-61 Gunn 823. "The root is the part used, and is regarded by those who are acquainted with its properties as a most powerful and valuable alterative in the cure of cancer, scrofula, and the venereal disease, or syphilis. . .In such diseases as these it is used in strong decoction, the patient drinking from a pint to a quart in a day; and in the case of ulcers, they are to be washed with the same. It is very highly recommended as a cure for cancer of the breast of females; the decoction of the root to be drunk daily. . .and apply to breast or cancer a poultice made of equal parts of Elm bark and the powdered root (or leaves). . .For ulcers, wounds, inflammations, and all affections which have a tendency to terminate in gangrene, it is thought this plant will prove to be among the most valuable remedies. It has also been recommended in dropsy. It seems to have long been an Indian remedy for scrofula, cancer and syphilis, from whom its wonderful properties were first obtained."

1892 Millspaugh 98. "The former uses of this plant were the same of those of *L. inflata* than which it is less active. . .Linnaeus thinking it justified its Indian reputation, gave the species its distinctive name *syphilitica*. The cause of failure may be the fact that the aborigines did not trust to this plant alone, but always used it in combination with may-apple roots [*Podophyllum peltatum*], the bark of the wild cherry. . .and dusted the ulcers with the powdered bark of New Jersey tea. Another chance of failure lay in the volatility of its active principle, as the dried herb was used."

1925 Wood & Ruddock. "The root is a most valuable remedy for the treatment of diarrhea and dysentery. . .physicians give it a high reputation for the cure of cancer of the breast."

1928 H. Smith MESKWAKI 194. "The flowers of *L. syphilitica* along with five other plants made up an inhalant for catarrh. 231. This is used as a love medicine and the roots are finely chopped and put into food of a quarrelsome pair, without their knowledge. This medicine averts divorce and makes the pair love each other again."

CARDINAL FLOWER   *Lobelia cardinalis* L.

The straight stem can be from 50-150 cm tall with alternate leaves mostly 3-5 times as long as wide. The lower ones have short stalks the upper none. The brilliant red flowers are on hairy stalks up the top part of the stem. One of our best known wild flowers.

Range. N.B. to Minn., s. to the Gulf of Mexico, July-Sept. in wet soil.

1830 Rafinesque 26. "The root has chiefly been employed in decoction by the Cherokee Indians in syphilis, and against worms. It is said to be equivalent to *Spigelia* or pinkroot. These properties deserve further inquiry, as the whole genus *Lobelia* appears to be more or less medical to us; other species have not yet been tried."

1859-61 Gunn 823. "This species of Lobelia is not much used or not very extensively used as medicine. The roots are said to be diuretic, anthelmintic, nervine and antispasmodic; and in large doses slightly emetic and cathartic. It has been used with some success in dropsy; also in diarrhea and dysentery, and as a remedy for worms.

1892 Millspaugh 97. "Shoepf mentions the use of the root of this species by the Cherokee Indians for syphilis; and Dr. Barton(1810) speaks of their successful use of it as an anthelmintic. . .seldom used now, *L. inflata* taking its place entirely. It is considered, however, to possess marked anthelmintic, nervine, and antispasmodic properties."

1928 H. Smith MESKWAKI 231. "Wm Davenport in explaining about 'shikatape' brought out a tobacco pouch of Indian tobacco, which is not for smoking at all. It was a maceration of the entire plant. When a storm portends this 'tobacco' dust is thrown into the air to dispel it. At the end of the funeral, it is thrown into the grave, much as we strew flowers. The roots are also used for a love medicine in the same way as those of the great blue lobelia."

1970 Krochmal, Wilkin & Chien. Ll. 33. Four Alkaloids found in *Lobelia cardinalis* which unexpectedly yielded as much lobeline as *L. inflata. L. syphilitica* had less lobeline.

Lobelia Kalmii growing on wet shores was used by the CREE of Hudson Bay as an emetic according to Haydon, 1884, who sent the plant to Holmes in London, England.

See *Lobelia inflata*, Indian tobacco, under dry open places.

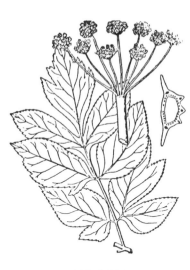

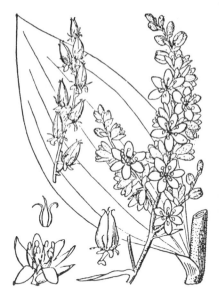

ANGELICA   AMERICAN VERATRUM

ANGELICA   *Angelica atropurpurea* L. Umbelliferae (Apiaceae).
A large plant to 2 m tall, smooth or nearly so up to the flowering tips. The lower leaves 10-30 cm
on long stalks whose ends form a sheath around the stem. The leaflets 4-10 cm with sharp teeth.
The white flowers in bunches 10-20 cm wide. The fruit 4-6.5 mm, smooth.
Range. Lab., to Minn., s. to Del., W. Va., and Ind. June-August in swamps and wet woods.
1633 Gerarde-Johnson 1000. "In an Island of the North, called Island, [Iceland] where it groweth very high. It is eaten of the inhabitants, the barke being pilled off, as we understand by some
that have travelled into Island, who were sometimes compelled to eate hereof for want of other
food; and they report that it has a good and pleasant taste to them that are hungry. . .The root of
the garden Angelica [*Angelica archangelica*], is a singular remedy against poison, and against the
plague, and all infections taken by evill and corrupt aire; if you do but take a piece of the root
and hold it in your mouth, or chew the same between your teeth. . .yet it driveth it out again by
urine and sweat, as Rue and Treacle . . .It openeth the liver and spleen: draweth downe the
termes . . .The decoction of the root made in wine, is good against the shivering of agues. It is
reported that the root is available against witchcraft and enchantments, if a man carry the same
about. . .It attentuateth and maketh thin, grosse and tough flegme; the root being used greene,
and while it is full of juice, helpeth them that be asthmaticke. . . but when it is dry it worketh not
so effectually. . .it cureth the bitings of mad dogges, and all other venomous beasts. The wilde
kindes are not of such force in working, albeit they have the same vertues attributed unto them."
1663 Boucher Quebec transl. 85. "There is angelica in the meadows."
1687 Clayton Virginia Indians 14-5. "I will now mention to you an herb though unknown, yet
worthy to be fetched from Virginia yielded the country nothing else, it is the herb called there
Angelica. . .the seeds are much like Angelica seeds . . .It stops the Flux and cures it to a wonder;
again it often loosens and purges the bodys of those that are bound and have the gripes especially if it proceed from cold; and prevents many unhappy distempers; I have reason to speak
well of it, for it is to it, under God, that I attribute the saving of my own life. . .I take it to be the
most sovereign remedy the world ever knew in the griping of the Guts and admirable against
Vapours, it is sudorific and very Aromatick, and will not be concealed for wherever it is mixed it
will have the predominant scent. It is mostly called by those who know it in Virginia by the name
of Angelica. But showing a piece of the root to a great Woodsman to see whether he knew it and
could tell me where it grew, he seemed suprized to see me have thereof, and told me that he kept

an Indian once for some weeks with him; because he was an excellent Woodsman, and going a hunting . . .they came where some of this root grew; The Indian rejoycing gathered some of it, but was very carefull to cut off the top of the root and replant it; He then asked him why he was so carefull, whereunto the Indian replyed, It was a very choice plant and very scarce for they sometimes travelled 100 or 200 miles without finding any of it. He then asked Him what use it was of, to which the Indian answered you shall see by and by. After some time they spyed 4 Deer at a distance, then the Indian contrary to his usual custom went to windward of them, and sitting down upon an old trunk of a Tree, began to rub the root betwixt his hands, at which the Deer toss up their heads and snuffing with their noses, they fed towards the place where the Indian satt, till they came within easy shot of him, whereupon he fired at them, and killed a large buck. . .I have often taken notice that the Indians smell generally strong of this herb. And I have since learned from others that the Indians call it the Hunting root. . .Another Gentleman, a White native of that Country, when I once pulled a piece of the root out of my pocket to bite thereof, for I frequently carry'd some of it about me, asked me if I loved fishing. . .said you have gotten some of the fishing root. . . when we were boys we used to get some of it to lay with our baits to invite the fish to bite."

1708 circa. Jussieu. List of plants sent from Quebec by Sarrazin to Paris, with notes on the use in Quebec of some of them. The whole list printed in unreadable form by Vallée, 1927, who apparently could read it, as he writes that Sarrazin's note on angelica states: "Here it is an angelica whose properties are interchangeable with those of cicuta and which can produce convulsions."

1743 Isham Hudson Bay 134. "Anchillico Vast quantity's of a great bigness, having some Eight or nine foot high, and about as thick as the Rist."

1830 Rafinesque 192. "*Angelica lucida* L. [a coastal species, L.I. to Lab. probably refers to *A. venenosa*] Angelic root, Belly-ache root. Nendo of the Virginian Indians. White root of the Southern tribes. Equivalent of Ginseng and officinal Angelica. Root like Ginseng, taste similar, smell like aniseed. Highly valued by the Southern Indians, and cultivated by them: used as a carminative, and in cookery. This root is said to give an excellent flavor to Virginia hams and pork when hogs feed on it. It is bitterish, subacrid, fragrant and aromatic, stomachic and tonic, useful in colics, hysterics, menstrual suppressions. . .The powdered seeds kill lice. Henry adds. . .useful to disperse tumours, and the root an antidote against yellow fever, chewed when visiting the sick. The Missouri tribes call it Lagonihah, and mix it with tobacco to smoke; they also eat it but it often produces indigestion."

1859-61 Gunn 736. "Angelica (*Angelica archangelica*) garden Angelica. . .cultivated in the gardens of this country. . .The root. . .calculated to remove spasmodic pain in the bowels, and flatulence or wind in the stomach. . .in the form of a tea or infusion, and may be used freely. It is also recommended in nervous headache, pains in the breast and stomach, and feeble digestion."

1892 Millspaugh 64. "*Angelica atropurpurea* When fresh the roots are poisonous, and are said to have been used for suicidal purposes by the Canadian Indians; when dried. . .they lose this quality, and are then considered carminative, diuretic, emmenagogue and stimulant. The dried root was often used. . .in various diseases of the urinary organs and alone in flatulent colic and suppressed menstruation. Dr. Schell (Fam, Guide to Health, 1856 corroborated in Am. Jour. Hom. Med. i 272) says that doses of 15 to 20 grains of the dried root will cause a disgust for all spirituous liquors. The stems were often made into a candied preserve in some sections of the country-a practice now nearly extinct. Its uses, all in all, have been greatly similar to those of the garden angelica. . .Its oils. . .may be, in all probability, compared with those of *Angelica archangelica*."

1901 Chesnut 371. "Angelica sp. Angelica root, as it is most commonly called both by the Indians and whites, is a most valued remedy and talisman. It is found in nearly every household and is frequently carried about the person for good luck in hunting and gambling. Those roots found in places where the plant does not ordinarily grow, especially cold places, are the more highly prized. The root, after thorough mastication, is sometimes rubbed on the legs to prevent rattlesnake bites, and it is also tied around the head and ears in bad cases of headache and nightmare. The juice mixed with saliva is used as a remedy for sore eyes. It is chewed and swallowed in cases of cold, colic, and especially fever. For cold and catarrh it is very frequently crushed up and smoked like tobacco. The fresh, young sprouts, being sweet and aromatic, are eaten raw with great relish."

1915 W. R. Harris Indian medicine 51. "In diseases of children the Angelica plant, boiled and strained, was frequently used. . .55. There are two common species on the dry and sandy lands throughout the United States. The 'villosa' [*A. venenosa*] seems to be the most widely distributed and was probably the species so popular among the Indians. The species 'atropurpurea' so common in our Canadian marshes does not seem, according to Hunter, to have been greatly prized by the western tribes, although all the species are known to be tonics, sudorifics and diuretics."

1923 H. Smith MENOMINI 55. "*A. atropurpurea*. This is a very important medicine to reduce swellings. The roots are cooked and pounded to a pulp. Then some bruised leaves of *Artemisia canadensis* are peppered over this pulp. With this mass and a piece of cloth, a hot plaster is made, that the Menomini claim is good for any pain in the chest or body. It is applied to the side of the body opposite the pain. This is done here because it is supposed to draw the pain through to the surface where it can make its escape."

1931 Grieve England 38-40. "Angelica [*A. archangelica*], is largely used in the grocery trade, as well as for medicine, and is a popular flavouring for confectionary and liqueurs. . .The flavour of Angelica suggests that of Juniper berries, and it is largely used in combination with Juniper berries, or in partial substitution for them by gin distillers. . .The seeds. . .in preparation of Vermouth. . . Chartreuse. . .*A. atropurpurea*. . .root has a strong odour and a warm aromatic taste. The juice of the fresh root is acrid and said to be poisonous, but the acridity is dissipated by drying. . .constituents, and the medicinal virtues of the whole plant are similar, so that it has been employed as a substitute for *A. archangelica*, but is inferior. . .being less aromatic."

1959 Mechling MALECITE of maritime provinces of Canada use the root for a cold in the head, sore throat and cough (the European *A. sylvestris* found around Louisburg)

A. archangelica. The drug is obtained from the roots which contain an essential oil. In large doses this has a bad effect on the central nervous system. Handling the drug may cause an allergic rash and irritation of the skin in some people. It contains a volatile oil that is poisonous in large doses (Stary & Jirasek 1973:72).

A. archangelica is rich in coumarin derivatives and considered a tonic to improve well-being and mental harmony (Lewis and Elvin-Lewis 1977:374).

AMERICAN VERATRUM   *Veratrum viride* Ait. Liliaceae

The poisonous root is erect, thick, with numerous rootlets. The stem stout, erect, leafy to the top, to 2 m tall. Leaves without stalks, sometimes clasping the stem, to 30 cm long and half as wide, the leaves have deep plaits like a half closed fan. The flowering stem 20-50 cm. hairy and branched, surrounded by yellowish green, hairy, 8-13 mm flowers on 2-4 mm long stalks. The seed pods 18-25 mm with many seeds.

Range. Lab., N.B., Que., Ont., Minn., s. to Tenn., and Ga. in grassy meadows, swamps and wet woods.

Common names. False hellebore, Indian poke, duck-retten, earth gall, devil's bite, bear-corn, itch-weed, tickle-weed, devil's tobacco.

Hellebore is the European plant, Christmas rose; green hellebore is *Helleborus viridis*, widely spread in U.S.; Poke usually means the shrub *Phytolacca* with long sprays of deep red berries, a native shrub in the south of our range. All three plants are poisonous in parts.

1628 De Rasieres New. Neth. 114. Young Indian in May. . . "He must then go out again every morning with the person who is ordered to take him in hand; he must go into the forest to seek wild herbs and roots, which they know to be the most poisonous and bitter; these they bruise in water and press the juice out of them, which he must drink and immediately have ready such herbs as will preserve him from death or vomiting; and if he cannot retain it, he must repeat the dose until he can support it, and until his constitution becomes accustomed to it so that he can retain it."

1638 Josselyn in his New England rarities informs us that the young Indians had a custom of electing their chiefs by a sort of ordeal using the root of white hellebore; "he whose stomach withstood its action the longest was decided to be the strongest of the party, and entitled to command the rest." [New Engl. Rar. 1672 cited Millspaugh 1892].

1633 Gerarde-Johnson 440-1. "White hellebore [*Veratrum album* of Europe]. The root. . .this strong medicine made of white hellebore, ought not to be given inwardly unto delicate bodies without great correction, but it may more safely be given unto Country people which feed grossely, and have hard, tough, strong bodies. The root of Hellebore cut in small pieces, such as may aptly and conveniently be conveid into Fistulaes doth mundifie [dissolve] them, and taketh away the callous matter which hindreth curation, and afterwards they may be healed up with some incarnative ungent,. . .The root given to drinke in the weight of two pence, taketh away the fits of agues, killeth Mice and rats being made up with honie and floure of wheat: Pliny addeth that it is a medicine against the Lousie evill."

1663 Boucher Quebec transl. 86. "For the wild herbs. . . Cicuta grows wonderfully well, as well as the Hellebore."

1672 Josselyn New England 42. "The Indians cure their wounds with it; annointing the wound first with raccoon's grease or wildcat's grease, and strewing upon it the powder of the roots: and, for aches, they scarify the grieved part, and annoint it with one of the foresaid oyls; then strew upon it the powder. The powder of the root, put into a hollow tooth, is good for the toothach. The root sliced thin and boyled in vinegar, is very good against herpes milliaris." [a skin disease].

1749 Kalm Philadelphia March 13th. 257. "*Veratrum album* [Hellebore] was very common in the marshes and in low places over all North America. [Kalm is here confusing the European species with the very similar american *V. viride*. . .the roots are boiled in water, into which the corn is put as soon as the water is cool; the corn must lie all night in it, and is then planted as usual. Then when the starlings, crows, or other birds, pick up or pluck out the grains of corn, their heads grow delirious, and they fall, which so frightens the rest that they never venture on the field again. When those which have tasted the grains recover, they leave the field, and are no more tempted to visit it again. By thus preparing the corn, one must be careful that no other creatures touch it; for when ducks or fowls eat a grain or two of the corn which is thus steeped, they become very sick, and if they swallow a considerable quantity they die. When the root is thrown away raw, no animal eats it; but when it is put out boiled, its sweet taste tempts the beasts. Dogs have been seen to eat a little of it and have become very sick; however they recover after a vomit . . .Some people boil the root for medicinal purposes, washing scorbutic parts with the water or decoction. This is said to cause some pain, and even a plentiful discharge of urine, but the patient is said to be cured thereby. When children are plagued with vermin, the women boil this root, put the comb into the decoction, and comb the head with it, and this kills the lice most effectually." [Waugh 1916:19. None of the medicines [for corn] described are poisonous, although Kalm records the use of the wild hellebore. . . by the Swedes and other colonists of the eastern states, possibly in imitation of the Indians.]

1796 Hahnemann Lesser Writings 302. Called for the use of *Veratrum album* in lung inflammation and the homeopaths used this remedy in various diseases characterized by fever and inflammation. (Coulter 1973:61).

1817-20 Bigelow 124-35. "As a medicine or as a poisonous plant, it has been known from an early period. The aborigines of the country were fully apprized of its activity. . .I have employed the American plant in dispensatory practice in the treatment of obstinate cases of chronic rheumatism. . .A course of experiments. . .was made some time since in the Boston Almshouse by Dr. John Ware. . .I am informed by several of our most respectable apothecaries, that for a long time, especially during the late war, when the white hellebore could not be obtained from Europe, the American plant was used in the preparation of medicine. . .Various gouty patients made use of it, and no difference was perceived by them, or their physicians; in its mode of operation or effect upon the disease. . .We have sufficient knowledge of the American green hellebore, to feel assured that it is a plant of great activity, closely resembling in its properties the *Veratrum album* of Europe. . .

1830 Rafinesque 273. "Poisonous active plant. . . dangerous article. . .Ointment used externally, has happened to cause emesis [vomiting] by application even on the legs. It is a poison for all insects in decoction, noxious to swine, sheep, geese, fowls. In gout it removes paroxysms, allays pains, procures rest and sleep, reduces pulse, and abates fevers. Keeps issues open in ulcers. . .Improper doses produce dimness, faintness, insensibility &c. Used once to poison arrows. Lately to tan leather very quick. It contains Veratrine, a narcotic alkali."

1840 Gosse Quebec 233. "Here is a rather handsome plant; do you know its name? it is called Poke, and its root is considered by the common people to be poisonous. . .it dies to the root every year, and in the spring sends up a large bulb of broad, lance-oval leaves sheathing each other. . .The plant is most common in the black swampy earth of the evergreen woods, and does not often grow in clearings except by the side of pools or water in low ground. . .The flowers have no beauty, but the large leaves give it rather a noble appearance."

1842 Christison 935. "White hellebore [*V. album*] is a violent irritant poison, which occasions, when snuffed into the nostrils, severe coryza, and when swallowed, urgent vomiting and profuse diarrhoea. When it proves fatal, narcotic symptons are superadded, such as stupor and convulsions. It was at one time used. . .in mental diseases. . .More recently. . .it came into general use as a remedy for arresting the paroxyms of gout. At present, however, it is little employed, partly on account of frequent complaints made of its uncertain actions, partly, in the arrestment of gout, it has been displaced by colchicum. Its principal use now is for the destruction of vermin that infest the skin. . .it forms part also of the London Unguentum sulphuris compositum [used for itch]."

1859-61 Gunn 876. "is a narcotic and acrid emetic in large doses; but used in medicine, that is in small doses, is a powerful arterial sedative. . .will reduce the action of the heart and frequency of the pulse. . .in disease of the heart, wherever there is too great an action or excitement. Also a valuable expectorant, diaphoretic, and nervine, in affections of the lungs. . .The best preparation is that called Norwood's tincture. . .Should an overdose be taken and unpleasant symptoms be produced, the free use of brandy with thirty or forty drops of Laudanum [opium] will soon afford relief."

1860 Cutter n.p. "Few remedies have so speedily attained such preeminence, not so much in the books as in the unwritten materia medica of the practical physician."

1880 Can. Horticulturist 95. "We have not found any inconvenience to result from the use of hellebore, which, though poisonous to man in considerable quantities, is washed off the currants and gooseberries long before they are fit for use. The saw-fly caterpillar makes its appearance very early in the season, and if the hellebore is promptly applied, they will all be gone many weeks before the fruit is ready for use, and the rains will have washed off all trace of the hellebore. We know of nothing that will meet these Saw-fly larvae so certainly and promptly as white hellebore."

1892 Millspaugh 176. "To Dr. Norwood of South Carolina goes the credit of establishing the proper method of administering the drug, and it was through his use in part that its employment began in England in 1862. . .from which time the drug gained gradually the prominence it now holds. . .The principal uses of the drug were as a depresser of the heart's action wherever it was deemed necessary; and an application and internal remedy in arthritic troubles of all kinds. . .The fresh root gathered after the leaves have fallen in the autumn is used. . .The action of the drug. . .is that of an arterial and nerve sedative; it paralyzes both the voluntary and involuntary muscles; it increases all secretions through its influence in paralyzing the vaso-motor system, allowing thus a great dilation of the capillaries."

1894 Household Guide Toronto 180-85. "How to use all kinds of Homeopathic remedies. . .for ague. . .chorea. . .cholera. . .diarrhoea . . .epilepsy. . .hiccough. . .whooping cough. . .remittent fever . . .sunstroke. . .typhus. . .use *Veratrum viride*."

1920 Fyles 25. "Hellebore is poisonous to all animals. Cattle and horses avoid eating it wherever possible, as they do not relish the acrid, burning taste of the fresh plant; but young animals sometimes eat it with fatal results. . .as hellebore is used in the preparation of certain medicines, cases of poisoning have occured from overdoses. . .In one case a whole family was poisoned by using the young leaves as greens in mistake for those of the marsh marigold. However, fatalities among humans are rare, as the drug induces spontaneous vomiting. . . .In general the symptoms of poisoning are salivation, vomiting, abdominal pain, diarrhoea, cold perspiration, depression of the heart, loss of sight, and finally death from paralysis of the heart. Professional advice should be obtained wherever possible. Treatment should be persued by heart stimulants, such as alcohol. . .and the external application of warmth. . .Young animals should be given warm water to assist vomiting and to wash out the stomach. Rest and quiet should be enforced."

1955 Mockle Quebec transl. 29. "*Veratrum viride*, American white hellebore. The rhizome is considered a specific in inflammatory, feverish affections and in particular pneumonia and puerperal fever. Its use in the form of a tincture provokes the rapid lowering of the temperature and the frequency of the pulse. This plant is considered toxic."

The plant is dug in the autumn, the leaves are cut off close to the crown, and the rhizomes is then usually halved or quartered to help it dry. The root contains the alkaloids germidine and germitrine which possess high hypotensive activity. (T. E. Wallis 1967: 365).

The alkaloids of *Veratrum* have a major effect on the heart and vessels. Blood pressure is lowered, arterioles are dilated. In severe cases of hypertension *Veratrum viride* is given in combination with *Rauwolfia*, reserpine. The blood pressure is lowered but there will be nausea and vomiting as well, so its use is limited (Lewis and Elvin-Lewis 1977: 188-9).

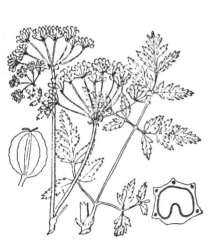

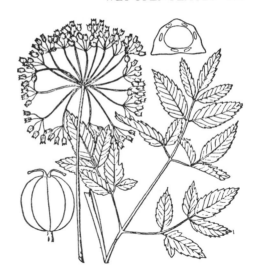

POISON HEMLOCK

WATER HEMLOCK

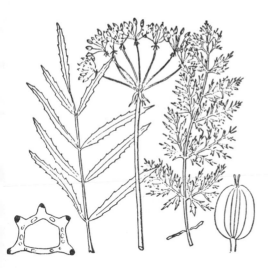

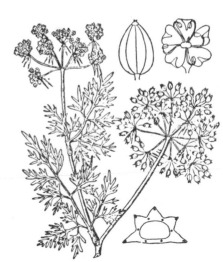

WATER PARSNIP

FOOL'S PARSLEY

POISON HEMLOCK   *Conium maculatum* L. Umbelliferae (Apiaceae)

The stem is straight, smooth, hollow, up to 300 cm tall with many branches, spotted with a purplish red and covered with a whitish bloom. These last two characteristics may not always be present. The leaves grow from sheathes around the stem. The lower leaves are large, 20-40 cm long, with stalks. They consist of many leaflets opposite each other, these in turn are cut up with teeth around their edges. They are thin and when crushed have an unpleasant mousy odor as does the whole fresh plant. The bunches of small white flowers are 4-6 cm wide. The fruit is 3 mm with prominent pale brown ribs, which become more noticeable when it is dry, the root is solid like the parsnip root and branched.

Range. Native of Eurasia, now widely introduced as a weed in waste places from Que., to Fla., w. to the Pacific. June-Sept. in dryish soil.

Common names. Snakeweed, poison or spotted parsley, wode-whistle, cashes, St. Bennet's herb. All parts of this plant are poisonous.

Poison hemlock has been used as a medicine and as a poison since at least 500 B.C. There is general agreement that it was this plant whose decoction Socrates drank when he was put to death by the Athenians. Dioscorides used it in skin diseases. The Anglo Saxons knew it as a useful medicine. The Romans called it Cicuta, using that name for several poisonous plants of the parsley family. In 1541 this name was applied to the European *Cicuta virosa* a quite different plant (see below).

1475 Bjornsson Icelandic mss. transl. Larsen. 48. "Cicuta. . .Cold as poison. If one drink it, he will die of it as of poison. But whoever dies of it is white spotted. And whoever gets harm from drinking it, he shall drink quickly hot, strong wine. Its leaves and juice crushed will help if applied to running eyes and for erysipelas. If a girl rubs her breasts with the juice of it, they stand evenly; and, if it comes upon the nipples, it will come about that the milk dries in them. Crushed and placed upon a man's genitals, it does away with the lust for women. And it cleanses the womb in which a child is to be got, and lets a woman have her flux. Crushed with quicksilver and tallow, it helps foot trouble."

1633 Gerarde-Johnson 1061-3. "Cicuta hath not only a loathsome smell, but his roots are great, thicke, and knobbly, like the roots of Myrrhis: [sweet cicely] the whole plant doth in a manner resemble the leaves, stalks and floures of *Myrrhis odorata*. . .It is therefore a very rash part to lay the leaves of Hemlocke to the stones of young boys or virgin brests, and by that means to keepe those parts from growing great; for it doth not only easily cause those members to pine away, but also hurteth the heart and liver, being outwardly applied: then must it of necessitie hurt more being inwardly taken; for it is one of the deadly poysons which killeth by his cold qualitie, as Dioscorides writeth, saying, Hemlocke is a very evil, dangerous, hurtful and poysonous herbe, insomuch that whosoever taketh of it into his body dieth remedilesse, except the party drinke from wine that is naturally hot, before the venom have taken the heart, as Pliny saith: but being drunke with wine the poison is with greatest speed caried to the heart, by reason whereof it killeth presently; therefore not to be applied outwardly, much less taken inwardly into the body. . .not to be used in physicke. . .1063-4. Water hemlocke, [*Cicuta virosa*] . . .riseth up with a thicke, fat and empty hollow stalke, full of knees or joynts, crested, chamfered or furrowed. . .of a sweet smell. . .temperature and faculties are answerable to the common hemlocke, which have no use in physicke, as we have said."

1681 Culpeper 182. "Hemlock (*Conium maculatum*). . . very dangerous, especially to be taken inwardly. It may safely be applied to inflammations, tumults, and swellings in any part of the body. . .leaves bruised and applied to the brow or forehead are good for red and swollen eyes; as also to take a pin or web growing there. . .Poisonous Water Hemlock, *Cicuta Virosa*, and Thick Water Hemlock, are but accidental variations which situation and soil naturally produce, they are thought to be poisonous, but there is nothing certain on this head."

1770 Stoerck wrote a book to demonstrate the medical uses of cicuta [conium].

1778 Johnson Pharm London 9. "Cicuta, herba, flos, semen, botanical name is *Conium maculatum*."

1805 Buchan 526. "Hemlock should always be begun in very small doses of one grain or less, and gradually increased as the consitution will bear. . .*Conium maculatum* is the botanical name."

1817-20 Bigelow 122. "In old syphilitic affections, it is occasionally useful. It has been recommended in hooping-cough, but it is not a perfectly safe medicine for children, owing to the difficulty of ascertaining when its constitutional effects take place in them. I am informed on the best medical authority, that it is of great use in some cases of hemicrania [migraine] which are not regularly intermittent. . .In some instances very great quantities have been taken without the least effect. The extract is apt to prove inert when the plant is gathered too young, when the evaporation is conducted with too much heat, when a decoction of the dried plant has been evaporated instead of the fresh leaves, and lastly when the extract itself has become old."

1820's Mat. Med. Edinburgh-Toronto mss. 2. "*Conium maculatum* leaves dried for medical use. It is a very powerful narcotic. It promotes the action of mercury. Dose 2 or 3 grains. It is used externally as a cataplasm, to painful or ill conditioned ulcers."

1828 Rafinesque 119. "It has since been found that these plants, like many other poisons, have valuable medical properties, nearly similar in all the deleterious species of this family. The

Conium maculatum is the most employed. . . The power of this plant varies exceedingly, according to the place and climate where it grows, the time it is collected, and the preparation of it. It is most powerful in warm climates, in the summer and when full grown. Some persons are hardly affected by it: while others are more susceptible; on these it produces dizziness, nausea, disturbed sight, faintness &c. which symptoms appear in half an hour and last half a day or more. A large dose produces worse symptoms, vertigo, paralysis, convulsions and death. There is little danger of being poisoned by this plant through mistake, owing to its bad smell; yet there are instances on record that children have taken it for parsley and the root for carrot; whereby sickness and death have been produced. In the United States, the *Cicuta maculata* is more dangerous on that score. . .It is never dangerous in very small doses often repeated, and gradually increased. It is also an effective anodyne, sedative and antispasmodic, useful to allay pain in acute diseases. . .such as cancer, epilepsy, mania, syphilis &c. but in those cases it acts only as a palliation to pain, like opium, to which it is often preferable, as less constipating. . .True Schirrus and Cancer cannot be cured by it; but obstinate scrofulous tumors or swelled testicles . . .have been removed by its use. . .In tic douleureux it has afforded relief or even effected a cure, when nothing else could avail. While highly extolled in jaundice, removing the yellowness in a short time, and curing the disease, when not too complicated. . .The best way to administer it, is that of the powdered leaves, beginning with two or three grains, and increasing the doses gradually. The leaves must preserve their green color to be efficient. . .An extract of the seeds is said to be stronger and produces giddiness very soon. Externally it has been used in cataplasms for carcinoma, syphilis, leprosy and obstructions. Vinegar and lemon juice are the antidotes for the poison or overdoses of this plant. . . substitutes. . .*Angelica atropurpurea*."

1859-61 Gunn 782. "Conium known as poison hemlock. . . The leaves and seeds are used, but mostly the extract made from the leaves, and found in drug-stores. Conium is a narcotic poison, and although a valuable medicine in certain cases, is to be used in small doses, and with caution. It acts specially on the nervous system, quieting the nerves, inducing sleep, and decreasing the action of the heart. It is therefore considered a valuable agent in enlargement of the heart, in palpitation, and inflammation of that organ, by allaying excitement and reducing the action."

1868 Can. Pharm. J. 6; 83-5. *Conium maculatum*, poison hemlock, the leaves and seeds included in list of Can. medicinal plants.

1892 Millspaugh 68. "Baron Stoerck. . .found it effectual in curing scirrhus, ulcers, cancer and many other chronic forms of disease. . .many physicians failed to get any effect whatsoever from this drug in diseases specified by Stoerck and others; so frequent were the failures that most careful and protracted experiments in gathering, curing, preserving, and preparing the drug were resorted to. . .A man ate a large quantity of Hemlock plant by mistake for parsley; soon afterwards there was loss of power in the lower extremities; but he apparantly suffered no pain. . .On being raised his legs dragged after him, or when his arms were lifted they fell like inert masses, and remained immovable; there was perfect paralysis of the upper and lower extremeties within two hours after he had taken the poison. . . Three hours after eating the hemlock the respiratory movements ceased. Death took place in three and one-quarter hours."

1904 Henkel 40. "The fruit should be collected while still green but full grown. . .It should be dried in dark but well ventilated places, and then stored in tight cans or boxes where it will not be exposed to the action of light and air . . .This very poisonous drug is used in rheumatism, neuralgia, asthma, and in cases where the nervous system is in an excited condition. The imports of conium or poison hemlock seed amount to about 20,000 pounds annually, and from 10,000 to 20,000 pounds of the leaves are imported. The price paid for the seed is about 3 cents per pound, and for the leaves about 4 cents."

1920 Fyles 68. "It is a question as to which part of the plant is most poisonous. . .it may well be said that the whole plant is deadly. It seems that early in the summer the poisonous properties are most abundant in the green leaves, and that later on the seeds are the most toxic, particularly just before ripening. . .small boys have been poisoned by making whistles out of the hollow stems of the plant."

1955 Mockle Quebec transl. 67. "The plant is narcotic and toxic. The leaves are used as a maturative in cataplasms and in an oily decoction for milky swellings and articulations. It contains the alkaloids coniine, methylconiine, conhydrine, pseudoconhydrine and coniceine."

1968 Forsyth (England) 68. "The most important of the alkaloids is coniine, which occurs in the largest amounts; it is particularly interesting because it was the first alkaloid to be produced synthetically in the laboratory. The others, no less poisonous but occuring in smaller amounts are methylconiine, coniceine, and conhydrine. The alkaloids are volatile liquids and are lost by slow drying or boiling, so the matured hay which contains hemlock is not likely to be dangerous to livestock. . .The alkaloids are excreted by the lungs and kidneys, and the typical mousy odor in the breath and urine of a poisoned animal is diagnostic. . .First aid treatment; give stimulants, alcohol. . .and coffee or tea in large quantities. Purgatives should only be prescribed by the medical attendant or veterinary surgeon, who may also administer such other alkaloids as strychnine or atropine, if necessary, and give oxygen by inhalation or subcutaneously. Artificial respiration may be used in man and in the smaller animals."

The amount of alkaloid in the plant changes from hour to hour and in different stages of its growth and varies with its habitat, those growing in the southern part of its range containing more than those in the northern (Kingsbury 1965:381).

Coniine is used in spasmodic and convulsive diseases, such as tetanus, chorea, and epilepsy and also in asthma and whooping cough. (TE. Wallis 1967:249).

WATER HEMLOCK
Cicuta maculata L. Umbelliferae (Apiaceae)

A stout stem to 200 cm tall, hollow except where the leaves grow; often with purple lines, many branches. The leaves 3-10 cm long consist of several leaflets, these again with several leaflets. These leaflets are usually well over 5 mm wide, their veins running to the notches between the teeth around each leaflet. The bunches of small white flowers 5-12 cm wide are followed by fruit 2-4 mm long with prominent, rounded, pale brown ribs separated by dark brown intervals. There are several thick roots except in weak or very young plants. The base of the stem and top of the roots is thickened. Cut these in half and the hollow at the base of the stem will be divided by tissue, then a space, another divider of tissue, one above the other, giving the effect of several chambers one above the other. The cut surfaces will ooze a yellow oil which is extremely poisonous, and smells of raw parsnip. If eaten it has the sweetish taste of parsnip. This is the most poisonous part of this plant. Water Hemlock is the most poisonous plant in eastern north America.

Range. Que., to Minn., and Wyo., s. to Fla., and Mex. June-Aug. in moist places, swamps and wet ditches.

Common names. Spotted cowbane, beaver poison, musquash root, wild parsnip.

1624 Sagard HURON 192. "They have likewise other plants of a very poisonous nature, which they call *ondachiera*; for this reason one must be careful, and not risk eating any kind of root there if one is not acquainted with it, and does not understand its effects, virtues, for fear of unexpected mischances. One day, we were put in great fear for a Frenchman who had eaten one of these and became at once very ill and pale as death, but he was cured by the emetics which the savages made him swallow."

1625 Wassenaer New Netherlands 81. "Poisonous plants have been found there, which those who cultivate the land should look out for. Hendrick Christiaensen carried thither, by order of his employers, bucks and goats, also rabbits, but they were found to be poisoned by the herbs."

1637 Jes. Rel. HURON 13;27. "They kill themselves by eating certain venomous herbs that they know to be poison, which married women much more often use to avenge themselves for the bad treatment of their husbands, leaving them to reproach themselves for their death."

1663 Boucher Quebec Transl. 84-6. "As to the native herbs, i.e. do not think I will write their names here, except for the most common which are met with here in the woods. . . Cicuta grows wonderfully well, as well as the Hellebore."

1708 Sarrazin-Vaillant, Quebec-Paris, Boivin 1978 transl. 15. "*Cicuta maculata.* This plant according to Mr. Sarrazin is worse than the 'cigue' [*Conium maculatum*]. It causes convulsions and death without remission. . .212. This plant is regarded as a 'cigue' in Canada because of the bad effects produced by the root. . .which is acrid in the autumn, for in the spring it tastes so good that children often eat too much of it. If they are not given a remedy before the first convulsion, they die without remission, because their tongue rolls in their mouth in such a way as not to allow anything to enter the esophagus, which is closed so exactly that if anything enters it comes out immediately. I saw 3 people die and I know of 12 or 15 who have done so in the last ten years. Last month a good workman aged 60 years ate a piece as big as a finger thinking it the root of Macedonian parsley. He died in an hour and a half, and if what a young man told me who did not wish to eat it [is true], he took some theriac as soon as he felt ill. Those who eat it raw die in horrible convulsions. Those who eat it cooked fall into a lethargic sleep, as happened last May, they were saved by an Emetic. . .The root is very resolutive and poisonous."

1710 Raudot Fort Pontchartrain Detroit HURON 409. "The women and girls. . .are very subject to poisoning themselves at the least grief that betakes them; the men also poison themselves sometimes. To leave this life they use the root of hemlock or of citron [mayapple], which they swallow."

1724 Lafitau 1;206. "An Indian at Michilimackinac cured, in a week, one of our missionaries of a general paralysis, which made all his members useless and forced him to have himself taken to Quebec for treatment. The secret of the cure was known but has been lost. All that I have been able to learn of it is that he went to the marshes to look for some root which he then mixed with water hemlock."

1779 Zeisberger DELAWARE 56. "In the use of poisonous roots the Indians are well versed, and there are many melancholy examples where they have by their use destroyed themselves or others. If a case of poisoning is taken in time, the effect of the poisonous root may be prevented by inducing vomiting. In case assistance is rendered too late, death follows, as a rule, in a few hours. There are poisonous roots that operate by slow degrees, in some cases illness may last a year or longer . . .83. Not every Indian, however, is indifferent to the light behaviour of his wife. Many a one takes her unfaithfulness so to heart that in the height of his despair he swallows a poisonous root, which generally causes death in two hours, unless an antidote be administered in good time; this is often done, the Indians knowing that the properties of certain herbs counteract each other and being able to judge from the effects, what poison has been taken, Women, also, have been known to destroy themselves on account of a husband's unfaithfulness."

1807 Pursh July 18th. reports that while at the Indian village at Onondaga that *Cicuta maculata* grows in great abundance. . .Indians use it to poison themselves. . .when they have eaten it they are lost without being able to get anything as a remedy and die. . .Elder bark or muskrat skin chopped fine with the hair on is reckoned a remedy if soon applied.

1828 Rafinesque 110. "A strong narcotic, solvent, and good substitute for the *Conium maculatum*, being more powerful, and requiring a lesser dose. A few grains of the dried leaves or extract have been given in schirrose and scrofulous tumors and ulcers with equal advantage; but larger doses produce nausea and vomiting: the doses should be very small often repeated and gradually increased. It has been used in gargle for sore throat, but safer substances ought to be prefered. The Indians when tired of life, are said to poison themselves with the roots of this plant and the purple Angelica, *A. atropurpurea*. . .265. Preferred to *Conium* in practice by some physicians as safer and less liable to lose its activity. The powder of the leaves gathered when the seeds are ripe, and dried in the shade is the best exhibition. . . 1830 209. The yellow juice of the root dyes yellow."

1829 Brockville Gazette (U.C.) 3 July. "On Saturday John. . .died from the effects of eating a poisonous root called the wild parsnip."

1833 Howard Quebec mss. 53. "To Cure Chronical Head Ache. Wear tender Hemlock leaves under your feet, changing them daily. . .253. To cure old ulcers and sores of every description in man. Pound a quantity of green hemlock to a mummy with the juice, then take the strings and stalks out and make the rest into small pills with flour. Take one every night and morning till cur'd. It cures if ever so bad."

1859-61 Gunn 470. "The Precipitated Carbonate of Iron and Extract of Cicuta, taken in the proportion of twenty grains of Iron to one of the Cicuta, twice a day for a length of time will both strengthen the tone of the system, and allay the irritability of the uterus or womb. This is a remedy for the whites. . .591. For neuralgia or nervous diseases. . .the cicuta is likewise equally beneficial, and by some preferred to the Valerian. One grain of the extract is the ordinary dose, given three times a day."

1878 Can. Pharm. J. 340. "Poisoning by *Cicuta bulbifera*. A week ago a sad case of poisoning occured in the vicinity of Teeswater. . .Two children were playing on the flats by the river, when one of them, a little boy aged seven, pulled up a root, ate a small quantity, and gave the rest to his sister. She merely tasted, and according to her own account did not swallow any of it. In a few minutes the boy was seized with convulsions and in half an hour was dead. The girl was affected in like manner but emetics were promptly administered and in twenty four hours the effects of the poison had disappeared . . .372. June. . .Since our last issue we have received some samples of the plant which gave rise to the poisoning. . . [It is] *Cicuta maculata*. . .373. Similar but more fatal case some few years ago. . .some residents on the hill above Davenport Road (Toronto). . .one of the children was found dead by the side of the house. . .found the plant growing in the potato patch where they had been at work." [There is a large pond at this place even today].

1884 Nor Wester (Calgary) 17 June. "Fifteen children of the Blackfeet were poisoned by eating wild parsnip and four of them died."

1892 Millspaugh 67. "A few practioners only using very small doses as a substitute for conium, and some of the laity, little knowing its toxic properties, as a gargle in sore throat. . .Later the powdered leaves were employed to a limited extent to alleviate the pain of scirrhus cancers."

1901 Morice DENE 19. "Scarifying. This is very commonly resorted to in all cases of rheumatism, local aching and *mal de raquettes*, or the spraining of the instep resulting from too severe snow shoeing. It is also regarded by many as a panacea against several other ills of a temporary nature. It consists in scratching numerous lines on the afflicted limb, followed in many cases, by a liberal application of the bruised root of the hemlock plant (*Conium maculatum*) 20.. . .[Saw] one of our women who since some time had been suffering from some nervous derangement, possibly catalepsy, bandaged about the head. . .she had undergone an almost identical operation in the vicinity of the temples with the addition, this time, of a poultice of bruised hemlock root." [Here Morice is using the name *Conium maculatum*, hemlock, for a plant which must be *Cicuta maculata* or water hemlock as *Conium maculatum* does not grow in the arctic. Cicuta relieves pain].

1920 Fyles 71. "Of all the poisonous plants in Canada, the water hemlocks are the most deadly and act most rapidly. All species of cicuta are exceedingly poisonous both to human beings and animals. . .The toxic principles are the alkaloid cicutine, with oil of cicuta and cicutoxine, a bitter resinous substance. . .The first symptoms usually occur within two hours after eating the plant. There is nervousness, twitching of the muscles of the mouth and ears, salivation, sometimes nausea and vomiting, bloating, intense pain, frenzied movements, dilated pupils, spasms and convulsions, frothing at the mouth and nose, twisting the head and neck backwards, rolling the eyeballs. The victim usually dies in the most violent spasm."

1922 Thomson & Sifton 74. "Parts of these are deadly in their effect. This fact was well known to the Indian by whom the root, the most poisonous part, was sometimes used for self destruction, being very rapid in its action. The roots have a sweetish and not unpleasant taste. Although the stems and leaves of the mature plant contain little poison, it has been repeatedly proved that the young plant, six inches or so in height, contains it in sufficient quantity to be the source of much danger. . .Some writers state that the plant is most poisonous in winter and spring. Others believe its effects in autumn are just as deadly. All agree, however, that during the hot summer season a larger quantity may be eaten without harmful results. Jacobson has discovered the reason for this, in his investigation of the properties of cicutoxin, the poisonous constituent, he found that it is very sensitive to rises in temperature, becoming polymerized by heat. The poison is very rapid in its action, and a very small quantity will produce death."

1923 H. Smith MENOMINI 55. "Musquash root not used. The Menomini say that this poisons the beaver."

1932 H. Smith OJIBWE 390. "Musquash root. The Pillager Ojibwe say that this root is used a little in their medicine, but did not know just how. It was smoked in hunting. . .432. The root of this is used in making a hunting medicine to be smoked to attract the buck deer near enough to shoot with bow and arrow."

1926-27 Densmore CHIPPEWA 377. "*Cicuta maculata* the seeds mixed with tobacco and smoked [as a charm].

1942 Fenton IROQUOIS 514. "Waterhemlock and its relatives, their physicians used the roots in poultices for reducing sprains and inflammations."

1955 Mockle Quebec transl. 66. "The plant is toxic. It is used as a gargle for sore throat." [Most of the chemical analysis has been done on *Cicuta virosa*, the species found in Europe. To the untrained eye this plant and our water hemlock are similar. One of the great dangers of the cicuta spp. is that the poison persists in the dried plants.]

1975 Robinson, Trevor. 108. "Cicutoxin in *C. virosa* owes its great toxicty to long chain acetylenic alcohols." [This presumably applies to the north American cicutas as well.]

BULB BEARING WATER HEMLOCK   *Cicuta bulbifera* L. Umbelliferae (Apiaceae)
A slender stem 100-300 cm tall, with many branches, round and hollow except where the broadened base of the leaf stalk joins it. The leaves are divided two or three times into narrow, saw-

toothed leaflets, not more than 5 mm wide. The whole plant has a fragile feathery look. As the plant matures tiny green bulbs appear in the angles formed by the leaf and the stem. Often there are no flowers, when they do appear they are in bunches rarely as wide as 5 cm of tiny white flowers. The base of the stem and the root may not be thickened. When cut open the stem will have less conspicuous divisions than the water hemlock. [not illustrated]

Range. Nfld., to B.C., s. to Pa., n. Ind., Io., and Oreg., and at higher altitudes to Va. July-Sept. in swamps, marshes, shores.

1724 Anon ILLINOIS MIAMI mss. 221-5. "For confined women who are not entirely delivered, they use the leaf of the sumac, with the root of an herb very common in the woods, and which has on its leaves a kind of ball. They call this herb by the generic name of Pallaganghy, which is to say Ocre; they take an equal quantity of the leaf of sumac and of the root of this herb, they crush the one and the other seperately; after each is in powder they mix them together and put them in a small kettle on a few embers; they add to it two times as much of sumac berries and make the confined woman drink the warm water in which the whole is soaked until she is entirely cured. That is to say, the space of two or three days, each day replacing in the kettle a similar dose, and giving some of it to the patient to drink a little before she eats at noon; at four o'clock and in the evening before retiring, the blood comes after the second or third taking, sometimes coagulated and as big as the fist, sometimes putrid, and at other times drop by drop. Those who have been wounded in the chest, head, or arm, and who lose much blood by the mouth take the same remedy with the same ingredients and are cured in a short time. The drop-sical ones find themselves well from it. They make them swallow the said drug with a little warm water in a spoon. The others above do not eat the medicine, they only drink the water in which it is soaked, but they give it all together to the dropsical ones. Those who have injured gums, be it from mal du Terre, be it from scurvy or other, are cured by holding this medicine on their gums a long time, without adding the sumac berries. . .Besides, those who are burned or frozen or who are attacked by a venereal disease use the same drug, applying it to the affected part without adding the berry of the said sumac." [Cicuta relieves pain, Gunn states it allays the irritability of the womb. However the herb Pallaganghy may be another plant than *Cicuta bulbifera*.]

1920 Fyles 73. "This species and the Western water hemlock (*C. vagans*) contain the same poisonous principle as (water hemlock). . .and are equally dangerous. . .In case of human poisoning an emetic may be given at once and a physician summoned."

1933 H. Smith POTAWATOMI 86. "The Forest Potawatomi have no name or use for this plant to our knowledge.'.

1955 Mockle Quebec Transl. 66. "Plant toxic, the toxicity attributed to cicutoxin."

WATER PARSNIP
Sium suave Walt. Umbelliferae (Apiaceae) (*S. cicutaefolium*)

Erect, furrowed, stout, branched stem up to 200 cm tall with stalked lower leaves that have 7-17 narrow leaflets, 5-10 cm long. The veins do not obviously run either to the notches or the teeth which are around their edge. The bunches of small white flowers are 3-12 cm wide. The fruit is somewhat flattened. The roots are fibrous, not like those of either *Conium* or *Cicuta*.

Range. Nfld. to B.C., s. to Fla. and Calif. July-Sept. in sunny wet meadows or swamps.

1892 Millspaugh 62. "The European Water Parsnip (*Sium latifolium* Linn.) an acrid narcotic poison." [This is the European species].

1920 Fyles 76. "This plant has long been held as suspicious and it has been reported as 'antiscorbutic, diuretic and poisonous', by Hyams of North Carolina. Pammel says it has been reported as poisonous from several different sources. As far as is known the toxic principles have not been investigated, but there is no doubt that it is poisonous. One of our correspondents in Ontario [Canada] recently lost several head of cattle from eating water parsnip. In writing of the effect of this plant upon his cows, he says; 'It seemed to affect the kidneys and back. First their water was red, then turned black as ink. They seemed to dry up. They did not bloat at all. Their milk dried up the first day'. A similar case was reported from Saskatchewan."

1932 H. Smith OJIBWE 432. "The seed of this is smoked over a fire by the Flambeau Ojibwe to drive away and blind Sokenau, the evil spirit that steals away one's hunting luck."

1943 Fernald & Kinsey. 291. Chippewayan and Cree ate the root of *Sium suave* but the authors question the significance of this plant for aboriginal subsistence.

1955 Mockle Quebec transl. 67. "*Sium latifolium*. The leaves and fruit eaten as an aperative and an antiscorbutic."

[The name *S. latifolium* was erroneously used by American authors for the North American *S. suave*. As a result there is confusion in the reports of poisoning due to different *Siums*.]

1976 Alex 112. "*Sium suave* Water Parsnip has been reported to be poisonous to livestock and, although experimental feeding trials have not proven it to be harmful, livestock growers should be cautioned against the potential danger of this native plant."

[Ontario Weeds is an excellent book to consult on the differences betwen *Cicuta*, *Conium*, *Sium* and *Heracleum* or, the water hemlocks, poison hemlock, water parsnip, cow parsnip, and also angelica]

FOOL'S PARSLEY   *Aethusa cynapium* L. Umbelliferae (Apiaceae)
A slender stem 20-70 cm tall with many branches. The leaves are shining, the botanical name Aethusa means burning from the shining foliage. This plant looks very much like parsley except for this shining foliage and the white flowers. Parsley has yellow flowers. Note the tufts of tiny leaflets that hang down from the base of the bunches of flowers.

Range. N.S. and Me. to Pa. and O. Native of Eurasia established as a weed here and there. June-Sept.

Common names. Dog-poison, lesser hemlock, false parsley.

1892 Millspaugh 65. "[There are] many cases of poisoning by the inadvertent use of this herb for parsley, from which it is easily distinguishable. . .By early writers it is so often confounded with *Conium*, that it is very difficult to trace its history. . .Its action has been generally considered like that of *Conium* but milder, and its principal, if not its only use, was in some forms of obstinate cutaneous disorders."

1931 Grieve (England) 614. "Poisoning from Fool's parsley showed symptons of heat in the mouth and throat. . .It is used medicinally as a stomachic and sedative for gastro-intestinal troubles in children, for summer diarrhoea and cholera infantum."

1968 Forsyth England 71. "Fool's Parsley contains two alkaloids, coniine and cynapine. The poisonous substances do not withstand drying and long storage; hay containing large quantities of the dried plant is harmless to livestock. . .The plant emits a repulsive odour, which becomes more marked when crushed or bruised." [The symptoms of poisoning by fool's parsley are similar to those produced by *Conium maculatum*].

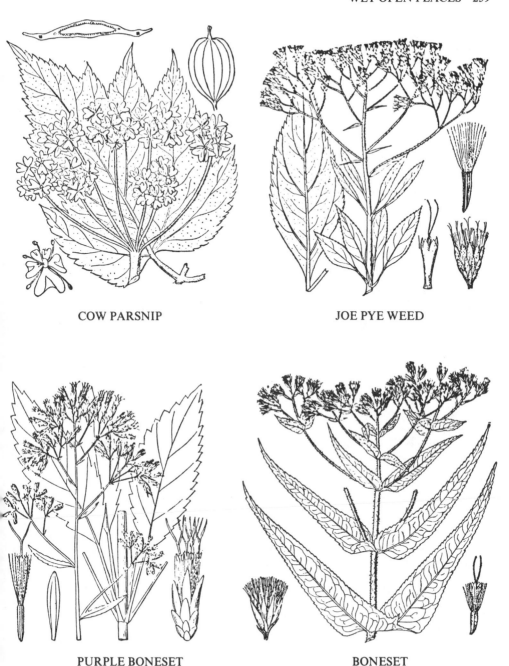

COW PARSNIP

JOE PYE WEED

PURPLE BONESET

BONESET

COW PARSNIP   *Heracleum lanatum* Michx. Umbelliferae (Apiaceae)
Stem very large and hollow up to 300 cm tall, grooved and often woolly. The leaf stalk has a
large sheath at its base which wraps the stem. The leaves are divided into three maple like leaflets
on one stalk. These are 10-30 (40) cm long and wide, dark green above, whitish below. The
bunches of white flowers are 10-20 cm across followed by flat fruit 7-12 mm long and nearly as
wide.

Range. Lab., to Alaska and Siberia, s. to Ga., and Ariz., June-July in rich damp soil.

Common names. Masterwort. In Europe this name is applied to *Imperatoria*.

1590 Harriot Virginia Indians 14. "There is an herbe which in Dutch is called Melden. Some of those that I describe it unto, take it to be a kind of Orage; it groweth about foure or five foote high; of the seed thereof they make a thicke broth, and pottage of a very good taste: of the stalke by burning into ashes they make a kind of salt earth, wherewithall many use sometimes to season their brothes; other salt they knowe not. Wee ourselves, used the leaves also for pothearbes." [see Chesnut below].

1633 Gerarde-Johnson 1009. "Cow Parsnip [*H. sphondylium* of Europe]. The leaves of this plant do consume and dissolve cold swellings if they be bruised and applied thereto. The people of Polonia and Lituania used to make a drinke with the decoction of this herbe, and leven or some other things made of meale, which is used instead of beere and other ordinarie drinke. The seede of Cow Parsnip drunken, scoureth out flegmaticke matter through the guts, it healeth the jaundice, the falling sicknesse, the strangling of the mother, and them that are short winded. Also if a man be falne into a dead sleepe or a swoune, the fume of the seed will waken him again. If a phrenticke or melancholicke man's head bee anointed with oile wherein the leaves and roots have been sodden, it helpeth him very much, and such as be troubled with the head-ache and the lethargie, or sicknesse called the forgetfull evil."

1830 Rafinesque 227. "Cow parsnep, masterwort. Root with a rank strong smell pungent caustic taste, it blisters the skin when fresh, dry it becomes aromatic. . .useful in cardialgy, dyspepsia and epilepsy. . .Leaves used as maturative in cataplasm. Seeds incisive. Roots and leaves used by empirics for many other complaints."

1859-61 Gunn. "The root and seeds are used, and are antispasmodic, carminative, and expectorant; also slightly stimulant. The seeds are used in the form of an infusion; in flatulent colic, to expel the wind from the stomach, and for dyspepsia or indigestion, being a rather pleasant aromatic stimulant and stomachic. A strong decoction of the dried root, taken daily for several weeks, has been found successful in curing epilepsy. The powdered root, in doses of one to two teaspoonfuls, given daily, has also been successfuly used for the same complaint. It is recommended in palsy, asthma, dysmenorrhea, in either decoction or in substance. The root should be dried before using, as it is said to be poison while green."

1868 Can Pharm. J. 6; 83-5. The root of masterwort, *Heracleum lanatum* included in list Can. medicinal plants.

1892 Millspaugh 62. "The European and North Asiatic Cowparsnip (*H. sphondylium*) an acrid vesicant." [Meaning it produces blisters when handled. Was this quality of the European plant attributed to the north American one, which apparantly is edible?]

1902 Chesnut 373. "*Heracleum lanatum*. . . is well known as the 'cow parsnip.' The tender leaf and flower stalk are sweet and very agreeably aromatic and are, therefore, much sought after for green food in spring and early summer before the flowers have expanded. In eating these, however, the outer skin is rejected. Mr George Grist. . .informed me that he has seen the hollow basal portion of the plant used as a substitute for salt. It was dried in short cylinders and eaten either in the dry state with other food or placed in the frying pan and cooked into the substance to be eaten. A strong decoction of the roots is said to have been used by the earlier Spaniards as a lotion for rheumatism."

1916 Waugh IROQUOIS 150-1. "Historical references are unanimous in stating that salt was seldom or never used by nearly all the eastern Indians at or immediately following the discovery. . .A desire for some saline material was shown by certain tribes. . .Beverly writes regarding the Indians of Virginia, that 'They have no Salt among them, but for seasoning, used the Ashes of Hiccory, stickweed, or some other Wood or Plant, affording a Salt Ash.' Hariot also reports that 'there is an hearbe which the Dutch called Melden.'"

1926-7 Densmore CHIPPEWA 301. "*Heracleum lanatum*. The leaves and roots are rubefacient; the root is said to be carminative and stimulant. . .342. Decoction of the root gargled for ulcerated sore throat or the dried root chewed. . . 350. For boils, boil the root and use as a drawing poultice. It was said that the dried root could be used without cooking. Dried root and flowers were pounded together and made into a poultice without boiling and applied to the boil."

1923 H. Smith MENOMINI 55. "An evil medicine used by the sorcerers. . .81. This herb is always found in the hunting bundle. It is a very personal sort of deer charm as only the owner of the bundle can handle it. If others touch it they will turn black and die. After the deer is killed, then it must be hung up and smudged for four days, after certain parts are removed. This plant and the leaves of Cynthia are burned in the smudge to take out the charm, by which the hunter was enabled to kill the deer. This smudge is also to drive away the evil spirit called sokenau, whose special mission is to steal one's hunting luck. On a deer hunt, as soon as the camp is established and the fire built, some of this cow parsnip is thrown on the fire, and the odor and smoke permeate the air for great distances, making it impossible for the sokenau to approach too closely under ordinary circumstances. But if the sokenau is desperate and determined to steal one's hunting luck, he may come right into camp, but the smoke of pikiwunus (cow parsnip) will cause him to go blind. In case a person is afflicted with bad hunting luck, a medicine made of pikiwunus seeds. . .is used. The whole hunting paraphenalia is smoked and smudged to drive away bad luck. The hunter must not eat any of the meat during this four days' smudging process, if he did, the Menomini believe that he would turn black and die. Wild ginger root is boiled with deer meat to remove the hunting charm."

1928 H. Smith MESKWAKI 249. "The root is a medicine for those who are sick with colic or any kind of cramps in the stomach. The seeds are used 'when they are almost crazed in the head'. It is used for severe pain in the head. The stem is used for a poultice to heal wounds. The root tea is used to cure erysipelas (doubtful identification). The fresh leaves and root of this plant will produce vesication, and have been used by the white man as a counterirritant. It is alleged to have a curative effect in epilepsy and to correct dyspeptic disorders. . .265. This is another of the Meskwaki potatoes, of which there is an unlimited supply on the reservation. It is cooked like rutabaga and tastes somewhat like it. We had always supposed the root to be poisonous, but they experience no ill effect from its use. The Meskwaki called our attention to the resemblance of the side roots to the ginseng root, and also to the fact that it smells the same as ginseng when fresh or dried. . .Many of the Meskwaki sold these side roots dried and tied like ginseng to the white buyer who used to visit the reservation buying ginseng, and he never discovered the difference. . .They say the roots are like sweet potatoes."

1932. H. Smith OJIBWE 390. "The Pillager Ojibwe pound the fresh root and apply it as a poultice to cure sores. . .432. According to the Flambeau Ojibwe there is a bad spirit 'sokenau' who is always trying to steal away one's luck in hunting game. He must be driven away from the camp of the hunter by smudging a fire with the roots of the Cow Parsnip. . .The Pillager. . .put the seed of the plant on a fire to drive away Sokenau. They boil the root to sprinkle their fishing nets and lure fish."

1945 Rousseau MOHAWK transl. 56. "Was used by the Indians of Loretta in the course of an epidemic of influenza. Marie-Victorin has already noted this use."

1955 Mockle transl. 67. "Used as an expectorant, diuretic, antidyspeptic, and antiepileptic. The Hurons of the village of Loretta (near Quebec) used with success it is said an infusion of this plant under the name of 'Poglus' to combat the Spanish influenza of the great epidemic of 1918 in their village."

[Some reports suggest that the fresh young shoots are eaten in salads and taste sweet. Others that the greens or the root should be boiled in 2 waters before using to prevent a disagreeable taste. The stems contain about 18% protein].

JOE PYE WEED
Eupatorium maculatum L. Compositae (Asteraceae)

Rough plants, 60-200 cm tall with stout stems that usually have purple spots and a whitish bloom. Four or five, stalked, leaves, rough with sharp teeth, occur at intervals around the main stem. The feathery flowers, lilac to deep purple, are in bunches of 9 to 22. The flowering top, flat in appearance, consists of many of these bunches.

Range. Nfld., to B.C., s. to Md., O., Ill., and N.M. July-Sept. in wet meadows.

Common names. Gravel root, trumpet weed, kidney root, king or queen of the meadows, skunk weed, marsh milk weed, quillwort.

PURPLE BONESET JOE PYE WEED
Eupatorium purpureum L.

Very like Joe pye weed except that the stem usually is full of pith and the purplish spots occur only where the leaves join it. The flowering top is rounded with 5 to 7 flowers in each bunch.

Range. s. N.H. to Pa. and in the mts. to Ga., w. to Wis., Io. and Okla. July-Sept. Rare in Canada; when found should not be picked, transplanted or disturbed. In drier habitats, open woods.

The Joe Pye Weeds and Boneset were given the botanical name of *Eupatorium* after Mithridates

Eupator, King of Pontus, Greece, who is said to have used a species of this genus in medicine in the first century B.C.

1799 Lewis Mat. Med. 143. [referring to *E. cannabinum* the very similar English plant]. "The leaves are greatly recommended for strengthening the tone of the viscera and as an aperient; and said to have excellent effects in the dropsy, jaundice. . .and scorbutic disorders. It is the common medicine of the turf diggers of Holland against the scurvy, foul ulcers and swellings of the feet, to which they are subject. The root is said to operate as a strong cathartic."

1785 Cutler. "Dr. Withering says an infusion of an handful of it vomits and purges smartly. An ounce of the root, in decoction, is a full dose. In smaller doses the Dutch peasants take it as an alterative and antiscorbutic."

1828 Rafinesque 176. "Joepye, gravel root has the same properties as boneset and has been used in fevers and gravel. The name Joepye is given to it from an Indian of that name, who cured typhus with it, by copious perspiration.'.

1859-61 Gunn 846. "The root is the part used, and is regarded by Botanic physicians as a valuable diuretic, while it is also somewhat tonic, stimulant, and astringent. It is highly esteemed in dropsical affections, in gravel, and affections of the kidneys and urinary organs. . .bruised roots in water. . .given in doses of from half to a teacupful three or four times a day. Eupurpuin. This is a concentrated resinous extract, obtained from the root and may generally be had at the Eclectic drug-stores and perhaps at others."

1868 Can. Pharm. J. 6; 83-5. The root of Queen of the Meadow, *Eupatorium purpureum*, included in list of Can. medicinal plants.

1876 Jackson Can. Pharm. J. 233. "It is diuretic, and one of the proper remedies for calculus."

1885 Mooney CHEROKEE 327. "Root used in decoction with a somewhat similar plant, not identified, for difficult urination."

1892 Millspaugh 78. "It proves useful in dropsy. . .gravel, gout and rheumatism; seeming to exert a special influence upon chronic renal and cystic trouble, especially when there is an excess of uric acid present."

1926-27 Densmore CHIPPEWA 348. Decoction of the root used lukewarm as a wash for inflammation of the joints, some put in a child's bath, if he is fretful this will make him go to sleep.

1923 H. Smith MENOMINI 30. "This is one of a large group of different plants known by the same Menomini name, but not all are for the same use. Most of them are used in diseases of the genito-urinary tract."

1928 H. Smith MESKWAKI 214. "Specimen 3620 of Dr. Jones collection is doubtfully identified as *Eupatorium purpureum* root. He gives it the name 'love medicine to be nibbled when speaking to women when they are in the wooing mood.'. . .It is said to have the power of 'fetching' them."

1932 H. Smith OJIBWE 364. "The Flambeau Ojibwe made a strong solution of the root, with which to wash a papoose up till the time he is six years old. This is supposed to strengthen him."

1933 H. Smith POTAWATOMI 52. "Fresh leaves of joe pye weed are used to make poultices for healing burns. Mrs. Spoon used the root as medicine to clear up after birth. . .117. The Forest Potawatomi use the flowering tops as a good luck talisman. When one is going to gamble he places the tops in his pocket and then is sure to win a lot of money."

1942 Fenton IROQUOIS 524. "The two purple flowered *Eupatoriums* were used for the kidneys."

1955 Mockle Quebec transl. 90. "The roots bitter, astringent, diuretic. They contain an acetyl-coumarin, euparine."

BONESET   *Eupatorium perfoliatum* L. Compositae (Asteraceae)
A hairy, straight, 40-150 cm stem with opposite leaves. These join around the stem making it appear the stem goes through the leaf. The leaves are rough, hairy beneath, with pointed ends. The bunches of white feathery flowers form a flat top, each bunch contains 9-23 flowers.
Range N.S., and Que., to Fla., w. to Minn., Nebr., Okla., and L. July-Sept in wet places.
Common names. Thoroughwort, agueweed, wild sage, feverwort, vegetable antimony, Indian sage.
1817-20 Bigelow 36. "A tonic stimulant. Given in moderate quantities, either in substance or in cold infusion or decoction, it promotes digestion, strengthens the viscera, and restores tone to the system. . .if given in large quantities, especially in warm infusion. . .it proves emetic, sudorific

and aperient. . .This plant has long been in use in different parts of the United States, for the same purposes for which the Peruvian bark. . .is employed. It has been found competent to the cure of intermittent fevers by various practitioners. . . when intended to act as an emetic, a strong decoction may be made from an ounce of the plant in a quart of water, boiled to a pint."

1828 Rafinesque 176. "Common in swamps, marshes and near streams. . .where it appears to have been stationed by the benevolence of nature, wherever men are liable to local fever. . .The whole plant, roots stems, leaves, and flowers are intensly bitter, but not astringent. . .It was one of the most powerful remedies of the native tribes for fevers, &c. It has been introduced extensively into practice all over the country. . .and inserted in all our medical works. . .It acts powerfully on the skin and removes obstinate cutaneous diseases. . .This plant may be so managed as to act as a tonic, a sudorific, a laxative or an emetic, as required. No other tonic of equal activity can be exhibited in fevers, with less danger of increasing the excitement or producing congestion; the only objection to its general use is its nauseous and disagreeable taste. . .Chapman relates that it cured the kind of influenza called Breakbone fever, acting as a diaphoretic, whence its popular name Boneset. . .Eberle says that catarrhal fevers may be removed by drinking a weak infusion of it going to bed. It is particularly useful in the indigestion of old people; and may be used as an auxiliary to other tonics and emetics in all cases."

1847 Winder Montreal. 11. "A favorite and well known remedy with the Aborigines is the *Eupatorium perfoliatum* . . .Its taste is intensly bitter, with a slight astringency, but no acrimony. . .The natives administer it with good effect in fever, and as a common drink in acute rheumatism, pouring a quart of boiling water on two drachms of the leaves, and drinking about three ounces three times a day."

1859-61 Gunn 744. "Boneset is a valuable plant and cannot be too highly prized as a medicine. . .An extract which may be made by boiling down a large quantity of the leaves and blossoms when fresh, straining, and then evaporating by slow heat, till it becomes a thick soft extract; or. . .by bruising the leaves and covering with alcohol or whisky and letting it stand a few days, then slowly evaporate. . .Both the leaves and Extract of Boneset can be had at the drug-stores."

1868 Can. Pharm. J. 6; 83-5. The leaves and tops of boneset, *E. perfoliatum*, included in list of Can. medicinal plants.

1876 Jackson Can. Pharm. J. 234. "Several species of *Eupatorium* are used medicinally in North America, foremost amongst them being the thoroughwort. . .the leaves and flowers reduced to a powder are purgative even in doses of from ten to twenty grains. It is said to have been prescribed with advantage in rheumatism, typhoid pneumonia, catarrhs, dropsy and influenza. . .thoroughwort tea is used by many physicians. . .is considered the very best of the indigenous antiperiodics as a substitute for quinine."

1892 Millspaugh 79. "There is probably no plant in American domestic practice that has more extensive or frequent use than this. The attic, or woodshed, of almost every country farm house, has its bunch of dried herb hanging, tops downward from the rafters during the whole year, ready for immediate use should some member of the family, or that of a neighbour, be taken with a cold. . .The use of a hot infusion of the tops and leaves to produce diaphoresis, was handed down to the early settlers of this country by the Aborigines, who called it by a name that is equivalent to ague-weed."

1894 Household Guide Toronto 116. "This is a good remedy for malarial diseases, chills, fevers and is also a tonic."

1915 Speck-Tantaquidgeon MOHEGAN 318. "Boneset tea. . .is drunk for many ailments, colds, fever, and general illness."

1926-27 Densmore CHIPPEWA 376. Root fibres combined with those of milkweed applied to whistle for calling deer.

1923 H. Smith MENOMINI 30. "This plant is used to brew tea which is used to dispel a fever. The Menomini name for this plant was not known to my informant. He thought it was a later one acquired from the white man."

1928 H. Smith MESKWAKI 214. "McIntosh uses the tea of the foliage and flowers to expel worms. The Meskwaki do not use it now, but say that long ago it was gathered for its root which was a sure cure for snake bites."

1924-25 Parker SENECA 11. Boneset a tonic.

1942 Fenton IROQUOIS 524. Boneset for colds and fevers.

1955 Mockle Quebec transl. 89. "The entire plant is used as a tonic and stimulant; the leaves and flowers as an emetic and to kill worms. It possesses as well as antibiotic properties, a glucoside, eupatorine."

1970 Jolicoeur Quebec 5. "Boneset steep and drink for colds, also relieves pain in the back and chest and gastric troubles."

1975 Antoine King Go-Home Bay Lake Huron, personal communication. Gathered boneset every fall to dry for the winter for use for colds and rheumatism. A bitter drink.

Several of the more southern Eupatoriums are being examined as anticancer chemotherapeutic drugs (Lewis and Elvin-Lewis 1977:134).

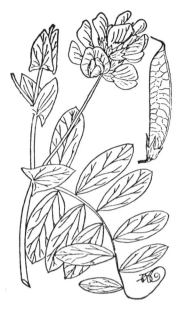

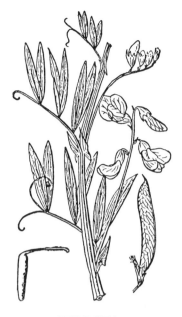

BEACH PEA   WILD PEA

BEACH PEA   *Lathyrus maritimus Fabaceae* (L.) Bigel. *(L. japonicus)*
An angled, smooth, strong stem to 100 cm lies on the ground. The leaflet at the base of the stalk
of the leaf (stipule) is 1.5-4 cm x 1-2.5 cm with two lobes at its base. The leaves consist of 3-6
pairs of leaflets 3-5 cm long and half as wide. There are usually 5-10 purple flowers about 2 cm
long. Pods 3.5 to 7.5 cm long containing small peas.
Range. Circumboreal, abundant on the Great Lakes, s. on the Atlantic coast to N.J. June Aug.
On coasts.
1534 Cartier transl. 33-4. "We found [on the Island of Brion in the St. Lawrence] that there it was
full of peas in flower, the same kind and as beautiful as those I saw in Brittany, they seem as if
sown by hand. . .[Cartier mentions seeing peas in P.E.I. and the Bay de Chaleurs in his second
voyage.]
1609 Lescarbot-Erondelle Port du Mouton [1606] Acadia 86. "We brought back in our ship wild
peas, which we found good. . ." 301-2 Port Royal. "And peas in great quantity along the sea-
shore, the leaves whereof we took in the springtime and put among our old peas, and so it did
seem unto us that we did eat green peas."
1632 Capt. James wintering in James Bay 140. "Here I am to remember God's goodness towards
us, in sending those aforementioned green vetches. For now our feeble sick men [scurvy] that
could not for their lives stir these two or three months, can endure the air and walk about the
house; our other sick men gather strength also, and it is wonderful to see how soon they were
recovered. We used them in this manner: Twice a day we went to gather the herb or leaf of these
vetches as they first appeared out of the ground; then did we wash and boil them, and so with oil
and vinegar that had been frozen, we did eat them. It was an excellent sustenance and refreshing; the most part of us ate nothing else. We would likewise bruise them and take the juice of
them, and mix that with our drink. We would eat them raw also with our bread. . .The fifteenth,
we did little but exercise ourselves seeing that by this time our men that were most feeble are
now grown strong, and can run about. The flesh of their gums became settled again, and their
teeth fastened, so that they can eat beef with their vetches."
1663 Boucher Quebec transl. 85. "There is found in the meadows a herb which is called 'Voisser-
on', which makes excellent hay, as well as another which is called Wild Peas, these are not found
at Three Rivers and Montreal where there are no tides." [Rousseau 1964:296 considers Vois-
seron to be *L. palustris*, see below, and wild peas to be *L. maritimus (japonicus)*].

WILD PEA   *Lathyrus palustris* L. Fabaceae
The stem usually is angled with wings extending out from it. It is slender, may be hairy and up to 100 cm long climbing over other plants. The var. *myrtifolius*(Muhl.) Gray is smooth and without wings and is found around the Great Lakes and from N.Y. to Wis. and Ill. The leaflet at the base of the leaf stem(stipule) has sharp lobes and is often toothed. The 2-6 red purple flowers are 12-20 mm long.
Range. Circumboreal, June-July in swamps, shores, wet meadows.
1910 Parker IROQUOIS 93. Ate the seeds.
1928 H. Smith MESKWAKI 273. "The root of this vetch is used as a lure to trap beaver and other game."
1932 H. Smith OJIBWE 373. "The Pillager feed this to a pony that is sick and claim it will make him fat. There is no record of its use as medicine by white men."
1933 Gilmore OJIBWA 133. Ate the seeds.

GARDEN PEA   *Pisum sativum* L. Fabaceae
1609 Lescarbot-Erondelle Acadia 1606 43. "For I may say (and that truly) that I never made so much bodily work for the pleasure that I did take in dressing and tilling my gardens, to enclose and hedge them against the gluttony of the hogs, to make knots, to draw out alleys, to build arbours, to sow wheat, rye, barley, oats, beans, peas, garden-herbs, and to water them. . .247 Our Souriquois did so anciently, and did till the ground, but since that Frenchmen do bring unto them kettles, beans, peas biscuits, and other food they are become slothful, and make no more account of these exercises."
1619 Champlain fac. ed. fourth voyage Ottawa River 1613 transl. 27. "To pass the rest of the day I walked in the gardens [of the Indians] which were filled with nothing but squashes, beans and our peas, which they are beginning to cultivate." (&de nos pois, qu'ils commencent à cultiver.)
1624 Sagard HURON 197. "They had planted peas secured at Quebec."
1628 Hennepin (1698) 596-7. "They had a hard winter of it at Quebec, for they wanted all sorts of Necessaries; and because the ships which brought Provisions were seized on by the English, they were therefore obliged to divide the small Provision that was left. Our Religious [Recollets] contended themselves with. . .the Pulse they had sown. Madame Herbers made them a Present of two Barrels of Pease, which are extraordinary good and large in Canada".
1632 Champlain-Bourne (1629) 48-9. "Nevertheless I had patience. . .waiting for the harvest of peas & grains which were growing on the ground cultivated by the widow Hebert & her son-in-law, who had 6 or 7 arpents of land sown." [at Quebec]
1632 Capt. James James Bay. "On the 15th [of May] I manured a little patch of ground that was bare of snow, and sowed it with peas, hoping to have some of the herbs of them shortly to eat, for, as yet, we can find no green things to comfort us."
See under woods for more vetches.

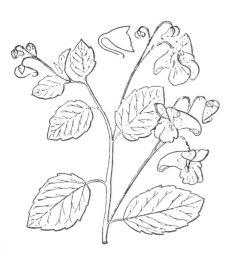

JEWEL WEED TOUCH ME NOT

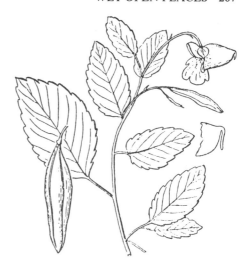

JEWEL WEED PALE TOUCH ME NOT

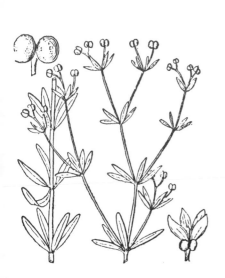

WILD MADDER

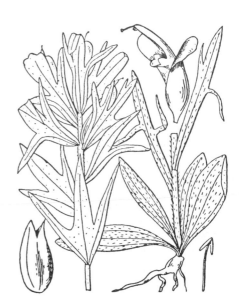

INDIAN PAINT BRUSH

WILD MADDER *Galium trifidum* L. var. *tinctorium* (L.) T.&G. Rubiaceae
Stems numerous, branched, slender, weak, often matted, sometimes with hooks. The leaves in whorls of 4-6 but nearly always some in a whorl of 5, their edges rough, tips rounded, 5-20 mm long with one nerve. The flowers on stalks that are rarely over 5 mm, 2-3 on each stalk. The fruit smooth, 1-2 mm long.
Range Can. and U.S. e. of the Rocky Mts. in moist places, May-July.
1663 Boucher Quebec transl. 167. "There are also some dye plants. . .which the Indians use: I will not give a full description, because I do not have complete knowledge, nevertheless there is a little root in the woods, which they use to dye color of fire, which gives a very live color." [This might also refer to the bloodroot which gives an orange red color].

1749 Kalm Fort St. Frederic July 15th. 380. "The *Galium tinctorium* is called Tisavojaune rouge by the French throughout all Canada and abounds in the woods round this place, growing in moist but fine soil. The roots of this plant are employed by the Indians in dying the quills of the American porcupines red, which they put into several pieces of their work; and air, sun or water seldom change this color. The French women in Canada sometimes dye their clothes red with these roots, which are small."

1830 Rafinesque 120. "The *Galium tinctorium* and *G. boreale*, called Savoyan in Canada, are useful plants, the creeping red roots dye a beautiful red like madder with acids; the Indians use them for their beautiful red dye. Schoepf says that *G. tinctorium* coagulates milk. . .and is useful for diseases of the skin."

1884 Holmes-Haydon CREE Hudson Bay 303. *Galium boreale* used as a diuretic. [The three nerved leaves are in whorls of four and the range is circumboreal].

1932 H. Smith OJIBWE 386-7. "The Flambeau Ojibwe make a medicinal tea from the whole plant of var. *tinctorium* for its beneficial effect upon the respiratory organs. Eclectic practioners [white] have used it for its nervine, antispasmodic, expectorant and diaphoretic properties. It has been successfully used in asthma, cough and chronic bronchitis. The plant has a pungent, aromatic, pleasant, persistent taste. . .*Galium trifidum*. . .in Ojibwe means male genetalia. The Pillager Ojibwe make a medicinal tea of this species for skin diseases such as eczema, ringworm and scrofula."

JEWEL WEED TOUCH ME NOT   *Impatiens biflora* Walt. Balsaminaceae
The stem is 50-150 cm tall, much branched, smooth, dark green and succulent. The leaves are 3-10 cm long, stalked and juicy when crushed. The flowers are like those of the snapdragon, orange yellow with reddish brown spots, 2-3 cm long with a tip at the end of their tubes that is 8 mm long and turns forward closely over the tube itself. The flowers hang from fine stems and are replaced by 2 cm long seed cases that burst open when touched.
Range. Nfld., and Que., to Sask., s. to S.C., Ala., and Okla. June-Sept. in moist woods, brooksides and springy places.

JEWEL WEED PALE TOUCH ME NOT   *Impatiens pallida* Nutt.
Very like touch me not except that the flowers are usually pale yellow with brown spots and the tip of their tubes is short, turns at right angles from the tube end and spreads out. This is really the best way to tell the two species apart as the colour of the flower is very variable.
Range. Que., and N.S., to Sask., s. to N.C., Tenn., and Mo. June-Sept. in wet places.

1749 Kalm Philadelphia October 14th. 105. "The flowers and leaves of the *Impatiens Nole tangere* or balsamine, likewise dye all woolen stuffs with a fine yellow color. . .868. Was called 'the crowing cock' by the Indians, because of the form of the flowers."

1830 Rafinesque 231. "Touchmenot, Jewel weed, Quickinthehand, Weathercocks. . .in common use for jaundice and asthma, as a tea. In large doses emetic, ecrocoptic [mildly purgative], and diuretic. Leaves used for piles and wash for wounds: they dye wool saffron color and yellow."

1859-61 Gunn 780. "*Impatiens pallida*, this herb is considered a good remedy in jaundice, and also a valuable diuretic in cases of dropsy, to be drank freely in decoction. The juice of the green herb, however, is most commonly used as a remedy for tetter, ringworm, and to remove warts, and for cleaning old and foul ulcers. A decoction of the herb is also said to be good applied to ringworm, salt-rheum and the like, and also as a poultice made by boiling in sweet milk."

1868 Can. Pharm. J. 6; 83-5. *Impatiens pallida* the herb included in list of Can. medicinal plants.

1915 Speck DELAWARE 320. "Balsam plant (*Impatiens biflora*) used for burns."

1923 H. Smith MENOMINI 78. "*I.biflora* the whole plant is used to make an orange yellow dye."

1928 H. Smith MESKWAKI 205. "Mc. Intosh used the fresh plant as a poultice to cure sores any place on the body, and the fresh juice to neutralize the sting of nettles."

1932 H. Smith OJIBWE 357. "Bearskin, the Flambeau medicine man said that the fresh juice of this plant rubbed on the head would cure headache. The leaves are steeped for a medicinal tea, but the ailment was undiscovered. The herbage of this plant. . .has been largely employed by homoeopathic physicians and eclectics. The chemical constituents are not known though the leaves apparently contain tannin. The medical value is questionable, though fresh applications of the juice appear to relieve skin irritations of various kinds, especially that of poison ivy. . .425. The whole plant is used by the Pillager Ojibwe to make a yellow dye and the material is boiled in the mixture with a few rusty nails."

1933 H. Smith POTAWATOMI 42. "*Impatiens biflora*. This is accounted a valuable medicine among the Forest Potawatomi who use the fresh juice of the plant to wash nettle stings or poison ivy infections. . .An infusion of the whole plant is drunk to cure colds in the chest or cramps in the stomach.. . .[They]also boil the infusion down to a thicker mass which they use as a liniment for treating sprains, bruises and soreness. . .116. The juice of the whole plant is boiled and the material placed in the pot while it is boiling to give an orange or deep yellow colour. Sometimes rusty nails are thrown into the solution when it is boiling and this deepens the color, making it somewhat reddish."

1955 Mockle Quebec transl. 53. "This plant is used as a diuretic, emetic and cathartic. It is used in infusion for jaundice. The crushed stems give abundant juice which is rubbed on eruptions caused by poison ivy to clear them up."

1978 Univ. Houston Dept. Pharm. was examining plants for antihistamine properties including *Impatiens*.

INDIAN PAINT BRUSH *Castilleja coccinea* (L.)Spreng. Scrophulariaceae
A straight, usually hairy stem 20-60cm tall with leaves deeply cut 3 to 5 times, the centre portion the longest. There may be uncut leaves near the base. The flowering stem crowded, the leaves at the base of the flower(bracts) bright scarlet, with three lobes or maybe five. The cup holding the flower 2-3 cm divided to the middle into two halves with rounded tops, scarlet, the flower greenish-yellow not much longer than its cup(calyx). Roots are often parasitic on other plants.
Range, Mass., to Ont., and Man., s. to S.C., Miss., and Okla. May-Aug. in damp sandy soil, meadows and moist prairies.
Common names. Wickawee, nose-bleed, red indians, bloody-warrior, prairie fire, scarlet painted cup, election posies.
1926-27 Densmore CHIPPEWA 288. "Indian name means 'Winabojo's grandmothers hair' and the plant was used for diseases of women and for rheumatism. . .362.The flowers were steeped and drunk for rheumatism either by themselves or in combination with other plants. It was said to be good for paralysis and for a cold."
1923 H. Smith MENOMINI 81. "This is a Menomini love charm. . .the scheme being to try to secrete some of the herb upon the person who is the object of the amour. . .The flowers and leaves of the Sessile paintbrush (a western species) are macerated in grease, such as bear oil or lard and after the virtues are extracted, the grease is set aside for use as a hair oil, invigorating the hair and making it glossy."

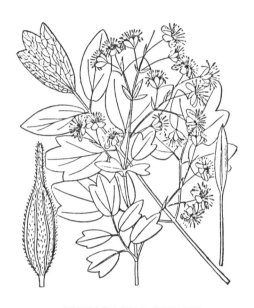

PURPLE MEADOW RUE

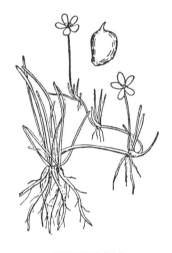

SPEARWORT

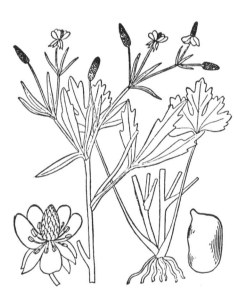

THE CURSED CROWFOOT

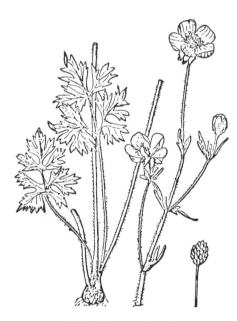

BULBOUS BUTTERCUP

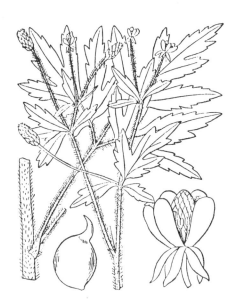

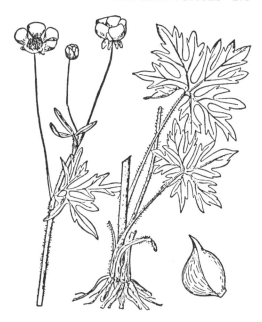

BRISTLY BUTTERCUP   TALL MEADOW BUTTERCUP

PURPLE MEADOW RUE   *Thalictrum dasycarpum* Fish. & Ave-Lall Ranunculaceae (*T. purpurascens*)

The stout purplish stem can be up to 90 cm tall and may be hairy. The leaves consist of several leaflets that are mostly more than 15 cm long. They have only three lobes at their ends and are hairy beneath. The flowers stand up, are feathery and purplish in color. The fruit is ridged and hairy.

Range. Que., Ont., James Bay, Man., Sask., Alta., s. to Ariz., Okla., Mo., Ind., and O. June-Aug. in wet meadows.

1633 Gerarde-Johnson 1252. *Thalictrum minus* [Great Britain]. . ."The leaves of Bastard Rhubarb with other pot-herbes do somewhat move the belly. The decoction of the root doth more effectually. Dioscorides saith, that the leaves being stamped do perfectly cure old ulcers."

1830 Rafinesque 267. "Roots of some species deemed useful for snake bites in Canada, leaves put sometimes in spruce beer, perhaps *Th. purpurascens*."

1928 H. Smith MESKWAKI 240. "This is love medicine used to reconcile a quarrelsome married couple. It is a hollow stemmed plant and as such is used by both tribes like a straw to drink water from a spring, hence it is called by two other names meaning hollow stemmed. . .Along with others of this family, Thalictrum contains a bitter tonic principle, berberine and has been used by the white man as a medicine."

1932 H. Smith OJIBWE 363. "Pillager Ojibwe have no Indian name for the purple meadow rue but use the root to make a tea to reduce fever."

1933 H. Smith POTOWATOMI 75. "The seed of the plant is used as a love medicine. When a man and his wife have been quarreling, the seeds are surreptitiously placed in their food to overcome the quarrelsome dispositions. The forest Potawatomi use the leaves and the seeds in combination with other materials to cure cramps. The seeds are peppered upon the surfaces of poultices to make them more effective. Among the whites, the root of Purple Meadow Rue is valued for its purgative and diuretic properties. The U.S. Dispensatory 1916 says that the Purple Meadow Rue contains berberine and has been used as a bitter and a tonic, especially useful in treating leucorrhea. . .123. Seeds are dried to smoke while hunting and are supposed to bring luck. In other circumstances, the seeds are mixed with tobacco and are the mark of a dandy. The young man will smoke this mixture when he is going to call upon some favorite lady friend."

1970 Willaman & Li 3975. "*Thalictrum dasycarpum* Fisch & Lall. the root contains berberine, thalictrucarpine, thalicarpine, thalidasine and magnoflorine. The stem bark contains thalicarpine and the whole plant above ground contains thalicarpine."
Currently under clinical trial as a cancer chemotherapeutic drug, *Thalictrum dasycarpum* (Lewis and Elvin-Lewis 1977:133).

SPEARWORT

Ranunculus flammula L. var. *filiformis* DC Ranunculaceae (*R. reptans*)

Spearwort resembles grass with leaves about 1.5 mm wide which sometimes have a few teeth. There is one flower with five yellow petals, at the end of a 3-15 cm tall stem, followed by tiny seeds with a minute beak.
Range. Circumboreal, s. to Mass., Pa., Mich., and Minn. and in the western cordillera, growing at the water's edge and creeping over moist sand or mud banks.

BULBOUS BUTTERCUP

Ranunculus bulbosus L.

A hairy erect stem 20-60 cm tall grows from a bulbous thickened base. Most of the leaves grow from the bulb on long hairy stalks. They are in three parts with the centre part on its own stalk, all the parts divided and cut up. The few stem leaves are not as divided. The five yellow petals are each 8-14 mm. The seeds are 2.5-3.5 mm with a distinct margin and stout outwardly curved beak.
Range. Native of Europe, naturalized in fields, meadows and lawns.

TALL MEADOW BUTTERCUP

Ranunculus acris L.

The slender hairy stem up to 1 m tall, leafy mostly below the middle. The hairy leaves from the root on long, hairy stalks are divided into three, each division again divided and cut and lobed. The upper leaves have just three divisions on short talks. There are many large yellow flowers the shining petals 8-16 mm. Pull off one and examine the honey gland at its base. The seeds are compressed with a short beak.
Range. Native Europe, naturalized in fields, meadows and roadsides, May-Sept. Double flowered forms occur.
Common names. Buttercup, yellow gowan, horse-gold, butter rose.

THE CURSED CROWFOOT

Ranunculus sceleratus L.

The thick hollow, branched stem is 20-60 cm tall, the whole plant is smooth. The leaves are deeply three parted, each part again divided, but all parts joined together at the base of the leaf. The upper leaves are smaller. The inconspicuous yellow petals of the flowers are only 2-3 mm, the cone shaped heads covered with seeds stand upright. The seeds have a minute beak.
Range. Circumboreal, In Am. s. to Va., Mo., N.M., and Calif. in marshes, swamps, wet meadows, ditch banks, April-Aug.
Common Names. Celery leaved crowfoot, ditch or marsh crowfoot, biting crowfoot, blisterwort, water celery.

BRISTLY BUTTERCUP

Ranunculus pensylvanicus L.f.

The erect, branched stem is 30-70 cm tall and hairy. The leaves are hairy, on short stems and are divided into 3 to 5 parts, each part on a short stalk, these stalks join together at the base of the leaf. There are few inconspicuous flowers with yellow 2-4 mm petals that are shorter than the turned down green sepals. The seed in a cone 10-15 mm tall, each seed with a beak one third its length.
Range. Lab., Nfld., N.B., P.E.I., N.S., Que., James Bay, Ont., Man., to B.C., s. to Wash., Ariz., N. Mex., Nebr., Ohio, Pa., and Del. and E. Asia. June-Aug. in marshes, ditches and wet meadows.
1633 Gerarde-Johnson 950. "There be divers sorts or kinds of these pernitious herbes comprehended under the name of *Ranunculus*, or Crowfoot, whereof most are very dangerous, to be taken into the body, and therefore they require a very exquisite moderation, with a most exact and due manner of tempering, not any of them to be taken alone by themselves, because they are

of most violent force, and therefore have the greater need of correction. The knowledge of these plants is necessary to the physician as of other herbes. . .For these dangerous Simples are likewise many times of themselves beneficial, and oftentimes profitable: for some of them are not so dangerous, but that they may in some sort, and oftentime in fit and due season profit and do good, if temperature and moderation be used. . .958. The chiefest vertue is in the root, which being stamped with salt is good for those that have plague sores, if it be presently in the beginning tied to the thigh. . .963. It is laid upon craggy warts, corrupt nails, and such like excrescences, to cause them fall away. . .Many do use to tie a little of the herb stamped with salt unto any of the fingers, against the pain of the teeth, which medicine seldom faileth, for it causeth greater paine in the finger than was in the tooth, by which meanes whereof, the greater paine taketh away the lesser. Cunning beggers do use to stampe the leaves, and lay it unto their legs and arms, which causeth such filthy ulcers as we daily see (among such wicked vagabonds) to move the people the more to pittie."

1791 Lewis ed. Aitkin 262. "The root and leaves of these plants taste highly acrid and fiery Taken internally they appear to be deleterious, even when so far freed from the caustic matter by boiling water. Oils in the air around the plants have occasioned headaches and anxieties. The leaves and roots applied externally inflame and ulcerate or vesicate the part, and are liable to affect also the adjacent parts to a considerable extent. They have sometimes, particularly among empirics and the common people, supplied the place of the far safer and not less effectual vesicatory, cantharides, for procuring an ulcer and discharge of serum, in sciaticas and some fixed pains in the head. Their pungency is diminished by drying, and by long keeping seems to be dissipated or destroyed."

1830 Rafinesque 73-5. "The whole plant, but chiefly the roots, of all those species, are of burning, acrid and corrosive taste when fresh. . .The acrid principle, like that of the *Arum*, is volatile, and disappears by the application of heat or even desication, but may be preserved by distillation. . .The acrimony of these plants is so powerful that it inflames and corrodes the lips and tongue of men and cattle, acts as a violent sternutatory, and if swallowed they bring on great pain, heat, inflammation of the stomach and even death. . .They act very differently on different individuals. . .Like the poison of the Rhus [poison ivy]. . .They have, however, often been used as external stimulants in rheumatism, hip disease, sciatica, piles, hemicrania, fixed pains &c; when applied to the scalp for hemicrania, it tumifies the hair without breaking the skin. A singular practice once existed in Europe, to cure intermittent fevers by applying them to the wrists or hands. They are useful to destroy warts, corns, and wens. In veterinary they are employed to cure the fistulous ulcers, and biles on the back of horses. Although very dangerous internally, the distilled water has been used as an instantaneous emetic. . .also a powerful but uncertain vermifuge. Henry mentions that the decoction thrown on the ground, makes the ground worms, used in angling, to come out of it."

1842 Christison 775. "The leaves and unripe germans [seeds] of both species (*R. acris, R. Flammula*) are acrid, occasioning when chewed a singular intense cutting sensation in the point of the tongue, which quickly ceases when the plant is spit out. . .According to my own frequent observation, the *R. acris* is far from being so energetic as to merit its specific name, and is often almost bland. *R. Flammula* and *sceleratus* are well named; and nothing can surpass the instant and intense pungency of the green unripe germens of the latter. *R. bulbosus*. . .less active than these last but much more so than *R. acris*. . .half an ounce of the juice of *R. sceleratus* will kill a dog."

1868 Can. Pharm. J. 6; 83-5. The corms of *R. bulbosus*, the bulbous buttercup, included in list of Can. medicinal plants.

1892 Millspaugh 3. "[Dr.] Withering. . .says 'It is an instantaneous emetic, as if nature had furnished an antidote to poison from among poisons of its own tribe; and it is to be preferred to almost any other vomit in promoting the instantaneous expulsion of deleterious substances from the stomach.' *R. sceleratus* is considered the most poisonous, its juice possessing remarkable caustic power, quickly raising a blister wherever applied, and a dose of two drops sometimes exciting fatal inflammation along the whole alimentary tract. . .A man at Bebay, France swallowed a glassful of the juice which had been kept for sometime, he was seized in four hours with violent colic and vomiting, and died the next day. . .A sailor who inhaled the fumes of the burning plant was attacked by epilepsy. . .terminated in death. . .The specific symptoms caused by this drug. . .show a decided irritant action upon the brain and spinal cord, as well as the mucous membranes generally."

1901 Morice DENE arctic 21. "Another appliance much in vogue among the Carriers, and which, though taken from the vegetable kingdom, is hardly less effective than fire, is a sort of blister made of the bruised green leaves and stems of a plant called *waltak* in Carrier, and of the botanical identity of which I am not quite sure, though I incline to belief that it is the *Ranunculus scleratus*. Its caustic properties are so great that it is seldom applied directly to the flesh, sometimes a thick covering of linen stuff being unequal to the task of rendering its application bearable for more than a few moments. It is used against almost any acute pain of local character."

1915 Speck MONTAGNAIS 306. "Pungent leaves of the buttercup, *Ranunculus acris*, when inhaled, produce local inflammation and sneezing which provides a 'vent' for the pent up feeling of a headache. . .315.[The] leaves are crushed and inhaled from the hands to relieve a headache."

1920 Fyles 35. "As its name implies, the cursed crowfoot is one of the most virulent of our native species. . .The chemical composition of the acrid and bitter juice of the buttercups is not well known, but it is thought that the substance is similar to the anemonine of the species *Anemone*. The toxic principle is volatile and the buttercups may be rendered harmless by drying. When dried with the hay they may be eaten by stock without injury. . .It is stated that in man a single flower of *R. scleratus* may give rise to poisonous symptoms similar to those caused by *Anemone* and *Colchicum*."

1923 H. Smith MENOMINI 79. "The root of the *Ranunculus recurvatus* Poir. is a coloring material for a shade of red. When it is boiled, the coloring matter is extracted and material is immersed in the tepid dye water."

1932 H. Smith OJIBWE 426. "The entire plant of bristly crowfoot is boiled by the Flambeau Ojibwe to yield a red coloring dye. Bur oak is added to set the colour. . .They smoke the seeds of this in their hunting medicine to lure the buck deer near enough for a shot with bow and arrow."

1933 H. Smith POTAWATOMI 75. "Mrs. Spoon uses the entire plant of the bristly crowfoot for an astringent medicine, disease unstated. . .The Forest Potawatomi use the entire plant boiled with rushes or flags which they wish to dye yellow, for making mats or baskets. To set the color they usually place a handful of clay in the pot."

1928 H. Smith MESKWAKI 239. "The centre of the flowers or stigma of the yellow water crowfoot are used for a snuff to cause sneezing. This buttercup floats in the water. [*R. flabellaris*]."

1945 Rousseau MOHAWK 42. "The Mohawk name means 'the plant which makes a hole,' that is to say which pierces a hole in the skin. When there is too much water in the blood, break up the plant and add to it a few pieces of poison ivy and after having placed on the patient an animal skin pierced with holes place on top of it the plants mixed with a little cold water. There will form a sore from which will run the surplus water in the blood. . .[According to F. Marie-Victorin] the Algonquins of Temiscaming take the flower and seed of the buttercup reduced to powder for a headache." [*R. acris*]

1955 Mockle Quebec transl. 43. "*Ranunculus abortivus* small-flowered buttercup, used in syphilis and also as a diaphoretic. [This buttercup has plain rounded leaves at its base, different from the cut and divided leaves on its stem]. . .*Ranunculus acris*, large flowered buttercup, the root rubefacient and vesicant. It contains an antibiotic principle, protoanemonine. *Ranunculus bulbosus*, the bulbous buttercup is used for skin disease. It contains protoanemonine."

1968 Forsyth England 35. "All members of the *Ranunculus* family so far described. . .contain an irritant poisonous substance, protoanemonin, which is a yellow volatile oil. It is present in its greatest concentration during the flowering period. . .Farmers have known for many generations that hay containing large quantities of buttercup is quite harmless. Had the animals eaten the same crop in its green state, they would have been severely ill or perhaps even died. . .First aid treatment, administer raw eggs and sugar, in skimmed milk, to allay the severe irritation of the mouth and stomach as early as possible. Further treatment should be prescribed only by the medical practitioner or veterinary surgeon."

1971 Jolicoeur 3. "Relieves headaches and together with honey from clover blossoms, other herbs and ingredients was used to treat cancer."

The use of various species of *Ranunculus* to treat cancer goes back to the oldest times and has continued in folk medicine right up to the present. Several secret 'cures' and formulas contain crowfoot. It has been used in Europe, Asia and America (Hartwell 1971:118).

[1972 Kinietz 223. In quoting the report in the Paris Archives of 1724 on the medicines used by the Illinois and Miami Dr. W. B. Hensdale is credited with considering a plant used for gun shot wounds and loss of blood by the mouth, as the crowfoot ranunculus. It has seemed to me much more likely that it was a geranium and so has been entered in that section, which follows.]

Ranunculus spp. contain anemonin and protoanemonin which are active against broad-spectrum bacteria. The plants are used in the treatment of abrasions, toothache and rheumatism (Lewis and Elvin-Lewis 1977:360).

[The name crowfoot comes from the fact that many of the leaves laid on wet sand leave a mark not unlike that left by the foot of a crow. The wild geraniums grow in the same places the crowfoots do, wet meadows and serpentines. Tufts of leaves, without flowering stalks, of both plants look much alike, the flowers and seed pods are different. To make things more confusing both ranunculus and geranium are called crowfoot, although the name crane's bill is the better name for the latter.]

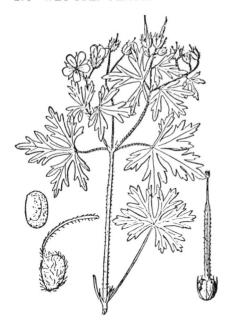

BICKNELL'S GERANIUM

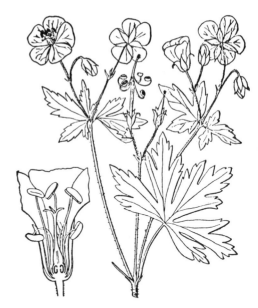

WILD or SPOTTED CRANE'S BILL

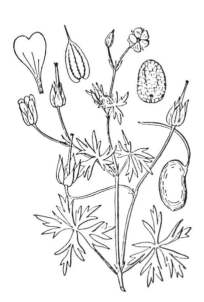

DOVE'S FOOT GERANIUM

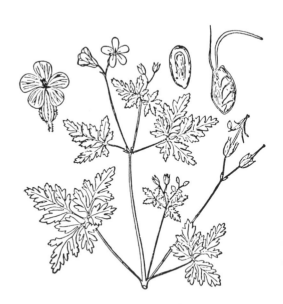

HERB ROBERT

BICKNELL'S GERANIUM   *Geranium bicknellii* Britt. Geraniaceae
Many ascending branches, to 50 cm covered with hairs. Some of the leaves will be on long stalks, growing from the root and looking much like those of the crowfoot (*Ranunculus acris*) or buttercup. The leaves are deeply cut into five lobed parts and are hairy. The flowering stem is covered with gland tipped hairs. It has two flowers, each with five pink-purple petals 7-9 mm long. These

are followed by a hairy tube 20-25 mm long with a sharp beak at its tip 4-5 mm long. The five seed cases split and roll up and out, so the whole resembles a candelabra. When the seed is ripe these cases curve round, turn down, their seed pods touch the tube and burst open hurling the seeds into the air.
Range. Nfld., N.S., N.B., to Yukon and B.C., s. to Io., Ind., Pa., and N.Y. May-Sept. in open woods, fields and moist meadows.

WILD OR SPOTTED CRANE'S BILL   *Geranium maculatum* L.

A few long stalked leaves grow from the roots. The stem, straight, hairy, 30-70 cm tall has a single pair of opposite, short stalked leaves near the top. These are cut into 5-7 sections but not as deeply as those of Bicknell's geranium. From this point grows the flowering stem bearing several conspicuous rose-purple or occasionally white flowers 2.5-4 cm wide, followed by a 3-4 cm tube with a 5-8 mm beak.
Range. Me., to S.C., and n. Ga., w. to Man., S.D., and Ark., Apr.-June. in woods.
Common names. Alum root, chocolate flower, american kino root, rockweed, shame-face, sailor's knot.

DOVE'S FOOT GERANIUM   *Geranium columbinum* L.

This geranium has purple flowers with petals only 8-10 mm long followed by a tube 2.5 cm with a beak of 4-5 mm.
Range. Native of Europe, established as a weed from N.Y., to O., s. to N.C.
1633 Gerarde-Johnson 938-9. Dove's foot cranesbill. "It seemeth, saith my Author to be good for greene and bleeding wounds, and aswageth inflammations or hot swellings. The herbe and root dried, beaten into most fine powder, and given halfe a spoonfulle fasting, and the like quantitie bedwards in red wine or old claret, for the space of one and twenty daies together, cureth miraculously ruptures or burstings, as my selfe have often proved, whereby I have gotten crownes and credit: if the rupture be in aged persons, it shall be needfull to add thereto the powder of red snailes (those without shells) dried in an oven, in number nine, which fortifies the herbs in such sort, that it never faileth, although the rupture be great and of long continuance: it likewise profiteth much those that are wounded into the body, and the decoction of the herbe made in wine, prevaileth mightily in healing wounds, as my selfe have likewise proved."
1724 Anon ILLINOIS-MIAMI mss. "When one is wounded by a gun shot, or arrow, or fall, or when one has been crushed under a tree and loses blood by the mouth, they use a root they call by the generic word ouissoucatcki, that is to say, with several feet; they crush this root and put four pinches of it with a quill in a little warm water that they make the patient swallow, who is marvelously strengthened by this medicine. If he is in delerium he returns to good sense, and the blood he vomits begins to stop; when he has breathed a little they give him some of that which we have shown above to stop the blood entirely and so the perfect cure." [Cited Kin. 222 who states that "The probable identification of the plants have been given through the courtesy of Dr. W.B. Hinsdale." his identification for this remedy is the crowfoot ranunculus. It seems an odd choice given the plants qualities, see under buttercups. I have placed this remedy under the geranium where it fits in with other recorded Indian use].
1785 Cutler. The root is astringent and frequently used in gargles for cankerous sores in the mouth and throat.
1791 Lewis ed Aitkins. One of our best indigenous astringents. . .Diarrhoea, chronic dysentery, cholera infantum in the latter stages and various hemorrhages are the forms of disease in which it is most commonly used. Also valuable as an application to indolent ulcers, and injection in gleet and leucorrhea, a gargle in relaxation of the uvula and apthous ulceration of the throat.
1817-20 Bigelow 86-7. "The root of the Geranium is the part to be used in medicine, is internally of a green colour, and when dry is exceedingly brittle and easily reduced to powder. It is one of the most powerful astringents we possess, and from its decided properties, as well as the ease of procuring it, it may well supersede in medicine many foreign articles of its class which are consumed among us. . .[it] has been repeatedly employed in medicine by various practitioners in this country. . .It is particularly suited to the treatment of such discharges as continue from debility after the removal of their exciting cause."
1828 Rafinesque 217. "Powerful astringent, vulnerary, subtonic and antiseptic. The root is the

officinal part. . .it is extensively used in the country for all bowel complaints; but sometimes improperly or too early. . .The infusion is a valuable lotion in unhealthy ulcers and passive hemorrhagy, also one of the best injections in gleet and leucorrhea. It was once deemed a styptic in bleeding hemorrhagy but has failed in many instances. United to our native Gentians or to *Frasera,* it forms one of the most effecient cures for intermittents. A decoction in milk is very good in looseness of bowels and diarrhea. Our Indians value this plant highly, and use it for wounds, gonorrhoea, ulcers of the legs, diabetes, bloody urine, involuntary dicharges of urine, immoderate menstruations &c. . .It is also used in Veterinary for diseases of cattle or horses, and cures the bloody water of cattle. The doses are one to two ounces in infusion or decoction, two to four drachms of the tincture."

1846 Winder Quebec 11. "Although the Indians, being without the advantages of science to guide them in their choice of remedies, and treatment of diseases, derive their principles from mere experience, it is certain we are indebted to their materia medica for many valuable articles of a vegetable kind: it is certain that they are frequently successful in their adaption of these to complaints of a formidable character. One of the remedies in great use amongst them is the *Geranium maculatum* which many eminent physicians of the United States rank as one of the most powerful vegetable astringents, being principally composed of tannin and gallic acid. In the second stage of dysentery, and diarrhoea, after evacuants; in hemorrhages of the alimentary canal; and as a styptic in external bleedings, it rarely fails of giving relief. . .With the Indians it is a favorite external styptic, the dried root being powdered and placed on the mouth of the bleeding vessel. It is also much used by them as a wash in leucorrhoea. Internally, in doses of half a teaspoonful in cold water they consider it very efficacious in haemoptysis, and in this opinion they are fully sustained by Thatcher, Mease, Bigelow and others."

1859-61. Gunn 795. "The root, which is the part used. . .has a sourish and very astringent taste, puckering up the mouth like alum. . .It is a pure and powerful astringent, and one that may always be used with safety and confidence. Useful in diarrhea, dysentery, cholera infantum or summer complaint of children, and in all cases where astringents are needed. . .For children a very good plan is to boil the root in sweet milk, until you have obtained the strength, sweeten with white sugar; and if you add a little nutmeg, Cloves and Cinnamon, you make it all the better. This is a splendid remedy for summer complaint and may be given freely."

1868 Can. Pharm. J. 6; 83-5. The root of *Geranium maculatum*, wild geranium, included in list of Can. medicinal plants.

1885 Mooney CHEROKEE 326. "Used in decoction with wild grapevine (*Vitis cordifolia*) to wash mouths of children in thrush; also used alone for the same purpose by blowing the chewed fiber into the mouth."

1892 Millspaugh 32. "The American Aborigines value the root of this plant as an astringent in looseness of the bowels, and exhaustive discharges of all kinds. . .in fact the uses of a decoction of the root have been great wherever an astringent or styptic seemed to be required."

1926-27 Densmore CHIPPEWA 342. The dried and finely powdered root put in the mouth when it is sore, used especially for children.

1923 H. Smith MENOMINI 36. "The Menomini claim that it has binding qualities in its roots, hence employ it in the treatment of flux and like troubles."

1928 H. Smith MESKWAKI 222. "This root is accounted a great medicine by McIntosh and also by the Meskwaki generally. It has many varied uses among them. It is used to cure sore gums and pyorrhoea, and to stop teeth from aching. It is also a cure for neuralgia. Its greatest use is in curing piles and hemorrhoids. A poultice of the pounded root is bound upon the anus to cause protruding piles to recede. The root of *G. maculatum* appears in three specimens in the Dr. Jones collection. . .Specimen 3657 is the root. . .and is used to relieve one with bloody piles. It is prepared for use by pounding the root in a bladder. Specimen 5057 is the base of the plant. . .It is boiled and made into a drink, or used as a poultice on a burn."

1932 H. Smith OJIBWE 370. "The Pillager Ojibwe use the astringent root for the treatment of flux, and also for healing a sore mouth."

1955 Mockle Quebec transl. 52. "The root, rich in tannin, is, because of its astringent properties, used for diarrhea, dysentery, cholera and externally for inflammations of the skin."

HERB ROBERT   *Geranium robertianum* L. Geraniaceae

A weak, hairy, reddish stem up to 60 cm tall with spreading branches. The hairy leaves are cut into 3 to 5 parts with at least the middle part on its own stalk but all joined together at the leaf stalk. All parts of the leaf are lobed and cut, sometimes with a reddish tinge to them. The pink to red purple flowers are 10-15 mm wide. It is the beak that separates with the seeds in this species. The whole plant has a heavy disagreeable scent when touched.

Range. Nfld., N.B., P.E.I., sQue., Ont., s to Ill., Ind., Ohio and Md. in damp rich woods, May-Sept.

Common names. Dragon's blood, jenny wren, red bird's eye, red robin.

1633 Gerarde-Johnson 939. "Herbe Robert. . .is good for wounds and ulcers of the dugs and secret parts; it is thought to staunch blood."

1785 Cutler. "Herb robert blossoms pale red. It is considered astringent and smells somewhat like musk. A decoction of the plant has been known to give relief in calculous cases. It is given to cattle when they make bloody water.

1828 Rafinesque 219. "The Geranium robertianum of Europe, grows also in north America from New England to Ohio, on stoney hills, and is the weak equivalent of *G. maculatum*; but it is also diuretic, and therefore more available in nephritis, gravel, and diseases of the bladder. . .1830 223. Good cataplasm for erysipelas, gargarism in sorethroat; used for disease of cattle called bloody water."

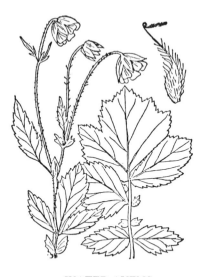

WATER AVENS

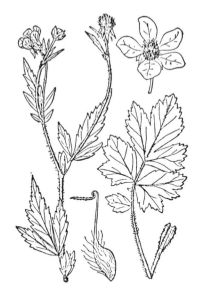

YELLOW AVENS

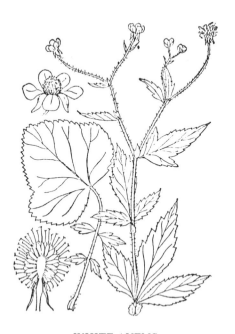

WHITE AVENS

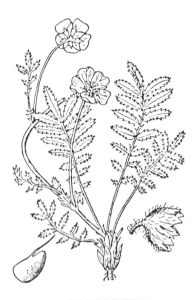

SILVERWEED

WATER AVENS *Geum rivale* L. Rosaceae

The hairy stem is from 30 to 60 cm tall. The outer petals [sepals] of the flower are purple, 7-10 mm long and upright. The inner petals are yellowish, suffused with purple and purple veined, shorter. The flowers nod at the end of their stem. The seeds have feathery hairs sticking out from them.

Range. Lab., Nfld., N.B., P.E.I., N.S., Que., Ungava Bay, Ont., Man., to B.C., s. to Wash., N. Mex., Mo., Ind., Pa., and N.C., Iceland, Europe and W. Asia, in swamps and wet places.

Common names. Purple Avens, Indian chocolate, throatwort, maiden-hair, chocolate root, cure-all.

YELLOW AVENS *Geum aleppicum* Jacq. (*G. strictum*)

The stems can be up to 30 cm tall covered with spreading brownish hairs. The leaves consist of many opposite leaflets of various shapes with tiny ones in between and always one large leaflet at the end of the stalk. They are green and hairy on both sides, having long stalks when at the base of the plant and none when near the top. The 1 to 2 cm, deep yellow to orange, five-petaled flowers are alone at the ends of their stems. They are followed by a brown 2 cm wide ball of hooked bristles. The very similar wood avens, *G. urbanum*, is introduced in America.

Range. Nfld., N.B., P.E.I., N.S., Que., Hudson Bay, Ont., Man., Yukon-Alaska, s. to Calif., N. Mex., Nebr., Pa., and N.J. in meadows, marshes, waste areas, open woods.

WHITE AVENS *Geum canadense* Jacq. (*G. album*)

A taller plant than the yellow avens, the white avens can grow from 40 to 100 cm. The stalks of the flowers are covered with small glandular hairs. The flowers are white, the petals broader at the tips than the base.

Range. N.B., N.S., Que., s. Ont., to Minn., N. Dak., s. to Tex., Okla., Ala., and S.C. in rich thickets and borders of woods.

1633 Gerarde-Johnson 996. Herbe Bennet and *Geum rivale*. "Avens is called Caryophyllata, so named of the smell of Cloves which is in the roots. . .The roots of. . .*Geum rivale* have the smell of Cinnamon. . .The decoction of Avens [*G. Urbanum*] made in wine is commended against the cruditie or rawnesse of the stomacke, paine of the Collicke, and the biting of venomous beasts. The same is likewise a remedie for stitches and griefe in the side, for stopping of the liver; it concocteth raw humours, scoureth away such things as cleave to the intrals, wasteth and dissolveth winde, especially being boyled with wine: but if it be boyled with pottage or broth it is of great efficacie, and of all other pot-herbes is chiefe, not only in physical broths, but commonly to be used in all. The leaves and roots taken in this manner dissolve and consume clottered bloud in any inward part of the body; and therefore they are mixed with potions which are drunk of those that are bruised, that are inwardly broken, or that have fallen from some high place. The roots taken up in Autumn and dried, do keep garments from being eaten with moths, and makes them to have an excellent good odour, and serve for all the physicall purposes that Cinkefoiles do."

1748 Kalm Philadelphia October 30th. 197. "The people who have settled on the Mohawk River in New York, both Indians and Europeans, collect the root of *Geum rivale*, and pound it. This powder some of them boil in water till it is a pretty strong decoction; others add only cold water to it and leave it so for a day; others mix it with brandy. Of this medicine the patient takes a wineglass full on the morning of the day when the fever does not come, before he has eaten anything. I was assured that this was one of the surest remedies, and more certain than the Jesuits' bark [ague remedy]."

1785 Cutler. Throatroot, cure-all, blossoms purplish, in boggy meadows. "The root is powerfully astringent. A decoction of it has been used, with good success, as a gargle, and a drink in inflamed and ulcerated sore throats and cankers. It is said, that the powdered root will cure the tertian agues, and that it is much used by the Canadians for that purpose. . .Common avens blossoms white or yellow by borders of fields. . .The roots gathered in the spring, before the stem grows up, and put into ale, gives it a pleasant flavour, and prevents its' growing sour. Infused in wine it is a good stomachic. When it grows in warm dry situations, its taste is mildly austere and aromatic."

1814 Clarke 72. "*Geum urbanum.* . .Common avens, Herb Bennet, Febrifuge, tonic. In intermittents, dysentery, chronic diarrhoea, debilities of the stomach and intestinal canal, &c. . .It i inferior in its febrifuge virtues to some species of the salix [willow]."

1828 McGregor Maritimes 23. "A decoction of the root, called chocolate root, is used by the Indians as a certain remedy for the severest attack of cholic."

1828 Rafinesque 222. "All the Avens have nearly the same properties, they are astringent, styptic, tonic, febrifuge, stomachic &c. They are used in the Northern States and Canada. In Connecticut they supersede the cinchona; but they are weaker, although less stimulant in fevers. They do not increase excitement and are therefor useful in hemoptysis and phthisis. They are decidedly excellent in dyspepsia and visceral affections; Ives states that its long use, restores to health the most shattered and enfeebled constitutions. They are often used in decoctions with sugar and milk like chocolate or coffee, to which they resemble: also for dysentery, chronic diarrhoea, colics, debility, asthma, sore throat, leucorrhea, uterine hemorrhage. They are the base of the Indian Chocolate of the Empirics. . .These roots are sometimes put in Ale as stomachics."

1841 Trousseau & Pidout Paris transl. Root used as base for astringent gargle.

1842 Christison 463. "The root of this common plant, [*G. urbanum*] is an old aromatic tonic and astringent remedy, now entirely abandoned in British practice. . .The root, which is brown externally and reddish in substance, has a fragrance like that of cloves while fresh; and when dry, i has an astringent, bitter, somewhat aromatic taste. It contains tannin, a little resin, and a trace o volatile oil, which is probably more abundant in the fresh root. Formerly it was used in frequen doses of thirty or sixty grains as an astringent and tonic in chronic mucous discharges. Mr. Pereira says it is employed in England for giving a clove like flavour to ale."

1868 Can. Pharm. J. 6; 83-5. The root of *Geum rivale* and the root of *Geum album*, the water and the white avens, included in list of Can. medicinal plants.

1885 Hoffman OJIBWA 200. "Yellow avens (*G. strictum*) [*aleppicum*], the roots are boiled and a weak decoction taken internally for soreness in the chest and cough."

1892 Millspaugh 54. "Though Geum has been dismissed from the U.S. Ph. it still retains a place in the Eclectic Materia Medica. . .An analysis of Avens by Buchner proves it to be very similar to the European *G. urbanum.*"

1920 Saunders 161. "Decoction of the fragrant rootstock of the water avens used as a beverage in Canada. The root said to be boiled and the water drunk with sugar and milk as a chocolate substitute. The best taste obtained from roots dug in fall or early spring."

1926-7 Densmore CHIPPEWA 356. The root of white avens is used for female weakness, manner of preparation not stated by Densmore.

1923 H. Smith MENOMINI 49. "None of the native Geums were known to be used."

1932 H. Smith OJIBWE 384. "*G. macrophyllum* Willd. The Flambeau Ojibwe used this for a female remedy." [The large-leaved avens differs from the yellow avens in having a larger, less cut leaflet at the end of each leaf].

1942 Fenton IROQUOIS 523. "To summarize this discussion of white borrowings from Indian medicine, we offer a partial list of the more important medicinal plants used by the Iroquois. . .524. Avens, (*Geum canadense, G. rivale, and G. strictum*) in fever and diarrhea. . .were common colonial remedies." [It seems the whites knew the uses of the geums before their contact with the Indians.]

1959 Mechling MALECITE of Maritime provinces of Canada used the root of the water avens for diarrhoea and that of the white avens for croup and cough.

1971 Palaiseul France transl. 74. "Herbe de Saint-Benoit was used by the army of the Republic when quinine was in short supply, and a large number of soldiers were cured of intermittent fevers by its use. It is given in an infusion of 30 to 40 gr. of the root to a litre of water, 3 cups a day, or in wine, 40 to 50 gr. of the root crushed and left for 8 days in a litre of good wine, filtered and 2 or 3 glasses drunk per day. This wine is tonic, digestive and cleansing. It has been written that it 'rejoices the heart, and brings from the eyes, nose, teeth, head and heart all that should not be there'."

SILVERWEED   *Potentilla anserina* L. Rosaceae (*Argentina anserina*)

The long reddish stem runs over the ground, rooting and starting new plants. The leaves can be up to 30 cm long, consisting of many opposite leaflets, some tiny, some to 4 cm in length. They are sharply toothed, dark green and smooth above and covered with silvery wool beneath. The yellow flowers, 2 cm across, are alone on their stalks.

Range. Iceland, Greenland, Nfld., N.B., P.E.I., N.S., Que., James Bay, northernmost Ont. to Yukon and Alaska s. to Calif., N. Mex., Ind., N.Y., and New Engl. on wet sandy beaches, along rivers in waste places.

Common names. Argentina. wild tansy, goose grass, silver feather.

1633 Gerarde-Johnson 993. "Wilde Tansie boiled in wine and drunk, stoppeth the laske and bloudy flix, and all other flux of bloud in man or women. The same boiled in water and salt and drunke, dissolveth clotted and congealed bloud in such as are hurt or bruised with falling from some high place. The decoction hereof made in water, cureth the ulcers and cankers of the mouth, if some honie and allom be added thereto in the boiling. Wilde Tansie hath many other good vertues especially against the stone, inward wounds, and wounds of the privie or secret parts, and closeth up all greene and fresh wounds. The distilled water taketh away freckles, spots, pimples in the face and Sun-burning; but the herbe laid to infuse or steepe in white wine is far better. But the best of all is to steepe it in strong white vineger, the face being often bathed and washed therewith."

1830 Rafinesque 253. "Antiseptic, used in gargles for loose teeth, spongy gums: by coction [cooking] becomes edible."

1945 Rousseau Quebec transl. 92. "When a person has a stoppage of urine, this makes it come. It is the leaves in infusion that are used."

1945 Porsild Arctic 16. "The thickened roots or fleshy, tuber-like branches are edible raw, cooked or roasted. The roots are best in early spring when they taste like sweet potato."

1955 Mockle Quebec transl. 59. "*P. anserina*, the leaves are astringent and diuretic. It is prescribed as an emmenagogue for dysmenorrhea. According to Youngken and Fischer the plant possesses a stimulant action on the uterine muscle. . .*P. argentea*, the same use is made of this plant as of silverweed."

P. anserina has been used since the middle ages in Europe in folk medicine in the treatment of cancer (Hartwell 1971)

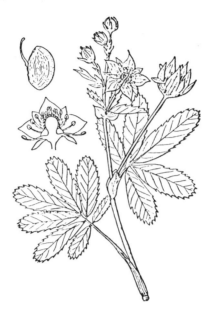

PURPLE OR MARSH CINQUEFOIL

PURPLE OR MARSH CINQUEFOIL   *Potentilla palustris* (L.) Scop. (*Comarum palustre*)
The smooth reddish brown stem may crawl or stand upright from the roots growing in the water
or marsh. The upper part of the stem is hairy. There may be 3 or as many as seven leaflets making up the leaf. All have deep teeth around the edges, each tooth ending in a sharp point. The
leaflets are green above and grayish below with a few hairs. The base of the leaf stalk sheathes
the main stem part way around it. The flowers stand up and are a showy reddish purple, 2 cm
across. There are usually several at the end of the stem. It is the sepals that are coloured not the
petals which are only half as long.
Range. Circumboreal, s. to N.J., O., Io., and Calif. June-Aug. in swamps, bogs and borders of
streams.
Common names. Purple marsh locks, cowberry, purplewort, meadownuts, bog strawberry.
1926-27 Densmore CHIPPEWA 344. A decoction of ½ a root to a quart of water drunk for
dysentery. . .302-303.The constituents are a bitter principle, mucilage and tannins. The roots are
bitter and astringent but do not appear to have been used in medicine by the whites.
1932 H. Smith OJIBWE 384. "The root was dug from the water by John Whitefeather's wife,
Flambeau Ojibwe, who said it was a cure for cramps in the stomach, and is used alone as one
medicine. Under the Pillager Ojibwe name of swamp root John Peper said that it was medicine
with them but that he did not know how to use it."

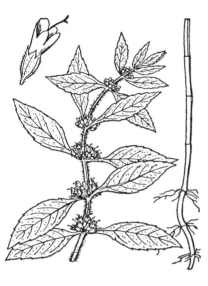

NATIVE FIELD MINT

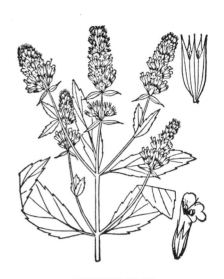

PEPPERMINT

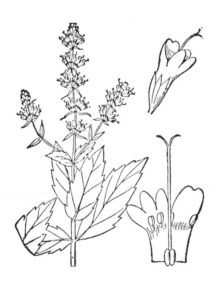

SPEARMINT

NATIVE FIELD MINT   *Mentha arvensis* L. var. *villosa* (Benth.) Stew. Labiatae (Lamiaceae) (*M. canadensis*)
Erect stems 20-80 cm tall, hairy at least on the angles of th square stem. The leaves with short stalks, toothed and pointed, 2-8 cm x 6-40 mm with several pairs of lateral veins. In this mint the flowers grow in the axils of the leaves, (where they grow from the stem) in tight bunches. The cup holding the flower(calyx) is hairy. The flowers are 4-7 mm long, usually bright lilac but may be white or pink. This mint is very aromatic when crushed.
Range. Circumboreal, in Am. s. to Va., Mo. and Calif. in wet places.
1475 Bjornsson Icelandic mss. transl. Larsen 83. "Mentha, mint. Dry and hot in the second degree. If a man drinks it, it digests food in his stomach and prevents vomiting and drives away

intestinal worms. Mint also helps the testicles against many things, if they are rubbed with its broth. If one crushes mint and applies it to the nipples, it purges burnt milk in them (translation difficult). If one crushes mint with salt it is good to drip in the ear for earache. If one rubs mint on his tongue, a sore will disappear therefrom. If a woman drinks it with must (fruit juice), it hurries her child-birth. Mint crushed with salt is good for the bite of a dog. Mint mixed with vinegar is good for a flux. If one washes cheese with mint juice, it will not rot. . .S17. Take a stem of mint and put it in the nose; then it takes away the offensive smell."

1884 Holmes-Haydon CREE Hudson Bay 303.*Mentha canadensis* L. in the form of a tea as a stomachic.

1916 Waugh IROQUOIS 149. "Monarda, horse-mint. . .represented the mint family which suggests that the other mints may also have been pressed into service."[as teas].

1919 Sturtevant 361. "The Indians of Maine eat mint roasted before the fire and salted and think it nourishing."

1923 H. Smith MENOMINI 39. "This is one of the three plants taken together to form a cure for pneumonia. The others used with it are (Catnip)*Nepeta cataria* and peppermint *Mentha piperita* L. The compound is drunk in the form of a tea and is also used as a poultice on the chest."

1932 H. Smith OJIBWE 371. "Among the Flambeau Ojibwe a tea is brewed from the entire plant, to be taken as a blood remedy. It is also used by them in the sweat bath, John Peper, Pillager Ojibwe, made a special trip to find this on the lake shore. . .and says that they use it as a tea to break fevers."

1933 H. Smith POTAWATOMI 61. "Use the leaves or the top of this plant for treating fevers and also make a stimulating tea for curing pleurisy."

1945 Rousseau MOHAWK transl. 58."An infusion is given to children for fever to dispel it."

1945 Raymond TETE-de-BOULE transl. 129. "Much used for fever. The Indian name means 'that which has a strong odor'."

[Menthol is obtained commercially from the high-numbered polypoid var. of this plant grown in Japan. The American wild plant also contains menthol used to flavor cigarettes]

1976 Parish. 377. "Menthol is used in numerous preparations for treating cough and common cold symptoms. It also relieves itching and is used in skin applications."

The introduced species, spearmint and peppermint are included here because they were so important in the households of America probably from their beginnings. Spearmint was collected by Clayton in 1739 in Virginia as a naturalised plant according to Gronovius. It seems reasonable to assume the reference from 1609 onwards to garden herbs being planted include spearmint. Too common to be worthy of note. See Dry open places for Pennyroyal and Monarda, two indigenous mints.

PEPPERMINT   *Mentha piperita* L. (*Mentha aquatica* L. x *Mentha spicata* L.)
An erect smooth, square stem 30-100 cm tall, may be glandular. In the black variety of peppermint the stem is often purple or reddish. The leaves are 3-6 x 1.5-3 cm on stalks mostly 4-15 mm long, they may be hairy on the veins beneath. The lavender flowers grow close together up a spike that is 2-7 cm tall. The cup that holds the flower (calyx) is 2.5-4 mm long. The tube of the flower is smooth, its lobes hairy.
Range. A European cultigen, often escaped in our range.

SPEARMINT   *Mentha spicata* L. (*M. viridis*)
Very like peppermint except that the stalks of the leaves are 0-3 mm long and the cups in which the flowers sit (calyx) is 1.5-2 mm long. The flowers grow at intervals up the slim spike. The taste of spearmint is distinctive as is that of peppermint. The mints hybridize freely so their identification is difficult.
Range. Native of Europe now found throughout our range. Both these mints like moist soil.
Spearmint was known to the Greeks and Romans and was brought to Britain by the latter. Peppermint was only recognized as a distinct species in 1696. Its medicinal properties were quickly recognized and it was admitted into the London Pharmocopoeia in 1721. The references that follow are to peppermint unless spearmint is indicated.

1789 Farrier's Disp. Mint is a strengthener of the stomach, restores lost appetite. It is used in baths to give vigor and spring to the nerves relaxed by hard riding and travel.

799 Lewis Mat. Med. 181. "For flatulent colics, languor, hysterical affections, retchings and other dyspeptic symptoms, acting as a cordial and often producing immediate relief, from its stomachic, antispasmodic and carminative qualities. It seems to act as soon as taken, and extend its effect through the whole system, instantly communicating a glowing warmth. Water extracts the whole pungency of this herb by infusion."

820's Mat. Med. Edinburgh-Toronto mss. 30. "This mint has a greater degree of pungency than the others. The leaves have a considerable degree of aromatic odour and taste. It is used as a stimulant and carminative. *M. viridis* much the same."

841 Trousseau & Pidoux Paris transl. "The tea for asiatic cholera [first case in Canada at Quebec 8th June 1832] made from peppermint; also for insomnia and nervousness. It is reputed an anaphrodisiac. It is used for typhoid, colds and to slow the coagulation of milk."

842 Christison 630. "It came into general use in the medicine of western Europe only about the middle of the last century and in the first instance in England. Essence of peppermint is one part of oil of peppermint and eight parts rectified spirit. Peppermint in its action a powerful diffusible stimulant, antispasmodic, carminative and stomachic. One of the most efficacious of carminative remedies."

854 Pharmacy Recipe Book Ontario Canada. Peppermint cordial made with oil of peppermint, wine, sugar and water to taste.

859-61 Gunn 819. "Peppermint is very extensively and profitably cultivated in some places for the purpose of distilling the oil, which is done from the green herb. . .The leaves are the part used, though the whole herb is medicinal. . .Used as a stimulant to promote perspiration, to relieve flatulent colic and griping pains. . .and to allay or prevent nausea and sickness at the stomach. . .Spearmint is used freely in infusion or tea, in fevers and is highly beneficial on account of its cooling effect, its action upon the kidneys, suppression of urine, high-colored, or scalding urine. . .A strong tincture of the green herb, made in Holland Gin, is also an excellent diuretic. . .to be taken in doses of a wineglassful three or four times a day."

868 Can. Pharm. J. 6; 83-5. Peppermint and spearmint, the whole plant, included in list of Can. medicinal plants.

871 Can. Pharm. J. 39. "A few years ago, when in China, I became acquainted with the fact that the natives, when suffering from facial neuralgia, applied oil of peppermint to the seat of the pain with a camel-hair pencil. Since then in my own practice I have frequently employed the oil of peppermint as a local anaesthetic not only in neuralgia but also in gout, with remarkably good results. I have found the relief of pain to be almost instantaneous."

892 Heebner Pharm. Toronto 190. "Menthol, found in most plants of the mint family, and extracted from oil of peppermint. . .used as a local anaesthetic, and to relieve the pain of burns. Oil of peppermint is often met with in commerce from which the menthol has been extracted. Test to detect the removal of pip-menthol from oil of peppermint. A test tube partially filled with the oil under examination is placed in a freezing mixture of snow and salt for 10 to 15 minutes. If the oil has not been tampered with, it will become cloudy, thick and of jelly-like consistence."

892 Millspaugh 116. "Facial and sciatic affections are greatly relieved by fomentations of the leaves, or rubbing the oil or menthol, directly over the course of the nerve itself; the action is temporary, but decidedly happy."

894 Household Guide Toronto 122. "Peppermint externally applied is an efficient remedy in neuralgia. It is good for sickness of the stomach, colic and cholera of children. Essence of peppermint may be given in doses of from ten to twenty-five drops in water, or on a lump of sugar."

915 Speck MONTAGNAIS 314. "'Peppermint leaf' the Montagnais name is taken from the French, steeped for headache medicine."

915 Speck-Tantaquidgeon MOHEGAN 318. "Spearmint made into a tea is good as a worm medicine. . .319.Peppermint tea is given to babies for worms and grown people drink it."

916 Waugh IROQUOIS 118.Other plants said to have been eaten raw, in some cases with salt. These include. . .Peppermint.

923 H. Smith MENOMINI 39. "Peppermint is one of the ingredients in a cure for pneumonia."

928 Parker SENECA 11. For croup cause the child to breathe vapour from crushed peppermint. Use skunk oil, twenty drops at a time, internally. Also use for coryza [bad cold].

949 Hobart & Melton. 96. "Menthol (from oil of peppermint or synthetic). Menthol applied externally produces a feeling of coldness by stimulation of the nerve endings associated with the sensation of cold. There follows a mild degree of anaesthesia due to paralysis of all sensory nerve ends. On this account menthol is rubbed into the skin to relieve frontal headache and neuralgia, and is a component of some analgesic liniments and balms for the relief of rheumatic and allied pain, the irritation of *herpes zoster, pruritus ani* etc. . .menthol vapour is inhaled, alone, or with steam, for the relief of respiratory catarrh and sinusitis, and it is a component of many oily nasal-spray solutions."

1955 Mockle Quebec transl. 81. "*Mentha piperita, M. spicata*, aromatic, stomachic and digestive."

1971 Jolicoeur Quebec 5. "Peppermint, one of the best herbs. For colds, colic, cramps, for babies, stomach pains, bringing out measles, diarrhoea, even in cattle, good for everyone."

1972 Palaiseul transl. 204. "Mint is one of the principal weapons in the war on vermin, it is put in beds, in sacks of grain to drive off mice. It has been in all epochs the mainstay of mothers of families. . .A monk in the 9th century wrote; 'if you wish to enumerate completely all the virtues, kinds and names of mint, you would be capable of saying how many fish swim in the Red Sea'."

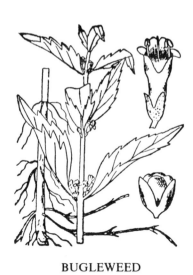

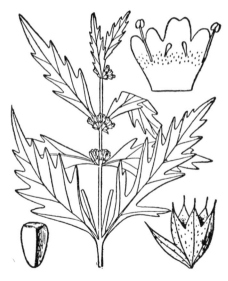

BUGLEWEED   CUT LEAVED WATER HOREHOUND

BUGLEWEED *Lycopus virginicus* L. Labiatae (Lamiaceae)
A slender square stem 16-60 cm tall, smooth or hairy. The leaves are 5-12 x 1.5-5 cm, dark green or purplish, with teeth, the lowest tooth far below the middle of the leaf. The insignificant flowers grow from the base of the leaf stalk. These are followed by nutlets, four meeting together to make one larger whole. This species is told from the northern bugle-weed (*L. uniflorus*) by the length of the angles of these nutlets. Both plants grow from roots which sometimes have tiny tubers on them.
Range e U.S.A. n. to Minn. and Maine July-Sept. in wet soil.
L. uniflorus Michx is found from Nfld., across Canada to Alas., s. to Cal., Ark., and N.C.
Common names. Water horehound, gipsy wort, Paul's betony.
1830 Rafinesque 29. "The *L. virginicus* is an excellent sedative. . .It has only lately been taken notice of. . .The whole plant is employed, it has a balsamic, terebinthaceous smell, peculiar to itself, when bruised, which is stronger in the seeds. The taste is pleasant, balsamic, and slightly bitter. . .one of the mildest and best narcotics in existence. It acts somewhat like Digitalis, and lowers the pulse, without producing any of its bad effects, nor accumulating in the system. . .I have made many experiments on this plant, and the results are, that although it does not cure the consumption, nor heal the lungs, it is very useful in hemoptysis, a plethoric habit, and internal inflammation. I consider it a very good substitute for all narcotics, Prussic acid, and even to bleeding, since it produces the same state of pulse and arterial system, without inducing any debility, nor acting on the heart or brain in any injurious manner. It may be used in many diseases, and whenever it is required to quell inordinate actions of the blood, or even other fluids. I am informed it is commonly used in New Jersey for diarrhoea and dysentery, which it helps cure. . .It is also peculiarly useful in inflammatory diseases of drunkards, in diseases of the heart, &c. I deem it the best sedative in almost all cases; it does not appear to act on the nervous system, but chiefly over the blood vessels. The usual way to take it has been in the form of a warm infusion, allowed to cool, taken as a diet drink, and without much nicety about the quantity. . .The *Lycopus vulgaris* has lately been extolled in Europe in fevers, and is said to have cured intermittents alone. As its qualities are very near alike those of *L. viginicus* being only a little more tonic and astringent, and a little less narcotic and sedative: they may, perhaps be tried as mutual equivalents in fevers and inflammatory disorders. All the species appear to have somewhat similar qualities and properties; but it is best to trust to *L. virginicus* alone as a sedative. The dried plants preserve their properties for many years."
1849 Stephen Williams 902. "One of the most valuable styptics we possess in our vegetable materia medica."

1859-61 Gunn 750. "When fresh it has a peculiar balsamic smell, somewhat like turpentine, and a slightly bitter, disagreable taste. The herb, or leaves and stems, are the parts used. It is astringent, tonic, and somewhat sedative. Used generally in infusion or tea, and is valuable in bleeding at the lungs, hemorrhages from the stomach or bowels, and in diabetes or excessive discharge of urine. Has cured this complaint when other means failed. To be drunk freely cold."

1868 Can. Pharm. J. 6; 83-5. *Lycopus virginicus*, the whole plant included in list of Can. medicinal plants.

1888 Delamare Island of Miquelon transl. 26. "*Lycopus virginicus* is very common on the plains of Miquelon. It is used in the U.S. for hemorrhages from the stomach."

1892 Millspaugh 117. "Most writers accept the idea that the plant is narcotic; we, however, infer, both from our own experience and that of others, that it is only sedative in that it removes, by checking hemorrhage, that nervous excitability and mental fear always accompanying such conditions. It is certainly an excellent hemostatic very useful in generous doses. . .Dr. King says Lycopus is decidedly beneficial in the treatment of diabetes."

1955 Mockle Quebec transl. 81. "*Lycopus virginicus* used in spitting of blood."

CUT LEAVED WATER HOREHOUND   *Lycopus americanus* Muhl.

The stiff, square stem can be smooth or hairy, from 30-60 cm tall. The leaves are 3-8 cm long, deeply cut into almost separate parts in the lower leaves or merely toothed in the upper. The rootlets do not have any tubers.

Range. Our most abundant sp. Nfld., and Que., to B.C., s. to Fla., and Calif. June-Oct in wet soil.

1785 Cutler. "*Lycopus americanus* is generally known by the name of Paul's betony. It is said the juice will give a permanent color to linen, wool and silk that will not wash out."

1928 H. Smith MESKWAKI 225. "Dr. Jones collection is the entire plant of this species used with a mixture of other medicines for cramps in the stomach. It is an unofficial herb sometimes used by the white man for its aromatic and bitter principles."

1926-27 Densmore CHIPPEWA 320. "*Lycopus asper* "These were called 'crow potatoes' and were dried and boiled." [Range of this species is Minn. and Io., w. B.C. and Cal., rare and probably adventitive eastward].

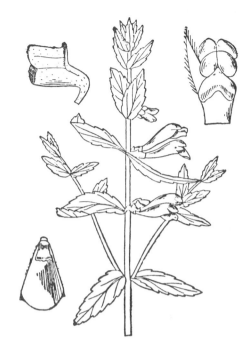

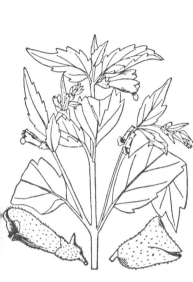

MAD DOG SCULLCAP   HOODED SCULLCAP

MAD DOG SCULLCAP   *Scutellaria lateriflora* L. Labiatae (Lamiaceae)
The slender, angled stem is 30-70 cm tall with many branches, hairy near the top. The thin stalked leaves are 3-8 x 1.5-5 cm with teeth. The flowering stem grows from where the leaf stalk joins the main stem. The flowers up this stem are each 5-8 mm long tubes, blue or rarely pink or white.
Range. Nfld., to B.C., s. to Ga., and Calif., July-Sept in wet places.
Common names. Blue scullcap, hoodwort, madweed, blue pimpernel.
1830 Rafinesque 81. "Is lately become famous as a cure and prophylactic against hydrophobia. This property was discovered by Dr. Vandesveer, towards 1772, who has used it with the utmost success, and is said to have till 1815, prevented 400 persons and 1000 cattle from becoming hydrophobus, after being bitten by mad dogs. . .Many empirics, and some enlightened physicians have employed it also successfully. But several sceptical physicians have since denied altogether these facts, and pronounced the plant totally inert, because it has no strong action on the system, and has failed in their hands. . .This plant has since been carefully analyzed by Cadet, in Paris, and found to contain many powerful chemical principles, which evince active properties. . .It has been used chiefly of late in all nervous diseases, convulsions, tetanus, St. Vitus' dance, tremors, &c. . .We lack, however, a series of scientific and conclusive experiments, made by well informed men; they have been discouraged by the ridiculous denial of sceptics. . .we have so few presumed remedies for this dreadful disease [hydrophobia] that it is desirable to confirm the properties of those supposedly available."
1859-61 Gunn 857. "Scull-cap is a valuable tonic nervine and antispasmodic. It is especially useful in St. Vitus' Dance, neuralgia, convulsions, delirium tremens; in nervous excitability, restlessness, and inability to sleep, and indeed in all nervous affections. It is also good in intermittent and nervous fevers. It is to be used freely in infusion, about half an ounce of the dry herb to a pint of boiling water. For nervous and spasmodic affections it is well to combine it with an equal quantity of the Lady Slipper root; and in fevers it may be combined with any of the diaphoretic or sweating herbs, such as Catnip, Sage, Pennyroyal, or Pleurisy root. The infusion may be taken either warm or cold. . .The scull-cap is by many considered to be a specific for the hydrophobia, or mad-dog bite-to be drunk freely in strong infusion. It may generally be had at the drug stores. The whole plant, leaves, stems and root, is medicinal."

1868 Can. Pharm. J. 6; 83-5. *Scutellaria lateriflora* the whole plant included in list of Can. medicinal plants.

1885 Mooney CHEROKEE 325. "A decoction of the four varieties of Gunigwaliski-*S. lateriflora, S. pilosa[elliptica], Hypericum corymbosum [punctatum]*, [see St. John's wort] and *Stylosanthes eliator* [pencil flower]- is drunk to promote menstruation, and the same decoction is also drunk and used as a wash to counteract the ill effects of eating food prepared by a woman in the menstrual condition, or when a woman by chance comes into a sick room or a house under the tabu; also drunk for diarrhea, and used with other herbs in decoction for breast pains." [*S. elliptica* and *Stylosanthes eliator* are in the southern limits of our range].

1892 Millspaugh 120. "Curative and prophylactic in canine rabies. . .Dr. S. W. Williams, whose cry of 'charlatan' and 'quack' was always raised upon the slightest pretext lends his support to the probable virtues of this plant. . .The plant has proved itself useful. . .when a tonic combining nervine powers might be deemed necessary; it is also considered diaphoretic and diuretic, Scutellaria is officinal in the U.S. Ph."

1901 Chesnut (California) 385. "*S. californica.* The leaves were known by the white man who was well versed in Indian lore, as being intensely bitter, and it was thought by him that the Indians use them as a substitute for quinine for chills and fever. This application was, however, disclaimed by all of the Indians consulted. The plant appears to be worthy of an investigation."

1924 Youngken 498. "This herb was long used by the Penobscot, Iroquois, Cherokee and other tribes, in decoction, as a remedy for numerous ailments." [Not listed by Speck as used by Penobscot, Montagnais, or Mohegans.]

1933 H. Smith POTAWATOMI 62. "The Forest Potawatomi did not know this plant and had no name or use for it to our knowledge."

1930 Am. Medical plants. The herb in reasonably constant demand.

HOODED SCULLCAP   *Scutellaria epilobilifolia* Ham. (*S. galericulata*)

The stem is weak, hairy on the angles, sometimes smooth or with glands, 20-80 cm tall. The leaves have almost no stalks, are 2-5 cm x 6-20 mm smooth above and hairy beneath with teeth. The flowers are conspicuous, each by itself where the leaf meets the stem, as the leaves are opposite, so there is usually a flower on each side of the stem. They are 1.5-2 cm long, blue or sometimes white.

Range. Transcontinental, s. to Del., Ind., Mo. and Calif. June-Aug. in wet soil.

Common names. Marsh scullcap, European scullcap, hooded willow herb.

1830 Rafinesque 82. "Schoepf states that *S. lateriflora, S. galericulata,* and *S. hyssopifolia,* to have similar properties, being abstergent and tonic; useful in intermittent fevers."

1923 H. Smith MENOMINI 40. Not used.

1932 H. Smith OJIBWE 372. "The Flambeau Ojibwe use this for medicine, having something to do with heart trouble, but we could get no definite information upon it."

1931 Grieve England 725. "The European species *S. galericulata* was at one time given for tertian ague, and was said to have proven beneficial where the fits were more obstinate than violent, 1 or 2 oz. of the expressed juice, or an infusion of a handful or two of the herb, being given. In England the remedy was not in use."

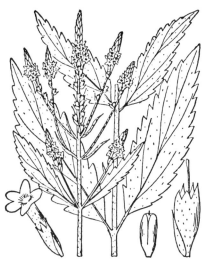

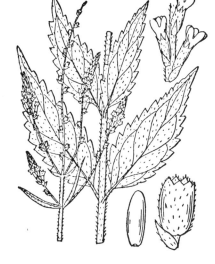

BLUE VERVAIN   WHITE VERVAIN

BLUE VERVAIN   *Verbena hastata L.* Verbenaceae
A hairy rough, square stem, 40-150 cm tall, with opposite, stalked leaves, 4-18 cm long with deep
teeth around their edges. There are several stiff narrow spikes crowded with 2.5-3 mm violet blue
flowers. The flowers come out one after the other up the spike and are followed by brown seeds
which overlap.
Range. N.S., to B.C., s. to Fla., Tex., Calif. June-Oct. in swamps, wet meadows, waste places.
Common names. False vervain, American vervain, wild hyssop, purvain, iron-weed.
The European *V. officinalis L* has leaves which are lobed as well as toothed and purplish to white
flowers. It is a weed in the U.S.
1475 Bjornson Icelandic mss. transl. Larsen 138. "Verbena iron-wort in Danish. It is of two kinds
and both work about the same. It is good to apply often to a poisonous bite. And with warm
juice of it, it is good to rinse one's mouth. If crushed and applied to new wounds, it draws them
together. If one crushes of it three roots and three leaves with water and drinks this before the
hour of the fever, that is good to do every second day. So also it helps for quartan fever if one
takes four roots and four leaves of it and drinks them boiled in wine. If one strews it between
people at the drinking, cheerfulness follows. If one bears this herb in his hand and ask a man
who is ill how he is getting on, and he answers 'Well' then he will improve. But if he answers 'ill',
there is no hope of life for him. If one makes a wreath of it and places upon a sick man's head, he
will get speedy help. . .S10. . .Item for stone of the bladder, take the root of the herb called
verbena and crush it with milk and drink it quickly. That does not at once cleanse the bladder,
but rather all that which injures and harms the urine in the bladder."
1633 Gerarde-Johnson 718-9. "Many old wives fables are written of Vervain tending to witchcraft and scorcerie, which you may read elsewhere, for I am not willing to trouble your ears with
reporting such trifles, as honest eares abhorre to heare.. . .a garland of Vervain for the head-ache,
when the cause of the infirmitie proceedeth of heat."
1672 Josselyn New. Engl. 205.*V. hastata* a wound herb not inferior to *V. officinalis.*
1741 Farrier's Disp. Cleansing obstruction of the liver, cataplasm for violent pains & stiffness in
joints.
1785 Cutler. "It is said that the surgeons of the American army, at a certain period when a supply of medicine could not be obtained, substituted a species of verbena for an emetic and expectorant and found its operation kind and beneficial."
1830 Rafinesque 274. "Our best medical sp. is *V. hastata* (simpler's joy). . .emetic expectorant,
tonic, a good substitute for *Eupatorium* [boneset], but much weaker, used in agues and fevers.

Said by Thompson to be next to *Lobelia* for an emetic in tea or powder, to check fevers and incipient phthisis. . .Was the holy herb of the Greeks and Druids, used as panacea, in incantations and to drive evil spirits."

1859-61 Gunn 875. "Wild hyssop, the root is the part used. . .It is an excellent emmenagogue, one of the best and safest known, in all cases of supressed menses; to be used freely in strong decoction, that is, say half a teaspoonful or more, three or four times a day. . .The warm decoction in large doses will vomit. A decoction of vervain root and boneset leaves, taken cold in doses of half a wineglass three or four times a day, is an excellent restorative, after having fever and ague."

1868 Can. Pharm. J. 6; 83-5. The roots of vervain, *Verbena hastata*, included in list of Can. medicinal plants.

1926-27 Densmore CHIPPEWA 356. "The flowers dried and snuffed up the nose to stop a nosebleed."

1923 H. Smith MENOMINI 58. "The root tea is used to clear up cloudy urine."

1928 H. Smith MESKWAKI 193. "The root of blue vervain with the root bark of sassafras is a remedy for fits. The root of blue vervain with that of the white avens (*Geum canadense*), golden seal (*Hydrastis canadensis*) and that of the white water lily (*Nymphaea odorata*) is a remedy for excema."

1945 Rousseau MOHAWK transl. 58. "'For refreshment cut the root into pieces, place on top of the head with a little cold water and sit in a current of air.' Whether one has vervain or not the other conditions will give the same result."

1955 Mockle Quebec transl. 80. "Vervain expectorant and emetic."

1970 Rimpler Ll. 33:4;491. New glycoside, hastatoside, isolated from *V. hastata* and *V. officinalis*.

WHITE VERVAIN   *Verbena urticifolia* L. Verbenaceae
The erect single, hairy, 40-150 cm tall stem has many branches. The stalked leaves are 8-20 cm long and toothed. The tiny white flowers are not crowded on their spikes.
Range. N.B., and Que.. to Ont., and Nebr., s. to Fla., and Tex. June-Oct. in moist fields and waste places.

1830 Rafinesque 274. "*V. urticifolia* herb useless, but root bitter, used against the erisypelas of Rhus [poison ivy] with milk and oak bark."

1923 H. Smith MENOMINI 58. "This is not used by the Menomini, though there are records of its aboriginal use by other Indians as an antidote to poison ivy. A bitter glucoside has been extracted from its leaves."

1928 H. Smith MESKWAKI 251. "The root tea is used to cure profuse menstruation. A specimen 3607 of Dr. Jones collection is the root of *V. urticifolia*. . .It is further described as 'they eat when they are on the point of death.' It is said that the eating of this medicine will revive the patient and restore him to health. Specimen 5173 of Dr. Jones collection is also the root of *V. urticifolia*, but it is used as a perfume and called 'fine haired woman'. Among white men, the white vervain has gained some repute as a treatment in cases of rhus-poisoning. . .195. The roots of white vervain with the berries of winter berry (*Ilex verticilata*) and those of the red cedar are made into a healing poultice for large external sores. A universal remedy for all sickness contains the roots of white vervain along with 7 other ingredients."

WOODS AND THICKETS

all kinds of wooded areas, ranging from climax forests, through open woods, to the edges of woods and including generally areas where plants are shaded by higher trees or shrubs and coniferous swamps. Also found in woods and thickets but discussed under other sections are jack in the pulpit, wood nettle, jewel weed, wild lettuce, columbine, cinquefoils, Indian hemp, chenopods, certain goldenrods, blackberries and raspberries

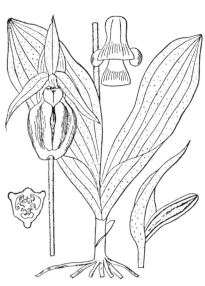

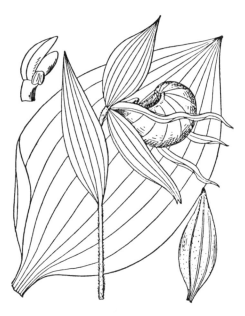

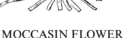

MOCCASIN FLOWER   YELLOW LADY'S SLIPPER

MOCCASIN FLOWER   *Cypripedium acaule* Ait. Orchidaceae
There are two stemless leaves, 10-20 cm long, hairy, pale beneath. The flowering stem is 20-40 cm high and hairy, there is a single narrow leaf (bract) arching over the solitary flower. The 3-6 cm long petals, pink with red veins fold inward to make the toe of the 'slipper' which has long white hairs inside. The greenish purple long petals (sepals) are 3-5 cm. The slipper may sometimes be white.
Range. Nfld. and Que. to Alta., s. to N.J. and n. Ind., and along the mts. and coastal plain to S.C. and Ala. Apr. June in acid soil, swamps and bogs to dry woods and sand dunes.
Common names. Stemless lady—slipper, nerve root, old-goose, squirrel's shoes, two-lips, Indian moccasin.

YELLOW LADY'S SLIPPER   *Cypripedium calceolus* L.var. *pubescens* (Willd.) Correll
The hairy 20-80 cm tall stem has leaves that wrap part of the stem and are 6-20 cm long and half as wide. The one or two flowers have toes that are yellow usually veined with purple and 2-6 cm long. The 3-8 cm long, narrow petals are yellowish green to purple brown, some twisted, the sepals are the same length and color.
Range. Circumboreal, s. to S.C., La. and N.M. May-June in bogs and moist woods.
Common names. Whip-poor-will's shoe, Indian shoe, yellows, American valerian.
1633 Gerarde-Johnson 443. "Calceolus, Our Lady's slipper. . .Touching the faculties of our Ladies Shoo we have nothing to write, it being not sufficiently knowne to the old Writers, no not to the new."
1749 Kalm Saratoga November 2nd. 611. "The moccasin flower (*Cypripedium*) which is found generally in the woods here, is said to be rather good for women in the throes of childbirth. I refer to the decoction made of the root."
1828 Rafinesque 141. "*Cyprepedium acaule* roots small and brownish, the roots the only medical part. It is with some satisfaction that I am able to introduce for the first time this beautiful genus to our Materia Medica; all species are equally medical; they have long been known to the Indians, who called them moccasin flower and were used by the Empirics of New England particu-

larly Samuel Thompson. Their properties have been tested and confirmed. . .They are sedative, nervine, antispasmodic &c. and the best American substitute for valerian in almost all cases. They produce beneficial effects in all nervous disease and hysterical affections by allaying pain, quieting the nerves and promoting sleep. They are also used in hemicrania, epilepsy, tremors, nervous fevers. They are preferable to opium in many cases, having no baneful nor narcotic effects. The dose is a teaspoonful of the powder diluted in sugar water. . .267 Favorites with Indian women to deck their hair."

1859-61 Gunn 815. "There are two or three varieties—perhaps more—all of which possess about the same medical properties; the two varieties, however, the one having yellow flowers, and the white and pink or red, are mostly used. . .The root is the part used. . .It is useful in all cases of nervous irritability, headache, hysteria, chorea, restlessness, and wherever a mild and safe nervine is needed. It is often combined with scullcap (*Scutellaria*) in severe nervous affections, the compound being more powerfully nervine and antispasmodic. . .The infusion is made by steeping about an ounce of the powdered root in a pint of boiling water; dose from a half to a teacupful every hour or two, or oftener, according to symptoms. . .It can always be found in drugstores."

1868 Can. Pharm. J. 6; 83-5. Lady's slipper, *Cypripedium pubescens*, the root included in list of Can. medicinal plants.

1885 Mooney CHEROKEE 327. "Yellow lady slipper. Decoction of the root used for worms in children. In the liquid are placed some stalks of the common chickweed or purslane (*Cerastium vulgatum*) which, from the appearance of its red fleshy stalks, is supposed to have some connection with worms."

1892 Millspaugh 170. "The. . .uses of the powdered root (given by Rafinesque) have been corroborated fully in domestic practice. Cypripedium acts as a sedative to the nerves in general, causing a sense of mental quiet and lassitude, and subduing nervous and mental irritation. It seems also to quiet spasms of voluntary muscles, and hysterical attacks, especially in women."

1915 Speck PENOBSCOT 310. "The plant of lady's slipper (*Cypripedium acaule*) 'many fine roots' is steeped as a medicine for nervousness."

1926-27 Densmore CHIPPEWA 342. "The dried, powdered root of *Cypripedium hirsutum* [*reginae*] is moistened and put on decayed teeth."

1923 H. Smith MENOMINI 44. "Moccasin flower (*C. acaule*) the root is used in male disorders. . .yellow lady's slipper is said to be used by the Menomini in female disorders. It has also been found in sacred bundles where its purpose is to induce dreams of the supernatural."

1928 H. Smith MESKWAKI 233. "Moccasin flower (*Cypripedium acaule*) Specimen 3641 of the Dr. Jones collection is the root of this species. . .It is part of a love medicine."

1932 H. Smith OJIBWE 377. "Yellow lady's slipper. . .Among the Pillager Ojibwe, the root of this species is said to be a good remedy for female troubles of all kinds."

1945 Rousseau MOHAWK transl. 69. "Yellow lady's slipper. An infusion of the roots alone when one has lots of wind in the chest, or mixed with *Dentaria* in the treatment of tuberculosis, or with dandelion to relieve kidney trouble when one leans over too often."

1945 Raymond TETE DE BOULE transl. 128. "Moccasin flower, the roots boiled in water make a tisane employed in stomach troubles either of men or women. It is equally good for the urinary system and controls children's kidneys. The Indian name translates 'that which has roots'."

1955 Mockle Quebec transl. 31. "The root is used as an infusion or extract for nervous excitement. It is praised also for epilepsy."

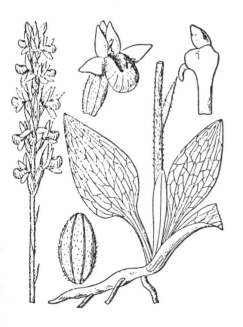

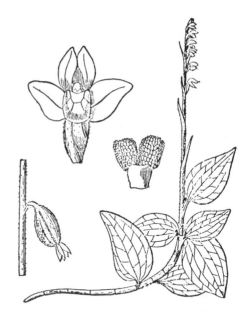

DOWNY RATTLESNAKE PLANTAIN   LESSER RATTLESNAKE PLANTAIN

DOWNY RATTLESNAKE PLANTAIN   *Goodyera pubescens* (Willd.) R.Br. Orchidaceae
(*Epipactis p.*)
The leaves are 3-6 cm long with 5 to 7 white veins and numerous cross veins in white. The flowering stem is 4-10 cm tall covered with gland tipped hairs. There are many greenish white flowers.
Range. Nfld. to Minn., s. to S.C., Ala., Tenn. and Mo. July-Aug. in dry woods.
Common names. Networt, adder's violet, scrofula weed, ratsbane, net leaf or spotted plantain.

LESSER RATTLESNAKE PLANTAIN   *Goodyera repens* (L.) R.Br.var.*ophioides* Fern.
The 3-6 cm tall stem is covered with gland tipped hairs, the leaves are net veined with white lines and the greenish white flowers grow only on one side of their stem.
Range. Circumboreal s. to N.Y., Mich. and Minn. and in the mts. to N.C. in dry woods.
1778 Carver 516. "Rattlesnake Plantain. . .the leaves of this herb are more efficacious than any other part of it for the bite of the reptile from which it receives its name; and being chewed and applied immediately to the wound, and some of the juice swallowed, seldom fails of averting every dangerous symptom. So convinced are the Indians of the power of this infallible antidote, that for a trifling bribe of spiritous liquor, they will at any time permit a rattle snake to drive his fangs into their flesh. It is to be remarked that during those months in which the bite of these creatures is most venomous, that this remedy for it is in its greatest perfection, and most luxurious growth. . .482. The bite of this reptile is more or less venemous according to the season of the year in which it is given. In the dog days, it often proves instantly mortal, and especially if the wound is made among the sinews situated in the back part of the leg above the heel, but in the spring, in autumn, or during a cool day which might happen in the summer, its bad effects are to be prevented by the immediate application of proper remedies; and these Providence has bounteously supplied by causing the Rattle Snake Plantain, an approved antidote to the poison of this creature, to grow in great profusion where ever they are to be met with."
1778 Carver 517. "Poor Robin's Plantain [*G. repens*] is of the same species as the last, but more diminutive in every respect; it receives its name from its size, and the poor land on which it

grows. It is a good medicinal herb, and often administered with success in fevers and internal weaknesses."

1830 Rafinesque 224. "Rattlesnake plantain deemed by some empirics a specific for the scrofula, the fresh leaves are applied to the sores, renewed every 3 hours, and the warm infusion used as a tea freely, also to wash the sores. It is employed by the Indians, and has effected some cures."

1868 Can. Pharm. J. 6; 83-5 *Goodyera pubescens*, net leaved plantain, the leaves included in list of Can. medicinal plants.

1915 Speck-Tantaquidgeon MOHEGAN 318. "The leaves of rattlesnake plantain (*Epipactis pubescens*) are made into a mash to prevent sore mouth in babies."

1928 Parker SENECA 12. Rattlesnake plantain used for nervousness.

1933 H. Smith POTAWATOMI 67. "Rattlesnake plantain (*Epipactis repens* var.*ophioides*) The Forest Potawatomi prize the root and leaves of this plant very highly because it is so hard to find and valuable to them in the treatment of stomach and bladder diseases. Captain John Carver traveled among the Forest Potawatomi. . .Perhaps his most curious reference to the efficacy of these plants is in connection with this Rattlesnake plantain. . .Among the whites the whole plant is esteemed for its demulcent, ophthalmic and anti-scrofulous properties. . .the leaves have been used in poultice form to cure severe cases of scrofula. Infusions of the leaves have been used by eclectic practioners as a wash to cure scrofula and as a wash for diseases of the eye."

1950 Wintemberg Waterloo County, Ontario 9. "There is a Canadian plant that if you step on it will cause you to lose your way. My mother told me that one day, about 50 or more years ago (when she was about 10), that she was sent into the woods by her employer to bring home the cows, and having stepped on one of these plants she got bewildered and lost her way. She wandered around the woods for some time, but always came back to her starting point, at length she emerged in a clearing and saw, as she supposed, a neighbour's barn. Seeing a man working in the field she went to him and inquired where her employer lived. As this man actually was her employer, he was amazed and thought she had become demented. . .Among Germans in Pennsylvania it is believed that 'You will lose your way in the woods if you step on rattlesnake plantain'. . .Plant known locally as err-kraut."

1955 Mockle Quebec transl. 31. "The large leaved is a vulnerary, lesser rattlesnake plantain antiscrofulous."

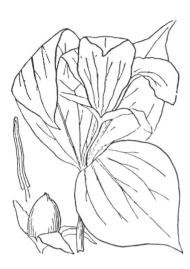

TRILLIUM

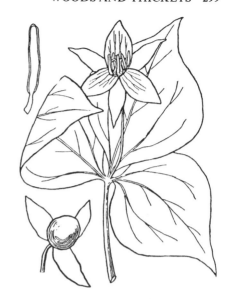

RED TRILLIUM

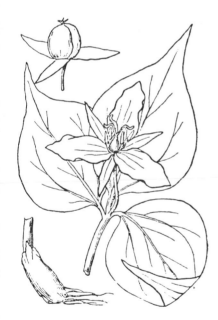

PAINTED TRILLIUM

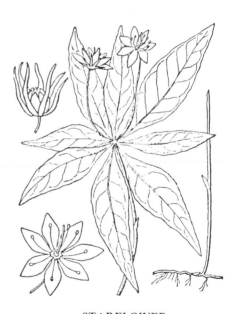

STARFLOWER

TRILLIUM *Trillium grandiflorum* (Michx.) Salisb. Liliacea
All trilliums have three leaves at the end of a 20-40 cm tall stem. The leaves in this species are broad, 8-12 cm long and painted at both ends. The flowering stalk, 5-8 cm tall grows from where the three leaves meet. The three white petals are 4-6 cm long and the three shorter green petals (sepals) are 3-5 cm long. There are many variations in the color of the petals.
Range. Me., s. Que., s. Ont., Minn. and Mich., s. to Ark., and Ga. in rich moist woods in May.
Common names. Trinity flower, large flowered wake robin, white lilies.

RED TRILLIUM
Trillium erectum L.

The stem is slender, the three leaves are about as wide as long, the 3-10 cm tall flowering stalk holds the red, or infrequently brownish, white, yellow or green flower erect. The three green petals (sepals) are about the same length as the three colored ones. The flower has an unpleasant scent.

Range. Mass., N.B., N.S., s. Que., s. Ont., se Man., s. to Tenn. and Ga. in moist woods in April-May.

Common names. Beth root, squaw flower, red benjamin, Indian balm, nose bleed, birth root, ill scented trillium.

PAINTED TRILLIUM
Trillium undulatum Willd.

The three thin leaves of this trillium have quite obvious stalks, 5-10 mm long. The three 2-4 cm long white petals have purplish blotches at their base and are longer that the three green ones. The fruit is three angled and bright shining red.

Range. N.B., P.E.I., N.S., s. Que., s. Ont., s. to Wisc., Mich., Tenn. and Ga. in moist or wet woods, May-June.

Common names. Wild pepper, sarah, benjamin.

There are other varieties of trilliums, they have all been used rather indiscriminately in medicine, Indian and white.

1800's Canniff 1894 Michilimachinac. Dr. William Lee, for a considerable time attached to the Indian Department there, reported that the Indians on the shores of Lake Superior used the trillium for childbirth and female diseases. While stationed at York, Dr. Lee not only dealt out medicine to the Indians visiting the place, but had to make long journeys to distant Indian settlements to prescribe for and administer medicine, even as far as Penetanguishene, which he did on horseback by bridle-paths, carrying the drugs in his saddle bag. Dr. Lee was an inhabitant of York from 1807 for a period of twenty six years."

1830 Rafinesque 102. "I have the pleasure to introduce this fine genus into Materia Medica. It has been neglected by all our writers, although well known to our herbalists. Schoepf merely says that the Indians considered the *T. cernum* (nodding trillium) as poisonous, which is not true; and that the acid berries of *T. sessile* [flowers without stalks] stain of a red color, or dye blue with alum. A popular remedy in the Northern States, and used also by the Shakers. The roots are the officinal parts; almost all the species may be used indifferently, although the Indians have a notion that those with red blossoms (which they call male) are the best, and those with white blossoms (called female) are best for women's complaints. . .Their roots. . .have a faint smell, somewhat like cedar, and a peculiar aromatic taste, somewhat like copaivi. Being chewed, they produce salivation and tears, with heat in the throat, and next a sensation of coolness over the whole system. These are indications of active properties. They have not yet been analyzed. They are employed internally in hematuria or bloody urine, uterine hemorrhage, immoderate menstrual discharge, bloody spitting, hectic fever, asthma, catarrhal cough, &c. either in powder, dose a teaspoonful, or in infusion. Externally they are very beneficial in tumors, indolent and putrid ulcers, carbuncles, and mortification, in a poultice by itself, or still better united with *Sanguinaria* [bloodroot]. . .It is said that they obviate or prevent gangrene and the need of cutting off mortified limbs. Even the leaves are useful applied to tumors. In female complaints, such as leucorrhea, menorrhea, and after parturition, they act as good restringents; the Indians value them much as such, both in Canada and in Missouri. They say in Canada that the roots chewed, will cure instantly the bite of rattle-snakes, both in men and cattle. Mr. Hawkins saw an Indian make an experiment for a gill of rum: how it acts was not stated. The Indians of Missouri call them Mochar Newachar, meaning heat and cold: it is their palliative for consumption. The sessile species are called Jewsharp in Kentucky, and used for sores and ulcers. The *T. tinctorium* [Raf?] is one of the red paints of the Western Indians; the roots stain the hands, and dye red with alum."

1830-54 There was much interest in, and publication on, the use of Trillium to treat cancers in the U.S. during this period according to Hartwell 1970.

1859-61 Gunn 886. "The root is astringent, antiseptic, and somewhat expectorant and tonic. Useful in all kinds of hemorrhages, and especially in the immoderate flow of the menses, flooding, and the like, also good in dysentery, diarrhea, cough, asthma and night sweats. Dose a teaspoonful of the pulverized root, repeated often; or the infusion may be used freely.'

1892 Millspaugh 175. "The use of the tubers as an external application in ulcers, inflamed swellings, sores, etc. is similar to that of liliacea in general. On account of the acridity of the roots, they have been used to promote pytalism, and are claimed to check epitaxis when a newly-cut root is held to the nose and the acridity inspired. Considerable doubt exists among our authors and pharmacists concerning which species of this genus should be used for our tinctures. . . .For use in disease, some definite, reliable tincture, made from a single species should be used. . .chemical constituents trilline. . .This is certainly a drug deserving full and careful study."

1926-27 Densmore CHIPPEWA 333. "An instrument for applying medicine beneath the skin consisted of several needles fastened at the end of a wooden handle. This was used in treating 'dizzy headaches', neuralgia, or rheumatism in any part of the body. In giving the treatment the medicine was 'worked in' with the needles. . . .A remedy for rheumatism was applied in a similar manner. The plant used was identified as *Trillium grandiflorum*, and it was used in the form of a decoction". . .362. Scrape the second layer of the bark of the root, put in hot water and boil, drop in the ear when sore.

1923 H. Smith MENOMINI 41. "This root was used to reduce the swelling of an eye. The raw root is grated and applied as a poultice to the eye. For cramps, it is grated, steeped and drunk as a tea. For irregularity of the menses, this root is grated and put into water to simmer and then drunk. It is drunk to remove the defilement entailed by intercourse with one during the menstrual period."

1933 H. Smith POTAWATOMI 63. "An infusion of the root is used for treating sore nipples. The infusion is drunk by the patient and the medicine man further hastens the action of the medicine by piercing the teats with a dog whisker."

1945 Rousseau MOHAWK transl. 66. "Infuse the roots of the red trillium and the flowers of the white clover (*Melilotus alba*) for pimples on the face or a too brown colour."

1945 Raymond TETE DE BOULE transl. 133. "The whole flower and leaves of the painted trillium are crushed and drunk to bring on childbirth."

1947 Marker et al. J. Am. Chem. Soc. 69; 2242. *Trillium erectum*; bethogenin, diosgenin, pennogenin, nologenin and fecogenin. J. Am. Chem. Soc. 1942 64; 1283-5. *Trillium grandiflorum*; diosgenin in roots.

1955 Mockle Quebec transl. 29. "*T. erectum*. The root is used in poultices for ulcers and tumors. It is also said to be emetic and emmenagogue. Boiled in milk, it is recommended for the treatment of dysentery and diarrhea. It contains a steroid saponoside, trillarine, with hydrolysis, diosgenin. Other species with the same properties are *T. grandiflorum, cernuum, undulatum*."

STARFLOWER   *Trientalis borealis* Raf. Primulaceae (*T. americana*)
From a creeping rootstock stands a 10-20 cm stem crowned by a whorl of narrow leaves 4-10 cm long, pointed at both ends and one third as wide. They are smooth with distinctive veining, where they join at the stem there is sometimes a little hair. From these leaves one or more thin stalks, 2-5 cm long arise bearing white or pink 5-9-petalled flowers 8-14 mm across.
Range. Lab., Nfld. and N.S. to Sask. s. to Pa., n. O, n. Ill. and Minn. also on coastal plain from Mass. to Va. May-June in rich woods and bogs.
Common names. Chickweed wintergreen, star anemone.
1915 Speck MONTAGNAIS 314. "For general sickness and incidentally for consumption, star anemone is steeped."
1932 H. Smith OJIBWE 431. "The root of this is mixed with many others to make the smoking scent that attracts deer to the hunter."

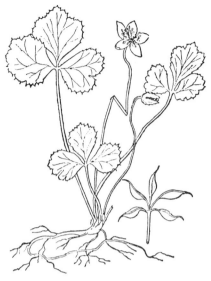

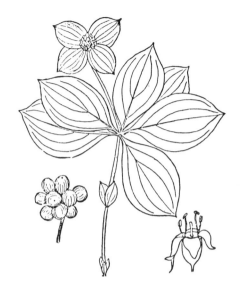

GOLD THREAD   BUNCHBERRY

GOLD THREAD   *Coptis trifolia* (L.) Salisb. var. *groenlandica* (Oeder) Fassett Ranunculaceae
The bright yellow thread like roots identify this plant. The evergreen leaves grow from them on
long stalks. They consist of three, toothed leaflets, rounded on the lower side. The flowering
stalk, 5-15 cm tall, holds one white, 5-7 petaled flower; 12-16 mm wide. It is followed by 3-7 long
beaked pods.
Range. Greenl. to Alaska and e. Asia, s. to N.J., N.C., n. Ind., Io. and Ida. in damp mossy woods
and bogs. May-Aug.
Common names. Yellow-root, canker-root, mouth root.
1739 Letters from Hudson Bay 290. "As to the Tysowian. . .it was very good and gathered in the
proper season. . .the Indians use to dye their quills with the root." [Cree; utesaweyan, dye root.]
1749 Kalm Quebec August the 13th. 461. "The three-leaved hellebore (*Helleborus trifolius*) grows
in great quantities in the woods, and in many places it covers the ground by itself. However, it
commonly chooses mossy places that are not very wet, and the wood sorrel (*Oxalis acetosella*L.),
with the mountain enchanter's nightshade (*Circaea alpina* L.) are its companions. Its seeds were
not yet ripe and most of the stalks had no seeds at all. The plant is called *Tissavoyanne jaune* by
the French in Canada. Its leaves and stalks are used by the Indians for giving a fine yellow color
to several kinds of work which they make of prepared skins. The French who have learnt this
from them, dye wool and other things yellow with this plant."
1778 Carver 513. "Gold Thread. This is a plant of the small vine kind, which grows in swampy
places, and lies on the ground. The roots spread themselves just under the surface of the morass,
and are easily drawn up by handfuls. They resemble a large entangled skain of thread of a fine
bright gold colour; and I am persuaded would yield a beautiful and permanent yellow dye. It is
also greatly esteemed both by the Indians and the colonists as a remedy for any soreness in the
mouth, but the taste of it is exquisitely bitter."
1785 Cutler. Mouth root. The roots, thread shaped, running, bright yellow. . .are astringent, and
of a bitterish taste, chewed in the mouth they cure apthous and cankerous sores. It is frequently
an ingredient in gargles for sore throats.
1807 Wenzel Letters 80. "The dyes made use of by the Indians to stain porcupine quills and
feathers, which are the only things they stain, are the roots of a plant which the Canadians call
Savoyan; its colour is of an orange caste."

1817-20 Bigelow 63. "Of this article larger quantities are sold in the druggist shops in Boston than of almost any indigenous production. The demand for it arises from its supposed efficacy as a local application in apthous and other ulcerations of the mouth. Its reputation however, in these cases is wholly unmerited. . .where benefit has attended its use, it is doubtless to be ascribed to other articles possessing the same properties with which it is usually combined. As a pure tonic bitter, capable of strengthening the viscera and promoting digestion, it is entitled to rank with most articles of the kind now in use. . .The tincture made by digesting half an ounce of the bruised root in eight ounces of diluted alcohol, forms a preparation of a fine yellow color, possessing the whole bitterness of the plant. I have given it in various instances to dyspeptics and convalescents, who have generally expressed satisfaction from its effects. . .A teaspoonful may be taken three times a day. . .It is, however, difficult to reduce to powder on account of the tenacity of its fibers."

1828 Rafinesque 266. "It is yet used extensively and alone for sore mouth and sore throat. It is also good for sore eyes. . .1830 212. Is the Tissavoyane jaune of the Canadians, the roots and leaves die skins, wool and flax yellow."

1859-61 Gunn 797. "The root can generally be found in drug stores. . .is a pure bitter tonic, very much resembling in its properties and uses, that of the Golden-seal. Good in dyspepsia, feeble digestion, weakness of the system, or in convalescence from fevers and wherever a bitter tonic and restorative is needed. . .It is mostly used however, as a gargle or wash for sore mouth and throat, for which it is very good."

1868 Can. Pharm. J. 1. "Gold thread is another dweller in swamps. It is very plentiful in this neighbourhood [Toronto]. The writer would not like to dig what would produce a pound of the dried root for any amount that could be obtained for it."

1868 Can. Pharm. J. 6; 83-5. The roots of *Coptis trifolia*, goldthread, included in list of Can. medicinal plants.

1879 Can. Pharm. J. 322. "'Yaller root', which is also known as golden-seal, is worth 7 cents a pound. It is used fur makin' washes for sore eyes an' mouths."

1892 Millspaugh 15. "Berberine exists in a number of other plants (besides barberry,) among which of particular interest to us are *Coptis trifoliata* and *Caulophyllum* (blue cohosh)."

1915 Speck PENOBSCOT 309. "Golden thread stems are chewed to allay canker or sores on the gums or in the mouth. It is good for mouths irritated by too much tobacco smoking."

1915 Speck-Tantaquidgeon MOHEGAN 319. "Golden thread is steeped for use as a mouth wash for babies."

1926-27 Densmore CHIPPEWA 374. Bright yellow dye formula; take a great many long slender roots and boil in hot water. Add material and boil.

1928 Parker SENECA 11. As an astringent use goldthread.

1923 H. Smith MENOMINI 48. "The roots yield an astringent mouth wash for sore throat of babies, and it is much used for teething babies. This wash also cures cankers in the mouth."

1932 H. Smith OJIBWE 383. "Use a decoction of the root to soothe and heal the baby's gums while it is teething. It is also used as a mouth wash for adults when their mouths are sore." [Same use by Forest Potawatomi]. . .426. Add the roots to other plant dyes to emphasize the yellow color."

1930 Grieve England 361. "It is stated to be good for dyspepsia and combined with other drugs is regarded as helpful in combating the drink habit."

1935 Jenness Parry Island OJIBWA Lake Huron 114. "Made yellow dye from boiled roots of gold-thread (*Coptis trifolia*)."

1945 Rousseau MOHAWK transl. 42. "An infusion of the root to facilitate digestion. Also for sore ears. . .60. The large branches of the white ash when heated, drip sap, which is collected and used for earaches. In cases of deafness it is mixed with an equal amount of a rich infusion of gold-thread. Only a few drops in the ear which is then closed with an animal skin. . .43. The French Canadian name is savoyane which comes from a Micmac word meaning dye for skins, tisavoyane."

1945 Raymond TETE DE BOULE transl. 126. "The boiled roots are used for serious colds and respiratory troubles. A linen is soaked in a tea of the plant and applied to the eyes. (Mere Dubé). The Canadians without doubt borrowed the knowledge of savoyane from the Indians. Our mothers, who called it sometimes fil-d'or (comté d'Iberville) patiently collected the roots in case of sore eyes or gums. The Potawatomi and Ojibwa used it for sore gums. The names in nearly every dialect as well as the popular English name, goldthread, allude to the yellow color of the roots."

1971 Jolicoeur Quebec 4. "For babies' sore mouth and confinement cases—eat it green: stimulates appetite: relieves colds, colic, heart disease, diabetes, stomach ulcer. For kidney trouble, use with six others: bunchberry leaves, ground hemlock, prince's pine, labrador, ganargues [?] (the seventh herb is forgotten)."

BUNCHBERRY   *Cornus canadensis* L. Cornaceae

Stem 10-20 cm tall with a cluster of 4-6 apparantly whorled leaves at the top and below them one to two pairs of scales. The leaves are 4-7 cm long with a distinctive veining, two or three pairs running from the centre vein below the middle of the leaf. The flowering stalk, 1-3 cm long grows from the top of the stem. There are white petals (bracts) each 1-2 cm long, the true flower is green, in the centre of these conspicuous white bracts. The berry is bright red and edible.

Range. Greenland to Alaska and e. Asia, s. to N.J., Pa., Ind. and Minn. and in the mts. to W. Va. and Calif. June-July in woods.

Common names. Dwarf cornel, cracker berry.

1624 Sagard HURON 326. "Several other kinds of small fruits and berries unknown here of which we ate delicious dishes when we could find them. There are some red ones which appear almost like coral, that grow almost on the ground in little bunches with two or three leaves, resembling laurel, which gives them charm; they seem like very fine bouquets and would serve as such if there were any here."

1708 Sarrazin-Vaillant, Quebec-Paris, Boivin 1978 transl. 59. "This plant grows everywhere in dry upland soils. It is called here *Matagon*. The Savages eat the fruit." [The description is that of *Cornus canadensis* according to Boivin].

1840 Gosse Quebec 299. "The course lying through a cedar swamp, the ground was mossy, and in some places wet; here the Scarlet Stoneberry was abundant. . .*Cornus canadensis* is a low and pretty plant, having a white flower, resembling that of a strawberry, and four large oval green leaves on the ground. At present they are crowned with a little cluster of bright red berries, which were ripe, and we ate many: they are farinaceous and agreeable. This plant is common in Newfoundland."

1888 Delamare Island of Miquelon transl. 20. "The children eat the red sweet berries with impunity."

1915 Speck MONTAGNAIS 315. "The plant of bunch-berry 'four seasons' is steeped for paralysis." [see Ice plant for same name and use.]

1926-27 Densmore CHIPPEWA 321. "Berries eaten raw."

1932 H. Smith OJIBWE 366. "The Flambeau Ojibwe make a tea from the root, which is used to cure babies of colic."

1933 H. Smith POTAWATOMI 98. "The Forest Potawatomi used to use the berries of this plant for food but claim they do not use them today. We could not ascertain how they used them, whether in the raw state or cooked."

1945 Raymond TETE DE BOULE transl. 128. "The plant boiled with wintergreen is part of the composition of a cold remedy. Mixed with the branches of yew (*Taxus canadensis*) it cures the stomach troubles of women (Willy Nemacic, Joseph Dubé)."

1959 Mechling MALECITE of maritime provinces of Canada used the whole plant for fits.

1971 Jolicoeur Quebec 4. "Used for heart disease."

One of the plants to be examined for cancer chemotheraputic use (Lewis and Elvin-Lewis 1977:135).

[See under Shrubs for the other dogwoods, *Cornus*.]

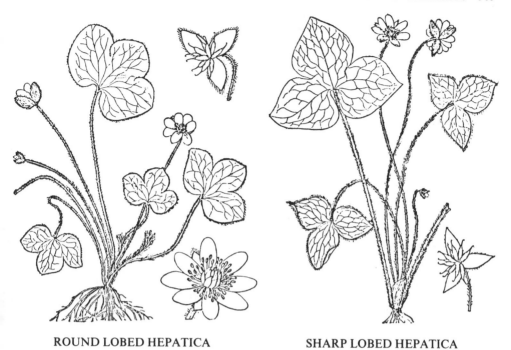

ROUND LOBED HEPATICA   SHARP LOBED HEPATICA

SHARP LOBED HEPATICA
Hepatica acutiloba DC. Ranunculaceae

A hairy stem grows from the roots bearing a leaf divided into three sharply pointed parts or occasionally 5 to 7 lobes. The hairy flowering stem, 5-15 cm tall, grows also from the roots, bearing one bluish white or pink flower, 12-25 mm wide usually hidden by the leaves.
Range. Que. to Minn., s. to Ga., Ala. and Mo. Mar.-April in dry or moist woods.

ROUND LOBED HEPATICA
Hepatica americana (DC.) Ker. (*H. triloba*)

Very like *H. acutiloba* except that the leaves are cut into three parts only to near the middle of the leaf and the ends are rounded.
Range. Que., and N.S. to Minn., s. to Ga., Tenn. and Mo. Mar.-April in acid soil in woods. Very similar to the European *H. nobilis* Schreb.

Common names for both species. Liverwort, mouse-ears, spring beauty, herb trinity.

1681 Culpeper 218. "[*H. nobilis*]. It is a singular good herb for all diseases of the liver, both to cool and cleanse it, and helps inflammation in any part, and the yellow jaundice; being bruised and boiled in small beer, if drank it cools the heat of the liver and kidneys, and helps the running of the reins in men, and the whites in women, it is a good remedy to stay the spreading of tetters, ringworm, and other fretting or running sores and scabs."

1799 Lewis Mat. Med. 158. "[*H. nobilis*]. The herb has a place in our gardens on account of the beauty and early appearance of its flowers. It is a cooling, gently refrigerant herb; and hence recommended in the lax state of the fibres as a corroborant."

1828 Rafinesque 240. "It was known to the ancients as a medical plant, and Linneaus has it in his Materia Medica; but it has fallen into disuse, its properties being very mild. It was formerly used in fevers, liver complaints, indigestion, cachexy, hypochondria and hernia. It has lately been brought to notice in America for hemoptysis and coughs, it has been used in Virginia with benefit in the form of a strong infusion, drunk cold. It may be serviceable in hepatitis and hepatic phthisis, as well as all complaints arising from dyspepsic and hypochondric affections; it may be used as a tea, warm or cold and adlibitum; but it has no effect on the lungs beyond that of a mild demulcent astringent. . .1830 227. Physicians disagree on the powers of these plants. Dr. Tully considers them of little use. Dr. Mease informs me that the leaves alone are useful, the roots and flowers useless. Dr. Lawrence has seen some good effects from them. . .They have failed to give even relief in many diseases of the lungs."

1859-61 Gunn 818. "It has acquired some reputation in lung affections, used in combination with Tar, in the form of a sirup, known as 'Dr Rogers' Liverwort and Tar.' It is an innocent herb and may be taken freely in infusion."

1868 Can. Pharm. J. 6; 83-5. The plant of hepatica, *H. triloba*, included in list of Can. medicinal plants.

1883 Can. Pharm. J. 16; 386. "Gehe's circular states that large quantities of liverwort have been bought up at advanced prices for the United States market, but nothing definite could be learned as to its use. We believe the greatest part of it is used for the manufacture of patent medicines—notably for making the so-called 'kidney cure.'"

1885 Mooney CHEROKEE 326. *H. acutiloba*. "Used for coughs either in tea or by chewing the root. Those who dream of snakes drink a decoction of this herb and the walking fern to produce vomiting, after which the dreams do not return. The traders buy large quantities of liverwort from the Cherokees, who may thus have learned to esteem it more highly than they otherwise would."

1892 Millspaugh 2. "The Liver-leaf has held a place among medicinal plants from ancient times until the present. It is now falling into disuse on account of its mild properties, forming as it does simply a slightly astringent, mucilaginous infusion. It was used in haemoptysis, coughs and other lung affections, as well as in all diseases of the liver, and in hemorrhoids; in the latter troubles its exhibition must have met with no very flattering success. . .Has been dismissed from the U.S. Ph."

1915 Speck DELAWARE 320. "Hepatica for fever and chills."

1926-27 Densmore CHIPPEWA 336 *H. americana*; a decoction of 1 root in 1 quart of water drunk for convulsions, used chiefly for children. . .376. *H. triloba* the root put on traps for fur bearing animals as a charm.

1928 Parker SENECA 11. Hepatica used as a tonic.

1923 H. Smith MENOMINI 48. *H. acutiloba*. "The roots are used with the roots of maidenhair fern in various female maladies, especially to cure leucorrhea.

1928 H. Smith MESKWAKI 238. *H. acutiloba*. "When the mouth gets twisted or crossed and the eyes get crossed, this root is brewed into a tea, and the face is washed with it until it returns to normal. At the same time the patient has to take two teaspoonfuls daily."

1933 H. Smith POTAWATOMI 75 *H. triloba* "The Forest Potawatomi use the root and the leaves to make a sweetish-tasting tea to relieve cases of vertigo. . .123. The roots are used to make a dye for mats and baskets."

1945 Rousseau MOHAWK transl. 52. "The coureurs de bois who had not much breath drank an infusion of the whole plant of hepatica and the bark of the sugar maple taken from the sunny side of the tree."

1955 Mockle Quebec transl. 41. "Used for its tonic properties, astringent, mucilaginous, pectoral, in fevers, in liver complaints, indigestion, cachexy hypochondria, hemoptysis and coughs."

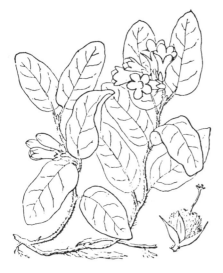

TRAILING ARBUTUS

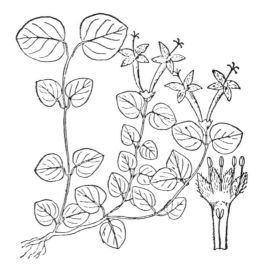

PARTRIDGE BERRY

TRAILING ARBUTUS *Epigaea repens* L. Ericaceae
The woody stems are covered with long reddish hairs that make them seem bristly. The plant creeps over the ground rooting here and there. The leaves, 2-10 cm long are hairy underneath, shining green and leathery on top and have stalks half as long as the leaves. In early spring the flowering stalk, 2-5 cm high, will hold a cluster of very fragrant white to pink flowers.
Range. Nfld., N.S., to Sask., s. to Fla., Ala., Ky. and Io. in sandy or rocky acid soil in the open or on the edge of woods. April to May.
Common names. Mayflower, winter or mountain pink, gravel plant, ground laurel, shadflower, crocus.
1792 Simcoe Diary Toronto 136. "I send you Mayflower seeds."
1868 Can. Pharm. J. 6; 83-5. The leaves of trailing arbutus, *Epigaea repens*, included in list of Can. medicinal plants.
1871 Dashwood 190. "In the early spring, may-flower picnics are got up, as the plant is by no means general, and only grows in certain localities."
1892 Millspaugh 101. "It is stated that in lithic acid gravel, and some forms of nephritis, cystitis and vesical catarrh, its use has often been of greater benefit than uva-ursi or buchu. Epigaea has no place in the U.S. Ph. . . .Chemical constituents, the three glucosides, urson, ericolin, and arbutin. . .formic acid and a body having properties similar to gallic acid have been determined in this plant." [See bearberry]
1925 Wood & Ruddock. "Tea of trailing arbutus used in gravel and other diseases of the urinary organs, drink freely."
1928 Parker SENECA 11. Used as a tonic. . .12 Flowers and leaves used for malaria.
1933 H. Smith POTAWATOMI 118. "This is the tribal flower of the Forest Potawatomi who consider that these flowers came direct from the hands of 'kitcimanitowwiwin', their divinity."
1942 Fenton IROQUOIS 524. "Used by Indians and settlers alike in western New York for blood and kidneys."
1955 Mockle Quebec transl. 70. "The leaves are prescribed for gravel. They contain arbutoside, ericoline and ursolic acid."
1970 Bye IROQUOIS mss. A popular domestic remedy for gravel. The Shakers sold medicine made from this plant under the name Gravel Plant.

PARTRIDGE BERRY

Mitchella repens L. Rubiaceae

The stem trails over the ground rooting here and there and often forming large mats. The leaves are dark green, opposite, shining, stalked, smooth and roundish, 1-2 cm long. In our range they usually have whitish veins and this is one way to identify them as they bear but few flowers and berries. Sitting in a small green cup are the twin white 10-14 mm tubes of the flowers which normally end in four lobes but which occasionally may have three, five or six.

They are followed by one sealing-wax-red berry with an indentation and two star-shaped marks, inside are about eight seeds. The leaves are evergreen and the berry persists all winter as food for partridges.

Range. N.S. to Ont. and Minn., s. to Fla. and Tex. May-July in woods.

Common names. Twin-berry, Squaw vine, two-eyed berry, winter clover, deer berry.

1830 Rafinesque 243. "Mild diuretic, tea used in New England to cure dropsy and gout. Red berries mild astringent, a popular remedy for diarrhea in the North, and for disury in Carolina."

1859-61 Gunn 780. "The whole plant is medicinal, but principally the vine only is used. It is diuretic, astringent, and parturient. A decoction of it used freely, it is said, will cure the dropsy. It is also highly valued by some as a remedy for diarrhea, dysentery, and the suppression or retention of urine. A tea or decoction of the berries is also said to be a sovereign cure for diarrhea. In females it seems to have a peculiar and special action on the uterus, and is highly recommended in the various affections of that organ. Among some tribes of Indians it seems to be regarded as a most valuable parturient. Dr. Smith, in his 'Botanic Physician', says, in speaking of it: 'This is an invaluable plant for child-bearing women. I first obtained knowledge of its use from a tribe of Indians in the West part of New York. The squaws drank it in decoction for two or three weeks previous to, and during delivery, and it was the use of it that rendered that generally dreaded event so remarkably safe and easy with them."

1868 Can. Pharm. J. 6; 83-5. The vine of *Mitchella repens*, partridge berry, included in list of Can. medicinal plants.

1892 Millspaugh 72. "Mitchella is one of the many plants used by the American Aborigines as a parturient, frequent doses of a decoction being taken during the few weeks just preceding confinement. It has also been found to be a valuable diuretic and astringent, and to have an especial affinity to various forms of uterine difficulties. The plant is not mentioned in the U.S. Ph. . . .The drug merits more extended proving." [It was listed in the National Formulary of the U.S. 1926-47. as an astringent, tonic and diuretic.]

1915 Speck PENOBSCOT 309. "The plants are a somewhat non-specific material to be steeped."

1915 Speck MONTAGNAIS 313. "The berries cooked into a jelly and used for fever."

1916 Waugh IROQUOIS 128. Partridge or squaw berry, the berry eaten.

1923 H. Smith MENOMINI 51. "The leaves of this plant are steeped to make a tea to cure insomnia."

1928 Reagan CHIPPEWA 239. "Much used by the Indians. . .Formerly he smoked kinnikinnik, which he obtained as the pulverized inner bark (or leaves) of several plants. Among these were the partridge berry (*Mitchella repens*)."

1933 Gilmore OJIBWA 41. Used for medicine.

1955 Mockle Quebec transl. 84. "Diuretic. The berries astringent."

1970 Bye IROQUOIS mss. "The berries eaten and used as a berry drink, and in many of their medical formulas, generally as a parturient to prevent severe labor pains."

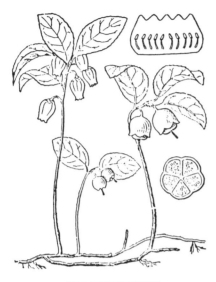

WINTERGREEN

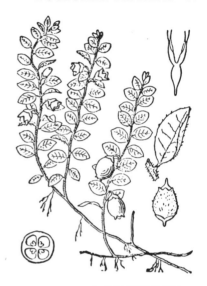

CREEPING SNOWBERRY

WINTERGREEN   *Gaultheria procumbens* L. Ericaceae
The true stem creeps just below the surface, resembling a root, the flowering stem stands upright,
5-15 cm with a few leaves crowded near its top. These are alternate, leathery, shining, evergreen
with finely cut edges, and are 2-5 cm long. The white bell shaped flowers hang down on 5-10 mm
stalks, and are followed by sealing-wax red berries that last all winter and taste of wintergreen
when chewed.
Range. Nfld. to Man., s. to Va., Ky., Minn. and in the mts. to Ga. in dry or moist woods in acid
soil, usually found just at the edges of the woods. July-Aug.
Common names. Tea berry, winterberry, partridge berry, mountain tea.
1778 Carver 509. "Winter Green. This is an evergreen of the species of the myrtle. . .in winter it is
full of red berries about the size of a sloe, which are smooth and round; these are preserved during the season by the snow, and are at that time in the highest perfection. The Indians eat these
berries, esteeming them very balsamic, and invigorating to the stomach. The people inhabiting
the interior colonies steep both the sprigs and berries in beer, and use it as a diet-drink for
cleansing the blood from scorbutick disorders."
1791 Long Lake Superior CHIPPEWA 45. "Proposed to adopt me as a brother warrior. . .When
the pipe has gone round, a sweating house is prepared. . .puts the person into a most profuse perspiration, and opens the pores to receive the other part of the ceremony. . .extended on his back,
the chief draws the figure he intends to make with a pointed stick, dipped in water in which gunpowder has been dissolved; after which, with ten needles dipped in vermilion, and fixed in a
small wooden frame, he pricks the delineated parts, and where the bolder outlines occur, he
incises the flesh with a gun flint; the vacant spaces, or those not marked with vermilion, are rubbed in with gunpowder, which produces the variety of red and blue; the wounds are then seared
with punk wood, to prevent them from festering. This operation, which is performed at intervals,
lasts two or three days. Every morning the parts are washed with cold water, in which is infused
an herb called Pockqueesegan, which resembles English box, and is mixed by the Indians with
the tobacco they smoke, to take off the strength. During the process, the war songs are sung,
accompanied by a rattle hung with hawk bells, called chessaquoy, which is kept shaking to stifle
the groans such pains must naturally occasion. . .I accordingly. . .gave them. . .vermilion, tobacco." [See Wilson below for Chippewa name for wintergreen, pahgezegun, also under Cedar].
1796 Simcoe Toronto 335. "Rode very pleasantly through the pine plains; gathered tea berries."
1817-20 Bigelow 30. "The aromatic flavour of the Partridge berry, which cannot easily be mis-

taken by those who have once tasted it, may be recognised in a variety of other plants. . .It is particularly distinct in the bark of the sweet birch, *Betula lenta*, one of our most useful and interesting trees. . .The leaves, the essence and the oil of this plant [partridge berry] are kept for use in the apothecaries' shops. An infusion of the leaves has been used to communicate an agreeable flavour to tea, also as a substitute for that article by people in the country. Some physicians have prescribed it medicinally as an emmenagogue, with success in cases attended with debility. It shares with oil of peppermint, the property of diminishing the sensibility of the nerve exposed by a carious tooth when repeatedly applied. The oil dissolved in alcohol is antispasmodic and diaphoretic. . .the tincture astringent and warm, useful in diarrhoea. A respectable physician of Boston informs me, that he has in various instances, found the influence of this plant very effectual in promoting mammary secretion, when deficient, and even in restoring that important function after it had been for some time suspended. Whether the medicine has any specific influence of this sort, independant of the general state of the patients health, I am not prepared to say."

1828 Rafinesque 204. "The whole plant has long been known and used as a pleasant common drink in the country by the name of mountain-tea. A popular remedy in many parts of the Country. . .The tea is used as a palliative in asthma, to restore strength, promote menstruation, also in cases of debility, in the secondary stage of diarrhoea, and to promote the lacteal secretion of the breast, &c. it is a very agreeable and refreshing beverage, much preferable to imported China Teas. . .The Indians made great use of this plant as a stimulant, restorative, cordial &c. It is injurious in fevers. . .They [the berries] are called Pollom by the Indians. The Oil of Gaultheria is now used in all the secret officinal Panaceas to disguise or cover the taste of the other ingredients. . .Berries, 1830 222. used in home beer in the North, gives it a fine flavor, they are good antiscorbutic, invigorate the stomach &c."

1846 Dr. Chase Mich. 158. "Films—to remove from the eye.—Wintergreen leaf, bruised and stewed in a suitable quantity of hen's oil to make the oil strong of the wintergreen—strain and apply twice daily. . .177. Wintergreen berries have been found a valuable corrector of Diarrhea brought on by the long-continued used of calomel [mercury] in cases of fever, eating a quart of them in 3 days time."

1857 Daniel Wilson 254. "During a visit to part of the Minnesota Territory at the head of Lake Superior, in 1855, it was my good fortune to fall in with a party of the Saultaux Indians, as the Chippeways of the far west are most frequently designated. . .The Indians accordingly make use of various herbs to mix with and dilute the tobacco, such as. . .the leaves of the winterberry, which receives the name of *pahgezegun*. . .The leaf of the winterberry, or tea berry. . .has a pleasant aroma which may have had some influence on its selection. The Indians of the north west ascribe to it the further property of giving them wind, and enabling them to hold out longer in running; but the main object of all such additions appears to be to dilute the tobacco, and thereby admit of its prolonged enjoyment. Having both chewed and smoked winterberry leaf prepared by the Indians, I am able to speak positively as to the absence of any narcotic qualities and I presume that with it and all the other additions to the tobacco, the main object is to provide a diluent, so as to moderate the effects and prolong the enjoyment of the luxury. . .Winterberry leaves are prepared by passing them through the top of the flame, or more leisurely drying them over the fire, without allowing them to burn."

1859-61 Gunn 883. "The leaves are. . .used in infusion or tea in chronic diarrhea and dysentery, stoppage of the urine, and in suppressed menses. The principal use of Winter-green, however, is in the manufacture of an essential Oil, by distillation of the herb, which is extensively employed for the purpose of flavoring sirups, mixtures and medical compounds. The infusion of the herb may be used freely."

1875 Can. Pharm J. 389. "Prof. Procter [Am. J. Pharm 14 211] of Philadelphia showed that our oil of wintergreen, *Gaultheria procumbens*, was really a salicylous ether and from this source salicylic acid was obtained by Cahours [Compt. Rendu T16 F 863]."

1876 Can. Pharm J. 13. "The preservation of health is the great question of the day. Many means are suggested by which the spread of disease may be prevented, but sanitary engineering, and all the other arrangements which town authorities are called upon to make, will not materially reduce the death rate unless people are more careful in their eating and drinking. We are accustomed to see cart-loads of aerated waters, lemonade, ginger ale etc. left at hotels, bar rooms, and private residences. The consumption of these liquids is enormous, and if the evils accruing from the system could be accurately ascertained and exposed, it would form a frightful cause of death. . .Ginger ale is even worse, while lemonade is hardly ever free from the poisonous influence of lead. People who are in the habit of drinking such preparations will do well to adopt the following formulas for making wholesome and agreeable summer beverages without a machine. . .To make Root Beer flavoring take Oil of wintergreen 4 drachms; Oil of Sassafras, 2 drachms; Oil of cloves, 1 drachm; alcohol 4 ounces. Mix and dissolve."

1882 Can. Pharm J. 263. "An interesting but lengthy paper was read by Mr. G.W. Kennedy. . .describing a visit to wintergreen oil distillery in Pennsylvania, where considerable quantities of the oil (about 30 pounds per week) are turned out, and yield a profit of about fifty dollars. The oil is sometimes obtained from teaberry leaves, but more frequently from the bark of the cherry, sweet or black birch, and from tests made by Mr. Kennedy the products appear to be identical."

1888 Delamare Island of Miquelon transl. 24. "The leaves are an agreeable aromatic tea which recalls the taste of anis tea. In the United States the essence called wintergreen is obtained from the plant. The fruit never comes to maturity until the spring."

1892 Millspaugh 102. "Distillation of the oil of wintergreen. . .is confined to men of limited means in those districts where its growth is most abundant. The apparatus used is simple and movable, being shifted when the supply of leaves gives out. It consists usually of a copper whiskey still. This is placed near some rivulet with a sufficient fall to keep the cooler filled. It is entirely invested by brick, with the exception of the cap, filled with leaves, covered with water, and heated by an open fire beneath. The volatile oil, together with the steam, passes through the condensing worm into the receiver, which is kept filled with water. The oil is collected by a separating funnel, placed in the bottom of the receiver, and the water used over and over again to economize the product. The average yield is ten pounds from a tun of the leaves; greater in dry seasons. Most of the oil of wintergreen is made from young birch trees in a similar manner. . .Chemical constituents Oil of Gaultheria. This body is a mixture of the volatile oil of the plant, salicylate of methyl, gaulthilene and gaultheric acid, forming the heaviest of the known essential oils. . .Salicylate of methyl constitutes the principal part of the compound oil."

1916 Waugh IROQUOIS 128. Berries eaten. . .148. The wintergreen. . .leaves were steeped [drunk as tea].

1923 H. Smith MENOMINI 35. "The leaf of this plant with the berry is steeped to make a tea, which is drunk for rheumatism."

1932 H. Smith OJIBWE 369. "The Flambeau Ojibwe use the leaves to brew a tea to cure rheumatism and 'to make one feel good'. The white man discovered the properties of this plant from the Indians. . .400. They also use the leaf tea from the youngest tenderest leaves as a beverage tea, and especially favor it because it 'makes them feel good'. They also eat the wintergreen berry."

1933 H. Smith POTAWATOMI 56. "The Potawatomi make a tea from the leaves of Wintergreen to break a fever. They also claim that the tea cures rheumatism and lumbago."

1926-27 Densmore CHIPPEWA 317. Leaves used for tea.

1928 Parker SENECA 11. Carminatives include wintergreen.

1945 Raymond TETE DE BOULE transl. 129. "The plant is applied as a poultice to the chest for tenacious colds. A tea made with the leaves is a veritable panacea: grippe, colds, stomach troubles, etc. The whites taught the Indians the evident virtues of gaultheria."

1942 Fenton IROQUOIS 524. "Wintergreen for blood and kidneys used by Indians and settlers alike in western New York."

1931 Grieve England 849. "The volatile oil obtained by distillation and to which all the medicinal qualities are due, contains 99 percent Methyl Salicylate. . .The oil of Gaultheria. . .has all the properties of the salicylates and therefore is most beneficial in acute rheumatism, but must be given internally in capsules, owing to its pungency, death from inflammation of the stomach having been known to result from frequent and large doses of it. It is readily absorbed by the skin, but is liable to give rise to an eruption, so it is advisable to use for external application the synthetic oil of wintergreen. . .or oil from the bark of *Betula lenta*. . .The leaves have found use as a substitute for tea and as a flavoring for genuine tea. . .The oil is a flavouring agent for tooth powders, liquid dentifrices, pastes, etc. especially if combined with menthol and eucalyptus."

1955 Mockle Quebec transl. 70. "The leaves prescribed as stimulant, diaphoretic, antidiarrhea and utilised as a paliative in asthma. The essence which is extracted is known by the name of essence of Wintergreen, and is used for rheumatism and diverse inflammations as a rub. The plant contains tannins and two primeverosides; gaultherioside, broken into primeverose and ethanol; monotropitoside, hydrolysable into primeverose and salicylate of methyl." [Salicylate of methyl is a tissue solvent see Willow]

1971 Jolicoeur (Quebec) 5. "For toothache, roll a leaf around the tooth."

1972 Assiniwi 73. "It can save a man from starvation. . .Strongly spiced, the fruit contains an oil that has been used as a medicine for over a thousand years by the Algonquins and Hurons. It is stimulant, it is an astringent so that it helps you to keep your breath while portaging heavy loads, and it is diuretic. It was Doctor Jean-Francois Gauthier of Quebec who, thinking he was the discoverer of wintergreen, named this plant. But four hundred years ago, Mother Marie de l'Incarnation mentioned it as a miracle drug, shown to her by the Indians. During the hunting season, many Algonquin guides from Maniwaki chew wintergreen leaves to improve their breathing. It also makes a good tea."

1975 Antoine King Go Home, Lake Huron personal communication. All his life has picked and used wintergreen as a tea and for rheumatism.

Wintergreen has lectinic, including mitogenic properties specifically for anti-M (RBC site), which makes it of interest in the future for cancer research. The roots chewed for 6 weeks each spring by children help to prevent tooth decay. (Lewis and Elvin-Lewis 1977)

CREEPING SNOWBERRY   *Gaultheria hispidula* (L.) Muhl. Ericaceae

The stem 20-40 cm long is bristly, especially when young, and creeps over decaying logs and mossy ground. The many 5-10 mm short stalked leaves are leathery, dark green and smooth on top, with stiff brownish hairs pressed against their undersides. The few flowers hang alone by the leaves. The berries are white, minutely bristly, 5-10 mm long with a crown.

Range. Nfld., and Lab., to B.C., s. to N.J., Pa., Mich., and Minn. and in the mts. to N.C., May-June in bogs and wet woods.

Common names. Moxie, ivory plums, mountain partridge berry, running birch, maidenhair berry.

1817-20 Bigelow 30. "The aromatic flavor of the Partridge berry, which cannot easily be mistaken by those who have once tasted it, may be recognised in a variety of other plants. . .It exists very exactly. . .particularly in *Gaultheria hispidula*."

1888 Delamare Island of Miquelon transl. 23. "The whole plant is aromatic, the berries are a beautiful white and sugary when mature. The leaves are used in infusion in place of tea and the berries are macerated in alcohol to make the 'liquer d'Anis'".

1926-27 Densmore CHIPPEWA 317. Leaves used for tea.

1955 Mockle Quebec 70 transl. "The plant is used for its stimulant and diaphoretic properties. As a tea it is given as a palliative in asthma. The extracted essence is reputed to be odontalgic [good for the teeth]."

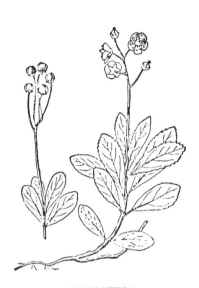

PIPSISSEWA

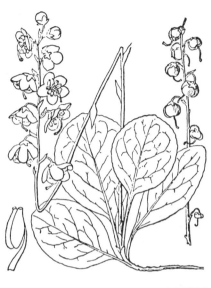

ROUND LEAVED WINTERGREEN

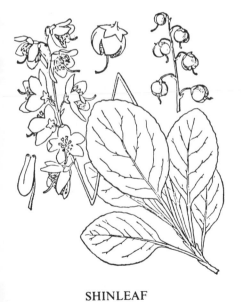

SHINLEAF

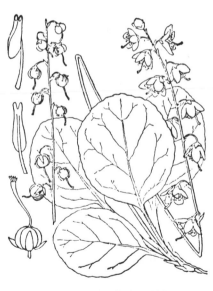

BOG WINTERGREEN

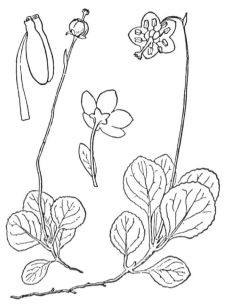

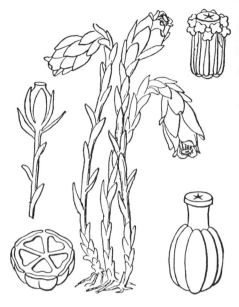

ONE FLOWERED WINTERGREEN   INDIAN PIPE

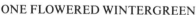

PIPSISSEWA   *Chimaphila umbellata* (L.) Bart. Ericaceae (*Pyrola u.*)
The stem creeps just under the ground sending up the flowering stem, 10-30 cm tall, bearing evergreen, bright and shining leaves 3-6 cm long on short stalks, their edges at the top with sharp teeth. At the top of the stem are 4-8 white or pinkish flowers 10-15 mm wide.
Range. Circumboreal, from Que. and N.S. to Minn., s. to Va., W.Va. and n. Ind. June-Aug. in dry woods especially in sandy soil.
Common names. Prince's pine, live-in-winter, [chimaphila means winter loving], ground-holly, noble-pine, king's cure, bitter wintergreen.

SPOTTED WINTERGREEN   *Chimaphila maculata* (L.) Pursh. (*Pyrola m.*)
Very like pipsissewa except that the leaves are striped white along the midvein and have pointed ends. [Not illustrated]
Range. Mass. to Mich., s. to S.C., Ga. and Ala. June-Aug. dry woods.
Common names. Rheumatism root, dragon's-tongue, wild arsenic, ratsbane.
RARE IN CANADA, ENDANGERED IN N.H., RARE IN MICH. PROTECTED BY LAW IN N.Y. OCCURS IN NEW ENGLAND IN DISJUNCT POPULATIONS OF FEW INDIVIDUALS. DO NOT DIG, PICK, GATHER SEED OR DISTURB HABITAT.
1633 Gerarde-Johnson 409. "Pyrola [Chimaphila] is a most singular wound hearbe, either given inwardly, or applied outwardly: the leaves whereof stamped and strained, and the juice made into an unguent, or healing salve, with waxe, oile, and turpentine, doth cure wounds, ulcers, and fistulas, that are mundified from the callous & tough matter, which keepeth the same from healing. The decoction hereof made with wine, is commended to close up and heale wounds of the entrailes, and inward parts: it is also good for ulcers of the kidnies, especially made with water, and the roots of Comfrey added thereto."
1785 Cutler. "Rheumatism weed. . .it is said to have been considered by the Indians as an effective remedy in rheumatism."
1817-20 Bigelow 19. "The leaves of *Pyrola umbellata*, when chewed, communicate to the mouth a taste which partakes of both sweet and bitter. As a diuretic in dropsy. As an external stimulant. . .The diuretic properties of the *Pyrola umbellata*. . .by Dr. W. Somerville in a paper on

this vegetable, published in the 5th. volume of the London Medico-Chirurigical transactions. . . .The most distinguished case. . .is that of Sir James Craig, the British governor in Canada, who was labouring under a general dropsy. . .and which was combined with different organic diseases, especially of the liver. After having tried with little or temporary success, almost every variety of diuretic and cathartic medicines. . .had recourse to a strong infusion of the Pyrola, in the quantity of a pint every twenty four hours. Although the case was altogether an unpromising one, yet the plant gave relief, not only in the first, but in subsequent instances of its use. . .Dr. Wolf. . .found it to alleviate altogether the ardor urinae attendant on gonorrhea. . .The Pyrola has been considerably employed as an external application to tumours and ulcers of various descriptions. It first acquired notice in consequence of some newspaper attestation of its efficacy in the cure of cancer. Those persons who know how seldom genuine cancers occur in comparison with reputed ones, will be more ready to allow it the character of curing ulcerous, than really cancerous affections. There are undoubtedly many ulcers, and those frequently of a malignant kind, which are benefitted by antiseptic stimulants; and to such the Pyrola may be useful. But of its effect in real cancer we require more evidence."

1830 Rafinesque 71. "Have the decided advantage of being grateful to the stomach while almost all other diuretics disagree with it; they invigorate the appetite, and strengthen the body, increase the flow of urine and all secretions. . .It was also used in typhus, and as a popular remedy for rheumatism in the United States. . .Externally decidedly useful in tumors, malignant ulcers, and chronic indurated swellings, acting as a topical stimulant, and sometimes they vesicate; but utterly useless in cancer and scrofula, for which the empirics have employed them. . .The Indian tribes of Canada and Missouri esteem highly these plants; they are called *Paigne* and *herb á pisser* in Canada. They are used chiefly for gravel and retention of urine, rheumatism and fevers. They dye urine of a greenish black color. The external application commonly produces redness, vesication, and desquamation of the skin. A drench of the leaves is used in veterinary for the diseases of horses unable to stale."

1830 Trans. Lit. & Hist. Soc. Quebec 94. "Pipsessawa is a small evergreen shrubby plant. . .one of the articles of Pharmacy among our aborigines."

1842 Christison 761. "This is a native North-American remedy, which in 1803 was introduced into medical practice by Dr. Mitchell of the United States, and afterwards to the notice of European practitioners by Dr. Somerville, now of Chelsea Hospital. . .The fresh plant is irritant, and acts as a rubefacient. It was introduced into medicine as a tonic and diuretic in scrofula and dropsy. It increases the flow of urine, and was therefore strongly recommended by Dr. Somerville in dropsies connected with debility. . . .It has likewise some diaphoretic action. It has been supposed, like uva-ursi, to have a soothing astringent effect on the urinary organs in catarrh of the bladder, chronic gonorrhoea, and chronic diseases of the kidneys. Its alleged virtues in scrofula are doubtful. It has not come into much use in this country [England]."

1868 Can. Pharm. J. 6; 83-5. The leaves of Prince's Pine included in list of Can. medicinal plants.

1892 Millspaugh 104. "It is used among the aborigines of this country as a tonic and diuretic, as well as for rheumatic and scrofulous disorders, and latterly as an application to scrofulous and other open sores. Chimaphila is still retained in the U.S. Ph."

1915 Harris ALGONQUIN 50. "Pipsisseway was held in great esteem by some Algonquin tribes as a sudorific and anodyne, especially in chest troubles, colds, etc. . .56. It is common around St. Catherines. It is a powerful astringent and also a diuretic."

1915 Speck PENOBSCOT 305. "Use of Prince's pine founded on its astringent quality. . .309. The name translates 'things for scorching' and the plant is steeped and applied to blisters. . .312. A concoction of seven herbs is taken as a sudorific [to produce sweat] before entering the sudatory [sweat bath]. It comprises sweet flag, fir twigs, lambkill, alder bark, witch hazel, cedar boughs, prince's pine and a kind of brake."

1915 Speck MONTAGNAIS 316. "Prince's pine is boiled and drunk to induce sweating."

1915 Speck-Tantaquidgeon MOHEGAN 318. "Pipsisseway is steeped and applied to blisters."

1915 Speck DELAWARE 320. "Pipsisseway for ague."

1923 H. Smith MENOMINI 35. "This is a valuable remedy in female troubles. It is used as a seasoner to make the medicine taste good."

1932 H. Smith OJIBWE 368. "A tea for treating stomach troubles."

1928 Parker SENECA 11. Diuretics, pipsissewa. . .12. For dropsy give pipsissewa tea.

1935 Jenness OJIBWA Parry Island Lake Huron 91. A decoction of Prince's pine is given to the baby to drink while its father is away hunting. If he were to merely wound an animal, whose body would suffer from the wound, the shadow of the baby would suffer in sympathy if it had not drunk the tea.

1955 Mockle Quebec transl. 70. "The leaves bitter and astringent are used in hydropsies, urinary affections and for scrofula and rheumatism. There is a belief that if you munch a leaf every day you will be protected from TB. Its chemical constituents are 4% tannins, glucosides; ericolin, chimaphilin and arbutoside and triterpenic acids."

1959 Mechling MALECITE maritime provinces of Canada used chimaphila for cold in the bladder, consumption, purification of the blood, smallpox and stomach trouble.

1971 Jolicoeur Quebec 4. "Drank a tea made of prince's pine, sarsaparilla, ground juniper and black cherry as a bitter and also as a spring tonic."

1975 Trevor Robinson 56. "Of all of these quinones (Vitamin K the most important) some are toxic and anti-microbial. Plants containing them have been used as drugs and poisons and since prehistoric times (e.g. chimaphilin, plumbagin, eleutherin) others have been equally important as dye stuffs. Chimaphilin is found in several species of Ericaceae."

1976 Antoine King, Go-Home Bay, Lake Huron personal communication. He collected Prince's pine when he was a child, there was a lot by Gloucester Pool. It is always used in his family as a tea for rheumatism. Very very bitter.

ROUND LEAVED WINTERGREEN *Pyrola rotundifolia* L. var. *americana* (Sweet) Fern. Ericaceae

The shining, round, firm leaves are 2.5-7 cm on stems from the roots. The flowering stem is 15-30 cm tall with one or two scale like leaves; at the top are the flowers with 8-10 mm white petals and outside of them 3-4 mm green leaves (sepals) that do not overlap at their base.

Range. Circumboreal, s. in Am. to N.C., Ky., Ind., and Minn in dry or moist woods and bogs. July-Aug. There is a smaller northern variety.

Common names. Consumption weed, Indian or canker lettuce.

SHINLEAF   *Pyrola elliptica* Nutt.

The leaves are 3-7 cm long, almost always longer than their stems. Their ends are rounded with fine teeth. The flowering stem is 15-30 cm tall with nodding white flowers that have green veins and are very fragrant. They have triangular small green leaves (sepals) at their base.

Range. Nfld., Que. to Minn and B.C., s. to Del., W.Va. and Io. in dry upland woods in rich soil. June-Aug.

BOG WINTERGREEN   *Pyrola asarifolia* Michx (*P. uliginosa*)

The leaves are mostly 3-6 cm, the flowering stem 15-30 cm with usually 1-3 scale like leaves. The petals are pink to pale purple 5-7 mm long. The triangular green leaves (sepals) at their bases are 2-3 mm and slightly overlap.

Range. Nfld. to Alas., s. to N.Y., n. Ind., Minn. and N.M. July-Aug. in moist woods and swamps.

ONE FLOWERED WINTERGREEN   *Moneses uniflora* (L.) Gray. (*Pyrola u.*) Ericaceae

The plants are only 3-10 cm tall with roundish 1-2 cm long leaves, finely toothed on 5-10 mm stalks. The one white flower is 12-20 mm and fragrant.

Range. Circumboreal, in Am. s. to Conn., N.Y., Mich., Minn. and N.M. July-Aug. in conifer woods and swamps.

1633 Gerarde-Johnson 409. "The leaves of Monophyllon, or Unifolium, are of the same force in wounds as Pyrola, especially in wounds among the nerves and sinewes. Moreover it is esteemed of some late writers a most perfect medicine against the pestilence, and all poisons, if a dram of the root be given in vinegar mixed with wine or water, and the sicke go to bed and sweat upon it."

1785 Cutler. "In wet meadows with deep purple flowers, this plant, [bog wintergreen] if it be eaten in large quantities, will occasion abortion in all kinds of herbivorous animals. . .separate from the hay."

1830 Rafinesque 72. "The *P. rotundifolia, P. elliptica* and *P. uniflora,* called vulgarly Wild Lettuce, Roundleaf, and Consumption Weed. They possess some of the above properties, but in a much less degree. [see under pipsissewa]. The Indians and empirics employ them as sudorific, astringent, anodyne, and nervine, in diseases of the breast, colds, wounds, ophthalmia, bad humours, weak nerves, and externally as blisters."

1868 Can. Pharm. J. 6; 83-5. The herb of *Pyrola rotundifolia* included in list of Can. medicinal plants.

1854-68 Reports of use of *Pyrola rotundifolia*, round leaved wintergreen, in decoction as a wash for cancerous sores and painful tumors in folk medicine (Hartwell 1970).

1915 Speck MONTAGNAIS 314. The plant of 'four seasons' (one flowered wintergreen) is steeped to make a medicine for paralysis. The Montagnais name for this is 'hauling'. . .The leaves (bog wintergreen) boiled in water and the water drunk for any kind of ailment. . .315. Roots (shinleaf) are boiled and drunk for weakness, 'back sickness'.

1915 Speck-Tantaquidgeon MOHEGAN 318. "'Canker lettuce', shin leaf is steeped and the liquid used as a gargle for sores or cankers in the mouth."

1915 Speck PENOBSCOT 311. Bog wintergreen. One of seven ingredients in a gonorrhea medicine.

1932 H. Smith OJIBWE 430. "Round leaved wintergreen. The Flambeau Ojibwe hunter makes a tea from the dried leaves of this plant and drinks it as a good luck potion in the morning before starting to hunt."

1933 Gilmore CHIPPEWA 138. Used for medicine.

1955 Mockle Quebec transl. 71 "The plant of one flowered wintergreen is astringent and vulnerary."

INDIAN PIPE   *Monotropa uniflora* L. Ericacea

Growing from decayed vegetation, the waxy white 10-20 cm tall stem has no green leaves. It is succulent and tender if handled, if rubbed it melts almost like ice. It has scales that are its leaves and one nodding, odorless white flower. When picked and dried the whole plant turns black or dark brown. Its seed pod is held upright. The plant may be pinkish in color.

Range. Nfld. to Wash., s. to Fla., Calif. and c. Am; also in e. Asia. June-Aug. in rich woods.

Common names. Ice plant, corpse plant, death plant, convulsion root, fit root, birds nest, fairy smoke.

1830 Rafinesque 243. "Ophthalmic and nervine. Used by Indians and herbalists, juice mixt with water deemed specific lotion for sore eyes. Dried roots in powder used in epilepsy and convulsions of children, dose a teaspoonful, often united to Valerian; cures also inveterate ophthalmia."

1859-61 Gunn 807. "The root is the part used in medicine, and should be gathered in September, and after being dried, should be kept in tight bottles, or it will lose its strength. It is nervine, antispasmodic, and sedative. It has been considered a great remedy for epileptic fits, especially in children. . .It is considered a good sedative and diaphoretic in intermittent fevers, and very valuable in nervous restlessness, pains and irritability, instead of Opium. It has been used with great success in cases of convulsions, spasms, fits and St. Vitus' Dance. . .It is no doubt a valuable plant, but too scarce to be of much general utility."

1868 Can. Pharm. J. 6; 83-5. The root of *Monotropa uniflora*, Indian pipe, included in list of Can. medicinal plants.

1892 Millspaugh 105. "The medical history of the plant begins with its use by the American Aborigines as an application in 'sore eyes;' they valued a mixture of the juice with water highly as a soothing and often curative measure. Of this property Dr. Kunze says in corroboration: 'This is a drug very highly recommended for overcoming nervous irritability, epilepsy, chorea, etc. when used in large doses—inwardly, of course, and for ophthalmic as well as other inflammations of delicate mucous surfaces outwardly applied, either in its fresh state or the preserved juice. I have myself used it very much in ordinary cases of inflamed eyes, both chronic and acute, and have never seen, or even heard of any evil effects following the most indiscriminate use. . .Dr. Stewart claimed that the dried herb was an excellent substitute for opium, 'easing pain, comforting the stomach, and causing sleep.'"

1933 H. Smith POTAWATOMI 57. "Used the roots of this plant to make a tea for female troubles."

1955 Mockle Quebec transl. 71. "The juice of the roots is mixed with water for an ophthalmic lotion."

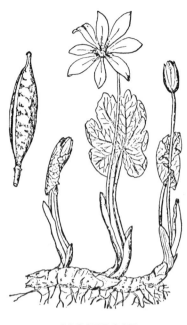

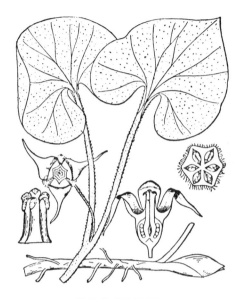

BLOODROOT   WILD GINGER

BLOODROOT   *Sanguinaria canadensis* L. Papaveraceae
The root is thick and covered with fine rootlets, from it grows the leaf stalk, 15-35 cm long. The leaves are smooth, prominently veined, scalloped around the edges and up to 20 cm wide. The 5-15 cm flowering stem is topped by white or pinkish flowers 2-5 cm wide. The seed pod is 3-5 cm long.
Range. N.B., N.S., sw. Gaspe pen. Que., Ont. n. to Thunder Bay, se. Man., s. to e. Tex. and n. Fla. April in rich woods.
Common names. Puccoon root, red-puccoon, red Indian paint, redroot, pauson, snake-bite.
1612 Capt. John Smith Virginia Indians 93. "Musquaspenne is a roote of the bignesse of a finger and as red as blood. In drying, it will wither almost to nothing. This they use to paint their Mattes, Targets, and such like."
1624 Wassenaer New Netherlands Indians 77. "The natives in the habit of clothing them selves with them [skins]; the fur or hair inside, the smooth side without, which, however, they paint so beautifully that at a distance, it resembles lace, They are so clever that they make use of the best for that purpose: what is poor of substance they deem unsuitable for their clothing."
1708 Sarrazin-Vaillant, Quebec-Paris, Boivin 1978 transl. 47. "The root is red and contains a juice that is like blood. It is acrid. I have been assured that it brings on the menses. . .Because the juice is red like blood, it has pleased our Savage women and some others who follow them, to believe that it can cause abortion. This I do not believe. I have used it myself often to bring on the menses, but I have not found anything that approaches what is said of it."
1724 Anon ILLINOIS MIAMI mss. 223. "To dye red, there is on the prairie of the Tamarcoua a plant they name the red Micousiouaki, they take the root, dry it, pulverize it in the mortar, and boil it with three times as many sumac berries. The red is very beautiful." [Could be *Lithospermum* also called puccoon root]
1778 Carver 515. "Blood Root. . .the root. . .when broken, the inside of it is of a deeper colour than the outside, and distills several drops of juice that looks very like blood. This is a strong emetic, but a very dangerous one."
1817-20 Bigelow 79. "The beautiful colour of the root seems to reside more in the resin than in any other principle, since the alcoholic solution has always more than twice as much colour as the aqueous. Papers dipt in these solutions receive a bright salmon colour from the tincture, but

a very faint one from the aqueous solution. This circumstance furnishes an impediment to the use of this article in dyeing. The medical properties of the Sanguinaria are those of an acrid narcotic. When taken in a large dose it irritates the fauces, leaving an impression in the throat for a considerable time after it is swallowed. It occasions heartburn, nausea, faintness, and frequently vertigo and diminished vision. At length it vomits, but in this operation it is less certain than other emetics in common use. The above effects are produced by a dose of from eight to twenty grains of the fresh powdered root. When given in smaller doses, such as to produce a nausea without vomiting, and repeated at frequent intervals, it lessens the frequency of the pulse in a manner somewhat analagous to the operation of Digitalis. This however is a secondary effect, since in its primary operation it seems to accelerate the circulation. . .Professor Smith of Hanover, New Hampshire, in a paper on this plant, published in the London Medical Transactions, vol. 1. states that he found the powder to operate violently as an emetic. . .Applied to fungous flesh it proved escharotic, and several polypi of the soft kind were cured by it in his hands. He found it of great use in the incipient stages of pulmonary consumption. . .Professor Ives of New Haven considers the Blood root as a remedy of importance in many diseases, particularly of the lungs and liver. . .Thinks highly of its use in influenza, in phthisis, and particularly in hooping cough. . .It has been given. . .for many years in the country, some physicians relying wholly on this remedy for the cure of croup."

1830 Rafinesque 79. "The root is the officinal part: it is one of the most valuable medical articles of our country, and already begins to be introduced into general practice. . .The Indians used the red juice to paint themselves, and dye or stain skins, baskets &c. It has not yet been much used in dyeing, although it stains wool of a fine orange colour; the mordants are alumine and muriosulphate of tin, for silk, cotton, &c. . .in powdering the dried root, the nose and throat are affected. . .When used as an emetic, it expels worms from the stomach. . .The juice being acrid and corrosive, was used for warts. Thatcher says it is the base of Rawson's bitters, a remedy for jaundice. . .Few medical plants unite so many useful properties; but it requires to be administered with skilful hands, and may become dangerous in empirical hands. . .Snuffed up the nose it excites sneezing. . .[drunk it lessens] the pulse from 112 to 80. . .Externally either in powder or as a wash, it has cured ill conditioned ulcers. . .it removes fungous tumors and excrescences, nay even soft polypus, by being used like snuff. . .It must not be given to pregnant women, since it is known to act on the uterus powerfully, and even cause abortions; whence its use in amenorrhea. . .It looses much of its strength by keeping, after powdering or preparing in any way; but the dried roots keep very well. . .The leaves have some of the same properties and are powerful, nay, deleterious stimulants. The farriers use them in diseases of horses, to make them sweat, shed their coats &c. The seeds are violent narcotics, similar to those of Stramonium [Datura sp.], producing fever, delirium, dilated pupils &c. They have been used as incitants, diaphoretics, and diuretics, but are dangerous and deleterious."

1836 Trail Backwoods of Can. 84- 5 "The blood-root. . .is worthy of attention from the root to the flower. . .a thick juicy fibrous root, which, on being broken, emits a quantity of liquor from its pores of a bright orange scarlet colour: this juice is used by the Indians as a dye, and also in the cure of rheumatic and cutaneous complaints. . .A rich black vegetable mould at the edges of the clearings seems the favourite soil for this plant."

1857 Fell A treatise on cancer London. Fell learned from Indian traders that the Indians of the shores of Lake Superior used the juice for treating cancers. He developed a treatment based on a paste of bloodroot extract, zinc chloride, flour and water. The paste, smeared on a cloth was put on the tumor until it became encrusted. Then cuts were made ½ inch apart into the tumor and filled with the paste. Generally the cancer fell out in about 6 weeks leaving a healthy sore. The Middlesex Hospital in London perfected the treatment and remissions occured in 25 breast cancer patients. Later the treatment was judged of very little use but was revived in 1962 for superficial cancers of the nose and external ear. (Lewis and Elvin-Lewis 1977:123-4.)

1859-61 Gunn 756. "Blood root is. . .a powerful medicine, and valuable in many cases. In small doses it excites the digestive organs, and stimulates the liver to healthy action; in large doses it depresses the pulse, lessens the action of the heart, and produces nausea and vomiting. It should never be given in very large doses. Its principal use should be in pulmonary and hepatic affections; that is in disease of the lungs. . .A little of the finely powdered root, mixed with as much of powdered Bayberry, is an excellent snuff for headaches, and cold in the head; and alone it is a good remedy for polypus of the nose, to be snuffed frequently. It is also good applied in the form of fine powder, to any fungous growths, to old and indolent ulcers, destroying the proud flesh and exciting them to healthy action. A strong tincture of the root made in vinegar, is often sufficient to cure ringworm, tetter, salt rheum and the like by being applied freely to the parts. For such purposes the tincture is best made of the fresh roots, first mashing them; and should be made as strong as possible. . .There is a concentrated preparation made from this article, called Sanguinarin; but I have not discovered that it is any case preferable to the root. . .it is a dark red powder and may be had at most of the drug stores."

1868 Can. Pharm. J. 6; 83-5. The root of *Sanguinaria canadensis* included in list of Can. medicinal plants.

1892 Millspaugh 22. "For many years it has been used by the aborigines of this country for painting their faces, clothing and implements of warfare, and by the laity as a domestic remedy in gastric trouble, compounded with podophyllum [may-apple] and kali tartaricum. Applied to a denuded surface it is quite a powerful escharotic. The root is still officinal in the U.S. Ph.. . . .Death has occured from overdoses, after the following sequence of symptoms; violent vomiting, followed by terrible thirst and great burning in the stomach and intestines, accompanied by soreness over the region of those organs; heaviness of the upper chest with difficult breathing; dilation of the pupils; great muscular prostration, faintness and coldness of the surface, showing that death follows from cardiac paralysis."

1915 Speck PENOBSCOT 311. "Bits of bloodroot dried and strung together into a necklace, were worn to prevent bleeding."

1915 Speck-Tantaquidgeon MOHEGAN 318. "Bloodroot is steeped and used as a blood medicine, and it is also regarded as an emetic."

1920 Fyles 51. "The whole plant contains an acrid, orange-red latex or milky juice, which is extremely irritating to the skin, particularly if the skin is bruised or broken. . .It is hardly likely to be eaten, as it has a repulsive appearance and a very bitter taste. It is used medicinally, and Johnson records fatal cases from overdoses."

1924 Youngken 498. "The rhizomes and roots of this plant constituted the 'Red Puccoon' of the Indians generally. . .The fresh rhizomes and roots containing a red milky juice were used for decorating their skin, while wearing apparel was often boiled with these parts. Bachelors of some of the tribes, after rubbing some of the red milky juice on their hands, would contrive to shake hands with girls they desired; if successful in this, after five or six days, these girls are said to have been found willing to marry them."

1926-27 Densmore CHIPPEWA 293. "Used as a charm. . .344. Mixed with equal parts of the root of blue cohosh (*Caulophyllum thalictroides*) and a decoction made and drunk for cramps in the stomach. . .371. Formula. . .used by Mrs. Razor for dyeing porcupine quills. . .the result was a brilliant scarlet which closely resembled analine dye. The quills were seen in the dye; bloodroot 2 handfuls; inner bark of wild plum, 1 handful; bark of red osier dogwood, 1 handful; bark of alder, 1 handful, boiled in 1 quart of hot water, all being boiled before the quills were put in the dye. Another formula 1 handful of bloodroot roots and 1 handful wild plum inner bark in 1 quart of water for a dark red. For a dark yellow double handful of shredded root of bloodroot and single handful of shredded root of wild plum in hot water boiled together. . .Another yellow formula the inner bark of the wild plum was scraped and it was said to set the colour: take sumac, inner bark, the root of bloodroot and the plum and boil."

1928 Reagan CHIPPEWA 231. "A very common Indian medicine, used as a blood medicine. It is also used in the jugglery performance of medicine. It blooms in April."

1928 Parker SENECA 11. Childbirth use Sanguinaria. Wash the uterus with water with a slight amount of lye [wood ashes].

1923 H. Smith MENOMINI 44. "This root is often added to medicines to strengthen their effect. . . .78. The fresh boiled root was often used to paint the face of a warrior. The boiled root furnished a dye that the Menomini women used in coloring their mats red or orange red."

1928 H. Smith MESKWAKI 234. "McIntosh used a tea of this root to bathe burns. Then too, the root is chewed and the spittle put upon burns to relieve the pain. It is called a great medicine and sometimes is prepared under water. It is then peeled under hot water. It is often added to other medicines to strengthen their effect. . .271. The Meskwaki cooked the root and made a red face paint long ago, and also used the fluid to dye baskets red. They also dye their rushes for mats with this root."

1932 H. Smith OJIBWE 377. "The Pillager Ojibwe use the orange red juice of the bloodroot to cure sore throat. The juice is squeezed out on a lump of maple sugar, and this is retained in the mouth until it has melted away. They also use the juice to paint the face for the medicine lodge ceremony or when on the warpath. . .426. The Ojibwe use this root in four or five combinations in dyeing various materials. It is not necessary to mix it with other materials to set the color and alone it gives a dark yellow or orange color. They use it to paint the face, also, making different clan marks with it. Either the fresh or dried root may be used."

1933 H. Smith POTAWATOMI 68. "The Forest Potawatomi steep the root for an infusion which is used to cure diptheria, which they recognize as a disease of the throat. . .121. As a facial paint root."

1945 Rousseau MOHAWK transl. 44 "For sore ears make an infusion of the dried roots broken into bits and place in a pot: one sees immediately 'the power coming out of the roots.' It only needs a few drops in the ear to make it better. For stomach troubles after a sumptuous repast, drink a decoction of the mashed root, after having soaked it in cold water for two nights. The color of the root used to be used to dye sheets an orange yellow and has the reputation of being nearly indelible. This color will not take on ash and other materials used in basketry."

1955 Mockle Quebec transl. 45. "The root is the part used, it is dark red, with a narcotic smell and persistent bitter taste; in small doses it is used as a stimulant, diaphoretic, and expectorant; in larger doses as a purgative and vomitive. The acrid juice is corrosive and is used as a rubefacient and vesicant. The powdered root is sternutatory. The root is said to be emmenagogue which is why it is frequently used as an abortifacient. It contains the alkaloids: protopine, allo-cryptopine, sanguinarine, oxysanguinarine, chelerythrine and homochelidonine."

1959 Mechling MALECITE maritime provinces of Canada, used the root for consumption with hemorrhage and for infected cuts.

Bloodroot contains protopine also found in opium. In full doses it depresses the action of the heart, and produces nausea and vomiting; in smaller doses it increases the appetite and improves digestion. It has been used in dyspepsia, croup, bronchitis and asthma. The powdered root is a powerful irritant of the respiratory passages (T.E. Wallis 1967:378).

WILD GINGER
Asarum canadense L. Aristolochiaceae

The creeping aromatic root grows terminally into a hairy stalk that divides at once into two hairy stems, 15-30 cm long, each supporting a velvety leaf with a heart shaped base, hairy on both sides and 8-15 cm broad. From between the stems, a short 2-5 cm hairy stalk arises from which hangs down the brownish red flower, creamy within, 2-4 cm across that is pollinated by ground insects.

Range. N.B., Que., Ont., se Man., s. to Kans., Tenn. and N.C. in rich woods, Apr.-May.

Common names. Canada snakeroot, false coltsfoot, colic root, Asarabacca, Indian ginger.

1475 Bjornsson Icelandic mss. Larsen transl. "Gingiber conditum [European ginger] is the name of an electuary which one may call Inifri. That helps man's nature to digest his food well. It is good for all chest troubles which are caused by the cold. And it is good for the loins and stirs a man mightily whether it be drunk or eaten with red wine."

1681 Culpeper 33. "European ginger, asarabaca. The common use hereof is to take the juice of five or seven leaves in a little drink to cause vomiting; the roots have also the same virtue, though they do not operate so forcibly; they are very effectual against the biting of serpents, and therefore are put as an ingredient both into Mithridate and Venice treacle. The leaves and root being boiled in lye, and the head often washed therewith while it is warm, comforteth the head and brain, that is ill affected by taking cold, and helpeth the memory. I shall desire ignorant people to forbear the use of the leaves: the roots purge more gently, and may prove beneficial to such as have cancers, or old purtrified ulcers, or fistulas upon their bodies, to take a dram of them in powder in a quarter of a pint of white wine in the morning. The truth is, I fancy purging and vomiting medicines as little as any man breathing doth, for they weaken nature, nor shall ever advise them to be used unless upon urgent necessity. If a physican be nature's servant, it is his duty to strengthen his mistress as much as he can, and weaken her as little as he can."

1687 Clayton Virginia Indians 12. "Again general report goes in favour of the Asarum. . .which many therefore particularly call Rattlesnake root." [Referring to the belief that the Indians possessed a root which when handled enabled them to hold rattlesnakes with impunity, it is the southern wild ginger. *A. virginicum*].

1724 Anon ILLINOIS MIAMI mss 224. "The root of ginger crushed in powder for putting stop to pains of a woman in childbirth. . .For scrofula they use the root of the herb of the rattlesnake which they call Akiskiouaraoui, they chew this root and apply it to the injured part and give the patient a little of the same root distilled in a little water to drink. This root is very good for the bite of the serpent, but orvietan and theriac [Venice treacle] have a faster and more certain effect."

1828 Rafinesque 71. "It has been called *Canadense* because it was first noticed in Canada. . .The whole plant, but particularly the root, has an agreeable aromatic bitterish taste, intermediate between Ginger and *Aristolachia serpentaria* (Virginia snakeroot) but more pleasant, warm and pungent. The smell is spicy and strong. . .Aromatic stimulant and diaphoretic cordial, emmenagogue, subtonic, errhine &c. but not properly emetic like *A. europeum* although often mentioned as such. It is a grateful substitute of the Serpentaria in many cases. It is useful in cachexia, melancholy, palpitations, low fevers, convalescence, obstructions, hooping-cough, &c. The dose must be small and often repeated, since it becomes nauseous in large doses. . .The dried leaves make a fine stimulating and cephalic snuff, when reduced to powder, which may be used in all disorders of the head and eyes. . .A grateful wine or beer may be made by the infusion of the whole plant, in fermenting wine or beer. . .264. The western Indians use it as a styptic for wounds, and an abortive also. In large doses produces pyrosis and water brash, besides nausea. It may be combined with tonics to advantage. . .1830 196. Dr. Firth says that he has cured the tetanus by the decoction of *A. canadense*. The Indians make a fine snuff with *A. virginicum*, the fresh leaves are used for wounds and scrofula."

1820's Materia Medica Edinburgh-Toronto mss 42. *A. Europeum* formerly used as an emetic but has fall into disuse. . .66. The leaves promise more errhine power. . .they are less acrid than some of this class and are upon the whole best adapted to the purpose for which errhines are used."

1834 Trail 107. "These persons who do not choose to employ medical advice on the subject dose themselves with ginger tea." [for the ague].

1849 Stephen Williams 883. A snuff made from the powdered root was useful in disorders of the head and eyes and was used for many complaints by Canadian Indians. When a party of them visited him at Deerfield [Mass.] in 1837, they were offended when he declined to accept from them a preparation of ginger root for the palpitation of the heart with which he was then afflicted (Vogel 1963:391).

1859-61 Gunn 879. "The root is the part used. . .It is a powerful emmenagogue; and if used in strong decoction, in large doses, it will produce abortion. There is no danger of this, however, if used in moderate quantities in infusion. May be used wherever a good diaphoretic or sweating tea is needed, either alone or combined with the Composition Powders."

1868 Can. Pharm. J. 6; 83-5. The root of wild ginger included in list of Can. medicinal plants.

1875 Balfour 576. Used as a spice in Canada.

1915 Speck MONTAGNAIS 314. "Wild ginger has general medicinal properties. Indian name means 'beaver his food.'"

1924 Youngken 490. "Canada snakeroot. The Indians of Canada and Maine employed the rhizome and roots as a remedy for stomach ills."

1926-27 Densmore CHIPPEWA 318. "The root of this plant was regarded as an appetizer', being put in any food as it was being cooked. It was also used for indigestion. . .342. The dried root was chewed for indigestion. . .334. The treatment of a fractured arm was described as follows: 'Wash the arm with warm water and apply grease. Then apply a warm poultice, cover with a cloth and bind with a thin cedar splint.' The roots used for the poultice were *Asarum canadense* L. (wild ginger) and *Aralia racemosa* L. (spikenard). These two were dried and mashed together in equal parts. The directions added 'when poultice becomes dry it should be renewed, or, if the arm is very tender, the poultice may be moistened with warm water without removing it.'"

1923 H. Smith MENOMINI 24. "The fresh or dried root of wild ginger is used by the Menomini as a mild stomachic. When the patient is weak or he has a weak stomach, and it might be fatal to eat something he craves, then he must eat part of this root. Whatever he wants then may be eaten with impunity."

1928 H. Smith MESKWAKI 196. "An internal medicine consists of seven herbs and wild ginger root. . .204. This is the medicine used for seasoning and used by one who has a sore throat. It was used by McIntosh in a mixture with other things for lung trouble. The Meskwaki give a fine reputation to this root, and use it for many things. The cooked root is put into the ear for earache or sore ears. . .When the root is chewed and the fisherman uses the spittle on the bait, it enables him to catch catfish. . .Mixed with Euphorbia and Monarda it is used for cramps in the stomach. . .255. The root of wild ginger is kept on hand at all times and it might be called their most important native seasoning. A good many mud catfish are caught in the Iowa river which flows through their reservation and the use of wild ginger in cooking them destroys the mud taste and renders them palatable. It is also used to cook some animal that has died, such as a hog or a cow, and has been given them by some farmer. When used in this way, they claim there is no danger of ptomaine poisoning."

1932 H. Smith OJIBWE 397. "Use this root in cookery to season food as do Meskwaki. . .The roots are processed in lye water for cookery on a large scale."

1933 H. Smith POTAWATOMI 41. "The Forest Potawatomi use Wild Ginger as a mild stomachic principally to flavor meat or fish and render them more edible."

1928 Parker SENECA 11. Wild ginger used as a carminative. . .12. Used for coughs.

1935 Jenness Parry Island OJIBWA Lake Huron 88. "So potent is this fear of witchcraft that every Parry Islander takes counter-measures for his own protection, and for the protection of his family. . .Since a sorcerer may visit a house by night and place evil medicine in dishes prepared for the following day some of the Indians regularly add a little wild ginger to their food. In the earlier days, they say, warriors always mixed this wild ginger with their war-rations of dried berries and dried meat, for it prevented the contagion of the food from several sources, from the touch of a little baby, of a woman in her seasons, and of a sorcerer or witch. . .97. While I was living with my foster-parents at Shawanaga one of their daughters reached maturity. My foster-mother put wild ginger in all our food to prevent any ill effect, and she gave me wild ginger to chew. Pegamagabow."

1942 Speck, Hassrick, Carpenter, RAPPAHANNOCK 25. Steeped leaves to reduce fever in typhoid. . .33. Treated asthma with a steeped infusion of red cedar berries and wild ginger. (Vogel 1963:175; 207).

1945 Rousseau MOHAWK transl. 41. "Used for children's convulsions and fevers."

1954 de Laszlo & Henshaw Science 626. Oral contraceptives thought to excite temporary sterility, decoction of boiled root and rhizome of wild ginger.

1955 Mockle Quebec transl. 36. "The roots are aromatic, stimulant, febrifuge and used for whooping cough. The powdered root and the dried leaves are sternutatory. There has been found in the root an antibacterial substance against gram positive pus-forming bacteria."

1967 Doskotch & Vanevenhoven Lloydia 30:141-144. Isolation of anti-tumor agent aristolchic acid from *Asarum canadense*.

1970 Willaman & Li. 770. *Asarum canadense* L. var. *reflexum* contains aristolochic acid.

Aristolochic acid has antimicrobial properties. Asarum canadense is an active agent against broad spectrum bacteria and fungi. (Lewis and Elvin-Lewis 1977:225; 360).

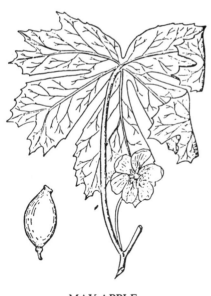

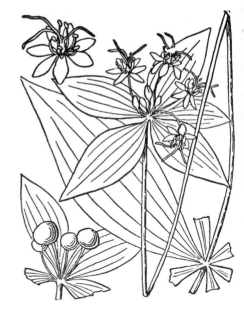

MAY APPLE   INDIAN CUCUMBER ROOT

MAY APPLE   *Podophyllum peltatum* L. Berberidaceae
The leaves are attached to the middle of the stout stems which grow from the root. They are 30-40 cm wide, deeply cut into 5-9 toothed lobes, smooth or slightly hairy, light green below, darker above. The flowering stem is 30-50 cm tall with a pair of smaller leaves, the 3-5 cm white flower hangs from a short stalk growing from this pair of leaves. The fruit is yellow, 4-5 cm and edible. The plant and seed are POISONOUS.
Range. N.S., sw. Que., s. Ont. (N to Stormont Co.) Minn., s. to Tex. and Fla. in rich woods, thickets, and pastures.
Common names. Mandrake, ground lemon, wild jalap, raccoon-berry, Indian apple.
1612 Capt. John Smith Virginia 92. "During somer there are either strawberries which ripen in april; or mulberries which ripen in May and June, Raspises, hurtes [blueberries], or a fruit that the Inhabitants call Maracocks, which is a pleasant wholesome fruit much like a lemond."
1613 Champlain fourth voyage fac. ed. transl. 35. [The Ottawas, in refusing to take Champlain north said]. . ."These people are sorcerers, & they have killed many of our people by sorcery and poisoning, & that is the reason they are not friends. . .[Champlain replied]. . .For myself, who have no other desire than to see these people, & become their friends, to see the Northern sea. . .as regards their sorceries, they have no power to harm me, & my God would preserve me; I know well their herbs, & therfor I will be careful in what I Eat." [He did not persuade the Ottawas to take him that year.]
1619 Champlain-Macklem. HURON Cahigue near Orilla Ontario 1616. 40. "One of their berries was new to us. It looked rather like a small lemon but tasted more like a fig. They grow on small plants not more than two and a half feet high. Each plant has only three or four leaves, shaped like a fig leaf, and each stem has only two flowers. In some parts of the country these berries are plentiful and they are extremely good to eat."
1628 de Rasieres New Netherland 113. "When there is a youth who begins to approach manhood, he is taken by his father, uncle, or nearest friend, and is conducted blindfolded into the wilderness, in order that he may not know the way, and is left there by night or otherwise, with a bow and arrows, and a hatchet and a knife. He must support himself there a whole winter. . .Towards spring they come again, and fetch him out of it, take him home and feed him up again until May. He must then go out again every morning with the person who is ordered to

take him in hand; he must go into the forest to seek wild herbs and roots, which they know to be the most poisonous and bitter; these they bruise in water and press the juice out of them, which he must drink, and immediately have ready such herbs as will preserve him from death or vomiting; for if he cannot retain it, he must repeat the dose until he can support it, and until his constitution becomes accustomed to it so that he can retain it."

1636 Brebeuf Jes. Rel. 10 HURON 199-209 "He dreamed, therefore, that there was only one certain kind of dance which would make him quite well. They call it akhrendoiaen inasmuch as those who take part in this dance give poison to one another. It had never been practised among this nation of the Bear."

1708 Sarrazin-Vaillant, Quebec-Paris, Boivin 1978 transl. 219. "This plant is one of the most beautiful that I can send you. [No. 2 of the year 1698]. . .The fruit of this plant which is called *citronier* in this country is ordinarily as big as a little pullet's egg. It is acid, good to eat, but feverish. The root is a very effective poison which the Savages use when they cannot bear their troubles."

1710 Raudot HURON 409. "They [women] are very subject to poisoning themselves at the least grief that betakes them; the men also poison themselve sometimes. To leave this life they use a root of hemlock [see *cicuta*] or of citron, which they swallow. This citron is a plant that grows in moist and shady spots and has only one stalk, where ripens a fruit rather like a small citron, and not disagreeable to the taste; it does not do any harm, but the root is a very subtle poison. These savages, however, cure themselves of it by making themselves vomit a great deal, which makes them throw out all this poison."

1779 Zeisberger DELAWARE 47. "Wild citrons or May apples, grow on stalks not over a foot high. The Indians enjoy eating the fruit, which has a sour but pleasant taste. The roots are a powerful poison, which, who eats, dies in a few hours' time unless promptly given an emetic. . .57. In the use of poisonous roots the Indians are well versed, and there are many melancholy examples where they have by their use destroyed themselves or others. If a case of poisoning is taken in time, the effect of the poisonous root may be prevented by inducing vomiting. In case assistance is rendered too late, death follows, as a rule, in a few hours."

1795 Simcoe Toronto 290. "The May apples are now a great luxury; I have some preserved and the hurtleberries [blueberries] are ripe. Baron La Hontan says the root of the May apple (or, as the French call them *citron sauvages*) is poisonous."

1817-20 Bigelow 36. "The dried root of the May apple is fragile and easily reduced to powder. It has a peculiar and rather unpleasant taste, but without much acrimony. . .The medicinal properties of the *Podophyllum peltatum* are those of a sure and active cathartic, in which character it deserves a high rank among our indigenous productions. We have hardly any native plant which answers better the common purposes of jalap. [*Ipomoea purgea* Hayne from Mexico], aloes and rhubarb. The root is the part employed, and should be given in substance in fine powder. I have commonly found twenty grains to operate with efficacy, and not to be attended with pain or inconvenience. . .The late Professor Barton informs us. . .the leaves are poisonous, and the whole plant has something of a narcotic quality. Its botanical affinities would justify, *a priori*, a suspicion of this kind. . .The root is said by some physicians to be a medicine particularly suited to dropsy. . .A physician in Albany informs me that the Shakers at Lebanon, N.Y. prepare an extract of the Podophyllum, which is much esteemed by medical practicioners as a mild cathartic. These people are well known to our druggists by the care and neatness with which they prepare a variety of medicines from native and naturalized pharmaceutical plants. For medicinal use the root of the May apple is advised to be dug in the cold season, when the vegetation is not active, viz. the autumn and winter. At this part of the year the secretions of perennial plants are concentrated in their roots. . .It is probable that those roots which constitute staple articles of commerce, as ipecac, gentian, rhubarb &c. are gathered indiscriminately for exportation at all seasons when they are found. Being collected by savages or by ignorant persons, who seek for them in their native wilds, and who are not much interested in their future efficacy; it is probable they would be gathered in greatest quantities when their vegetation was most luxuriant, because at this time their shoots and tops would be most conspicuous. We know this to be the case with our Ginseng, spigelia, snake-root, &c. which form considerable articles of exportation and which would be difficult to find at any other than the vegetating season."

1830 Rafinesque 60. "One of the best native cathartics. . .The medical properties of this article have been well ascertained, and are admitted by all physicians; many use it frequently in the country; the extract is very good, even better than the powder. Those who employ mercurial preparations, use it united to calomel, twenty grains of the powder with ten of calomel being a strong dose: but from five to twenty grains of the extract alone is equally good. In smaller doses, it proves a gradual and easy laxative. Ten grains of the powder alone, taken at night, purges next morning. . .The Cherokee use it against worms, which are expelled by its drastic effects. . .The leaves are said to be narcotic. . .A drench of the whole fresh plant in decoction, will purge a horse completely. Two ounces of the leaves in decoction killed a dog. The Cherokees employ the fresh juice of the root for the cure of deafness, by putting a few drops in the ear. The Osage Indians consider it a cure for poisons, by driving them through the bowels. They are very fond of the fruit, like all the Indian tribes. A fine preserve is made of them in Louisiana. To me, this fruit is hardly palatable, and the root is so nauseous that I employ a syrup of it like the Cherokees, which becomes then a mild and not unpleasant purgative, two spoonsful being a dose. Small doses of it, or of the extract, lower the pulse from 77 to 64, and are useful in cough and pleurisy."

1855 Trail 85. "Mandrake or May-Apple ripe in august. This was the first native fruit that I tasted, after my arrival in Canada. It attracted my attention as I was journeying through the wood to my forest home. The driver of the team plucked it for me, and told me it was good to eat, bidding me throw aside the outer rind, which he said was not fit to be eaten. The May-apple when ripe is about the size of an egg-plum which it resembles in shape and colour. The pulp of the fruit is of a fine sub-acid flavour, but it is better not gathered too ripe. . .The time of ripening is in August: the rich moist lands at the edge of the forest, and just within its shade, is the place where the May-apple abounds. . .Gather the fruit as soon as it begins to shew any yellow tint on the green rind: lay them by in a sunny window for a day or two; cut them in quarters and throw them into a syrup of white sugar, in which ginger sliced and cloves have been boiled: boil the fruit till the outer rind is tender: take the fruit out, lay them in a basin, sift a handful of pounded sugar over them, and let them lie till cold. Next day boil your syrup a second time, pour it over the fruit, and when cold put it into jars or glasses, and tie down. It should not be used till a month or six weeks after making: if well spiced this preserve is more like some foreign fruit. It is very fine. Some only use the soft acid pulp, but though the outer part is not fit to be eaten in a raw state, it is very good when preserved, and may safely be made use of, boiled with sugar and spices. The fruit might I think be introduced into garden culture and prove a valuable addition to our tables: but in the event of planting it in the garden, a very rich light mould must be given to feed the plant, which grows by nature in the rich vegetable leaf-mould."

1859-61 Gunn 827. "The root is the part used. . .valuable in active doses in all forms of dropsy, and internal or local inflammations. . .The powdered root was formerly very much used as a cathartic; but latterly, since the introduction of the *Podophyllin*, which is made from this root, the substance is not so much used. . .In small doses, that is what is termed alterative doses, the May apple is an excellent hepatic, that is, liver medicine, acting as a stimulant to the liver, as well as the whole glandular system, and as a valuable alterative in scrofulous diseases, in syphilis, mercurial taints, and the like. . .Podophyllin. . .is the Samson among vegetable remedies, and may be regarded as the substitute for Calomel. . .It will be found to have quite all the beneficial effects of mercury, without any of its injurious effects. . .is one of the remedies that should always be kept in the house."

1868 Can. Pharm. J. 1; 4. "Before closing this subject I must advert to an effect of Podophyllin on the system which I have never seen mentioned. If ever so small a particle should reach the eye—in eight or ten hours a violent inflammation ensues. The eyelids become swollen and red and the ball of the eye so suffused with blood as to cause loss of vision, for sometimes two days—I need not say the pain is most intense, and as I have been myself a subject I can speak very feelingly. By the application of tepid milk and water, which, coupled with the avoidance of light, I have found the best treatment, the inflammation may be reduced in three days. I have seen three men similarly affected, during the past two years, one of them while grinding the root. . .In concluding this paper I have to express my regret at not being able, from lack of time, to prepare a more systematic essay. But I hope the subject will not drop, and that some member will pursue further investigation on this very interesting substance."

1868 Can. Pharm. J. 1; 4. *Podophyllum peltatum*—"Mandrake—is so well known as to require but little notice. The consumption of the various preparations from the root is rapidly increasing, and sensibly affects the sale of Jalap, Scammony [Convolvulus Scamonia] and calomel [a preparation of mercury].'"

1868 Can. Pharm J. 6; 83-5. The root of mandrake, *Podophyllum peltatum* included in list Can. medicinal plants.

1892 Millspaugh 17. "This plant constitutes one of the principal remedies used by the American aborigines, by whom it is especially valued on account of its cathartic action. Their use of the drug as an anthelmintic seems to have been successful only as far as purging is concerned; specifically, it has no anthelmintic power. The use of podophyllum as a component of cathartic pills is very general. . .Podophyllin—a resin mass, first observed and used by Prof. John King (1835)."

1916 Waugh IROQUOIS 18. "When all is ready for planting, the corn is soaked in a decoction made of certain herbal ingredients. The moisture causes the corn to germinate slightly, though the utility of the added materials is not so evident. There is possibly some connexion with sympathetic magic, the other plants contributing their vitality or otherwise assisting and protecting the corn. Regarding what appeared to be the oldest or, at any rate, the most important of these preparations, it was stated by a Cayuga informant that it prevented the worms and birds from bothering. A sort of halo was also said to be sometimes seen around the plants. . .19. Quite different materials from those named are used in some localities. Peter John, Onondaga, employed the leaves of the mandrake (*Podophyllum peltatum*). These were simply placed in water". . .125. Fruits used as food referred to in the Jesuit Relations, 38:243, the mandrake. . .129. Principal varieties of fruit eaten. . .mandrake.

1928 Parker SENECA 11. Used as a laxative. . .12. As a cathartic. . .for nervousness.

1923 H. Smith MENOMINI 25. "This is not a medicine for the Menomini but his substitute for Paris green [acito-arsenate of copper a poison]. The whole plant is boiled and the resulting liquid is sprinkled on potato plants to kill potato bugs. The Menomini claim that it kills the eggs of the potato bugs in the ground as well as the bugs. . .62. The fresh ripe fruits of the Mandrake are prized as a food. The writer has seen them gathered by the peck and taken home to eat or preserve."

1928 H. Smith MESKWAKI 207. "This is a valuable remedy to the Meskwaki, and is always used in mixtures, never alone. The root is recognised as a physic and is also used in treating rheumatism. . .It is boiled and drunk as a tea for an emetic. . .193. One of the nine herbs in a mixture for a poultice for snakebite; also used as a tea to cure dropsy. . .The fruit is eaten raw or cooked."

1949 Hobart & Melton Pharm 54. "Drastic purgatives. . .Jalap, Scammony, Podophyllin. . .their use is contraindicated in inflammatory, ulcerative, and haemorrhoidal conditions of the bowel, or for habitual constipation. . .a 25% solution of podophyllin suspension in oil by local application has been found useful against condylomata acuminata [venereal warts]."

1955 Mockle Quebec transl. 45. "The root is used as a purgative, cathartic, cholagogue. It is as well used as an antihydropic associated with cream of tartar, and for scrofulous conditions. rheumatism and syphillis; externally used as an epipastic. The resin, podophyllin is used as an antivenereal ointment. The root contains quercetol, 3-10% of resin or podophyllin which contains 40% of podophyllotoxine, a lactone whose composition is well known."

The roots of *Podophyllum peltatum* are collected in the autum from plants growing wild in Virginia, north Carolina, Kentucky, Indiana and Tennessee. They are washed, cut into lengths of about 10 cm and carefully dried. . .The roots contain two purgative substances as well as quercetin. Podophyllin is a gastro-intestinal irritant. In large doses it produces inflammation of the stomach and intestines, which has proved fatal. It is used to paint venereal warts (T.E. Wallis 1967).

1970 Bye IROQUOIS mss "Useful to the Iroquois, possibly cultivated by them as it was later by the white settlers. Iroquois ate and made a drink from the yellow fruit 'wild citron'. The root poisonous, may have been used for Iroquois suicides. When the root is cooked it is safer and used as a cathartic. . .The Iroquois used the leaves of this plant along with the flowers of the elder to make a corn medicine."

1974 Farnsworth Lynn Index 8 70. "Akaloids are absent from *Podophyllum*, which is unique in this family as containing cytotoxic and antitumor lignans."

May apple a potential new cash crop plant of eastern north America. The medicinal use of the plant as a purgative and anthelmintic was already known to the Indians before the white settlers arrived. Pohl & Paeschke considered that because of its low side effects Podophyllin extract should be given right after radiation treatment in cancer. May apple is collected in the wild, the supplies are bought up by the Abbott Laboratories in North Chicago where 300,000 lbs are needed yearly. It is desirable to cultivate may apples on a commercial scale. Little is known about growing them. It is difficult to germinate the seeds in Kentucky. In India *P. hexandrum* Royle (*P. emodi*) seeds need 2 or 3 winters to ripen. It has been found there that it is best to sow them with fruit pulp when ripe, they still requires 9 to 10 months dormancy. The northern boundary of natural growth area in north America is where the average January temperature does not fall below 20°F.; where the last freezing day in spring is about April 30th-May 10; where there is a frost free growing season of at least 150 days. Possibly may apple is conditioned to a winter rest period induced by coldness. The distribution is like that of *Quercus alba*. It might be argued that part of the area of may apple distribution in s. Canada was possibly brought about by man. In several reports from Canadian Herbaria it was mentioned that may apple occurs in the sites of old Indian villages. Whatever the Indians might have done with the plants they merely brought it to its natural limits (Meijer 1974).

1976 Trevor Robinson 268. "*Podophyllum peltatum*, podophyllin is a resinous extract used as a powerful cathartic. It is a complex mixture of lignins, the constituent podophyllotoxin is of interest, having partially napthalene nucleus. It has shown some promise in treatment of certain types of neoplasms." [Cancers.]

INDIAN CUCUMBER ROOT   *Medeola virginiana* L. Liliaceae

A white, crisp root the size of a little finger sends up a stem 14-45 cm high. At the top is a whorl of 5-11 leaves, their veins running parallel pointed at both ends 6-12 cm long and a fourth to a third as wide. At the spot where they all join the stem there will be some fine wool. Most plants will look like this. When they flower the flowering stem grows up from this whorl of leaves another 14-45 cm to produce another whorl of usually 3-5 leaves 3-6 cm long and often having a dark purple to red stain at their bases. Stalks 15-25 mm grow from this whorl bearing yellowish green flowers which are followed by dark purple berries.

Range. N.S. and Que. to n. L. Superior and Minn., s. to Va. and Mo., and in the mts. to Ga. and Ala; to Fla. and La. May-July in rich woods.

1708 Sarrazin-Vaillant, Quebec-Paris, Boivin transl. 206. "This is called *Jarnotte* in Canada. . .A Jesuit thought that one could make bread with its root."

1785 Cutler. "The roots, which are of a conic form, are excellent and of an agreeable taste. The Indians made them a part of their food."

1830 Rafinesque 242. "Root succulent, eaten by the Indians like cucumbers, good taste, when much is eaten acts as a diuretic and hydragogue, but not emetic as supposed by Schoepf."

1892 Millspaugh 175. "The Indian cucumber, has been used as a diuretic."

1895 Havard 114. "Indian cucumber. . .more medicinal than nutritious. Eaten by the Indians of the n. eastern states."

1955 Mockle Quebec transl. 28. "The root is diuretic and purgative. It is eaten by the Indians like cucumbers.

VIOLETS Violaceae

There are a great many varieties of violets in eastern north America. Some have their leaves and flowers, each on their own stalks, growing directly from the roots. Others have stems that bear both leaves and flowers. Most species produce normal flowers in the spring and cleistogamous flowers in the summer. Cleistogamous means self-fertilising; these flowers are permanently closed and without petals. The violets cross breed and their identification is often difficult. Here follows the general uses of violets both in the old world before and as the first white explorers and settlers arrived in America, and those uses that followed in America, where the variety of violet is not specified.

1475 Bjornsson Icelandic mss. transl. Larsen 135. "Viola is wet and cold in the first degree and is of three kinds. . .And they all have about one strength in leechdom. if one crushes it, that is good to apply to burns. If a man's head is heavy from meat or drink, then it is good to drink violets. If one has on his head a wreath of violets, it drives away vipers with its smell. . .If drunk with water, the root of violets crushed with myrrh and saffron is good to apply for eyes in which is great heat. Leaves of violet crushed with honey are good to rub upon boils of the head. . .If one drinks violets it is good for a hot stomach and dry. . .Oil of violets or roses is good for a cough and many kinds of disease. It is good to put in the ears which ring and ache. It is good for all kinds of heat in the head. . .If one crushes roots of violets with vinegar it is good to apply for swelling of the feet, cools sweetly the body and gives sleep. . .180. Oil which is made of violets or of the stems of violets or of the berries of violet which men in Norse call hof-gras, and rub a man over the liver, that takes away all the heat of the fever or other disease. But if the navel is rubbed, that speedily produces sweating."

1612 Capt. John Smith Virginia 92. "Many herbes in the spring time there are commonly dispersed throughout the woods, good for broths and sallets, as Violets, Purslin, Sorrell &c. Besides many we used whose names we know not."

1633 Gerarde-Johnson 852. "The floures are good for all inflammations especially of the sides and lungs; they take away the hoarsenesse of the chest, the ruggednesse of the winde-pipe and jaws, allay the extream heate of the liver, kidneys and bladder; mitigate the fierie heate of burning agues; temper the sharpness of choler, and take away thirst. There is an oyl made of Violet, which is likewise cold and moist.The same being annointed upon the testicles, doth gently provoke sleepe which is hindered by a hot and dry distemper: mixed or laboured together in a woodden dish with the yelke of an egge, it asswageth the pain of the fundament and hemorrhoides: it is likewise good to be put into cooling clisters, and into pultesses that coole and ease pain. . .The later Physitians do thinke it good to mix dry Violets with medicines that are to comfort and strengthen the heart."

1799 Lewis Mat. Med. 260. "The flowers officinal, syrup from infusion useful laxative for children. Seeds more purgative, sometimes emetic."

1820 Heckewelder 229. Indeed it is in the cure of external wounds that they particularly excel. . .I once for two days suffered the most excruciating pain from a felon or whitlow on one of my fingers, which deprived me entirely of sleep. I had recourse to an Indian woman who in less than half an hour relieved me entirely by the simple application of a poultice made of the root of the common blue violet.

1830 Rafinesque 275. "Prolific genus, we have nearly 40 native species. Properties more or less alike in all. Roots commonly mild emetic and cathartic, leaves emollient laxative, blossoms and seeds laxative, pectoral, &c. All the parts contain the *Violine*, a peculiar kind of Emetine. Flowers of the fragrant *V. odorata* cult. much used for a grateful tea and syrup, used for cough, sorethroat, constipation, often given to children. We have only two fragrant wild [species that are equivalent] *V. canadensis* and *blanda*, smell sweeter but fainter. Roots bitterish acrid, tonic in doses of 10 grains, purgative 25 to 30, emetic 40-50, also used as depurative in diseases of the skin. *V. tricolor, arvensis* and *calcarata* used in Europe, their leaves also purgative. We use chiefly *V. clandestina, rotundifolia, palmata, heterophylla*, sometimes called Healall. Leaves emollient, suppurative, used for wounds, and sores, bruised or in poultices. Elliot says that the negroes eat the leaves of the two last in soups.

1833 Howard Quebec mss. 107. "To cure the Stone take a teaspoonful of Violet seed morning and evening."

1841 Trousseau & Pidoux France transl. Homeopathic medicine uses violet flowers to allay inflammation. . .do not bleed, purge gently with violets. They are also emetic.

1842 Christison 944. "Take of fresh violet petals two pounds; boiling water five pints, infuse for twenty four hours; strain liquor through a fine cloth without expression; and then add 15 lbs of sugar to make a syrup,. . .violet is principally used as a test of alkalinity and acidity, being rendered green by alkalis and red by acids. It is sometimes also employed for imparting colour or fragrance to mixtures of other drugs. . .its syrup is laxative to children. . .the roots of this and other species of the genus *Viola*, they all contain a principle analogous in external character to the emeta of ipecacuan, and possessing, like that alkaloid, powerful emetic properties. (Boullay). It has not been particularly examined, but seems an alkaloid, and is termed Violina. This observation accounts for the emetic virtues long ascribed to the roots of various species of violet,—virtues so remarkable in the opinion of some, as to deserve more attention than the subject has hitherto received."

1892 Millspaugh 27. "Salicylic Acid. This acid, so far in its history, has been rarely extracted under its own form from plants. . .Mandelin. . .[after]careful analysis of *Viola tricolor*, reports. . .a proportion of from 0.43 per cent in cultivated plants to .107 per cent in var. *arvensis*. He finds it in all parts of the fresh plants and principally in the roots, stems and leaves. Violin,. . .was found in *V. odorata*. . .and *V. tricolor*. . .as well as in *Viola pedata*. . .A mixture of one part of the juice of this plant [V. *odorata*] with ten parts of water, will form a jelly like mass. . .This property has given various uses to *Viola* as an expectorant, emollient, and infusion for coughs and bronchial affections. . .The emetic effect of some of the violets, due to the presence of violin. . .The most characteristic symptom of its action is an offensive odor of the urine, like that of the cat. . .On the skin it causes burning, stinging and itching, followed by. . .eruptions."

1929 Brooks 529. "Diaphoretics were in very general use. . .such a practice is, as you know, very common with us and is especially used by many of the best French clinicians in the form of decoctions or infusions of violet flowers."

1931 Grieve England 839. "Of late years, preparations of fresh violet leaves have been used both internally and externally in the treatment of cancer, and though the British Pharmacopoeia does not uphold the treatment, it specifies how they are employed. From other sources it is stated that violet leaves have been used with benefit to allay the pain in cancerous growths, especially in the throat, which no other treatment relieved. . .An infusion of the leaves in boiling water (1 in 5) has been administered in dose of 1 to 2 fluid ounces. A syrup of the petals and a liquid extract of the fresh leaves are also used, the latter taken in teaspoonful doses, or rubbed in locally. The fresh leaves are also prepared as a compress for local application. . .A continuous daily supply of fresh leaves is necessary, and a considerable quantity is required."

1955 Mockle Quebec 50. "The flowers of different kinds of violets are used for coughs and the leaves for emollients. The roots are emetic and cathartic due to the presence of saponosides. There are numerous species in Canada; the most popular is without doubt the Field pansy (*V. tricolor* var *arvensis*)"

Viola odorata and *viola* sp. have been used for cancer from very early times in Europe. From 1901 to 1906 there were five different articles in British medical journals on the use of violets in cancer. The National Cancer Institute of the U.S. received many reports on the folk use of violets for cancer. One from Michigan in 1958 cites the use of a decoction of the flowers, plant and root as an 'old Indian cure for cancer.' (Hartwell 1971.)

The roots and seeds of the cultivated sweet violet, *V. odorata* can cause severe stomach upset, nervousness, trouble with breathing and the circulation of the blood that can be serious if a large dose has been taken. (Lewis and Elvin-Lewis 1977:35)

The roots of *V. odorata* are collected in the wild in Europe for the drug trade. They are used in cough syrup and for rheumatic diseases. (Stary and Jirasek 1973.)

1978 Globe and Mail 6th. Feb. "A five year Canada wide study under Dr. Henry Barnett, head of neurology at the University of Western Ontario, London, found that ASA (Acetosalicylic acid or aspirin) is effective, particularly among males, in preventing major strokes among patients who have already had little strokes. . .However no scientifically controlled studies have been done among apparently healthy people to see if taking ASA might reduce initial heart attacks.

The salicylic acid found in violets is an active disinfectant and tissue solvent rarely given by mouth. It is applied externally in ointments to soften hard skin, corns and warts, it is also fungicidal. ASA is thought to owe its ability to relieve pain to the acetyl group it contains. See willow and wintergreen.

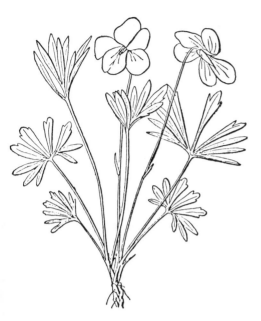

BIRD'S FOOT VIOLET

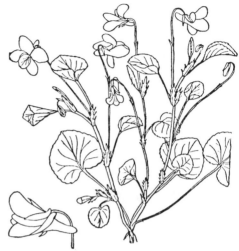

AMERICAN DOG VIOLET

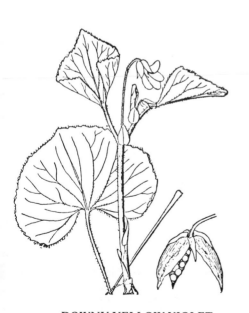

DOWNY YELLOW VIOLET

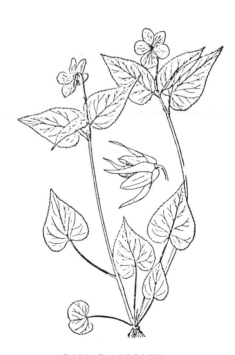

CANADA VIOLET

BIRD'S FOOT VIOLET
Viola pedata L. Violaceae

The smooth leaves on their own stalks are cut into many segments, often with a few teeth at their tips. The flowers also on their own stalks are 2-4 cm wide, dark violet with conspicuous orange stamens. There are no cleistogamous flowers. the seeds are copper colored.

Range. N.H., N.Y., s. Ont. Minn., Mich., Wisc. and Kans. s. to e. Tex. and Fla. in dry open places and woods.

Common names. Pansy violet, crowfoot violet, snake violet, velvets, horse violet.

1859-61 Gunn 878. "Both the herb and the root are used in medicine. Mucilaginous, alterative, diuretic, and slightly laxative. Used in infusion in affections of the lungs, coughs, consumption and the like, and in diseases of the kidneys and urinary organs, where a mucilaginous diuretic is needed. Said to be a powerful antisyphilitic remedy."

1868 Can. Pharm. J. 6; 83-5. The plant of blue violet, *V. pedata* included in the list of Can. medicinal plants.

AMERICAN DOG VIOLET
Viola conspersa Reichenb.

Many stems on a much branched root, smooth, up to 20 cm tall in full growth. Stem leaves 2-4 cm, the leaflets at the base of their stalks bristly toothed, usually over half their length. The flowers may begin to bloom when their stalks are only 1-2 cm tall. Their petals are light violet blue with darker veins. Seeds light brown.

Range. N.B., N.S., Que., Ont., s. Man. s. to Tenn., Ala. and Ga. in meadows, damp woods and low grounds.

1932 H. Smith OJIBWE 392. "The whole plant is used by the Flambeau Ojibwe to make a tea for heart trouble."

DOWNY YELLOW VIOLET
Viola pubescens Ait.

The soft hairy stems are 10-45 cm tall from a short stout root. There are 2-4 leaves near the top, 4-10 cm long and usually a little wider. There may be a stalked leaf growing from the root. The flower bearing stalks grow from the axils of the leaves near the top of the stem. The flowers are yellow with brown purple veins near their base. The seeds are pale brown.

Range. Me., Que., Ont., s. Man., s. to Nebr., Mo., Tenn. and Va. in rich deciduous woods.

1785 Cutler. Violets with yellow flowers. "It is said the Indians applied the bruised leaves of violets to boils and painful swellings for the purpose of easing the pain and producing suppuration."

1885 Hoffman OJIBWA 201. "A decoction is made of the roots, of which small doses are taken at intervals for sore throat.

1933 H. Smith POTAWATOMI 87. "Make a medicine from the root for treating various heart diseases."

CANADA VIOLET
Viola canadensis L.

Numerous stems, 20-40 cm tall, usualy smooth but may be finely hairy. Several leaves growing on their own stalks from the root. The stem leaves 5-10 cm. Single flowers on stalks growing from the axils of the upper leaves. The inner surface of the petals white above, bright yellow at the base, the outside more or less tinged with violet, the three lower petals striped with fine dark lines. The seeds brown.

Range. N.B., N.S., Que., Ont. to B.C., s. to Ariz., N. Mex., Tex., Tenn., Alas. and S.C. in woods, thickets, and rocky slopes.

Common names. Tall white violet, American sweet violet, hens.

1885 Hoffman OJIBWA 201. The decoction made of the root used for pains in the region of the bladder."

The common blue violet of the southern part of our range, *V. papilionacea*, its basal leaves when collected in the spring have been found to contain 264 mg of [Vitamin C] ascorbic acid per 100 grams of leaves in comparison to oranges which contain 50 mg per 100 grms of orange; and 20,000 mg per 100 grams of Vitamin A. in comparison to spinach which contains 8,100 mg per 100 grams of spinach. (Zennie and Ogzewalla 1977.)

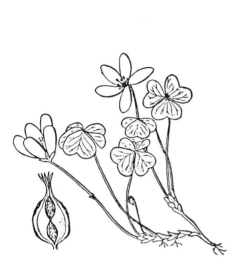

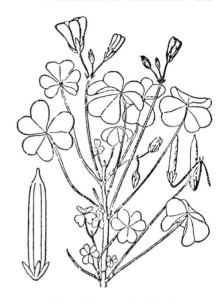

WOOD SORREL   YELLOW WOOD SORREL

WOOD SORREL   *Oxalis acetosella* L. Oxalidaceae
There are no stems on this small plant. The few clover like leaves grow on stalks from the scaly root. There are single, white veined with pink or purple, flowers on stalks 6-15 cm long.
Range. Nfld. and N.S. to Sask., N.Y. to Mich., Wisc., s. in mts. to N.C. and Tenn. May-July in cold damp woods.
Common names. White or true wood-sorrel, sleeping beauty, cuckoo flower, sour trefoil, hearts, shamrock.
1633 Gerarde-Johnson 1202. "Sorrell du Bois or wood Sorrell stamped and used for greene sauce, is good for them that have sicke and feeble stomackes; for it strengtheneth the stomacke, procureth appetite, and of all Sorrel sauces is the best, not only in vertue, but also in the pleas-antnesse of his taste. It is a remedie against putrified and stinking ulcers of the mouth, it quen-cheth thirst, and cooleth mightily an hot pestilentiall fever, especially being made in a syrup with sugar."
1612 Capt. John Smith Virginia 92. "Many hearbes in the spring time there are commonly dis-persed throughout the woods, good for brothes and sallets, as Violet, Purslin, Sorrell, &c. . .The [Indians] chiefe root they have for food. . .sliced and dried in the sun, mixed with sorrell and meale or such like."
1820's Mat. Med. Edinburgh-Toronto mss 79. "Refrigerants are medicine which diminish the circulation and reduce the heat of the body without occasioning any diminution of sensibility or nervous energy. . .*Oxalis Acetosella* infused in water has been used as a refrigerant or by boiling with milk & drinking when cool."
1830 Rafinesque 47-48. "Useful in decoction as a cooling drink in inflammatory disorders, fevers, piles, putrid diseases, &c. Boiled in milk they form a good acid whey, very cooling. They may also be eaten in sallad; they are peculiarly useful in diseases of the kidneys, bladder, and urethra, when they are inflamed and painful, acting as cooling diuretics. They are often substi-tuted to common sorrel and sheep sorrel; but they must not be eaten to excess, because they con-tain a violent poison, the oxalic acid. . .100 lbs of the leaves give only 30 lbs of juice and this only 10 ounces of the super oxalate of potash, which is sold and used by the wrong name of Salt of Lemons, for making a bad and dangerous imitation of lemonade and for taking off ink stains from linen, cloth and paper. A good conserve and syrup of oxalis leaves [can be] made, which are pleasant medical preparations; they are now, however, superseded by currant jelly and other preparations of acid fruits."

1842 Christison 2. "The leaves have a pleasant acid taste, strongest in spring, weaker and united with some bitterness in autumn. Their acidity is impaired by drying and keeping them. It depends on binoxalate of potash, which may be extracted from them to the amount of two ounces and a quarter of pure salt, and rather more of an impure crystalline mass, from twenty pounds. . .In the form of infusion wood-sorrel leaves are still used in domestic practice, and were once in request in regular practice also, as a refrigerant drink in fever, and an antiscorbutic in scurvy. They are now little employed, and in this part of the kingdom never. [England] The plant is a needless article of the Materia Medica."

1859-61 Gunn 860. "There are several varieties of sorrel. . .The properties of each are about the same—being refrigerant or cooling, diuretic, and antiseptic. To be used in infusion, or the fresh leaves bruised and macerated in cold water to make a pleasant acid drink, like lemonade; or the leaves may be eaten. It should not be taken in too great a quantity, however, on account of the Oxalic acid it contains. It is good as a cooling article in fevers, and as a diuretic and antiseptic in chronic affections of the urinary organs, and in scurvy. Sorrel is mostly celebrated, however, as a remedy for cancer, to be used in the form of a plaster made by expressing the juice of the green herb, and evaporating it in the sun till of proper consistence, and then applying it to the cancer, renewing it once or twice a day. It is sometimes mixed with the juice of red clover leaves and heads, and may be thickened with the ashes of white oak bark, or any other article desired. It was long kept a secret, as a great cancer remedy, and has been known to cure numerous cancers of the female breast, as well as other kinds."

1868 Can. Pharm. J. 6; 83-5. The herb wood sorrel, *Oxalis Acetosella*, included in list of Can. medicinal plants.

1928 Parker SENECA 12. Treat cancer with a salve made by boiling sheep sorrel (oxalis) in bear grease.

1933 H. Smith POTAWATOMI 68. "The Forest Potawatomi do not use this as a medicine but rather as a food. . .cooked and sugar added to make a desert which they eat with considerable relish."

1931 Grieve (England) 752. "The juice of the leaves turns red when clarified and makes a fine, clear syrup. . .The juice used as a gargle is a remedy for ulcers in the mouth, and is good to heal wounds and to staunch bleeding. Sponges and linen clothes saturated with the juice and applied, were held to be effective in the reduction of swellings and inflammation. An excellent conserve, *Conserva Ligulae*, used to be made by beating the fresh leaves up with three times their weight of sugar and orange peel, and this was the basis of the cooling and acid drink that was long a favourite remedy in malignant fevers and scurvy. . .Salts of Lemon, as well as Oxalic acid can be obtained from the plant: 20 lbs of fresh herb yield about 6 lb of juice, from which by crystallization, between 2 and 3 oz of Salts of Lemon can be obtained."

1955 Mockle Quebec transl. 52. "The leaves refreshing, antiscorbutic and diuretic."

1972 Assiniwi 99. "Wood sorrel has a delicate flavor, and is good for satisfying your thirst in the woods. It is a tasty seasoning for beaver, muskrat or porcupine meat. It is also good in salads, with watercress and wild onions. . .The Algonquin Indians consider it an aphrodisiac."

In Europe involuntary emmision of semen has long been treated by a tea of the seeds. (Lewis and Elvin-Lewis 1977:326)

YELLOW WOOD SORREL   *Oxalis stricta* L. Oxalidaceae (*O. corniculata*)

The slender stem to 50 cm is covered with blunt tipped hairs. The clover like leaflets are 1-2 cm wide usually smooth with an edging of hairs. There are 2-7 flowers on each stem, the petals yellow 4-9 mm followed by seeds pods 8-15 mm long.

Range. Nearly cosmopolitan weed, often in natural habitats as well, probably originally native to N.Am.

Common names. Sour grass, sheep or poison sorrel, toad sorrel.

1785 Cutler. "Dr. Withering says, the expressed juice depurated, properly corporated, and set in a cool place, affords a crystalline salt in considerable quantity, which may be used whenever vegetable acids are wanted. The London College directs a conserve to be made with the leaves beaten with thrice their weight of fine sugar."

1894 Household Guide Toronto 157. "The following treatment has completely cured several persons of cancer, and is vouched for; Take sheep-sorrel, the variety with yellow flowers, bruise the whole, stalks, flower and all, and press out the juice. Boil it down to one half and bottle.

Apply with a quill three or four times a day. Wash the sore with castile soap between applications. Drink red clover blossom tea."

1916 Waugh IROQUOIS 118. Other plants are said to have been eaten raw, in some cases with salt. These include. . .Oxalis, *Oxalis corniculata*, the sour plant.

1928 H. Smith MESKWAKI 271. "*Oxalis stricta* The common sorrel was often eaten by the Meskwaki for its acidity. In former times, the whole plant was boiled to obtain an orange dye."

1955 Mockle Quebec transl. 52. "The leaves refreshing, antiscorbutic and diuretic."

There are records of the use of wood sorrels for the treatment of cancer by folk medicine from Europe, Asia and North America. (Hartwell 1970).

See under Dry, Open places for Sheep sorrel a *Rumex*.

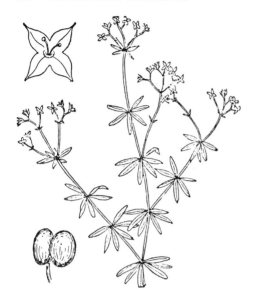

SHINING BEDSTRAW

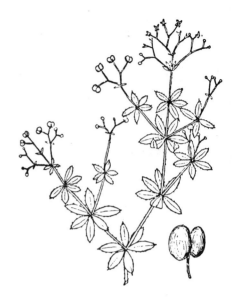

ROUGH BEDSTRAW

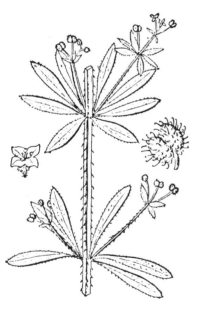

CLEAVERS

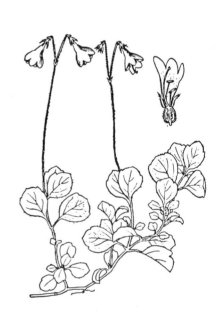

TWINFLOWER

SHINING BEDSTRAW   *Galium concinnum* T.&.G. Rubiaceae
Shining and smooth, branched, leaves in 6's or those on the branches in 4's, 1-2 cm long their
edges with backward turned hooks. Flowers with four tiny white petals, the fruit smooth 2 mm.
Range. N.J. to Minn. and Kan. se to Tenn. and Ark. in dry woods.

ROUGH BEDSTRAW *Gàlium asprellum* Michx.
Many branching stem; hooked on the angles, up to 200 cm long. Leaves in sixes on the main stem or in fours or fives on the branches, hooked on their edges with sharp pointed tips, 20 x 6 mm long. The fruit smooth, 2 mm long.
Range. Nfld. to Minn. s. to N.C. and Mo., wet woods and thickets June-Aug.

CLEAVERS *Galium aparine* L.
Weak stems, square with hooks on the angles that enable cleavers to clamber over other plants. The leaves are 8 together around the stem (occasionally 6) narrow and with only one nerve, 1-8 cm long, rough on the edges and on the veins beneath. Flowers tiny, followed by fruit that is usally 2-4 mm long covered with short hooked bristles.
Range. Circumpolar and found in most of temperate N. Am. May-Sept in damp ground.
Common names. Goose-grass, scratch weed, loveman, sweathearts, poor robin.
1070-1320 Juntunen site Mich. Yarnell 1964:35. Seeds of Cleavers (*Galium* sp) found in seven different locations at this site.
1500 Yarnell, Parmalee, Paul, & Munson, 1970. Subsistence ecology of Scovil, a terminal middle woodland village in west central Ill. Cleaver seeds found, no evidence of corn, garden beans, sunflower or tobacco.
1633 Gerarde-Johnson 1123. "The juice which is pressed out of the seeds, stalks, and leaves, as Dioscorides writeth, is a remedie for them that are bitten by the poisonous spiders. . .and of vipers if it be drunke with wine. And the herbe stamped with swines grease wasteth away the kernels by the throte. Pliny teacheth that the leaves being applied do also stay the aboundance of bloud issuing out of wounds. Women do usually make pottage of Clevers with a little mutton and Otemeale, to cause lanknesse, and keep them from fatnesse."
1833 Howard Quebec mss 14. To cure a Cancer in the Breasts. Drink twice a day a quarter of a pint of the juice of Cleavers or goose grasse, and cover the bleeding around with the bruised leaves."
1830 Rafinesque 120. "The *G. verum* and also *G. aparine* are ancient medical plants; the whole plants are used. . .Although neglected lately by medical writers, because apparently inert; they are by no means so. The taste is bitterish and acid. . .Externally applied in poultice, it is a good discutient for indolent tumors, strumous swellings and tumors of the breast. Internally used in decoction sweetened with honey, for suppression of urine and gravelly complaints, in scurvy, dropsy, hysterics, epilepsy, gout &c. There are instances on record of having cured these diseases. Useful also in bleeding of the nose and stomach. Lately found peculiarly beneficial in scorbutic, scofulous, and dropiscal complaints, acting mildly, but effectually."
1859-61 Gunn 776. "Cleavers is regarded as a most valuable cooling diuretic, useful in most diseases of the urinary organs. In suppression or retention of urine, it is a most admirable remedy: also in inflammation of the kidneys, inflammation of the bladder, scalding of urine, as in gonorrhea, it is one of our best remedies. It is also said to be a solvent of stone in the bladder, and a most admirable remedy in all cases of gravel. The whole herb is used. It yields its virtues readily to warm or cold water, and is always to be used in infusion, and may be drank freely. Cleavers must never be boiled or scalded, as that will destroy its properties. An ounce of the dry herb may be infused for two hours in a pint of warm water. . .An infusion of equal parts of Cleavers and Elder blossoms is a good drink in scarlet fever, small pox, and eruptive diseases; and it is said that a cold infusion of the Cleavers drank three times a day, and the parts washed with the same, will remove freckles from the skin, if continued for two or three months."
1868 Can. Pharm. J. 6; 83-5 Cleavers, *Galium aparine*, the whole plant included in list of Can. medicinal plants.
1915 Speck PENOBSCOT 311. The following concoction was obtained in confidence from an old Indian healer who claimed to have used it effectively a number of times. The cure is for gonorrhea primarily, although he used it for kidney trouble and for spitting up blood, but he could not explain how the two were connected. Cleavers vine (*Galium aparine*) is mixed with six other plants. A small quantity of each is steeped in water and about half a cupful drunk three times a day in a quart of water. It is further claimed to be an excellent tonic by the possessor.
1919 Sturtevant 285. "The seeds form one of the best substitutes for coffee. . .The dried plant is sometimes used as a tea." [Galium is in the same botanical family as coffee.]

1925 Wood & Ruddock. It has recently been successfully used in treating children for bed wetting. Drink three times a day, 3 oz. of herb in 2 pints of water, steeped for 3 or 4 hours.

1928 H. Smith MESKWAKI 243. *G. Aparine*, Specimen 5066 of the Dr. Jones collection is the whole plant of this species. . .It is boiled and drunk as an emetic. . .244. The whole plant of *G. concinnum* is brewed to make a tea for bladder and kidney trouble. The tea is also used to cure the ague. McIntosh cited the case of John Jensen, who had been very sick but was well and seen working on the section that very day.

1932 H. Smith OJIBWE 386. "The whole plant [*G. aparine*] is used by the Flambeau Ojibwe to make a tea used as a diuretic, in kidney trouble, gravel, stoppage of urine, and allied ailments. Other species are used in much the same way for the same purposes."

1955 Mockle Quebec transl. 83. *G. Aparine*. "Used as an astringent, antiscorbutic, diuretic. Herissey has isolated a glucoside, asperuloside from it. . .84. *G. asprellum*. Popular remedy for kidney trouble."

Cleavers has been used since the time of the Greeks in Europe as a domestic remedy for cancers, particularly in Germany. In the United States it was used for this purpose in the nineteenth century. (Hartwell 1971:147-8).

See Wet Open Places for other bedstraws.

TWINFLOWER   *Linnaea borealis* L. var. *americana* (Forbes) Rehd. Caprifoliaceae
The slender root creeps along the floor of the woods sending up hairy stems to 10 cm tall. The short hairy stalked leaves are 1-2 cm long with a few teeth at their ends. The flowering stems are up to 10 cm long with two nodding white to pink flowers at the top, each on its own stalk. The berries are brown.

Range. Circumboreal s. in Am. to N.J., W.Va., n. Ind., Minn. and Calif. in moist or dry woods and cold swamps. June-July.

Common names. Deer vine, ground vine, twin sisters.

1830 Rafinesque 239. "Bitterish, subastringent, diuretic, *eq.* of *Arbutus*, used also for rheumatism and disorders of the skin."

1888 Delamare Island of Miquelon transl. 21. "Stem and leaves bitter, sudorific and diuretic according to Provencher(?)."

1915 Speck MONTAGNAIS 314. "A mash made of the plant of *Linnaea borealis americana* will cure inflammation of the limbs."

1923 H. Smith MENOMINI 27. "The leaves of this plant are steeped to make a tea to cure insomnia."

1933 H. Smith POTAWATOMI 45. "Mrs. Spoon used the entire plant of this as a squaw medicine, although just what type of female trouble it was supposed to cure was not plainly explained."

1955 Mockle Quebec transl. 84. "The stems and leaves diuretic and antipyretic."

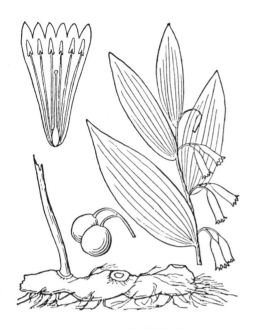

SOLOMON'S SEAL

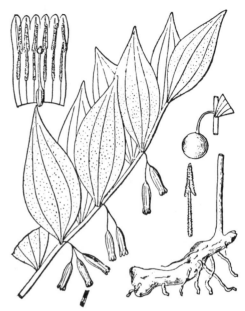

HAIRY SOLOMON'S SEAL

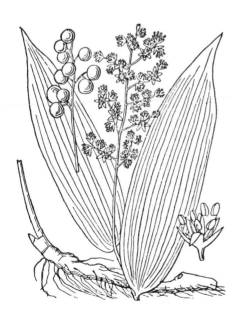

FALSE SOLOMON'S SEAL

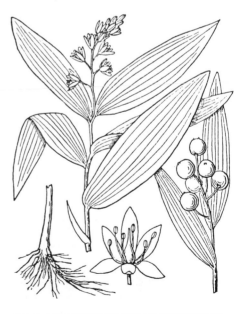

STAR FLOWERED SOLOMON'S SEAL

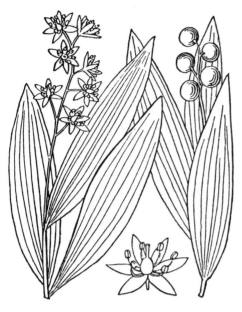

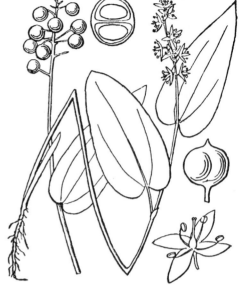

THREE LEAVED SOLOMON'S SEAL   WILD LILY OF THE VALLEY

SOLOMON'S SEAL   *Polygonatum biflorum* (Walt.) Ell. Liliaceae
From a stout, whitish, scarred root grows a 40-120 cm tall, straight or bending stem. The 5-15 x
1-8 cm leaves are smooth, paler beneath, with 1-19 prominent veins and nearly always clasp the
stem. Under the leaves where they join the stem hang, in pairs, the slender stalks that carry white
to yellow flowers and later the dark blue berries.
Range. Mass. s. N.H., N.Y., Conn., sw. Que. s. Ont. to s. Man. s. to n. Mex., Tex. and Fla. in
woods, on stream banks, May-July.
Common names. Sealwort, smooth solomon's seal.

HAIRY SOLOMON'S SEAL   *Polygonatum pubescens* (Willd.) Pursh.
The 50-90 cm stem has 4-12 x 1-6 cm stalked leaves, narrowed at both ends, that are hairy on the
veins beneath. There are 3-9 prominent veins. The flowers are yellowish green and the berries
blue.
Range. N.S. to se Man., s. to Pa., Ind. and Minn. and in the mts. to n. Ga. May-July in moist
woods.
Common names. Conquer-john, dwarf solomon's seal.
All the sources cited below apply equally to both the smooth and the hairy true solomon's seals.
1633 Gerarde-Johnson 906. "The root of Solomons seal stamped while it is fresh and greene, and
applied, taketh away in one night, or two at the most, any bruise, black or blew spots gotten by
falls or womens wilfulnesse, in stumbling upon their hasty husbands fists, or such like. . .Note
what experience hath found out, and of late days, especially among the vulgar sort of people in
Hampshire. . .if any of what sex or age soever chance to have any bones broken, in what part of
their bodies soever; their refuge is to stampe the roots hereof, and give it unto the patient in ale
to drink; which sodoreth and glues together the bones in very short space. . .Moreover, the said
people do give it in like manner unto their cattell, if they chance to have any bones broken, with
good success; which they do stampe and apply outwardly in manner of a pultesse, as well unto
themselves as their cattell. The root stamped and applied in manner of a pultesse, and layd upon
members that have been out of joynt, and newly restored to their places, driveth away the paine,
and knitteth the joynt very firmely, and taketh away the inflammation, if there chance to be
any. . .common experience teacheth, that in the world there is not to be found another herbe

comparable to it for the purposes aforesaid. . .The water drawn out of the roots, wherewith the women of Italy use to scoure their faces from sunne-burning, freckles, morphew, or any such deformities of the skinne. . .905. There is kept in our gardens, and said to be brought from some part of America another *Polygonatum*, which sends up a stalk some foot or more high. . .bearing at the very top thereof, above the highest leaf, upon little foot-stalks, some eight or nine little white floures, consisting of six leaves apiece, which are succeeded by berries." [probably *Smilacina stellata*.]

1687 Clayton Virginia Indians. 17. "There are likewise many others which bear some analogy to the European plants, such as *Solomons Seal, Wood Sage*, much better I think than the English, which the Indians use much for infusions, and which they take as we do diet drinks."

1778 Carver 514. "It is greatly valued on account of its being a fine purifier of the blood."

1785 Cutler. Sweet smelling solomon's seal. . .The young shoots may be eaten as asparagus. The roots are nutritious and are used in diet drinks.

1791 Lewis ed. Aitkin 367. The roots are recommended externally as refrigerants; and internally as. . .mild corroborants. Cullen in his Mat. Med. says they have been used with success in haemorrhages.

1830 Rafinesque 85. [Discussing the different solomon's seals.] "The roots of those plants are chiefly used. . .Their smell is vapid, the taste rather mucilaginous and sweetish; they contain gum, sugar, mucilage and fecula. Their properties are so mild that they can be eaten, particularly when dry or cooked. In Sweden a flour and good bread is made with them. Our Indians collected them as an article of food. . .Schoepf says that the bruised root is employed for. . .sore eyes. They are also useful in poultice, for piles, wounds, and inflammations of the skin. A vinous infusion of them with Comfrey roots is useful as a restringent in fluor albus, leucorrhea and immoderate flow of menses. The powdered roots purify the blood; their extract has been used by Dr. Arnold for coughs and pains in the breast. They appear to be equivalent of *Ulmus fulva* [*U. rubra*], slippery elm and may perhaps be used in bowel complaints."

1859-61 Gunn 860. "A mucilaginous tonic, mildly astringent, and very healing and restorative. Very useful in female weakness and diseases, as in leucorrhea or whites, and excessive and painful menstruation. Also good in affections of the lungs, in irritable conditions of the stomach and bowels, in piles, and in general debility. Used freely in decoction; also in the form of a sirup or cordial. It is said that in erysipelas, and in poison from the poison vine [poison ivy] as well as in other skin diseases, a decoction of the root drank freely, and the parts bathed with the same will soon effect a cure. . .There is another variety with speckled berries (*Smilacina racemos* false solomon's seal). . .both varieties are the same in medical properties."

1885 Mooney CHEROKEE 327. "Root heated and bruised and applied as a poultice to remove an ulcerating swelling called tusti, resembling a boil or carbuncle. The U.S. Dispensatory 1877 says that this species acts like *P. uniflorum* which is said to be emetic. In former times it was used externally in bruises, especially those about the eyes, in tumors, wounds, and cutaneaous eruptions and was highly esteemed as a cosmetic. At present it is not employed though recommended by Hermann as a good remedy in gout and rheumatism. This species in decoction has been found to produce 'nausea, a cathartic effect and either diaphoresis or diuresis' and is useful 'as an internal remedy in piles, and externally in the form of a decoction, in the affections of the skin resulting from the poisonous exhalations of certain plants'."

1916 Waugh IROQUOIS 119. "The roots of. . .Solomon's seal. . .are referred to as having been used as food in the Iroquois area, but have been practically forgotten by present day Iroquois."

1926-27 Densmore CHIPPEWA 336. A decoction was made of the roots of solomon's seal and sprinkled on hot stones and the steam inhaled for a headache.

1923 H. Smith MENOMINI 41. "The root is dried and pulverized. Then it is mixed with cedar (the twigs and leaves) and burned as a smudge to revive one who has become unconscious. If they suppose the patient is about to die, then smoke of this smudge is blown into his nostrils to bring him back to life." Used as a reviver of consciousness by the Meskwaki also.

1932 H. Smith OJIBWE 374. "The Pillager Ojibwe use the root as a physic and it is also cooked to yield a tea to treat a cough."

1931 Grieve England 750. "The flowers and roots are used as snuff celebrated for their power of inducing sneezing and thereby relieving head affections. They also have a wide vogue as aphrodisiacs, for love philtres and potions. The properties of these roots have not been very fully investigated. . .The berries are stated to excite vomiting, and even the leaves nausea, if chewed."

1955 Mockle Quebec transl. 29. "The root is used as a vulnerary and astringent; reduced to pulp

it is applied on bruises, contusions, boils, etc. The berries and the roots are emetic."
1970 Bye IROQUOIS mss. Rootstock used as food, raw or cooked or as flour.

FALSE SOLOMON'S SEAL — *Smilacina racemosa* (L.) Desf. Liliaceae (*Convallaria r.*)

FALSE SOLOMON'S SEAL   *Smilacina racemosa* (L.) Desf. Liliaceae (*Convallaria r.*)
From a rather thick fleshy root a usually twisted stem, 40-60 cm tall bears alternate leaves, narrowed at both ends, 7-15 x 2-7 cm, finely hairy beneath, with very short stalks or none. The feathery flowers are on 3-5 mm long stalks on stems growing alternately from the end of the main stem. They do *not* grow directly from the main stem as they do in the star flowered solomon's seal. There are about nine of these flowering stalks and each one bears several flowers. These have six white petals and are followed by berries, first white then turning red speckled with purple.
Range. N.S. through n. Ont. to B.C., s. to Ga. and Ariz. May-June in rich woods and in the open.
Common names. Wild or false spikenard, small or zigzag solomon's seal.

STAR FLOWERED SOLOMON'S SEAL   *Smilacina stellata* (L.) Desf.
Very like false solomon's seal but usually shorter. The clear difference is the flowers, which are on a short stalk growing directly from the main stem. See illustration. The flowers are larger, 8-10 mm across. The berries are at first green with blackish stripes becoming dark red or black.
Range. Lab. Nfld., N.B., P.E.I., N.S., Que., James Bay, northernmost Ont. to Yukon and s. Alaska, s. to Calif., N. Mex., Ohio and Va. in thickets, meadows, or gravelly shores. Grown in Gerarde's garden, London England in 1597.

THREE LEAVED SOLOMON'S SEAL   *Smilacina trifolia* (L.) Desf.
A slender erect 10-40 cm stem with usually 3 but maybe 2-4 leaves 6-12 x 1-4 cm pointed at both ends, without hairs. The 3-8 flowers are spaced up the end of the stem. They have 6 petals each and are 8 mm wide. The berries are dark red and not recommended for eating.
Range. Lab., Nfld., N.B., P.E.I., N.S., Que., northernmost Ont. to southernmost Yukon, s. to Alta., Minn., n. Ill., Pa. and N.J. in bogs, mossy woods, and peaty shores.
This plant is very like false or wild lily of the valley, *Maianthemum canadense* below. Three leaved solomon's seal is found in wet places, has few flowers and berries which are spaced far apart. It has a wider flower with six petals. All sources cited below refer to *Smilacina racemosa*, false solomon's seal, unless one of the other plants is named. Rafinesque, Gunn and the Indians used the true and the false solomon's seal indiscriminately, regarding the properties of both as being the same, and probably used some of the other plants discussed in this section in the same way also.
1672 Josselyn 87 note. "Treacle berries having the perfect taste of treacle, when they are ripe—and will keep good for a long while. Certainly a very wholesome berry and medicinal."
1830 Rafinesque 85. "The berries are cephalic and cardiacal."
1868 Can. Pharm. J. 6; 83-5 The root of Solomon's seal, *Convallaria racemosa* included in list of Can. medicinal plants.
1885 Hoffman OJIBWA 199. "Indian name snake weed or snake vine, a warm decoction of the leaves used by lying in women. The roots are placed upon a red-hot stone, the patient with a blanket thrown over his head, inhaling the fumes, to relieve a headache. The fresh leaves are crushed and applied to cuts to stop bleeding."
1915 Speck-Tantaquidgeon MOHEGAN 318. "The leaves steeped to make a cough medicine. The root is steeped for a medicine to strengthen the stomach."
1925 Anderson 145. "*Smilacina racemosa* root in conjunction with the roots of *Epilobium angustifolium* (fireweed) were used by the French Canadians for scrofulous cases. The roots were dried, broken up and mixed together with some water, became mucilaginous and were put on sores."
1926-27 Densmore CHIPPEWA 356. The root is steeped and the decoction drunk for pain in the back and female weakness.
1923 H. Smith MENOMINI 41. "The root is ground up and soaked to furnish a liquid that is put on a hot stove. The fumes that arise are inhaled by a person who is suffering from catarrh."
1928 H. Smith MESKWAKI 230. "The smudge of this is used to hush a crying child. It is also used as a smudge in severe illness. Cover the head with a shawl and smoke the patient for five minutes, then he will revive and talk to you. . .the root is burned and smudged for one who has had a fit or for insanity. . .Specimen 3624 of the Dr. Jones collection is the stem-base of

Smilacina racemosa referred in his notes to *Acorus calamus* [sweet flag]. . .This is said to be the conjurer's root, used in the meetings of the medicine society when the medicine man wants to perform tricks, or cast spells. Specimen 3665 of the Dr. Jones collection consists of the root of *Smilacina racemosa* and the wood of *Fraxinus nigra* [black ash] and. . .is used to loosen the bowels. Specimen 5147. . .is the root. . .alone. . .It was put into the cooking kettle during the time of plague to prevent sickness. It was also put into the food that was fed to hogs to prevent hog cholera. The white man has used it in the same manner as his drugs containing convallarin, that is, as a substitute for digitalis. It is less powerful and was thought more efficient in treating dropsy. It strengthens the contractions of the heart muscle, reduces the number of heart beats, increases blood pressure, stimulates respiration, and frequently increases the appetite and digestion. . .Solomon's Seal, *Polygonatum biflorum*, has also been used by the white man as a substitute for digitalis, though it is much less powerful. As it augments the flow of urine, it was formerly used for dropsy."

1932 H. Smith OJIBWE 374. "The Flambeau Ojibwe use this root in combination with that of the dogbane (*Apocynum androsaemifolium*) to keep the kidneys open during pregnancy, to cure sore throat and headache. It is also used as a reviver. . .407. They also prepare and eat the root. It is soaked in lye water and parboiled to get rid of the lye, then cooked like potatoes. The Pillager Ojibwe use this root added to oats to make a pony grow fat."

1933 H. Smith POTAWATOMI 63. "The Prairie Potawatomi stated that they sometimes ate the berries as a food but the Forest Potawatomi knew nothing about this practice. The smoke or smudge from the burning root, placed upon a pan of live coals, was used to revive a patient who had sunk into a coma. It was fanned toward the nostrils and a paper cone was placed over the nose to make sure that the fumes reached them."

1947 Marker 69:2242. *Smilacina racemosa* contains sitosterol.

1954 De Lazlo and Henshaw Science 3097. The root infusion of star flowered solomon's seal, *S. stellata*, was used by the Nevada Indians to regulate menstrual disorders. Conception was prevented by drinking half a cup of the leaf tea daily for one week.

1962 Montgomery 17. "The red berries are conspicuous in the fall, tasteless or slightly bitter and should not be eaten in quantity since they are cathartic."

1966 Campbell, Best & Budd 70. "Star Flowered Solomon's seal, its occurrence is more common in moist meadows and around groves of trees. . .very little is known of the usefulness of this plant except that it is grazed readily by all classes of livestock. Its early spring growth is particularly attractive to sheep and cattle, and even dry leaves of this plant are eaten by sheep."

WILD LILY OF THE VALLEY   *Maianthemum canadense* Desf. Liliaceae (*Smilacina c.*)
One of the commonest plants, often carpeting large parts of the woods. Most of the plants will consist of a stem 5-20 cm tall and one or two leaves, broad at the stem end 3-10 cm long, sometimes clasping the stem, sometimes with short stalks. There may be 1-4 leaves. The flowers have four white petals are 4-6 mm wide and are crowded together up the tip of the stem. They are followed by berries that may be white, or pale red or mottled.

Range. Lab. and Nfld. to Mack. to B.C., s. to Iowa, Tenn. and Ga. Probably occurs in each Province of Canada north to the north limits of black and white spruce. It is hard to distinguish from three leaved solomon's Seal until you have held both plants in your hand. If in flower it is easy, wild lily of the valley has four petals, the three leaved solomon's seal has six; its leaves are pointed at both ends, whereas those of wild lily of the valley are wide at the stem end.

1915 Speck MONTAGNAIS 314. "A tea of this plant is drunk for headache."

1932 H. Smith OJIBWE 373. "The Flambeau Ojibwe recognise that this [plant] is somewhat different from Spikenard (*Smilacena racemosa*) but give it the same name and uses, namely to keep the kidneys open during pregnancy, to cure sore throat and headaches. It is also used to make smoke for inhaling. The Pillager Ojibwe do not know or use it."

1933 H. Smith POTAWATOMI 62. "The Forest Potawatomi use the root of this plant to make a medicine for curing sore throat. Among the whites the root has been used for its stimulant properties for diseases of the head, to produce sneezing, as an expectorant and for its mucilaginous properties. . .105. The Forest Potawatomi insist that they eat the berries. . .but just how they are prepared as a food was not discovered. Certainly the berries as they come from the plant would hardly be considered esculent by the whites."

1962 Montgomery 19. "Berries not recommended for eating."

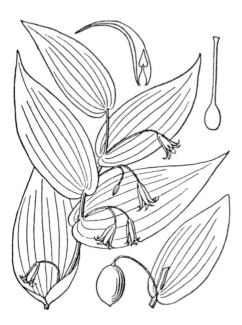

LIVERBERRY

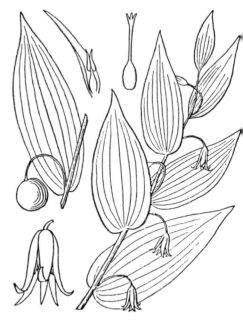

TWISTED STALK

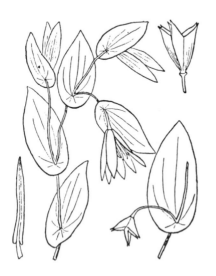

WILD OAT

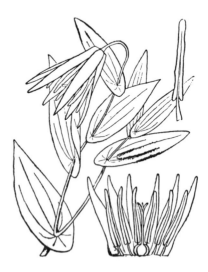

BELLWORT

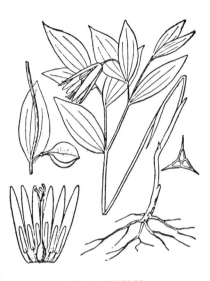

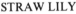

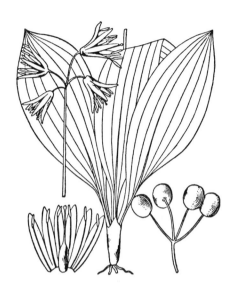

STRAW LILY   YELLOW CLINTONIA

LIVERBERRY   *Streptopus amplexifolius* (L.) DC Liliaceae
A smooth twisted 40-100 cm stem, branching, with leaves clasping around the stem at one end
and pointed at the other, the main ones 6-12 x 2-5.5 cm. From where they join the stem the long
slender bent stalks hang, holding the greenish white to purplish flowers 15 mm long. Followed by
red berries.
Range. Circumboreal, in Am. s. to Mass., N.Y., Mich., Wis., and Minn. and in the mts. to N.C.
and Ariz. June-July in rich woods.
Common names. Clasping leaved twisted stalk.
1915 Speck PENOBSCOT 311. A mixture of eight herbs, one of which was identified by Speck as
Streptopus amplexifolius, but called solomon's seal by the Penobscot, was steeped and drunk as a
cure for gonorrhea primarily, although the old Indian healer who gave Speck the recipe used it
also for kidney trouble and for spitting of blood.
1915 Speck MONTAGNAIS 314. "For sickness in general the berries and stems of Solomon's
seal (*Streptopus amplexifolius*) are steeped and taken. Snakes are thought to eat the berries and
roots of this plant."

TWISTED STALK   *Streptopus roseus* Michx. var. *perspectus* Fassett
The hairy stem 30-80 cm tall has stalkless leaves, pointed at one end and rounded to where they
join but do not clasp the stem. The main ones are 5-9 x 2-3.5 cm with finely hairy edges. A single
rose colored flower 1 cm long hangs from a hairy stalk growing from the leaf axil. The berries are
red.
Range. se Lab., Nfld., N.B., P.E.I., N.S., Que., Ont., Man., s. to Minn., Mich., Pa., N.J. and in the
mts. of N.C. in moist woods and thickets.
Common names. Sessile leaved twisted stalk.
1915 Speck MONTAGNAIS 314. "The blossoms of the plant are steeped to make a medicine to
produce a sweat."
1926-27 Densmore CHIPPEWA 360. The steeped root was used as a poultice for a stye on the
eye.

1932 H. Smith OJIBWE 374. "This plant is called by the same Indian name as *Polygonatum biflorum* among the Pillager Ojibwe, but this particular one is always referred to as the squaw, while *Polygonatum* [see Solomon's seal] has always been called the man. It is used as a physic or to make a tea for a cough."

1933 H. Smith POTAWATOMI 63. "Mrs. Spoon. . .used the root to make a cough syrup or tea."

WILD OAT   *Uvularia perfoliata* L. Liliaceae

The 20-40 cm stem forks near the top, bearing 2-4 leaves below the fork. The stem goes through the leaf. These are smooth up to 9 cm long. The flowers are pale yellow, 17-25 mm long. There are three angled capsules holding the seeds, no berries. RARE IN CANADA ENDANGERED IN NEW HAMPSHIRE EXTREMELY RARE IN NEW YORK.

Range. Vt., Mass., s. Ont., s. Man., s. to La. and nw. Fla., in rich woods and thickets.

BELLWORT   *Uvularia grandiflora* Sm.

The smooth 20-50 cm branching stem goes through the leaves. These are up to 12 cm long, minutely hairy beneath. There are yellow flowers 2.5-5 cm long, hanging on stalks growing from where the leaves join the stem. No berries.

Range. Me., s. Que., s. Ont., s. to Okla., Ark., Ala., and Ga. April-May in rich woods.

STRAW LILY   *Uvularia sessilifolia* L.

The leaves are attached directly to the 10-30 cm tall stem. The straw colored flowers are 12-25 mm long followed by three angled capsules.

Range. N.B., N.S., s. Que., s. Ont., s. Man., s. to Ark., Ala. and Ga. in rich woods, April-May.

1708 Sarrazin-Vaillant, Quebec-Paris, Boivin 1978 transl. 139. "The roots are used in Canada for hernia. It is said the remedy came from the Savages." *U. perfoliata*

1830 Rafinesque 272. "All sp. eq. although *U. perfoliata* and *grandiflora* mostly used. Root subacid when fresh, with a fine mucilage. Eq. to Cypripedium as a nervine, but much less efficient. When chewed and the saliva swallowed, it cures sorethroat. Said to equal *Hieracium nervosum* [*venosum*?] in bites of rattlesnakes. Useful in wounds and sores. Decoction of the plant in sore mouth, inflamed larynx and gums. Shoots edible like Asparagus, roots edible when dry and cooked. . .85. Schoepf says that one species (more probably *Uvularia grandiflora*) is employed in Pennsylvania against the bites of rattle snakes."

1923 H. Smith MENOMINI 41. "The Menomini name for this unknown to my informant, who, however, knew that it was used by the Menomini to reduce swellings.

1932 H. Smith OJIBWE 375. "The Pillager Ojibwe use the root [bellwort] for stomach trouble. The trouble is described as a pain in the solar plexus, which may mean pleurisy. It has been used by eclectic practitioners [whites] for erysipelas, ulcerated mouth, etc. . .430. The Flambeau Ojibwe use the root of this plant [straw lily] as part of their hunting medicine to bring a buck deer near the hunter."

1933 H. Smith POTAWATOMI 64. "The Forest Potawatomi use the root of this plant [bellwort] for two purposes. In an infusion, it is used to cure a backache. When it is boiled down and added to lard it is used as salve to massage sore muscles and tendons. Among the whites the entire plant is used as a tonic, demulcent, nervine and hepatic. It has also been used to prevent the bad effects of poison inwardly."

YELLOW CLINTONIA   *Clintonia borealis* (Ait.) Raf. (*Smilacina b.*) Liliaceae

Growing from the root are two to five dark green, shiny, stalked leaves, narrowed at both ends, up to 30 cm long. The flowering stem, 14-40 cm tall is usually hairy at the top. It bears 3-8 yellow flowers on stalks 1-3 cm long. The berries are a bright silvery blue, 8 mm thick.

Range. Lab., Nfld., N.B., P.E.I., N.S., Que., James Bay, Ont., Man. s. to Minn., Tenn and Ga. in coniferous forests.

Common names. Wild corn, dogberry, northern lily, healall.

1708 Sarrazin-Vaillant, Quebec-Paris, Boivin transl. 204. "The Savages use it for the suppuration of tumors. Name in the country, pas de cheval."

1830 Rafinesque 211. "Algic tribes [Algonkians], leaves used by them as a plaster for bruises, and old sores, applied wet or bruised. Berries sweetish, edible."

1915 Slippy 111 2-3. Dextrose, levulose, citric, tartaric and acetic acid and fatty oil in fruits.

1915 Speck MICMAC-MONTAGNAIS 317. "Expressed juice of the root drank a gill at a time for gravel. *Smilacina borealis.*"

1932 H. Smith OJIBWE 373. "The Flambeau Ojibwe use the root tea as a remedy to help parturition. John Peper. . .said that the dogs use it to poison their teeth so that they can kill their prey. Should they bite a person, then it would be necessary to procure the same root and put it on the bite to draw out the poison. This curious superstition was also encountered in. . .the Menomini."

1933 H. Smith POTAWATOMI 62. "This Forest Potawatomi name sounds as though it should be a plant used in midwifery and our informant told us that it was employed in medicine but did not explain its exact use."

1942 Marker 24: 1283-5. Diosgenin in the roots of *Clintonia borealis*.

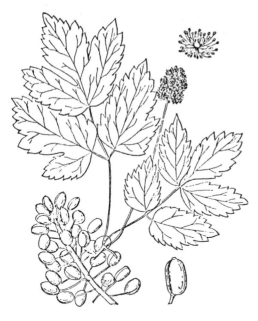

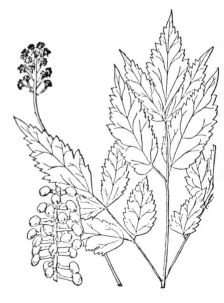

RED BANEBERRY   WHITE BANEBERRY

WHITE BANEBERRY   *Actaea pachypoda* Ell. Ranunculaceae (*A. alba*)
A tall, bushy, smooth erect plant 40-80 cm tall, from the same place on the stem the leaf and the flowering stalk grow. The leaf is divided into three leaflets each of which is divided into 3-7 leaflets with teeth around their edges. The flowering stem is long and thick with feathery white flowers. These are followed by white berries with a black spot on their ends, resembling an eye. They grow on red stalks which thicken as they mature. There are plants that bear red berries on thickened red stalks but they are rare. The berries are POISONOUS.
Range. N.B., P.E.I., N.S., Que. and Ont. s. to Okla. La. and Ga. in rich woods and thickets.
Common names. White cohosh, doll's eyes, necklace weed, white beads, snake root.

RED BANEBERRY   *Actaea rubra* (Ait.) Willd. (*A. spicata* var. *rubra*)
Very like white baneberry except that the leaflets may have hairs on the veins beneath and the flowers and red berries are on thin, 11-14 mm long stalks that are green. There is a white berried form of this plant, easily told by the berries growing on thin green stalks. The berries are POISONOUS.
Range. Lab. Nfld., N.B., P.E.I., N.S. Que., Hudson Bay, Ont. to Yukon, Alaska, s. to Calif., Ariz., N. Mex., S. Dak., Ohio and N.J.
Common names. Red cohosh, coral, pearl or redberry, poison berry, herb christopher, rattlesnake herb, grapewort, snake berry.
Actaea spicata L. is the species found in Europe but not in N. America. It bears almost black berries. The botanical name *Actaea* used to be given to the elders.
1633 Gerarde-Johnson 980. "I finde little or nothing extant in the ancient or later writers, of any good properties wherewith any part of this plant is possessed; therefore I wish those that love new medicines to take heed that this be none of them, because it is thought to be of a venomous and deadly qualitie. . . .I have received plants thereof from Robinus of Paris, for my garden where they flourish." [Robin probably received them from Canada.]
1708 Sarrazin-Vaillant Quebec-Paris, Boivin 1978 transl. 54. "These plants grow everywhere. . .It is thought that the fruit is a poison, which I don't believe, at least I know of no bad effects. This belief is perhaps founded on the name of aconite given them by Cornuti." [A. *rubra* according to Boivin.]

1785 Cutler. The berries are exceedingly poisonous. . .the plant is powerfully repellant and the root is useful in some nervous cases, but it must be administered with caution.

1830 Rafinesque 186. "Roots, bitter, repellant, nervine used for debility in Canada. Equivalent of Botrophis. Plant and berries poisonous."

1868 Can. Pharm. J. 6; 83-5. The rhizome of both red and white baneberry included in list of Can. medicinal plants.

1884 Holmes-Haydon CREE Hudson's Bay 303. "*Actaea spicata* L. as a purgative." [Here is one of several instances where Holmes in London England applies the European species' name and uses to the plants sent him by Haydon, who brought them from Hudson's Bay. If the Cree did indeed use an Actaea it would have had to have been the red berried *Actaea rubra*.]

1885 Hoffman OJIBWA 201. *A rubra*. "A decoction of the root, which has a sweet taste, is used for stomachic pains caused by having swallowed hair (mythic). Used also in conjunction with Ginseng. This plant, according to some peculiarities, is considered the male plant at certain seasons of the year, and is given only to men and boys, while the same plant at other seasons, because of size, color of fruit, or something else, is termed female, and is prepared for women and girls in the following manner, viz: the roots are rolled in basswood leaves and baked, when they become black, an infusion is then prepared, and used in a similar manner as above."

1892 Millspaugh 10. "This white species, white cohosh, together with red cohosh has received the attention of many writers upon medical botany. The two species vary principally in the color of the berries and thickness of the pedicles; probably slightly only in their properties and action. . .Just how much our species of *Actaea* differ from the European *Actaea spicata* Linn. still remains to be proven. This much we know that the American species are much milder in their properties. . .The white cohosh. . .will, however, often be found useful in many forms of reflex uterine headache, some types of chronic fleeting rheumatism, congestion in the female especially, and reflex uterine gastralgia."

1920 Fyles 42. White Baneberry. "The European baneberry, *A spicata* L., is classified in the group of plants containing poisons which act upon the heart, of which group A.B. Smith gives the following symptoms: numbness and tingling in the mouth, abdominal pain, vertigo, purging, tremor, occasional delerium, paralysis, dyspnoea, ending in syncope. . .Warn children against eating unknown fruit in the woods. Should poisoning occur, the usual emetic may be given and the advice of a doctor obtained as soon as possible. . .Red baneberry. . .Sayre says the rootstock is a violent purgative irritant and emetic."

1925 Wood & Ruddock. "*A. alba* the root is a specific in controlling after pains and for this purpose there is probably no remedy known that surpasses it. It is also useful in neuralgia of the womb and painful menstruation. A strong tincture of the root to one pint of 96% alcohol is made, the dose 15 drops three times a day."

1926-27 Densmore CHIPPEWA 358. "Take the root of the plant which has white berries and make a decoction to be drunk for excessive flowing of the menses. There was said to be another variety of this plant which had red berries and was used for diseases of men." *Actaea rubra* 299. The rhizome is said to be emeto-purgative and parasiticide.

1928 H. Smith MESKWAKI 237. "*Actaea alba*. The Meskwaki name translates as sweet or squaw root. The latter name is the same as that for Blue Cohosh (*Caulophyllum thalictroides*) and the root is used in the same manner as a genito-urinary remedy for men and women. Specimen in the Dr. Jones collection is the root of *A. alba*. . .It is said to revive and rally a patient when he is at the point of death. The root is also boiled and made into a drink to relieve the pain of childbirth."

1932 H. Smith OJIBWE 382. "*A rubra* The Pillager Ojibwe make a tea from the root to be drunk by women after childbirth. It is to clear up the system. A man also eats the root for stomach troubles. White men use the root as a substitute for black cohosh (*Cimicifuga racemosa*). . .It has been used in treating ovarian neuralgia, uterine tenderness, subinvolution and amenorrhea. It has also been used as a substitute for digitalis in fatty or irritable heart, but only after other remedies have failed. Headache due to eyestrain has also been cured by this root."

1933 H. Smith POTAWATOMI 74. "*A rubra*. The Forest Potawatomi use the root to make a tea administered to purge the patient of after-birth."

1933 Gilmore CHIPPEWA 130. *Actaea alba* used as a medicine.

1955 Mockle Quebec transl. 40. "*Actaea alba*. The root is a violent irritant purgative and an emetic. The berries are poisonous. *A. rubra* has the same properties."

1970 Willaman and Li. 3863 *Actaea rubra*. The seed contains an unamed alkaloid.

There seems to be an unknown essential oil in all parts of the plant that is poisonous. Eating even a few of the berries can result in quickening of the heart, dizziness and stomach upset. The symptoms usually disappear after a few hours. (Lewis and Elvin-Lewis 1977:30.)

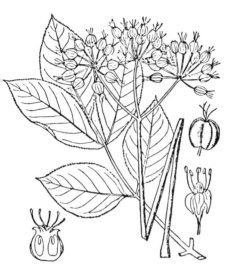

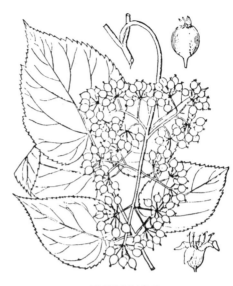

WILD SARSAPARILLA   SPIKENARD

WILD SARSAPARILLA   *Aralia nudicaulis* L Araliaceae
A long, narrow brown root sends up a short stem from which grows three long stalks, each bearing three to five leaflets, up to 15 x 8 cm each, with fine teeth around the edges. The leaflets are pale yellow green above, whitish green beneath and sometimes hairy on the veins. The woods may be carpeted with these leaves. Occasionally there will grow from the short main stem a longer stalk with usually three balls of many small greenish white flowers. These are followed by purplish black berries.
Range. Nfld., to B.C., s. to D.C., Ind., Nebr., and Colo. and in the mts. to Ga. May-June in moist or dry woods.
Common names. False sarsaparilla, american sarsaparilla, wild liquorice, rabbit root, small spikenard.
1624 Sagard HURON 192. "I inquired of them respecting the chief plants and roots which they use for curing their illnesses and among others they highly esteem the one called *oscar*, which does wonders in healing all kinds of wounds, ulcers and sores."
1708 Sarrazin-Vaillant, Quebec-Paris, Boivin 1978 transl. A. 22. "The plant passes here for a sarsaparilla [Mexican smilax] because its root is something like it and has the same vertues almost as powerfully. . .I treated a patient. . .who two years ago was cured of dropsy by using a drink made of the root of this plant."
1724 Anon ILLINOIS-MIAMI mss 224. "The root of sarsaparilla, for sores and cuts."
1778 Carver 512. "Sarsaparilla. The root of this plant, which is the most estimable part of it, is about the size of a goose quill, and runs in different directions, twined and crooked, to a great length in the ground; and from the principal stem of it springs many smaller fibres, all of which are tough and flexible. . .The bark of the root, which alone should be used in medicine, is of a bitterish flavour, but aromatic. It is deservedly esteemed for its medicinal virtues, being a gentle sudorific, and very powerful in attenuating the blood when impeded by gross humours."
1785 Cutler. The roots are aromatic and nutritious. They have been found beneficial in debilitated habits. It is said the Indians would subsist upon them, for a long time, in their war and hunting excursions. They make an ingredient in diet drinks."
1779 Zeisberger DELAWARE 149. "After the flow of blood. . .from a fresh wound [is stopped]. . .other roots must be applied, such as the great sarsaparilla."
1828 Rafinesque 53. "Two other American species *A. racemosa* and *A. hispida* have the same properties as this, and may be used for each other. . .It is often called Sarsaparilla, the root being similar to that article [*Smilax officinalis* of Mexico] and having similar properties. . .The whole

plant is balsamic, fragrant, and has a warm aromatic sweetish taste; most unfolded in the root and berries. All the Spikenards or Aralias are popular medical plants throughout the United States; they made part of the Materia Medica of the native tribes, and are extensively used by country practitioners. . .The roots and berries are most efficient. The roots bruised, or chewed, or in poultice, are used for all kinds of wounds and ulcers by the Indians. Fomentations and cataplasms are useful for cutaneous affections, erysipelas and ring-worm. An infusion or a decoction of the same, are efficient substitutes for those of Sarsaparilla (and more powerful) in all diseases of the blood, syphilitic complaints, chronical rheumatism, local pains, cardialogy, bellyache &c. As a pectoral both roots and berries may be used in syrups, cordials, decoctions. . .The roots are also nutritious. . .a kind of beer can be made with them. The berries give a fine flavor to beer, and a wine similar to elder wine can be made with them. The fresh roots and leaves chewed and applied to wounds, heal them speedily; Dr. Sp. informed me that he was once cured by them alone of a desperate accidental wound by a broad axe. . .1830. 195. Used for bilious complaints as a ptisan [little tea] in Canada."

1859-61 Gunn 886. "It is alterative, and somewhat stimulant, and used in the form of a decoction and syrup, as a substitute for the foreign or Smilax sarsaparilla, and by many is considered fully as good. Indeed some physicians consider it better. Useful in constitutional disease, such as scrofula, syphilis, skin diseases, and wherever an alterative and purifying medicine is needed. Dose of the decoction or syrup, half a wineglassful three times a day."

1868 Can. Pharm. J. 6; 83-5. *Aralia nudicaulis*, small spikenard, the root included in list of Can. medicinal plants.

1876 Can. Pharm. J. 15. New Orleans Mead: Take 8 ozs. each of the contused roots of sarsaparilla, licorice, cassia and ginger, 2 ozs. of cloves and 3 ozs. of coriander seeds. Boil for fifteen minutes in eight gallons of water; let it stand until cold. . .Then strain through flannel and add to it in the soda-fountain; syrup 12 pints [thick sugar syrup], honey 4 pints, tincture of ginger 4 ozs. and solution of citric acid 4 ozs. [See under wintergreen for a root beer recipe.]

1879 Can. Pharm. J. 322. Sarsaparilla root, a 'blood purifier', brings 5 cents a lb. when collected for sale.

1888 Delamare Island of Miquelon transl. 20. "The root esteemed in Miquelon because it has depurative [to free of impurities] properties."

1915 Speck PENOBSCOT 310. "Root dried and crushed to powder and sweet flag root steeped together for coughs."

1915 Speck MONTAGNAIS 315. "Roots steeped in case of weakness. The dark berries are made into a kind of wine by the Montagnais and used as a tonic. . .Women cut up pieces of the root, tie them on a string and keep them in their tents until needed. The same is done by the Penobscot. The berries are put into cold water and allowed to ferment in making the wine referred to."

1915 Speck-Tantaquidgeon MOHEGAN 320. A spring tonic is made by steeping together the following: wild cherry bark, sassafras root, sarsaparilla root, false sarsaparilla root (*Smilacina racemosa*), sweet flag root, burdock, and dandelion leaves, blossoms of the white daisy, boneset and motherwort and black birch bark.

1926-27 Densmore CHIPPEWA 340. A decoction of the root drunk for 'Humor in the blood'. . .350. The fresh root was mashed and applied as a poultice to sores. . .356. For nosebleed the dried and powdered root, or the fresh chewed was inserted in the nostril. . .358. For stoppage of periods the root of sarsaparilla and spikenard and the stalk of the red currant were made into a decoction and drunk. Sarsaparilla was sometimes omitted from this combination. It could also be used alone. This remedy was used if the difficulty threatened to lead to consumption.

1928 Reagan CHIPPEWA 231. "Another remedy for fainting and fits, also used as a blood medicine is sarsaparilla (*Aralia nudicaulis*) tea made from the leaves of this plant. The owner of the receipts advised the writer that this remedy is called 'Eastern Medicine', as it is the medicine of the Wabena (Eastern) Society of his people."

1923 H. Smith MENOMINI 24. "Not used as medicine."

1928 H. Smith MESKWAKI 195. A remedy for interior troubles, for lungs and for fevers, a mixture of six other herbs and the root of sarsaparilla. . .203. The root is pounded to make a poultice to cure burns and sores. Boiled with two other herbs given to give strength to one who is weak.

1932 H. Smith OJIBWE 356. "The Flambeau Ojibwe recognise the root of this plant as strong medicine, but do not steep it to make a tea. The fresh root is pounded and applied as a poultice to bring a boil to a head or to cure a carbuncle. . .428. This root is mixed with sweet flag root to make a tea to soak a gill net before setting it to catch fish during the night. Big George Skye, at Lac de Flambeau, was quite successful in catching them."

1933 H. Smith POTAWATOMI 40. "This is a valued root among the Forest Potawatomi, and they pound it into a mass to be used as a poultice to reduce swelling and cure infections."

1940 Stowe CHIPPEWA 8. "The roots used for their stimulating properties."

1954 Rousseau Quebec transl. 96. "Make a wine of the fruit."

1945 Raymond TETE DE BOULE transl. 119. "The mashed root is put into sore ears. All Indians tribes use it for one illness or another."

1955 Mockle Quebec transl. 67. "The plant is reputed to be depurative, emetic and cathartic."

1971 Jolicoeur Quebec 5. "Mixed with molasses for a spring tonic; with certain leaves and mandrake roots, helps rheumatism."

1970 Bye IROQUOIS mss. "Seeds used as a beverage."

SPIKENARD   *Aralia racemosa* L. Araliaceae

Like a small shrub, the main stem has many branches and grows to 2 m tall. The few leaves can be 80 cm long, they consist of three branching stems each with several stalks bearing 5 stalked and toothed leaflets, 2 pairs and one at the end. These leaflets can be as long as 15 cm and almost as broad, with sharp pointed tips. The flowering stem grows from the main stem where the main leaves do. It will have several stalks on each side, each covered with many stalked greenish white flowers. The berries are many, small, dark red and rather hard.

Range. Que. and N.B., Ont., to Minn., and S.D., s. to N.C. and N. Mex. in rich woods. Susceptible to late frosts in the spring, dies to the ground in the fall.

Common names. Spicebush, spignet, petty morel, life of man, old maid's root.

1380 Crawford Lake site Ontario. One seed found archeologically, personal communication by J.H. McAndrews 1978.

1778 Carver 511. "Spikenard vulgarly called in the colonies Petty-Morrell. The plant appears to be exactly the same as the Asiatic spikenard, so much valued by the ancients. Its berries are of such a balsamic nature, that when infused in spirits, they make a most palatable and reviving cordial."

1785 Cutler. "It is aromatic. The berries give to spirits an agreeable flavour. The bark of the root and the berries are a good stomachic. It is said to have been much used by the Indians for medical purposes."

1828 Rafinesque 53. [Read what he says of sarsaparilla in the previous pages it also applies to spikenard.] "The cordial of spikenard berries is recommended for the gout. . .1830 195. Used by the Indians as carminative, pectoral and antiseptic, in coughs, pains in the breast, mortification; the root with horseradish, made in poultice for the feet in general dropsy. The juice of the berries and oil of the seeds is said to cure ear ache and deafness poured in the ears."

1855 Trail 207. "Dysentery in Children. I lost two infants who were under the care of the most careful medical men; but saved another by the use of a wild herb, that was given me by a Yankee settler's wife. A plant called spikenard (or spignet, as she called it,) that grows in the forest with a long spindle root, scraped, and a small quantity boiled in milk, thickens it, as if flour had been put in: it has a sweet astringent taste, slightly bitter. A teaspoonful, thrice given in one day, cured the child, who was wasting fast under the disease. The spikenard belongs to the same family of plants as the sarsaparilla: it bears black berries, not unlike the elderberry in size and taste. There are many old settlers who know the plant. No one should use the wild herbs without the experience of a careful person, to whom their sanatory or hurtful qualities are well known. The old Canadian settlers are often well skilled in the use of the native plants—they may, possibly, have learned the value of them from the Indians, or from long experience, taught by necessity, in a country where, formerly, educated doctors were far from being as commonly met with, even in towns, as they now are."

1858-61 Gunn 862 "The root is considered an excellent substitute for Sarsaparila (*Smilax officinalis*) as an alterative in all constitutional diseases, and as an important remedy in consumption, breast complaint, and all female complaints. May be used in decoction, sirup or bitters. . .303. Cough mixture. This medicine has a wide reputation and must possess great merit from the success which attends it. Mix 1 oz of spikenard with 2 teaspoonfuls of salt petre in 1 quart of the best whiskey. Dose half a wineglassful, more or less, as necessary, three times a day."

1892 Millspaugh 69. "In domestic practice it has been made into a composite syrup with the root of *Inula helenium* (elecampane) and used as a remedy in chronic coughs, asthma and rheumatism: a tincture of the root and fruit has also been used as a stomachic."

1915 Harris HURON 48. "When a child was attacked by whooping cough they gave liberal doses of an infusion of spikenard, which was also administered for asthma and pains in the breast."

1915 Speck PENOBSCOT 311. One of the ingredients of a cure for gonorrhea.

1922 Wallis MICMAC 26. Root was used for colds, sore eyes and wounds.

1926-27 Densmore CHIPPEWA 334. The roots of spikenard and wild ginger were dried and mashed together in equal parts. . .and were used in a warm poultice on a fractured arm [see wild ginger for details]. . .340. A decoction of the root drunk for a cough. . .350. The root pounded in a cloth and applied as a poultice to boils. This poultice was said to be healing as well as 'drawing'. . .358. The root of sarsaparilla and stalk of red currant in a decoction for stoppage of periods. This remedy was used if the difficulty threatened to lead to consumption. . . .362. Dried root in decoction or fresh root pounded and applied as a poultice for sprain or strained muscles.

1923 H. Smith MENOMINI 24. "The root of this species is used in cases of blood poisoning and as a poultice for sores. A drink is also said to be made from the root which is said to be good for the stomach ache. . .This medicinal root is also edible. An aboriginal Menomini dish was spikenard root, wild onion, wild gooseberry and sugar. This is described as being very fine."

1928 H. Smith MESKWAKI 203. "Specimen 3627 of the Dr. Jones collection. The root chewed and the saliva showered or sprayed from the mouth upon the head of mothers when they are giving birth. . .The split root was used as a seasoner for other medicines."

1932 H. Smith OJIBWE 356. "They use it [the root of A. racemosa Smith thinks] as a special squaw remedy for blood purification during pregnancy. The root was pounded in a mortar, then boiled in hot water. . .prepared the same way and the tea was used to cure a cough."

1933 H. Smith POTAWATOMI 41. "The Forest Potawatomi pound the root unto a pulp to be used as a hot poultice on inflammations. . .96. They relish the young tips of the Indian spikenard in soups. Soup was a favorite aboriginal dish and still is among the Indians. Being expandable, it fits in well with the well-known Indian hospitality. After a meal is started several more guests may arrive and they are always welcome."

1928 Reagan CHIPPEWA 237. "One very old Ojibwa man cultivates a patch of spikenard near his house."

1955 Mockle Quebec transl. 68. "This species is used as a carminative, cough medicine and antiseptic in colds. The roots are used to flavor little beers. Holden found in it a saponiside which he called aralioside."

American ginseng is a member of this genus.

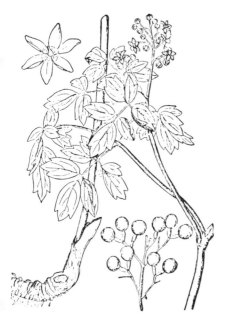

BLUE COHOSH

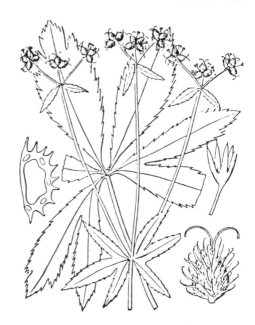

BLACK SNAKEROOT

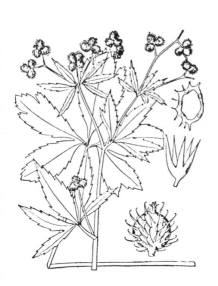

CANADA SANICLE

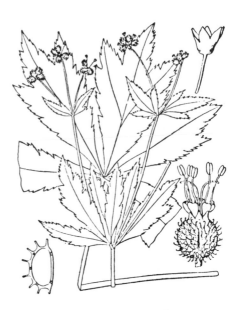

CLUSTERED SNAKEROOT

BLUE COHOSH   *Caulophyllum thalictroides* (L.) Michx. Berberidaceae

Growing from a thick, long root, the smooth 30-80 cm tall stem is sheathed at its base. There is one main leaf about half way up this stem. This leaf consists of three stalked leaflets, each of which is further divided into three to five leaflets. These leaflets are lobed at their ends and can be from 5-8 cm long when full grown. The whole plant has a peculiar dark greenish purple bloom when young. The loose cluster of flowers are in bloom before the leaves are fully open. These flowers are yellowish green or greenish purple, nearly 1 cm across and are followed by dark blue berries.

Range. N.B., N.S., s. Que. Ont., se. Man., to S.C., Ala and Mo. April-May in rich woods.

Common names. Squaw root, pappoose root, blue ginseng, blueberry root. Cohosh is an Algonquin name and has also been used for *Cimicufuga racemosa*, black cohosh; and *Actaea pachypoda*, white cohosh.

1828 Rafinesque 98. "The berries are ripe in summer; they are dry, sweetish, insipid, similar to huckle berries, but larger. This is a medical plant of the Indians, and although not yet introduced into our officinal books, deserves to be better known. I have often found it used in the country and by Indian doctors; Smith and Henry extol it. . .The root is the only part used: in smell and taste, it partakes of Ginseng and Seneca root, and is sometimes mistaken for both. It is sweetish, a little pungent and aromatic. . .It is used by the Indians and their imitators for rheumatism, dropsy, cholic, sore throat, cramp, hiccup, epilepsy, hysterics, inflammation of uterus, &c. It appears to be particularly suited to female diseases, and Smith asserts that the Indian women owe the facility of their parturition, to a constant use of a tea of the root for two or three weeks before their time. As a powerful emmenagogue it promotes delivery, menstruation, and dropsical discharges. It may by used in warm infusion, decoction, syrup or cordial."

1844 *Caulophyllum thalictroides*, blue cohosh used by the Eclectic physicians in a number of female complaints since it seemed to exert its action on the uterus. It was introduced into homeopathic practice in 1858. The Dispensatory of the U.S. in 1867 states. "It is deemed especially an emmenagogue and is thought also to promote the contractions of the uterus for which purposes it is much employed by the 'eclectic' practioners who consider it also possessed of diaphoretic and various other remedial properties" (Coulter 1973).

1858-61 Gunn 743. "This is an Indian remedy, and considered by them as one of great value, principally used by the squaws as a parturient—that is to facilitate child-birth; hence the name Pappoose root. It is said that they drink a tea of this root for two or three weeks before the expected time of labor. . .owing to this, the 'confinement' of the Indian women is a matter of but short duration and small concern. It has been abundantly proved as a valuable article in this respect by our white women. It is also considered by many as one of the most valuable antispasmodics, that is to relieve cramps, spasms, convulsions, and nervous derangements. . .in hysteria, and in all cases connected with the uterus or womb—that is known. It is recommended also in colic—especially cramp colic—in fits, in cholera-morbus, especially if there be cramps, in profuse and painful menstruation, inflammation of the womb, in suppressed menses, and in worm complaints of children. It is diuretic, emmenagogue, and antispasmodic, and may be used with safety in almost any moderate quantity. It is used in the form of a strong infusion or tea, in the proportion of an ounce of the root, powdered or bruised, to a pint of boiling water. Dose, from a half to a teacupful several times during the day. It can always be found at Botanic drug-stores, and often at others—either crude or in powder—caulophyllin—This is the active, resinous principle, obtained from the root of the Blue Cohosh. . .Dose, from one to three grains."

1868 Can. Pharm. J. 6; 83-5. The root of blue cohosh, *Caulophyllum thalictroides*, included in list of Can. medicinal plants.

1892 Millspaugh 16. "The berries are mawkish, insipid, and without special flavor. The seeds are said to resemble coffee when roasted. . .The dust of the powdered root is extremely irritating to the mucous membranes with which it comes in contact. . .This irritation follows administration of the drug throughout the body, but especially upon the female generative organs. It also exhibits the power of causing contractions of both voluntary and involuntary muscular fibres, the latter showing in the gravid uterus especially; here it does not cause the long lasting contractions of ergot, but intermittent and more successful ones."

1920 Fyles 47. "Blue cohosh contains the poisonous glucosidal *saponine*, a peculiar substance which, when stirred in water, creates a froth like soap suds. The plant is extremely bitter to the taste. . .The rootstock is said to contain *saponin* and the alkaloid *caulophylline*."

1926-27 Densmore CHIPPEWA 340. Decoction made of two roots and one quart of water and drunk a swallow at a time for lung trouble. . .344. Decoction of equal amounts of the roots of blue cohosh and bloodroot drunk for cramps. . .342. Equal parts of the roots of blue cohosh and coneflower steeped in water and drunk for indigestion and biliousness. . .346. As an emetic scrape the root fine, tie a small quantity in a white cloth and squeeze it in warm water and drink the water.

1923 H. Smith MENOMINI 25. "The root of this plant is boiled to obtain a tea which is drunk for the supression of profuse menstruation. It is accounted a very valuable female remedy."

1928 H. Smith MESKWAKI 205. "The root is called a woman and it is nearly like the sycamore bark in action. The roots are boiled and the tea taken as a remedy for profuse menstruation. It is also a genito-urinary remedy for man."

1932 H. Smith OJIBWE 358. "The Pillager Ojibwe use the root for female troubles espcially for cramps in the stomach during painful menstruation. The fine roots are also boiled to make a tea for emetic purposes."

1933 H. Smith POTAWATOMI 43. "This is known to the Forest Potawatomi as the Squaw Root and it seems to be of rather universal use amongst our Indian tribes to furnish a tea which suppresses profuse menstruation and aids in childbirth."

1955 Mockle Quebec transl. 45. "The rhizome and roots are used as an antineuralgic, antirheumatic and above all as an emmenagogue, facilitating delivery and menstruation; this latter action is due to a saponine, caulosaponine, which provokes strong uterine contractions recalling those provoked by ergot. The Indians attributed the facility of their parturition to the use of a tea of these roots, taken for two or three weeks before the birth. The roasted seeds have had a certain vogue as a substitute for coffee. Davy and Chu have isolated, besides the caulosaponine, methylcystine which is identical to the caulophyllin of the ancient writers."

Blue cohosh considered an abortifacient. The leaves and seeds contain methylcystine. Children have been poisoned by eating the berries (Lewis and Elvin-Lewis 1977:31, 325).

BLACK SNAKEROOT
Sanicula marilandica L. Umbelliferae (Apiaceae)

A stout stem, 45-120 cm tall, with leaves around it at intervals. These consist of 3 to 7 leaflets each 4-15 cm long, joined together where they meet at the stem. They have long stalks at the bottom and are without stalks at the top of the plant. They have large teeth, themselves toothed, around their edges. There is a small divided leaf on each side of the stem where the flowering stalk grows. The flowers are greenish white in balls of 12 to 25. The fruit is 4-6 mm long with two slender antennas (styles) coming from its top. It is covered with fine hooked bristles.

Range. Que. and Nfld. to B.C., s. to n. Fla., Mo. and N.M. June-Aug. In rich woods.

Common names. Sanicle.

CANADA SANICLE
Sanicula canadensis L.

Canada sanicle is very like blacksnakeroot except that there are only 2 to 7 flowers in each ball and they are white. The fruit does not appear to have antennas (styles) sticking out from its top as they are shorter than the bristles on the fruit.

Range. Vt. and s. Ont. to Minn. and S.D., s. to Fla. and Tex. June-Aug. in wood.

CLUSTERED SNAKEROOT
Sanicula gregaria Bickn.

Slender stems usually several in a clump. Leaves with five leaflets. Flowers 12-25 in one head, yellowish. Fruit longer than the petals (sepals), 3-5 mm.

Range. N.S., and Que. to Minn., S.D.,s. to Fla. and Tex. in woods.

1633 Gerarde-Johnson 949. "Sanicle [*S. Europea*]. The juice being inwardly taken is good to heal wounds. The decoction of it also made in wine or water is given against spitting of bloud, and the bloudie flix: also foul and filthy ulcers be cured by being bathed therewith. The herbe boyled in water, and applied in manner of a pultesse, doth dissolve and waste away cold swellings; it is used in potions which are called Vulnerarie potions, or wound drinkes, which maketh whole and sound all inward wounds and outward hurts: it also helpeth the ulcerations of the kidneys, ruptures, or burstings."

1778 Carver 516. "A tea is made of the root is vulnery and balsamick." [*S. marilandica*]

1795 Michaux Journ. 68. "A decoction of *Sanicula marilandica* roots were a sovereign remedy for long continued Venereal diseases." [Identification questioned.]

1830 Rafinesque 261. "Subtonic, astringent, antisyphilitic. Useful for leucorrhea, gonorrhea and syphilis, hemorrhagy, dysentery &c. whole plant used in decoction, also vulnerary and balsamic, root for tumors and wounds of horses." [*S. marilandica*]

1859-61 Gunn 755. "This article is regarded as an excellent nervine—that is, it quiets, as well as strengthens the nerves. It is also tonic, astringent, and somewhat anodyne, being very similar to Valerian root, and also the Ladyslipper root. It is a good remedy in chorea, or St. Vitus' Dance; and is also considered good in intermittent fevers, in the form of decoction, as well as in croup, sorethroat, and hives. It is also good in all nervous diseases, and has been used with advantage in hemorrhages from the womb, in leucorrhea (or whites) and in dysentery. The dose of the powdered root is from twenty grains to a drachm, or a teaspoonful, three times a day, according to age; but it is most used in decoction, from a half a pint to a pint or more of which may be taken, warm or cold, during the day. It is by some considered a sure cure for snake-bites, in which case a strong decoction is to be drank freely, and the same applied freely to the bite." [*S. marilandica*]

1868 Can. Pharm J. 6; 83-5. The root of *S. marilandica* included in list of Can. medicinal plants.

1915 Harris ALGONQUIN 55. "'Black Snake Root', an umbelliferous plant (parsley family) of the genus 'sanicula' so called from the Latin 'sanare' to heal, on account of its medicinal properties. Very common around Toronto, growing in rich woods amongst our wild Canadian lilies, violets and mitreworts. . . .There are, I might say, two plants in our Canadian woods popularly known as the Black Snake Root: one is of the crowfoot family, '*Cimicifuga racemosa*' or bugbane, and the other of the parsley family, '*Sanicula Canadensis*' or the sanicle, mentioned above. The latter, 'Canadensis' is the black snakeroot of the Indians. . .51. For swellings and inflammation they bruised and applied the leaves of the black snake root, which in almost all cases gave immediate relief."

1925 Wood & Ruddock. Black cankeroot, the Indians regard this as a sovereign remedy for rattlesnake bites. Take a handful of the roots and boil in about a pint of water, divide in half, drink each half hour. At the same time a decoction of the leaves is applied to the bitten part. Universally regarded as a great blood purifier and often taken as spring bitters. It is also valuable as a cure for hives, sore throat and croup and intermittent fevers. It is excellent to quiet and strengthen the nerves [*S. marilandica*].

1926-27 Densmore CHIPPEWA 358. A decoction [*S. canadensis*] made from a handful of the powdered root and 1 quart of water, drunk for stoppage of periods. . .360. A decoction of the roots of canada snakeroot and cowslip (*Caltha palustris*) drunk during confinement. . .302. The root is said to be astringent, antispasmodic and antiperiodic."

1923 H. Smith MENOMINI 55. "This [*S. marilandica*] root was not used by the Menomini, which is somewhat strange as it has been a noted aboriginal remedy with other Indians, and possesses rather active aromatic, bitter principles. When pressed for information, my informant thought it might be used by the sorcerers for some evil purpose. . .Clustered snakeroot (*Sanicula gregaria* Bick.) The same comment may be made on this species as in the preceding, for it was often used without distinguishing the difference in the species for the same purpose."

1928 H. Smith MESKWAKI 250. "Clustered snakeroot. . .This plant is used by the Indians as an astringent, and to stop nosebleed. They burn the plant upon hot stones, and inhale the fumes or steam up the nostril to stop the nosebleed. The Meskwaki did not know this plant although they had a name for it, but McIntosh knew it and gave the use."

1932 H. Smith OJIBWE 391. "The Flambeau Ojibwe use the root [*S. marilandica*] pounded as a poultice to cure rattlesnake bite or any snake bite. Bearskin, chief Flambeau medicine man said that if this root be chewed, it would cause eruptions on the epithelial lining of the mouth. They consider it a very potent remedy. The Pillager Ojibwe. . .make a root tea that is used to cure fevers of various kinds."

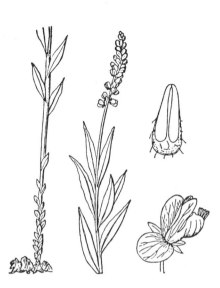

SENECA SNAKEROOT

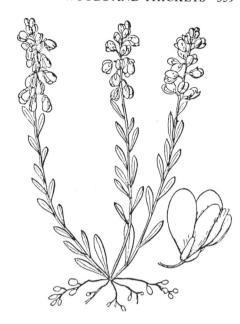

RACEMED MILKWORT

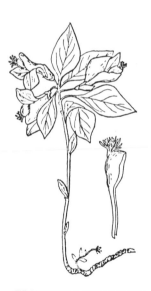

FRINGED MILKWORT

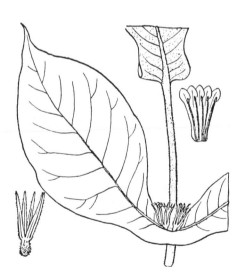

FEVERWORT

SENECA SNAKEROOT *Polygala senega* L. Polygalaceae
From a stout root grows a cluster of straight, slightly hairy stems 10-50 cm tall, with alternate stalkless leaves 3-8 x 3-30 mm. The lowest leaves are merely scales. On the upper part of the stem the flowers are tightly packed. They have five white petals (calyx), two of them larger, like wings, 3-3.5 mm. The inner true flower is inconspicuous. There are two hairy seeds with white appendages on the concave side.

Range. N.B., Que., Ont., James Bay, Man. to s. Alta. s. to S.Dak., Ark., Tenn. and Ga. in dry or moist woods, prairies and rocky places.

Common names. Senega root, rattlesnake root, mountain flax.

1687 Clayton Virginia Indians 12. "Among their herbs I have had 40 several sorts or near that number showed me as great secrets, for the *Rattle-snake root*, or that kind of *snake root* which is good for curing the bite of the *rattlesnake*. But I have no reason to believe that any of them are able to effect the cure."

1698 Hennepin 222. "We named it *The River of the Grave*, or *Mausoleum*, because the Savages bury'd there one of their Men, who was bitten by a Rattle-Snake."

1705 Beverley Virginia 217. "Their Priests are always Physicians, and by the method of their Education in the Priesthood, are made very knowing in the hidden qualities of Plants, and other Natural things, which they count a part of their Religion to conceal from everybody, but from those that are to succeed them in their holy Function. They tell us, their God will be angry with them, if they should discover that part of their knowledge; so they suffer only the Rattle Snake Root to be known, and such other Antidotes, as must be immediately apply'd; because their Doctors can't be always at hand to remedy those sudden misfortunes, which generally happen in their Hunting or Travelling."

1737 Tennent London Sept. 28th. Letter to Sir Hans Sloane. "Sir, The Rattlesnake root you had from me being of a Small size, I send you some larger, with a Copper plate cut of the Plant, that thereby you may see that it is quite different from the Serpentaria [*Aristolochia s.*] of the Shops, or any Rattle Snake root of Chelsea Physick Garden. I presume that Collo Byrd has notified you that this root really cures the bite of a Rattle Snake, and that the Evidence you have had of its great Efficacy in Pleurisys and Peripneumonys is satisfactory. Therefore I doubt not of your introducing a Medicine of this kind, as it is for the Publick benefit, and as you have notably given demonstration of your earnest desire to forward things calculated for that purpose. I send some of the decoction of the root, as it is given after the bite of a Rattle Snake, and in a Pleurisy or Peripneumony, which if you please to taste, you will then discover the activity of the particles of the root, and thence may be convinced that it is a powerfull medicine and may be applied to excellent purposes in several Diseases. The operation of this root is Emetick, Cathartic, Diuretick and Diaphoretick, and may with a little discretion be made to operate altogether in any of these ways, exclusive of its restrictive property upon the Fibres. I am Sir with all great respect, your most obed't humble serv't, Jno. Tenn [ent. Sir Hans Sloane gave the land for the Chelsea Physick Garden in London, England. Collo Byrd is William Byrd, a settler in Virginia in the first half of the eighteenth century and an enthusiastic advocate of the value of *Polygala senega*, being convinced among other things that it would cure gout].

1736 Tennent Williamsberg. Essay on Pleurisy, on the virtues of a plant obtained from the Indians, the Seneca snakeroot, which Tennant extolled as a sovereign remedy for pulmonary ailments. For his services the Virginia Assembly awarded him one hundred pounds.

1817-20 Bigelow 13. "The Seneca snake root has attracted so general an attention from the medical public, as to have become an article of exportation to Europe, and one which holds a regular place in the druggist stores. . .[it] has a firm, hard, branching perennial root, consisting of a moderately solid wood, and a thick bark. . .The root. . .has an unpleasant and somewhat acid taste. After chewing, it leaves a sensation of acrimony in the mouth, and still more in the fauces, if it has been swallowed. . .Medicinally administered, the Seneca snake root is sudorific and expectorant in small doses, and emetic and cathartic in large ones. . .Its most usual mode of exhibition is in decoction, which may be made of suitable strength by boiling an ounce of the root in a pint and a half of water, till it is reduced to a pint. . .The first reputation of the Seneca root was one which it divides with a multitude of other plants, that of curing the bite of the Rattlesnake. . .When, however, we consider the number of cases of recovery from the bite of this serpent, under every variety of treatment, we cannot avoid the conclusion, that these injuries are not necessarily dangerous, and that spontaneous recoveries are perhaps as frequent as those which are promoted by medicine. More certain success attends the use of the Seneca in pneumonia and some diseases related to it. . .I have often found a decoction of the Seneca root to afford a very marked relief by promoting expectoration, and relieving the tightness and oppression of the chest. . .Benefit has been derived in asthma from the use of this plant. . .eminently useful. . .administered to old people, but in the paroxysms of young persons, I have found it too irritating. . .In various forms of dropsy, the Seneca root has been resorted to with advantage. . .A man labouring under severe rheumatism was ordered to take at intervals a wine glass full of a strong decoction of the Senega made from an ounce of the root, in a pint of water. The patient, from a desire to expedite the cure, thought it proper to drink the whole quantity at once. The consequence was the most violent vomiting and purging, which lasted the whole night accompanied with profuse diaphoresis. The patient, as might have been hoped from the violence of the operation, was radically relieved of his disorder."

1820's Mat. Med. Edinburgh-Toronto mss 61."*Polygala Senega* has been employed as an Expectorant in Pneumonia & also in pertussis & catarrh chronic, the dose in substance is from 10 to 20 grains but it is usually employed in Decoction. . .It is however little used."

1830 Rafinesque 64. "The common officinal Senega Snake-root, well known in materia medica, and kept in all the shops. . .The Indians use it besides snake bites, for syphilis and malignant sore throat. . .The taste and smell is very pungent and nauseating. A resin and the Senegine, a peculiar substance, are the most active constituents. Ten grains of the powder is a dose; a larger one will often prove emetic. . .It is injurious in consumption and inflammatory disorders, Some compare its action to calomel, and consider it a general alterative, In croups, it often disengages the morbid membrane. It is very beneficial in chronic rheumatism, the asthma of old people, and inveterate dropsy; small and moderate doses prove sudorific."

1842 Christison 842. "Senega. . .has been chiefly commended as a local stimulant in relaxed sore throat—as an expectorant in chronic catarrh, and in protracted pneumonia where bleeding ceases to be admissible, and as a diaphoretic-diuretic in rheumatism. It has been thought also useful in dropsy. It is of no use as an antidote to snake poison. Six grains of its active principle will kill a dog in three hours, with symptoms of irritant poisoning."

1846 Winder Quebec 11. "The *polygala senega* is too well known to need description. It is much used by the Indians, who give it in cold infusion during remission of fevers, attended with great prostration of strength, and in diseases of the pulmonary organs. They also esteem it highly in female complaints, and in this agree with Dr. Chapman, who considers it the most efficacious emmenagogue, and useful in all forms of amenorrhoea."

1859-61 Gunn 856. "It is mostly used for its expectorant properties, in coughs, colds and lung affections. . .It is also used in suppressed menses, in combination with other emmenagogues. . .is one of the principal ingredients in the celebrated Hive Sirup, which is much used in croup."

1868 Can. Pharm. J. 6; 83-5. The root of *Polygala senega* included in list of Can. medicinal plants.

1885 Hoffman OJIBWA 199. "A decoction of the roots is used for colds and cough. An infusion of the leaves is given for sore throat; also to destroy water-bugs that have been swallowed."

1892 Millspaugh 45. "About the year 1735, John Tennent, a Scotch physician, noted that the Seneca Indians obtained excellent effects from a certain plant as a remedy for the bite of the rattlesnake; after considerable painstaking and much bribing, he was shown the roots and given to understand that what is now known to be Seneca Snakeroot was the agent used. Noting, then, that the symptoms of the bite were similar in some respects to those of pleurisy and the latter stages of peripneumonia, he conceived the idea of using this root also in those diseases. . .His epistle was printed in Edinburgh in 1738, and the new drug favorably received throughout Europe, and cultivated in England in 1739. . .Chemical constituents Polygalic Acid. . .This acid forms a frothing, saponaceous solution in boiling water. . .tends to prove at least a similarity between this acid and Saponin."

1915 Harris HURON 50. "The Seneca snake-root was considered a valuable remedy by the Hurons and cognate tribes. It was prepared and used sometimes as a powder, at other time as an infusion and given warm to induce sweating or to help in the discharge of mucus from the throat and lungs. It was given to children when suffering from difficulty of breathing, and drunk generously by consumptives. . .51. Children. . .For colds, asthma and pleurisy they drank bear's oil and Seneca snake root steeped for hours in an extract of wild liquorice. . .56. Common in Ontario, growing abundantly all over Canada and throughout the western and south-western States."

1926-27 Densmore CHIPPEWA 336. For convulsions drink a decoction of the roots of seneca snake root, wild rose, ground plum and prairie sage. . .338. For the heart: scrape off the inner bark of the bur oak, red oak and aspen, dry and powder in the hands, add equal amounts of root, bud and blossom of the balsam poplar. "A pail was made ready containing about a pint of water. A little of the mixed bark was placed on the water at the eastern side, the medicine man saying. . .'eastward'; the same was repeated at the south, west, and north with similar words. He then placed on top of these piles a smaller portion of the powdered *Polygala senega* root, saying the same words. The medicine was then allowed to steep. It was said to be very powerful so that care must be used not to take too much of it. The dose was measured in a small receptacle made of birch bark and marked with the symbol of the remedy, or 'one swallow' was taken, the dose being repeated in an hour"...365. Taken dry as a tonic or the dried root pounded and kept separately. Equal parts of the roots of prairie sage, ground plum and wild rose are pounded together until powdered. "A quart of water is heated and about a 1/3 of a teaspoon of the mixed ingredients is placed on the surface of the water of the 4 sides of the pail. A very little of the first (principal ingredient) is placed on top of each. The ingredients soon dissolve. A stronger decoction was secured by boiling. This medicine was taken 4 times a day, the dose being small at first, and gradually increased to about a tablespoonful. A measure made of birch bark was used for this remedy"...376. The root was carried on one's person for general health and safety on a journey.

1928 H. Smith MESKWAKI 193. An emetic; for eczema sores, etc. A Menomini remedy. Polygala senega and nine other ingredients...A poultice for snake-bite; also used as a tea to cure dropsy. Senega and eight other ingredients...196. Pile medicine, senega and seven other ingredients...A universal remedy for all sickness...senega and eight other ingredients...236. "This is the chief remedy of both tribes in cases of heart trouble. Specimen 5174 of the Dr. Jones collection is the root of *Polygala senega*...The root is boiled and made into a drink to be used for heart trouble."

1933 Can. Formulary 107. Stokes' Expectorant...1 fl. oz of Tincture of Senega, 1 fl. oz tincture of Squill, 1 fl. oz camphorated tincture of opium with Ammonium Carbonate, Syrup of Tolu and distilled water.

1955 Mockle Quebec transl. 56. "Base of stem and roots have expectorant properties and are used in pulmonary affections, bronchitis, asthma, and as an emetic in large doses. This plant contains terpenic saponosides; senegine and polygalic acid."

1959 Mechling MALECITE maritime provinces of Canada used the root for colds.

1964 Yarnell 159. Menomini and Iroquois used the plant for food. The root is collected in the wild in western U.S. It has a distinct odor recalling that of wintergreen. The taste is sweet at first but soon sour and acrid. The powdered root is very irritating to the throat and nostrils when inhaled. It makes water froth.

Contains about 4% senegin, and 5.5% polygalic acid, glucosides belonging to a group of saponins. Senegin is toxic. The drug contains a small percentage of methyl salicylate. Senega is used as a stimulant expectorant in bronchitis (T.F. Wallis 1967:419).

RACEMED MILKWORT   *Polygala polygama* Walt. var. *obtusata* Chod. Polygalaceae
A cluster of smooth stems, 10-25 cm tall that are sparingly branched. The crowded leaves, 1-3 cm x 2-7 mm grow gradually smaller towards the bottom of the stem. At the top of the stem the rose-purple to white flowers are spaced apart. There are cleistogamous (closed) flowers under ground.
Range. Me. to s. Ont., Mich. and Minn., s. to N.J., w.Va., O., Ind. and Io. also along the coastal plain from e. Va. to Fla. and Tex. in dry usually sandy soil, May-June.
1830 Rafinesque 65. Bitter and tonic, although likewise stimulant and expectorant."
1868 Can. Pharm. J. 6; 83-5 The root and herb of *Polygala polygama* included in the list of Can. medicinal plants.
1915 Speck MONTAGNAIS 314. "Indian name means 'blue-berry flower,' it is boiled for cough medicine."
1955 Mockle Quebec transl. 56. "A bitter tonic."

FRINGED MILKWORT   *Polygala paucifolia* Willd. Polygalaceae
From a small root grow thin 8-15 cm stems with 3-6 leaves at the top, each 1.5-4 cm long, of a dull dark green with a noticeable midvein and finely pointed tips. There are scale like 2-8 mm leaves on the stem. The flowers, on short stalks, are conspicuous, of a rich rosy-purple and fringed.
Range. s. Que. and N.B. to Sask., s. to Conn., N.Y., and Wis. and in the mts. to Ga. May-June in large patches in moist rich woods.
Common names. Flowering wintergreen, evergreen snakeroot, may-wings, Indian pink, little pollom, dwarf, milkwort, bird-on-the wing.
1830 Rafinesque 64. "The whole plant, but chiefly the root, has a sweet pungent taste, and somewhat the smell of *Gautiera* [wintergreen]. Its properties are similar to it, and to *Polygala senega*. It

is stimulant, sudorific, restorative, &c. It may be used in tea or decoction: being milder than either; it may be very useful when the Senega would be too stimulant, and it may perhaps answer all its effects in asthma, rheumatism, dropsy, &c"
1955 Mockle Quebec transl. 56. "The plant is used as a stimulant, tonic and sudorific."

FEVERWORT
Triosteum perfoliatum Caprifoliaceae

A coarse plant up to 130 cm tall with hairy stems. The leaves, softly hairy beneath, are 10-22 x 4-12 cm and in var. *perfoliatum* meet at the stem which appears to grow through them. In var. *aurantiacum* they merely touch the stem. There the 1-4 flowers grow, they are purplish brown or dull red followed by orange red or yellow fruits which contain usually 3 bony nutlets.
Range. N.B., Que., Ont. to Minn., s. to N.C. KY., and Kan in dry or moist woods.
Common names. Horse-gentian, tinkers-weed, wild coffee, horse-ginseng, fever root, wild or wood ipecac.
1687 Clayton Virginia Indians 9-10. "When they design to give a Purge they make use of the following herbs. . .There is another herb which they call the Indian purge, this plant has several woody stalks, growing near 3 feet tall, and as I remember perfoliat, it bears yellow berries, round about the joynts, they only use the Root of this plant."
1830 Rafinesque 269. "Fever root, Tinker weed, Horse Ginseng, Ipecac, Wild Coffee, White Ginseng, Sincky of Indians. Root purgative, emetic, diuretic, tonic, &c. taste bitter and nauseous, 5 lbs. give 2 lb. of extract, yields no resin nor oil. A mild purge, eq. of jalap in doses of 20 to 30 grains in powder, or half of extract. In larger doses emetic. Impaired by age. Useful in fevers, agues, pleuritis, &c. Leaves diaphoretic, seeds used as coffee by the Germans near Lancaster."
1859-61 Gunn 794. "Gentian—(*Triosteum Perfoliatum*)—This is a well known plant. . .The root is light-brown, long, round, tapering and bunchy, and of a pungent, bitter taste. Both the root and berries are used as medicine. Gentian root is an excellent bitter tonic and restorative, laxative, somewhat stimulant, and in large doses cathartic. . .Useful in intermittent fevers, especially as a restorative tonic after the fever and ague have been broken. The ripe berries also make an excellent bitter, tinctured in whisky or gin. . .Seldom used alone."
1868 Can. Pharm. J. 6; 83-5. Fever root, *Triosteum perfoliatum*, bark of the root included in list of Can. medicinal plants.
1892 Millspaugh 74. "The feverwort is indigenous to North America. . .not really plentiful in any locality. . .Dr. Tinker was the first who put to use its roots as an emetic. . .A decoction is said to have been used by the Cherokee Indians in the cure of fevers (Porcher). . .Dr. J. Kneeland calls attention to this plant as an application to painful swellings, regarding which he says [1859] 'My attention was first called to it by a gentleman. . .who derived his knowlege of its value indirectly from the Onondaga Indians. . .I applied the bruised root, moistened, to. . .[a] young man. . .had not slept much for two nights. The whole hand was much swollen. . .We applied *Triosteum* and nothing else. After six hours application he slept; the throbbing and tensive pain gradually diminished after the first application; in two days time the swelling disappeared from the forearm and hand. . .*Triosteum* is one of the drugs dismissed from the U.S. Ph.[armacopoeia], at the last revision."
1928 H. Smith MESKWAKI 207-8. "Tinker's Weed. . .The root is used in several ways by the Meskwaki, and in many combinations, one of which is the cure of snake bite. It is also applied to the healing of old raw sores. Specimen 5122 in Dr. Jones collection is the root. . .It is used by the Meskwaki on a new-born infant with a sore head. . .boiled and applied to old sores. It is also used as a drink for cleansing the system. The white man uses it, under the names Wild Ipecac and feveroot, during convalescence from low fevers, in hysteria and hypochrondia, in intermittent fever and chronic rheumatism. It has emetic and cathartic properties and may be substituted for ipecac."
1955 Mockle Quebec transl. 85. "The root emetic, cathartic, and vulnerary."

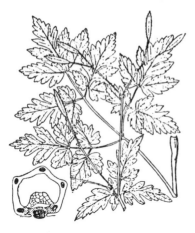

WOOLY SWEET CICELY

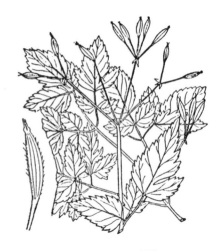

WILD CHERVIL

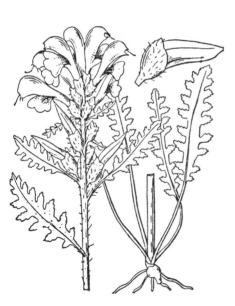

WOOD BETONY

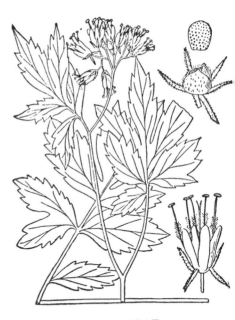

WATERLEAF

WOOLY SWEET CICELY *Osmorhiza claytoni* (Michx.) Clarke Umbelliferae (Apiaceae)
A tall hairy plant with the leaves growing from the upper parts of the stem. They consist of opposite leaflets, each cut into segments, with deep teeth around their edges, hairy on both sides. The long flowering stem is topped by a cluster of small white flowers, followed by 15-22 mm long thin, brown seed pods that have styles 1.2-1.5 mm long at their ends.
Range. Gaspe and N.S. to s. Sask., s. to N.C., Ala., and Ark. May-June in moist woods.

WILD CHERVIL   *Osmorhiza longistylis* (Torr.) DC.
Similar to wooly sweet cicely but the leaves are less deeply cut. The points on the seed pods are 3-4 mm long. The roots and plant are anise scented.
Range. Que. to Sask., s. to Ga., Tex. and Colo. in moist woods, May-June.
1619 Champlain-Macklem HURON 1616 77. "The average lodge will have a dozen fires and two dozen families. The smoke inside is thick and blinding and diseases of the eyes are common, in fact many of the older people have lost their sight altogether. The trouble is that there are no windows and so there is no way for the smoke to escape except through a single hole in the roof."
1724 Anon ILLINOIS-MIAMI mss 221-5. "The root of the wild chervil is marvelous for the ills of the eyes, by dropping in the eye the water in which this root is steeped, in the Month of May when the vine is in sap."
1830 Rafinesque 249. "Root fusiform, with a sweet smell and taste, near aniseed, edible, carminative, expectorant, demulcent, useful for coughs with Malva, for flatulent bowels with Heracleum. . .Children are fond of this root, may be poisoned by mistaking for it, two sp. of the same genus." [see *Conium*.]
1868 Can. Pharm. J. 6; 83-5. The root of Sweet Cicely, *Osmorrhiza longistylus* included in list Can. medicinal plants.
1925 Youngken 184. "*O. longistylis*. The roots were pounded by the Omaha and Ponca to make poultices for boils. The Winnebago medicine men used the same remedy for wounds. A decoction of the roots was employed by several tribes for weakness and debility and by the Cheyenne for disordered stomach. The last named also employed a decoction of the roots stems and leaves for kidney trouble."
1926-27 Densmore CHIPPEWA 342. *O. Claytoni*; the root chewed for a sore throat or made into a decoction. . .354. The root dried and pounded moistened with warm water and applied externally to ulcers and especially to running sores.
1923 H. Smith MENOMINI 55. *O. Claytoni*. "This is the remedy to enable one to put on flesh. The root has the taste of carrots and only one piece or branch must be eaten at one time."
1928 H. Smith MESKWAKI 249. "*O. longistylis*. This is a medicine imported by the Meskwaki from Wisconsin and they say it is a good medicine for everything. It is chiefly used as an eye medicine. It is a horse medicine too, the root is grated and mixed with salt for distemper. When hunting they fed a pony with the root and he was thus able to catch the buffalo. . .The leaves of this plant and bark of *Gleditsia triacanthos*, the honey locust, are mixed to make a tea which is drunk to regain flesh and strength."
1932 H. Smith OJIBWE 391. "Evidently they did not distinguish between the two species. A tea for making parturition easier is prepared from the roots. The licorice flavor of the tea is said to be good for a sore throat."
1933 H. Smith POTAWATOMI 86. "*O. longistylis*. The root is used to make an eye lotion and also to make a tea which is used as a stomachic. . .124. Chop root into fine bits and add to oats or other seeds which they give to their ponies to make them fat and sleek."
1966 Campbell, Best & Budd 89. "All portions of sweet cicely plants are relished by sheep and cattle and will be eaten by horses and deer. However its palatability and nutritive value will be destroyed by frost. Because it stores its food reserves in its fleshy root, it can be grazed fairly intensively without killing individual plants or overgrazing stands."

WOOD BETONY   *Pedicularis canadensis* L. Scrophulariaceae
This plant has stalked, much segmented leaves that grow tufted from the roots. The several stems, 15-40 cm tall are hairy as are the leaves. The flowers grow tightly up the top of the stem, yellowish to reddish purple, rather like foxgloves, producing long brown seed capsules.
Range. Que. and Me. to Man., s. to Fla. and Tex. also Colo. to n. Mex. April-June in upland woods and prairies.
Common names. Lousewort, high heal-all, beefsteak plant, snaffles.
1708 Sarrazin-Vaillant, Quebec-Paris, Boivin 1978 transl. 129. "Eaten in the soup." (Probably *P. canadensis*). [By the inhabitants of New France].
1830 Rafinesque 251. "This is one of the vulnerary plants called Healall. *P. canadensis* deemed by the Indians to cure Rattlesnake bites."
1916 Waugh IROQUOIS 118. Many of them are still in use. . .cooked like spinach. . .wood betony, *P. canadensis* and *P. lanceolata*, usually collected in the earliest part of the season.

1923 H. Smith MENOMINI 53. "The root is chopped fine and put into oats that are fed to the pony. . .will make him fat and vicious to all but his owner. . .81. 'Enticer root', the root is carried on the person of the Menomini who is contemplating making love advances."

1928 H. Smith MESKWAKI 247. "The whole plant is boiled to make a tea to reduce any internal swellings. For external swellings the root is made into a poultice. Tumors are supposed to be healed by this according to McIntosh. . .273. This is not the ordinary love charm but the root is used to make married people congenial again after they have been estranged. It is placed as is the *Lobelia* root in some dish that they are going to eat in common. It makes them love each other again."

1932 H. Smith OJIBWE 389. "According to John Peper this root was a bad kind of medicine, an aphrodisiac, when cut fine and placed in some dish of food without the knowledge of those who were going to eat it. . .432. He said it was too often put to bad uses."

1933 H. Smith POTAWATOMI 83. "The use of the root of this plant is rather different in the two tribes. The Forest Potawatomi use it as a physic, whereas the Prairie Potawatomi use it for reducing both internal and external swellings. Among the whites the entire plant is used by eclectic practitioners for its tonic, sedative, astringent and vulnerary properties. . .124. The Forest Potawatomi mix the roots with oats to make their ponies fat."

1968 Forsyth England 94. "The Scrophularia family includes the Foxglove (*Digitalis purpurea*). . .Lousewort (*Pedicularis* spp.) all of which are known to contain sufficient poisonous glucosides to cause acute illness or death to any animal which eats a quantity of them. That few recorded cases of poisoning by the growing plant in man or animals are to be found in either medical or veterinary literature of the last fifty years, is due to several factors, the most important of these being that animals will not eat them."

WATERLEAF   *Hydrophyllum virginianum* L. Hydrophyllaceae
The stem is 30-80 cm the upper part hairy. The lower leaves long stalked, with 5(7-9) leaflets or divisions, all with wide sharp teeth and smooth. The flowering stalk grows from the top of the plant bearing many hairy 7-10 mm white to violet flowers.
Range. Que. to N.D., s. to N.C., Ala. and Ark. May-June in moist or wet woods or open wet places.
Common names. Indian salad, John's cabbage, brook-flower.
1778 Cartwright Labrador Journal 11 319. "Indian salad now springing up."
1818 Barton 2; xiii. Root of *H. canadense* eaten by Indians in times of scarcity.
1822 de Serra Tran. Hort. Soc. London 4; 445. Indian salad eaten by Indians when young and tender. Some of the first settlers ate the plant.
1830 Rafinesque 229. "Schoepf says that the *H. canadense* is used against the bite of snakes and the poisonous erysipelas produced by *Rhus* [poison ivy]." [*H. Canadense*, the broad leaved water leaf, has a leaf more like the maple, with flowering stalks that are short, whitish flowers and a more southerly distribution.]
1885 Hoffman OJIBWA 201. "The roots are boiled, the liquor then taken for pains in the chest, back, etc."
1892 Millspaugh 122. "The young leaves serve in some localities as a salad,. . .and are eaten as potage in other places, under the name of John's Cabbage. We have no previous medical history of this plant, or any other species of this order."
1916 Waugh IROQUOIS 117. Many are still in use. . .cooked like spinach and seasoned with salt, pepper or butter. . .Waterleaf, *Hydrophyllum virginianum*.
1925 Youngken 178. "The root was used as an astringent by several tribes."
1923 H. Smith MENOMINI 37. "The root of this plant 'puckering root' is known as a remedy for flux, because of its astringent properties. . .68. The leaves are eaten as greens. First they are wilted like lettuce in vinegar made from the last run of maple sap, then simmered in a kettle. The first water is thrown away. They are then boiled with pork and fine meal until ready to serve."
1932 H. Smith OJIBWE 371. "John Peper. . .it furnishes a root that may be used to keep flux in check. He states that it is good for man, woman or child. It was used for the same purpose among the Meskwaki Indians, but there is no record of its use by whites. . .405. The Pillager Ojibwe use the root as feed for ponies to make them fatten rapidly."

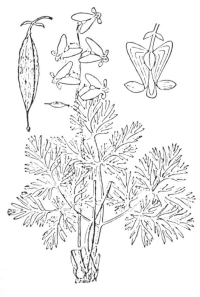

DUTCHMAN'S BREECHES

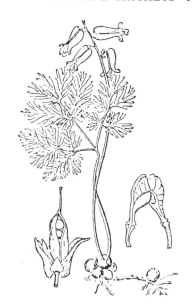

TURKEY CORN

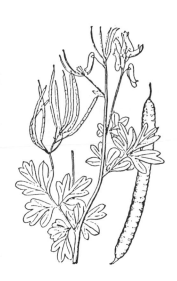

PALE CORYDALIS

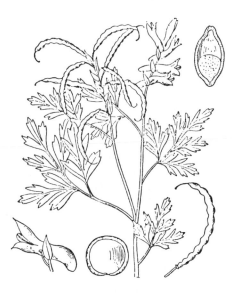

GOLDEN CORYDALIS

DUTCHMAN'S BREECHES   *Dicentra cucullaria* (L.) Bernh. Fumariaceae (*Fumaria c.*)
The whole plant has a lacy appearance. The very finely cut, blue-toned leaves are on their own
stems growing from minute grain like bulblets. The flowering stem, 10-30 cm tall, has flowers
hanging from one side only. These resemble insects alighting on the stem, or a pair of breeches
hung up to dry. They are yellowish white and are followed by brown seed pods with long pointed
ends.

Range. N.B., N.S., Que., Ont., s. to e. Kans., Mo., Ala. and Ga. in rich woods.
Common names. Indian boys and girls, colic weed, kitten breeches, monk's hood.

TURKEY CORN   *Dicentra canadensis* (Goldie) Walp. (*Corydalis c.*)
The leaves grow from yellowish-brown tubers the size of grains of corn, about twice as large as
the grains of Dutchman's breeches. The leaves look alike but the flowers are purplish-pink, without a long spur, their wings appearing closed. They can be greenish white with a purple tinge.
Range. New Engl. s. Que., s. Ont., Minn., s. to Mo., Tenn., and N.C. in rich woods.
Common names. Squirrel corn, bleeding heart.
1633 Gerarde-Johnson 1089. "Fumitorie [*Fumaria officinalis* of Europe] is good for all them that
have either scabs or any other filth growing on the skinne, and for them also that have the
French disease syphilis."
1830 Rafinesque 216. "Dutchman's breeches several species. Root. . .used for tumours, when
eaten gives the colic, the decoction purifies the blood."
1859-61 Gunn 872. "Turkey corn, corydalis, is a powerful and very valuable alterative and tonic.
It is regarded by Eclectic physicians as very nearly a specific in syphilis, and some other constitutional diseases, where a powerful alterative and tonic is needed. . .As a purifier in syphilitic and
scrofulous diseases, it probably has no superior. The only obstacle to its more general use is the
difficulty of procuring it, as the top disappears so soon that there is but a short time, in the early
spring, when it can be found. In consequence of this, but little is gathered, and it is generally
difficult to find in the drug stores. . .Dose of the powder from five to ten grains. . .of the extract (a
fine powder called Corydalia) from half a grain."
1923 H. Smith MENOMINI 81. "Dutchman's breeches. This is one of the most important love
charms of the Menomini. The young swain tries to throw it at his intended and hit her with it.
Another way is for him to chew the root, breathing out so that the scent will carry to her. He
then circles around the girl, and when she catches the scent, she will follow him wherever he
goes, even against her will."
1925 Wood & Ruddock Dutchman's breeches. For syphilis one of the best blood purifiers.
1931 Grieve 822. Turkey corn. This plant is essentially indigenous to America. . .The amount of
alkaloids in the dried tubers is about 5%. . .Corydine is a strong base found in the mother liquor
of Bulbocapnine. . .All these alkaloids have narcotic action. Protopine, first isolated from opium,
has been found in several species of *Dicentra* and *Corydalis*. . .The corydalin sold by druggists is
often impure."
1955 Mockle Quebec transl. 47. "*Dicentra canadensis*, squirrel corn, the tuberous root used for
syphilis and certain skin affections. According to Manske it contains the alkaloids: protopine,
corydine, isocorydine, bulbocapnine. . .*Dicentra cucullaria*. Dutchman's breeches, is used in the
same manner. According to Manske it contains the alkaloids protopine, biscuculline, cryptopine,
allocryptopine, corlumine, cularine, cularidine and ochotensine."
Bulbocapnine is presumed to be hallucinogenic. Cryptopine has a slowing action on the myocar-
dium of the heart but has not been used clinically as an antiarrythmic drug (Lewis and Elvin-
Lewis 1977:191).

PALE CORYDALIS   *Corydalis sempervirens* (L.) Pers. Fumariaceae (*Fumaria s.*)
An upright, bluish, much branched plant. The stem is 30-80 cm tall, the lower leaves stalked, the
upper ones not stalked. The flowering stem bears a cluster of pale pink flowers with yellow tips
(may be white with yellow tip). The 2-4 cm capsule full of seeds is erect.
Range. Lab., Nfld., N.B., P.E.I., N.S., Que., Ungava Bay, Ont. to Yukon, Alaska, s. to B.C., n.
Mont., Minn., and n. Ga. in rocky places, particularly recent burns and clearings. Discussed here
because its chemistry is so similar to the Dicentras.
Common names Rock-harlequin, roman wormwood.
1955 Mockle Quebec transl. 47. *Corydalis sempervirens*, pale Corydalis. "The root is bitter and
astringent and used as an anthelmintic and emmenagogue. It contains the alkaloids: protopine,
cryptopine, 1-adlumine, biscuculline, capnoidine."

GOLDEN CORYDALIS *Corydal⁩s aurea* Willd.

The 20-50 cm tall, many branched stem may recline or stand erect. The flowering stem is 10-30 cm tall with many bright yellow, 13-16 mm long flowers. The 1.5-2.5 cm seed pods spread out and droop.

Range. s. Que., s. Ont., Man. to Yukon, Alaska, s. to Calif., Mex., Tex., Mo., Ohio and Vt. in moist or dry sandy or rocky places.

1932 H. Smith OJIBWE 370. "The Pillager Ojibwe place the root on coals and inhale the smoke for clearing the head and reviving the patient."

1955 Mockle Quebec transl. 47. *Corydalis aurea*, golden corydalis. The root is bitter and astringent and used as an anthelmintic and emmenagogue. According to Manske this plant contains the numerous following alkaloids: protopine, allocryptopine, corydaline, aurotensine, bicucine, biscuculline, capauridine, capaurine, cordrastine, corypalline, corpaverine."

There have not been any cases of human fatalities recorded from eating *Dicentra* or *Corydalis* species in America but if large quantities are eaten the symptoms would be trembling, staggering and convulsions. Use emetics and gastric lavage (Hardin 1974).

Because the alkaloids of Corydalis and Dicentra species are related to those found in the opium poppy, they have been intensively investigated.

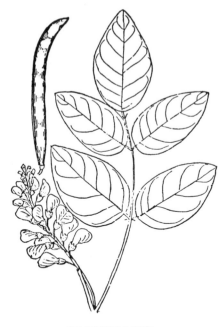

GROUND NUT

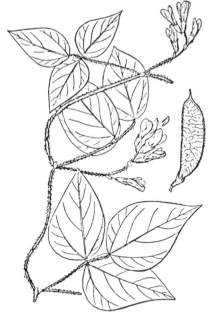

HOG PEANUT

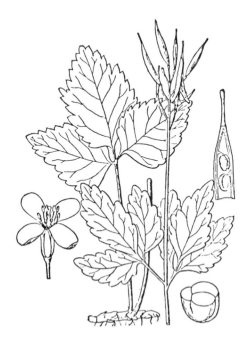

PEPPER ROOT

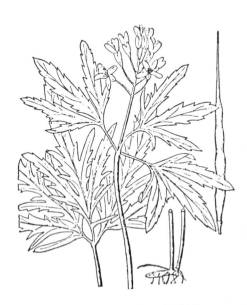

CUT LEAVED TOOTHWORT

GROUND NUT *Apios americana* Medic. Fabaceae (*A. tuberosa, Glycine Apios*)
A slender stem that climbs over bushes and that can be hairy or smooth. The leaves have 5-7 leaflets each 4-6 cm long, smooth or short hairy underneath. The brown-purple flowers are 10-13 mm long, usually many on one stem and very fragrant. The stems contain a milky juice, the roots have a string of tubers.
Range. N.B., N.S., s. Que., s. Ont., s. to Tex., La. and Fla. in rich thickets, moist woods, borders of ponds and marshes. July-Aug.
1590 Harriot Virginia Indians 16. "Openask are a kind of roots or round form, some of the bignes of walnuts, some far greater, which are found in moist and marish grounds growing many together one by another in ropes, or as though they were fastened with a string. Being boiled or sodden they are very good meate."
1604 Champlain-Hakluyt 181. "Wee anchored as high as Saint Croix, which is distant from Quebec fifteen leagues. . .[found] certain small Roots of the bignesse of a little Nut, resembling Musherooms in taste, which are very good roasted and sod [boiled]."
1609 Lescarbot-Erondelle Port Royal 299. "There is yet in the land of the Armouchiquois certain kind of roots as big as a loaf of bread, most excellent for to be eaten, having a taste like the stalks of artichokes but much more pleasant, which being planted do multiply in such sort that it is wonderful. I believe that they be those which be called afrodilles, according to the description that Pliny maketh of them. These roots (saith he) are made after the fashion of small turnips, and there is no plant that hath so many roots as this hath; for sometimes one shall find four score afrodilles tied together. They are good roasted under the embers or eaten raw with pepper, or oil, and salt."
1624 Sagard HURON 330. "They eat them raw as well as cooked, likewise another sort of root, resembling parsnips, which they call Sondhratates, which are in truth far better; but they very seldom gave us any, and that only when they had received some present from us, or when we visited them in their cabins."
1660 Perrot POTAWATOMI Blair 1; 115. "That country also produces potatoes; some as large as an egg, others are the size of one's fist, or a little more. They boil these in water by a slow fire, during twenty four hours; when they are thoroughly cooked, you will find in them an excellent flavor, much resembling that of prunes which are cooked the same way in France, to be served as a desert."
1698 Hennepin 346. Tonti and Father Zenobe: "They were then in such want of provisions, that they had nothing to feed upon but Potatoes, Wild Garlick, and some small roots they had scratched out of the ground with their own fingers."
1749 Kalm Philadelphia March 17th. 259. "Hopniss or Hapniss was the Indian name of a wild plant, which they ate at that time. . .The roots resemble potatoes, and are boiled by the Indians who eat them instead of bread. Some of the Swedes at that time likewise ate this root for want of bread. Some of the English still eat it instead of potatoes. Mr. Bartram told me that the Indians who live farther in the country do not only eat these roots, which have as good a taste as potatoes, but likewise take the peas which lie in the pods of this plant, and prepare them like common peas. Dr. Linne calls this plant *Glycine Apios.*"
1778 Carver 100. "The River St. Pierre. . . the meadows are covered with hops, and many sorts of vegetables; whiles the ground is stored with useful roots, with angelica, spikenard, and ground nuts as large as hen's eggs."
1779 Zeisberger DELAWARE 47. "Of roots, wild potatoes and wild parsnip are found. Bread is baked of both, which one may be driven to eat by pangs of hunger. The Indians look for both when famine threatens and supply of corn runs low, sometimes sustaining life with them for a considerable period."
1791 Long Nipigon 50. "The land affords abundance of wild roots. . .We lived on animal food and roots, reserving our corn and hard grease for the winter."
1882 Can. Hort. 5; 66. "The *Apios tuberosa* or ground nut. This is a little gem; in July and August it is one mass of chocolate colored, pea shaped flowers, which is a very unusual color in flowers. Its leaflets are very pretty also. It grows upon the low bushes of the Northern woods, and often lends a beauty to a hazel bush, which is rarely very fine in itself. The Apios has a tuber, or a number of them, to one plant, like a potato, but smaller. They are nutritious, and would be a good substitute for some of the things we eat. This can be grown in a window, and would be a fine ornament if the tubers were started late in summer so as to throw its flowering season late in

the fall, but as a garden climber it would be fine planted amongst tall-growing summer roses, as it would do them no harm, but lend a beauty to them after they had done blooming."

1916 Waugh IROQUOIS 120. "The common potato, although a native to America, was a comparatively recent introduction among the eastern woodland tribes, arriving there with the general adoption of European products. The tubers of *Apios tuberosa* are often referred to as potatoes and sometimes planted in suitable locations, though they are not, strictly speaking cultivated."

1923 H. Smith MENOMINI 68. "It is difficult to connect the root of this very important 'potato' with its above ground portion. . .The tuberous enlargements of beads are very numerous. . .They run from marble size to three inches in diameter. These 'potatoes' are sweet and starchy and quite palatable raw. they are peeled, parboiled, sliced and dried for winter use. When cooked, maple sugar is used until it thickens to a sticky syrup and the resulting flavor is superior to candied yams."

1928 H. Smith MESKWAKI 259. "This is one of the chief wild potatoes with all of our northern forest Indians. . .The substance is quite white and elastic, and cuts more like a turnip than a potato. . .They are cooked with meat in the winter time."

1933 H. Smith POTAWATOMI 103. "The roots run in a mat through the ground, some of the individual roots running as far as twenty feet."

1955 Mockle Quebec transl. 63. "The tuberous rhizome is farinaceous and the seeds resembling peas are edible."

HOG PEANUT
Amphicarpa bracteata (L.) Fern. Fabaceae

A slender, sparingly branched, hairy, climbing stem bears leaves with three leaflets. The 2-10 pale purple or white flowers are followed by pods that are mostly three seeded. Down near the roots of the plant, on threadlike creeping branches appear tiny blossoms without petals. These flowers are self fertile and produce pods that contain one big light brown seed about the size and shape of a peanut.

Range N.B., N.S., s. Que., s. Ont., s. Man., e. Sask., Mont. S. to Fla. and Tex. Aug-Sept. in woods and thickets.

Common names. Wild peanut, american licorice, pea vine.

1779 Zeisberger DELAWARE 47. "A kind of bean, called by the Indians earth bean, because it grows close to the ground, is also found and tastes when boiled like a chestnut."

1926-27 Densmore CHIPPEWA 320. The root of this plant was boiled and eaten. . .346. The root was used in combination with other roots in a decoction drunk as a general physic.

1928 H. Smith MESKWAKI 259. "When the mice gather these small nuts from underground, in the fall and store them in heaps, the Meskwaki collect these heaps and take them home to eat."

1932 H. Smith OJIBWE 405. "Ojibwe name translates 'unusual red bean'. The Pillager Ojibwe cook the beans and are very fond of the unusual flavor imparted to their cooking in this way. They also cook the roots, although they are really too small to be considered of much importance."

1939 Medsger 189. "The underground seed is more agreeable than a raw peanut, in fact it is very pleasant eating. These large seeds are often quite abundant and appear beneath the dead leaves, generally just under the surface of the ground [see Hennepin under groundnut]. . .The Dakota nations when taking these seeds from the nests of animals left corn or other food in exchange." Hog peanuts are approximately 25% protein. . .The tough outer shell is easily removed by boiling. . .soak beans in warm water or water with hardwood ashes added if eating raw" (Weiner 1972: 53)

CUT LEAVED TOOTHWORT
Dentaria laciniata Muhl. Cruciferae (Brassicaceae)

The root narrows in places, making finely joined segments each 2-3 cm long. The stem is 20-40 cm tall, its top part hairy, the hairs each 0.2-0.3 mm. The leaves are deeply three parted, the parts cut so as to appear there are five.

Range. s. Que., s. Ont., Minn., s. to Fla., La. and Okla. Apr.-May in moist rich woods.

Common names. Pepper root, purple flowered toothwort.

PEPPER ROOT
Dentaria diphylla Michx.

This plant has a long root all in one piece and often branched, from it grows a 20-40 cm tall stem with two stalked, opposite leaves. These leaves each have three leaflets, their teeth large, the edges hairy, the hairs 0.1 mm long. The white flowers have 4 petals, 11-17 mm long followed by long upright seed pods.

Range. N.B., N.S., s. Que., s. Ont., s. to Mich., Ky. and S.C. in rich woods.

Common names. Crinkle root, white flowered toothwort.

Dentaria maxima resembles *diphylla* except that its root is thicker in places, its flowers are pale purple, and there are more leaves. It is found in s. Que. and s. Ont. to Wisc. s. to Tenn. and Pa.

1070-1320 Juntunen site Mich. Carbonized tubers of *D. laciniata* including *D. maxima*, found at three locations archeologically in the site. Yarnell 1964:36.

1916 Waugh IROQUOIS 120. "Crinkle root, *Dentaria diphylla*. . .the roots eaten raw with salt. Some boil them. A Mohawk recipe is to wash the roots and add vinegar, also *Dentaria laciniata* [roots were eaten]."

1923 H. Smith MENOMINI 65. "The running rootstock of this cress [*D. maxima*] literally mats the ground where there is a rich forest loam, wet by a spring. The tiny thread root that connects the main stem with the rootstock is so frail that it is difficult to associate the subterranean root with the leaf and flower, but finally we were able to dig one in the spring of the year, with a flower that had just withered and determined its genus and species. It is a 'potato' much relished by the Menomini, but has a pungent, acrid taste when it is freshly dug. The mass of cleaned roots is accordingly heaped on a blanket and covered to exclude the air. Then there is a natural process of fermentation for four or five days, following which the roots are found to be sweet. The Menomini cook it with corn, and say that, besides being good to eat, it is a good medicine for the stomach."

1932 H. Smith OJIBWE 399. "The rootstocks of this cress are very abundant in wet, springy ground in the forest. The white man can only identify this plant in the spring of the year when the flower and leaf are found, but the Ojibwe knows the root and where it grows so gathers it when it has matured. It is a favored wild potato, but has a very pungent acrid taste when freshly dug."

[The roots have a mustard and cress flavor and can be used as a relish]

1945 Rousseau MOHAWK trans. 45. "An infusion of the roots of pepperoot and those of yellow lady's slipper was given in the begining of tuberculosis. In the spring the whole plant is eaten to 'reinforce the chest' (strengthen the lungs?). . .Most of the Cruciferae [now Brassicaceae], an important source of vitamins for populations at the stage of gatherers, are antiscorbutic. One understands their use as tonics when they are fresh, but it is doubtful that the boiled roots contain any vitamins."

1974 Antoine King Go-Home Bay Lake Huron personal communication. Used root for food.

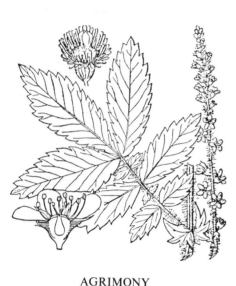

AGRIMONY

TALL HAIRY AGRIMONY

TALL HAIRY AGRIMONY

Agrimonia gryposepala Wallr. Rosaceae

The 50 to 150 cm tall stem is covered with short, gland tipped hairs. The main leaves have 5 to 9 pairs of leaflets opposite each other on each stalk. These leaflets have broad teeth, are almost smooth on top and hairy beneath on their veins. Where the flower stalk grows from the stem there are long spreading hairs. The little yellow, rose-like flowers, 6-12 mm across, grow one above the other up this flowering stalk. The five yellow petals when in bud and when faded are enclosed by green outer petals (sepals) that fold over them, making a tiny, turban shaped dome. This dome sits on a rim from which stand out two rows of hooked bristles.

Range. N.B., P.E.I., N.S., Que., Ont., N. Dak., s. to Kans., Mo., Tenn. and N.C. in thickets and borders of woods.

Common names. Feverfew, beggar's -ticks, cockle-bur, stickseed.

A. Eupatoria the European plant introduced in n. America. Early reports of the use of this herb refer to the indigenous *A. striata*

AGRIMONY

Agrimonia striata Michx

The whole plant is softly downy. The stout stem to 1 m tall hairy and with glands on the top part. The larger leaves consist of 7-11 leaflets which are conspicuously covered with glands beneath. Flowers crowded together.

Range. Nfld., N.B., P.E.I., N.S., Que., Ont., Man., S. to Ariz., N. Mex., Nebr. Io., Ohio., and N.J. in thickets and borders of woods.

1475 Bjornnson Icelandic mss Larsen transl. 56. "Eupatorium. . .has power to make one thin and to cleanse, and therefore it lessens pain of the liver and purges it thoroughly and opens what is stopped up. Its seed crushed with paunch-fat of swine is good for old wounds and such as grow poorly. It helps also for fever. . ."

1633 Gerarde-Johnson 712. "The decoction of the leaves of agrimony is good for them that have naughty livers, and for such as pisse bloud upon the diseases of the kidnies. The seed being drunke in wine. . .doth help the bloudy flixe. . .a remedy for such as are bitten with serpents."

1650 Representation New Neth. 298. "The medicinal plants found in New Netherlands up to the present time, by little search, as far as they have come to our knowledge. . .agrimony." [One of more than 30 listed].

1785 Cutler. "It is said the Indians used an infusion of the roots in inflammatory fevers, with great success. Dr. Hill says an infusion of six ounces of the crown of the root in a quart of boiling water, sweetened with honey, and a half a pint drank three times a day, is an effectual cure for the jaundice."

1799 Lewis Mat. Med. 81. "The leaves said to be aperient, detergent and to strengthen the tone of the viscera; hence it is recommended in scorbutic disorders, a debility and laxity of the intestines, &c. Digested in whey it forms a useful diet drink for the spring season, not ungrateful to the palate or stomach, attenuent and tonic."

1812 Peter Smith. "Agrimony is a valuable medicine both the herb and the root. It is a tonic or strengthener of the system and affects most sensibly the regions of the kidneys and bladder. A tea or powder of this simple is a remedy for diabetes, or involuntary emission of the urine. I conclude it is very advisable to give it either as a tea for breakfast and supper, or as a diet drink, whenever we wish to promote nervous strength. The roots may be boiled in milk or water, and given in dysentery and other fluxes. It is the high Canadian agrimony that I recommend. . .An old man of my acquaintance. . .was for several months unable to retain his urine. . .He was advised by Dr. George Faulk to drink agrimony tea. This tea, being the only medicine he used, he became a well man in a few days, being as free from this complaint as in his youth and he was then above 80 years of age."

1828 Rafinesque 36. "A mild astringent, tonic and corroborant. Useful in coughs, and bowel complaints. Being a very mild astringent, it may be given in diarrhea, dysentery and relaxed bowels. It has been recommended for many other complaints, and is said to have cured asthma. The best way to take it, is in a strong decoction sweetened with honey or Maidenhair syrup. The dose is four cups every day. Both the roots and the plant may be boiled. . .262. The roots and the whole plant boiled in milk are used by herbalists for diabetes and incontinence of urine. One of their remedies for the tape-worm is agrimony tea, with alum and honey. The roots are said to be more astringent than the leaves, the Indians use them in fever, and some empirics for jaundice with honey. It is said to be diuretic and vulnerary."

1833 Howard Quebec 95. "To cure a Rupture—Take Agrimony, spleen wort, Solomon's seal and strawberry root of each a handful—pick and well wash them—stamp and boil them 2 hours in 2 quarts of white wine in a vessel closely stopt down—strain it and drink a large glass of it every morning, and drink another in an hour after. It commonly cures in a fortnight. . .123. To cure bloody urine. Take twice a day a pint of decoction of agrimony or of yarrow.124. To cure involuntary urine. Take a tablespoon of powdered agrimony in a little water morning and evening."

1859-61 Gunn 735. "Both the root and the leaves are used but mostly usually the leaves only. It is a mild and safe astringent and somewhat tonic, and is used in the form of a tea or decoction in bowel complaints, fevers. . .may be used freely. It can generally be found in drug-stores."

1868 Can. Pharm. J. 6; 83-5. The root and leaves of *Agrimonia Eupatoria* [*A. striata*] included in list of Can. medicinal plants.

1928 H. Smith MESKWAKI 241. "*A. gryposepela*, the root of this is used as a styptic to stop nosebleed."

1932 H. Smith OJIBWE 384. "*A. gryposepala*, the Flambeau Ojibwe use the root with other ingredients as a medicine for urinary troubles."

1933 H. Smith POTAWATOMI 76. "*Agrimonia gryposepala*. The Forest Potawatomi have no medical use for this plant to our knowledge, but the Prairie Potawatomi. . .use the plant as a styptic and snuff an infusion up the nostrils to stop nosebleed. . .The U.S. Dispensatory 1916 says that Indians in Canada and the United States have used the root for reducing fevers."

1955 Mockle Quebec transl. 58. "The leaves are used in infusion and as a gargle for their astringent properties in light diarrhea and inflammation of the throat; they are also used in renal infections such as nephritis."

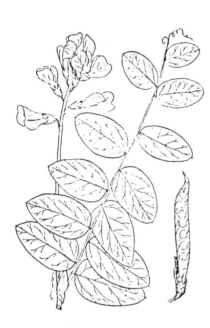

VEINY PEA

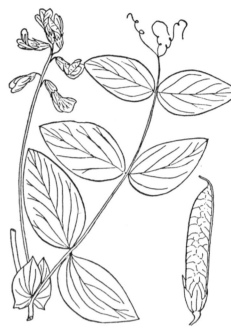

CREAM COLORED VETCHLING

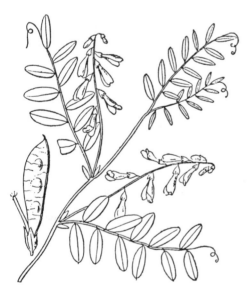

WOOD VETCH

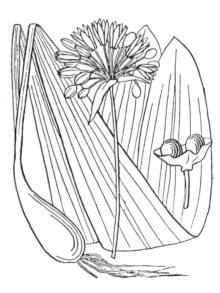

WILD LEEK

VEINY PEA *Lathyrus venosus* Muhl. var. *intonsus* Butters & St. John Fabaceae

The stems are strongly four angled and hairy, up to 100 cm long. The leaflets at the base of the leaf stem (stipules) are narrow with sharp basal lobes. There are 8-12 leaflets each 3-6 cm long with a pointed tip at their ends. The purple flowers are 12-20 mm long with 10-20 flowers on each stem. The pods are 4-7.5 cm long.

Range. s. Ont. to Minn. and Sask., s. to Ind. and Mo. as well as in the mts. of e. W. Va., w. Va., N.C. and Tenn. and one station in e. Que. June-July in moist woods, thickets and drywoods.

1624 Sagard HURON 90. Saw them eat wild peas.

1646 HURON Jes. Rel. 31; 91. Gave the Jesuits "certain seeds to eat, but so insipid and dangerous that they served as a very quick poison to those who knew not how to prepare them". [Could refer to wild peas which have caused distress when eaten in Europe.]

1926-27 Densmore CHIPPEWA 336. The root, dried and rubbed into powder, taken in decoction for convulsions. If the convulsions were so severe that only a little of the decoction could be forced into the patients mouth, the decoction was sprinkled on the chest and applied to the palms of the hands and soles of the feet. When the decoction was made from the veiny pea, and dogbane, the pea root was so strong that the amount used was measured from the last joint to the tip of the little finger. The amount of dogbane was about one foot of root. There were said to be 8 varieties of pea plants that were equally good. . .356. The root was boiled and used as a poultice for hemorrhages from wounds. Also the decoction was drunk, this was said to act as an emetic if blood from a wound had accumulated inside a patient. . .364. A decoction of the root was drunk as a tonic and stimulant. One dose of this had no effect, results being obtained only by considerable quantity of the remedy. . .376. The root was carried on the person as a charm to insure success, especially when the person was in extreme anxiety concerning the outcome of circumstances. . .290. Seeds eaten as food.

CREAM COLORED VETCHLING *Lathyrus ochroleucus* Hook. Fabaceae

A slender, somewhat angled, smooth stem up to 80 cm long, the leaflets at the base of the leaf stem (stipule) are 1.5-3 cm with only one lobe at their base which is often toothed. There are 3-5 pairs of thin leaflets. 2.5-5 cm long. There are 5-10 yellowish white flowers 12-15 mm long. The pods are from 2.5 to 5 cm long.

Range. w. Que. to B.C., Vt. s. to Pa., Ill., Io., and Wash. May-July in dry upland woods and thickets, and on river banks.

1919 Sturtevant 327. "The seeds of (*L. aphaca*) the European yellow flowered pea are sometimes served at table while young and tender but if eaten abundantly in the ripe state are narcotic, producing severe headache."

1932 H. Smith OJIBWE 372. "John Peper, Pillager Ojibwe, said that the foliage was fed to a pony to make him lively for a race. The Flambeau Ojibwe. . .say it is used for stomach trouble. By white men, it is considered one of the loco weeds, bad for horses. . .406. The Pillager Ojibwe use the root of this plant as a sort of Indian potato, and store it in deep pits in the garden, as they do their regular potatoes."

1966 Campbell, Best & Budd. 87. "Vetches have characters similar to many other legumes. They produce nodules on their roots which contain bacteria to synthesize atmospheric nitrogen. . .They are useful for green manuring, and are fair to good bee pasture. However, it is doubtful if vetches generally are as palatable to livestock as most other legumes. . .Chemical analyses reveal a high spring and early summer protein content and a relatively low crude fibre percentage."

1968 Forsyth England 62. "In America a cyanogenetic glycoside has been found in the seeds of common vetch. The toxicity of the seeds of most species of Lathyrus, particularly for horses has long been recognised. . .During exercise the horse became suddenly. . .near suffocation, and fell to the ground apparently suffering from paralysis of the hind quarters. . .A very similar condition. . .known as lathyrism affects human beings."

1975 Trevor Robinson 233. "The neurotoxic effects of eating certain species of *Lathyrus* can be attributed to their content of certain peculiar amino acids."

WOOD VETCH *Vicia caroliniana* Walt. Fabaceae.

A slender trailing or climbing stem up to 1 m long. The leaflets usually in 5-9 pairs, each one 1-2 cm long. The flowering stalks 6-10 cm long with 7-20 white flowers each 7.5 to 12 mm long tipped with blue sometimes. Pods 1.5-3 cm long.

Range. N.Y., Ont., Minn., Wis., s. to Tex. and Fla. in open woods in the spring.

1885 Mooney CHEROKEE 325. "*Vicia Caroliniana*—Decoction drunk for dyspepsia and pains in the back, rubbed on the stomach for cramp; also rubbed on ball-players after scratching to render their muscles tough, and used in the same way after scratching, in the disease. . .in which one side becomes black in spots, with partial paralysis; also used in same manner in decoction with *Gnaphalium decurrens*, life everlasting, for rheumatism; considered one of their most valuable medicinal herbs."

See wet open places for other wild peas.

WILD LEEK
Allium tricoccum Ait. Liliaceae

The 2-6 cm long conical white bulb sends up a furled pencil of two or three leaves. These will attain a total length of 20-30 cm including a slender stalk and a flat blade 10-20 cm long and from 2-6 cm wide. The 15-60 cm tall flowering stalk has at its end a cluster of white flowers which are followed by three lobed seed cases. The leaves disappear before the flowers are produced.

Range. s. Que. and N. Engl. to Minn., s. to N.C., Tenn. and Va. June-July in rich woods, often in large colonies.

Common names. Ramps, three seeded leek, wild garlic.

1624 Sagard HURON 239. "They also have little onions named anonque, which put out only two leaves like those of the lily-of-the-valley, they smell of garlic as much as of onion. We used them for putting into our sagamite to give it a flavour. . .The savages eat them baked in ashes when quite ripe and full grown, but never in soup any more than all other kinds of herbs, of which they make very little account although purslane is very common and grows naturally."

1649 Rageneau Jes. Rel. 34. In time of famine. . ."those who have none [other food], live partly on garlic baked under the ashes, or cooked in water without sauce."

1660 Perrot 1; 115. "These tribes of the prairies also find in certain places lands that are fertile, and kept moist by the streams that water them, whereon grow onions of the size of one's thumb. . .One imagines that it is a certain wild garlic, which is quite common in the same places, and has also an insupportable acridness. When the savages lay in a store of these onions, with which the ground is covered, they first build an oven, upon which they place the onions, covering them with a thick layer of grass, and by means of the heat which the fire communicates to them, the acrid quality leaves them, nor are they damaged by the flame; and after they have been dried in the sun, they become an excellent article of food. Their abundance, however, counts for nothing, although the agreeable taste which one finds in them often induces him to satisfy his appetite with them; for nothing in the world is more indigestible and less nourishing. You feel a load on your chest, your belly is as hard as a drum, and colic pains which last two or three days. When one is forewarned of this effect, he refrains from eating much of this root. I speak from experience having been taken unawares by it; after the distress I experienced I have no longer any desire to taste it."

1698 Hennepin HURON 579. "Our common food was the same as the savages, viz. Sagamite, or Pottage made of Water and Indian Corn with Gourds; To give it Relish we put into it Marjoram, and a sort of Balm, with wild Onions which we found in the Woods and Fields."

1710 Raudot Quebec 386. "This country produces a quantity of roots and kinds of onions of which these savages eat a great deal."

1775-76 Long St. Lawrence 20. "I was immediately ordered on a scout at the head of ten Connecedaga or Rondaxe Indians, with Captain La Motte, a Canadian gentleman. . .We were out six days and nights, with very little provisions, living chiefly on the scrapings of the inner bark of trees and wild roots, particularly onions, which grow in great abundance, and are not disagreeable to the palate. Hunger reconciles us to everything that will support nature, and makes the most indifferent food acceptable. From my own woeful experience I can assert that what at any other time would have been unpleasant and even nauseous, under the pressure of hunger is not only greedily eaten, but relished as a luxury."

1829 Head Kempenfeldt Bay, Ont. 11th. April. 242. "I discovered a quantity of wild leeks just shooting up out of the earth, of which I gathered a good many. I was unfortunate in this, my first essay on vegetable diet, for they heated me to such a degree, that I was for some time afraid they had possessed some deleterious quality; but the intolerable high flavour of the plant quieted my apprehensions. I was in a burning fever, at the same time quite sure that I had eaten nothing but leeks. Though they abounded all over the woods, for a long time afterwards I was too well satisfied with my first dose ever to try another."

1916 Waugh IROQUOIS 118. Eaten while young and tender.

1926-27 Densmore CHIPPEWA 346. As an emetic make a decoction of one root, the proper amount for a dose. It is quick in its effect.

1923 H. Smith MENOMINI 69. "This is the larger wild onion known as the hero's onion, or the one pointed out by Manapus for food. It is very highly esteemed by the Menomini and sought especially in the spring. It is then much rounder and plumper than in the fall when it is shrunken. It is also gathered and dried for future use. It is somewhat bitter to the taste." The Ojibwe and Potawatomi also use this leek for food, fresh and dried for storage.

1928 H. Smith MESKWAKI 262. "Cook it with deer meat."

1955 Mockle Quebec transl. 28. "Substitute for cultivated garlic. Marker and his collaborators isolated a saponin, tigogenin in the proportion of 0.1 gr/kg. of the dried material from this onion."

1970 Dore 35. "The species gathered most in the East—at least, the one talked-up the most, is the broad-leaved wild leek. . .often referred to, lovingly but usually whimsically, as 'ramps'. The flavour of ramps is strong and the pervading odour they expel is so overwhelming that it provokes such descriptions as 'the kind of spring tonic that everybody needs,' 'the true test of friendship'. . .Farmers, of course, detest this plant of their pastureland; it taints the cattle's milk."

1970 Bye IROQUOIS mss. Possibly cultivated by the Iroquois.

1979 Maugh Science 204; 293. "Onions and their close cousin garlic, have long been reputed to have almost mystical medical powers. Among those alleged powers are the ability to stimulate bile production, to lower blood sugar, to alleviate hypertension, to speed healing of gunshot wounds, and to cure scorpion bites, freckles, and the common cold. Moses Attrep Jr. of East Texas State University was intrigued by the reports that onions could lower blood pressure and guessed. . .that this effect might be produced by a prostaglandin. . .He isolated the compound. . .and primarily by mass spectroscopy, identified it as prostaglandin A_1, which is known to be antihypertensive. . .present at a concentration of only about 1 part per million, in *Allium cepa*, suggesting it might have a therapeutic effect only if very large quantities of onions are consumed."

Allium cepa is the common garden onion. Whether *A. tricoccum* contains prostaglandin A, is not known.

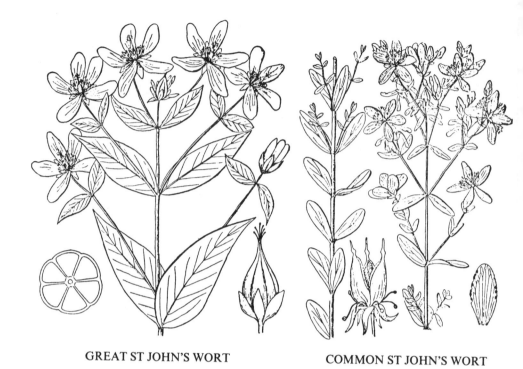

GREAT ST JOHN'S WORT

COMMON ST JOHN'S WORT

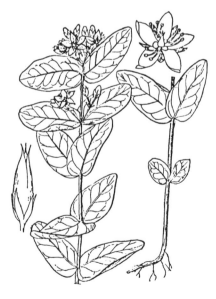

SPOTTED ST JOHN'S WORT

MARSH ST JOHN'S WORT

GREAT ST JOHN'S WORT   *Hypericum pyramidatum* Ait. Hypericaceae (*H. ascyron*)
Stem 50-150 cm tall with branches. The leaves partly clasping the stem 4-9 cm long. The yellow
petals 2.5 cm long. The pods 2-3 cm long; five-celled.
Range. n. Me., Que., s. Ont., s. to Kans., Mo., O. and Md. in rich thickets and moist ground.

COMMON ST JOHN'S WORT   *Hypericum perforatum* L.
A somewhat 2-edged stem with many branches. Leaves without stalks, covered with black dots
seen when held against the light. These contain an essential oil. The bright yellow petals of the
flowers are black dotted only on their edges. Pod three-celled.
Range. Native of Europe now found from Nfld., N.B., P.E.I., N.S., Que., Ont., throughout U.S.
in meadows and roadsides.

SPOTTED ST JOHN'S WORT   *Hypericum punctatum* Lam.
The stem round with few branches. The leaves conspicuously covered with black dots. The
flowers crowded together, the petals pale yellow marked with dark lines and dots. Pods three-
celled.
Range. N.S., Que., Ont., to Minn., s. to Tex. and Fla. in thickets and damp grounds.

MARSH ST JOHN'S WORT   *Hypericum virginicum* L. (*Elodea v., Triadenum v.*)
Small erect marsh plant, the leaves clasping the stem are black dotted. Flowers with red-purple
petals, the entire plant often looks red or purple.
Range. Lab. Nfld., N.B., N.S., Que., Ont., Man., Sask. s. to Nebr., Ark., Ala. and Ga. in wet
sands, boggy and swampy ground.
1633 Gerarde-Johnson 541. "St. Johns wort [*H. perforatum*] with his floures and seed byled and
drunken, provoketh urine, and is right good against the stone in the bladder, and stoppeth the
laske. The leaves stamped are good to be layd upon burnings, scaldings, and all wounds; and
also for rotten and filthy ulcers. The leaves, floures, and seeds stamped, and put into a glasse
with oyle olive, and set in the hot Sunne for certaine weekes together, and then strained from
those herbes, and the like quantitie of new put in, and sunned in like manner, doth make an oyle
of the colour of bloud, which is a most precious remedy for deepe wounds, and those that are
thorow the body, for sinewes that are prickt, or any wound made with a venomed weapon. . .The
seed drunke for the space of forty days together cureth the Sciatica, and all aches that happen to
the hips."
1785 Cutler St. John's wort, blossoms yellow. "The small dots upon the leaves, which appear like
so many perforations are said to contain an essential oil. The leaves are given to destroy worms.
The flowers tinge spirits and oil of a fine purple colour."
1799 Lewis Mat. Med. 160. "Hypericum has long been celebrated. . .in maniacal disorders; it has
been reckoned of such efficacy in the latter as to have thence received the name fuga daemonum.
It was also recommended internally for wounds, bruises, ulcers, spitting of blood, bloody urine,
agues and worms. . .however it is now rarely brought into practice."
1830 Rafinesque 229-30. "*H. perforatum* bad weed in fields. . .Blossoms chiefly used, although
yellow they dye oils red, infused in sweet oil or bears grease, they make a fine red balsamic ointment for wounds, sores, swellings, ulcers, tumors, rough skin, &c. The tea of the leaves gives
relief in diseases of the breast and lungs. Used for many disorders by empirics. . .A syrup made
with sage, specific for croup, dose a tablespoon full for a 12 months child, half if 6 months old.
Used with *Iris* and *Sanguinaria* for sore mouths and throat. An ointment of it with bittersweet,
elder bark and Datura, said to be a specific for hard breast and tumors. Other sp. are mostly
equal. . .*H. virginicum* Tincture of flowers used in cholics, against vomiting, &c."
1849-61 Gunn 866. "*H. perforatum*. . .The leaves and blossoms are the part used. . .a strong
tea. . .in suppression of urine, and in chronic affections of the urinary organs."
1868 Can. Pharm. J. 6; 83-5. St. John's wort, *H. perforatum*, tops and flowers included in list of
Can. medicinal plants.
1892 Millspaugh 30. "This European emigrant [*H. perforatum*] has become so thoroughly naturalized with us as to become a very troublesome weed upon our farm-lands. . .The great use of

Hypericum in wounds where the nerves are involved to any extent is the rightful discovery of the true science of medicine. . .Many cases of injury to the cranium and spinal column are reported benefited by its use; and every homeopathic physician of at least three months practice can attest to its merits."

1915 Speck MONTAGNAIS 314. "St. John's wort, (*H. perforatum*) 'goldenwood' is boiled to make a cough medicine."

1923 H. Smith MENOMINI 38. "Great St. John's Wort. This is a very important Menomini remedy. The root is used in connection with others for weak lungs, and if taken in the first stages of consumption, it is thought by the Menominis to be specific. In compound with blackcap raspberry root, it is used for kidney troubles. The leaves of this species have been formerly employed by the white man as a laxative, alterative and vulnerary. It has also been used by him internally as an emmenagogue, diuretic and stimulating expectorant. The fresh drug is given internally in the treatment of chronic catarrhal conditions of the respiratory, intestinal and urinary apparatuses, thus paralleling the Menomni use."

1928 H. Smith MESKWAKI 223. "Great St. John's wort. The Meskwaki use this root in connection with others to cure tuberculosis. McIntosh said that if it was used in the first stages of consumption it was a cure. . .The Meskwaki boil the root and use it for a dusting powder to place upon the bite of a water moccasin, to draw the poison and heal it."

1933 H. Smith POTAWATOMI 60. "Marsh St. John's wort. The Forest Potawatomi claim that this plant contains three different kinds of medicine. In one of these the leaves are used to make a tea to cure fevers. Among the white people this plant is considered to have aromatic, astringent, resolvent and nervine properties. . .The tea of the flowers supresses urine. . .Externally it has been used in a fomentation or used as an ointment to dispel hard tumors, caked breasts, bruises, etc."

1955 Mockle Quebec transl. 51. "*H. perforatum*. The leaves and flowers resolutive, vulnerary and vermifuge. The essence of the flowering tops is used in the external treatment of contusions, burns, ulcers."

In eastern north America *H. perforatum* is reported to produce photosensitization in domestic cattle. Since the pigment that causes this reaction is contained in the pigment found in the glandular dots it is reasonable to assume that *H. punctatum* also probably has the same properties. A very tiny amount of hypericin will cause reaction in white skinned animals. Ordinary window glass or a layer of water will not protect them. Black skinned animals are rarely affected. In Holstein cattle the white skin hangs in rags and the black skin is soft and supple. The animals develop intense itching and become almost demented. Dried hay containing St. John's wort is just as dangerous as fresh. Touching the plants will not affect the animals they must eat it. In California, where the ranges were full of St. John's wort, a beetle that feeds specifically on this plant was imported, and now only scattered stands of it remain (Kingsbury 1964:171-5).

The flowering tops are gathered as they start to flower, no seeds can be included. They are dried as quickly as possible. It is taken internally to improve blood circulation, and the basic metabolism, it also heals and reduces inflammation. It is used in the treatment of depression and disturbed sleep and as a specific for gastric and intestinal catarrh accompanied by diarrhoea. Externally it is chopped up in oil and put on wounds, burns and hemorrhoids. It should be cultivated (Stary & Jirasek 1973:138).

One of the most interesting quinones both chemically and physiologically is the substance hypericin which is found in the petals, stems, and leaves of St. John's Wort. Animals eating these plants become highly sensitized to light as a result of this compound becoming concentrated in the skin. The biochemistry of this sensitization is unknown. Possibly the actual irritants are peroxides formed in the presence of light. Other species of *Hypericum* contain a second, similar pigment named pseudohypericin (Trevor Robinson 1975:124).

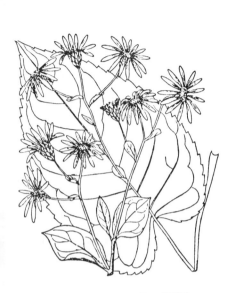

LARGE LEAVED ASTER

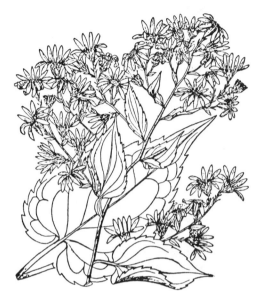

COMMON BLUE WOOD ASTER

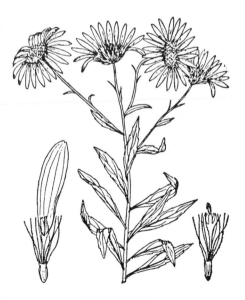

BOG ASTER

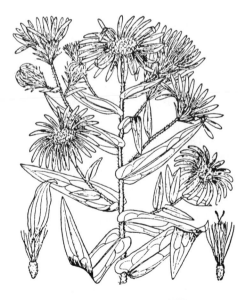

NEW ENGLAND ASTER

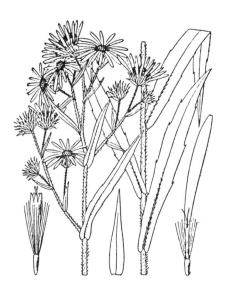

**RED STALKED OR
PURPLE STEMMED ASTER**

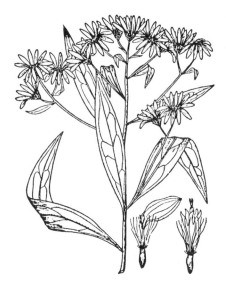

FLAT TOPPED WHITE ASTER

LARGE LEAVED ASTER   *Aster macrophyllus* L. Compositae (Asteraceae)
The large green leaves growing on the forest floor are those of this aster. The plants with
flowering stems are often found at the edges of the wood. The leaves have a heart shaped base,
are rough, thick with broad teeth. The flowers at the top of the sometimes reddish angular stem
have stalks covered with brown, gland-tipped hairs. The 9-20 pale violet rays (petals) are 7-15
mm long. The centre disk is brown.
Range. N.B., Que., to Wis., and Minn., s. to Pa., and Ind., and in the mts to Ga. in woods, and
dry shaded places.

COMMON BLUE WOOD ASTER   *Aster cordifolius* L.
The smooth 20-120 cm tall stem may have loose hairs in lines and many bushy branches. The
leaves are thin, rough, hairy beneath. Very many small violet or blue flowers on stalks without
hairs. They have 8-20 rays (petals) 5-10 mm long.
Range. N.S., to Minn., s. to Ga. and Mo. in woods and thickets.
Common names. Tongue, bee-weed.

BOG ASTER   *Aster nemoralis* Ait.
A slender upright 10-60 cm stem covered with slightly sticky hairs. The many narrow stalkless
leaves, 12-50 mm x 12 mm are rough above with a conspicuous centre vein their edges often curling under, with sticky hairs on the veins beneath. There is a fine fringe of hair around the edge
of the leaf. The flowers are usually solitary on long thin stalks. There are 13-27 bright purplish
pink rays (petals) 9-15 mm long around a golden centre. A beautiful little flower.
Range. Nfld. to Lake Superior, s. to N.J., N.Y. and Mich. in acid bogs, or on sandy or peaty
shores of lakes and ponds.

NEW ENGLAND ASTER   *Aster novae-angliae* L.
A cluster of strong, 30-200 cm tall stems covered with hairs that carry glands on those near the

top of the plant. The leaves clasp the stem with a lobe on each side. They are longer than wide, without teeth, hairy and roughish. There are many large conspicuous violet-purple flowers with 45-100, 1-2 cm long rays. The stalks of the flowers are covered with glands.

Range. Vt., Mass., s. Que., Ont. to Alta. s. to Wyo., N.M., Ark. and Ala. in moist open or wooded places.

RED STALKED OR PURPLE STEMMED ASTER   *Aster puniceus* L.

The stout, red or purple stem is 0.4-2.5 m tall and obviously covered with white hairs. The leaves clasp it with lobes on each side. They are toothed, rough on top, rub a finger along the top of the leaf towards the stem, and have hairs on the veins beneath. There are no glands on any of the hairs. The 30-60 blue or rose or white rays (petals) are 7-18 mm long. The aster found in moist places that looks like this one is the Great Northern Aster, *Aster modestus*, which has glands on the green leaflets under the rays of the flowers. Its range is more western and overlaps in the northern part of the range.

Range. Nfld., New Engl. to s. Man., s. to Iowa, Ala. in swamps and moist places.

FLAT TOPPED WHITE ASTER   *Aster umbellatus* Mill. (*Doellingeria u., Diplopappus u.*) The

usually smooth stem is 20-30 cm tall with many flowers on branching stems at the top, but the top of the whole plant looks flat. The leaves are long, narrow, without teeth but with an edge of fine hairs. The upper surface is dark green, the under lighter with fine cross veining. There are 30-300 heads of white flowers, the 7-14 rays each 5-8 mm long around a golden centre.

Range. Nfld. to s. Alta., s. to Neb., Ga. and Ken. in most low places.

1708 Sarrazin-Vaillant, Quebec-Paris, Boivin 1978 transl. 26. "The physicians of Canada have always considered this plant a Betony [the European *Betonica officinalis* cultivated in gardens] and use it as one." Aster Coronae solis folio, Sarrac. sent in 1698. Boivin notes *Aster* (*?macrophyllus*).

1708 circa, Jussieu Paris. List of plants sent him by Sarrazin from Quebec with Sarrazin's comments on the plants. This list is reproduced in an unreadable form in Vallée's book on Sarrazin who states on p. 59 that Sarrazin wrote "*Aster corona* is used by certain people in the same way betony is, whose emetic and purgative properties are praised, although its action is revulsive and its use known since Galen in epilepsy and convulsions."

1830 Rafinesque 198. "Aster, Starwort. . .Never before introduced in Materia Medica. I am indebted to Dr. Lawrence, of New Lebanon, for the following indications. The *Aster novae angliae* is employed in decoction internally, with a strong decoction externally, in many eruptive diseases of the skin: it removes also the poisonous state of the skin caused by Rhus [poison ivy] or Shumac [poison sumac]. The *A. cordifolius* is an excellent aromatic nervine, in many cases preferable to Valerian. Many other species must be equally good, such as *A. puniceus* and those with a strong scent: they ought to be tried as equivalents of Valerian in epilepsy, spasms, hysterics, &c."

1915 Speck MOHEGAN 319. "Indian tea, *Aster umbellatus*, steep the dried leaves for tea."

1926-27 Densmore CHIPPEWA 320. "Aster species doubtful. This plant grows near Lake Superior. The leaves are boiled with fish and eaten with fish. . .360. *A. nemoralis*. A decoction of the plant is dropped in the ear or applied on a warm cloth for soreness in the ear. Use lukewarm water. . .376. *A. novae-angliae* the root is smoked in a pipe to attract game. *A. puniceus*, the fine tendrils of the root are smoked with tobacco to attract game." [Unable to find that Densmore wrote 1928-287 that powdered root of *A. novae-angliae* smoked by Ojibwa "in earliest times" Yarnell 1964:181.]

1928 H. Smith MESKWAKI 211-12. "The smooth aster (*A. laevis*) The entire plant is used to furnish smoke in the sweat bath, and it is also smudged as a reviver of consciousness for one who is ill. A paper cone is fitted over the nostrils of the unconscious one and this smoke forced into the nostrils to revive him. The calico or starved aster (*A. lateriflorus*), the entire plant is used as a smoke or steam in the sweat bath. The blossoms only are smudged to cure a crazy person who has lost his mind. White wreath aster (*A multiflorus*) is used as a reviver of consciousness in the sweat bath as are some of the other asters."

1932 H. Smith OJIBWE 363. "Large leaved aster (*A. macrophyllus*). The Flambeau Ojibwe consider this a feeble remedy but also good as a charm in hunting. Young roots were used to make a tea to bathe the head for headache. . .398. The leaves of this aster are eaten when young and tender. The Flambeau Ojibwe declare that they are fine flavored and good to eat, because they act as medicine at the same time that they are food. Among the Pillager Ojibwe they use the root of this same aster as a soup material. . .429. This is one of the Flambeau Ojibwe hunting charms. It is smoked to attract deer. Blue Wood aster (*A. cordifolius*), the root of this aster is but one of nineteen that can be used to make a smoke or incense when smoked in a pipe, which attracts the deer near enough to shoot it with a bow and arrow. The deer carries its scent or spoor in between its toes, and wherever the foot is impressed into the ground, other animals can detect its presence. . .It is a peculiar scent and the Ojibwe tries successfully to counterfeit it with roots and herbs."

1933 H. Smith POTAWATOMI 49-50. "Forking aster (*A. furcatus*) The basal leaves of this aster are the ones used and they are much larger than the stem leaves and more apt to be found than the fertile part of the plant. The leaves are steeped and the solution is rubbed on the head to cure a severe headache. . .Short's aster. The Potawatomi used the flowering tops of this species for a medicinal tea. The National Dispensatory states that the flowers have been used by the whites as a mild carminative, anti-spasmodic and intestinal astringent. Flat top white aster (*A. umbellatus*), the Potawatomi use the flowers of this species as a smudge to drive away evil spirits working against patient's recovery. Nickell records that it has been used among the whites as an expectorant and an emmenagogue. It has also been used to cure croup. The New England aster was used as one of the fumigating agents."

1945 Rousseau MOHAWK transl. 65. "New England Aster, the Indian name is perhaps given to other species of aster as well. An infusion of the entire plant with the rhyzome of the Lady fern for mothers who have a fever in their intestines. My informatrice distinguished apparently between two kinds of asters, the blue one, this one and the white ones or the panicled aster (*A. paniculatus*) which is used in infusion with the blue aster for the treatment of fever. This last name probably applies to all aster with white flowers."

DRY OPEN PLACES

fields, fence rows, sides of roads, recently burnt-over land, pockets of soil in crevices in open rock and generally areas that are unshaded and dry in summer conditions. Also found in dry open places but discussed in other sections are some of the St. John's worts, asters, rattlesnake plantains, seneca snakeroot, racemed milkwort, golden and pale corydalis

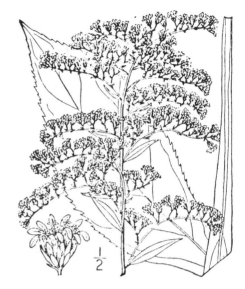

SHOWY GOLDENROD

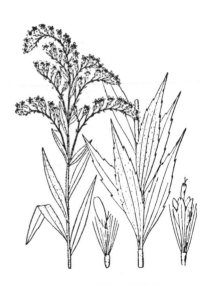

EARLY GOLDENROD

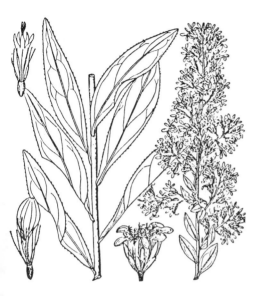

CANADA GOLDENROD

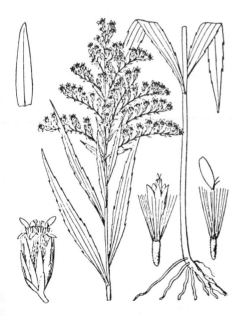

TALL GOLDENROD

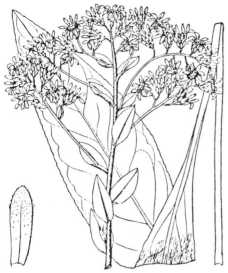

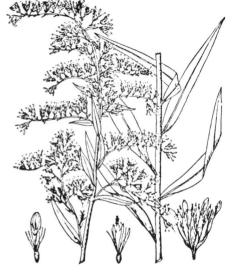

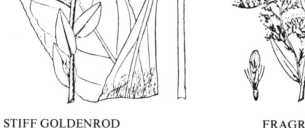

STIFF GOLDENROD   FRAGRANT GOLDENROD

SHOWY GOLDENROD   *Solidago speciosa* Nutt. var. *rigidiuscula* T.& G. Compositae (Asteraceae)

From a thick woody root grows a slender stem usually smooth below and rough above. Numerous leaves, thick, firm with hairy margins, seldom over 2 cm wide, the lower generally falling off. The plant looks like a candle with its tall narrow flowering top, the stalks filled with flowers all around it.

Range. Mass., s. N.H., N.Y., s. Ont., Minn., Ohio, to Wyo., s. to Ga., Ark., and Tex. in dry soil. This goldenrod is like *S. spathulata* ssp *Randii* which in the nineteenth century was also called *S. virga aurea.* Early writers seem to have referred to many American goldenrods by this European name.

EARLY GOLDENROD   *Solidago juncea* Ait.

Stem 30-120 cm tall, smooth, growing from a basal tuft of large leaves, each 15-40 x 2-7.5 cm tapering to a long stalk, their edges hairy. The upper leaves progressively smaller and stalkless. The many flower bearing branches make the flowering top of the plant about as broad as long. The flowers are only on one side of their branches.

Range. Nfld., N.B., P.E.I., N.S., Que., Ont., s. Man., s. to Ga., Mo., Tenn. in dry or moist places and thickets.

CANADA GOLDENROD   *Solidago canadensis* L.

This is conspicuous with a large flowering top. The leaves have three distinct nerves. Its basal leaves soon fall off, the upper leaves are numerous, hairy on the veins beneath. The flowers are on one side of their bending branches only.

Range. Lab., Nfld., N.B., P.E.I., N.S., Que., Ont., se. James Bay to Yukon, Alaska to Sask., s. to Calif. N. Mex. Tex. & Fla., Tenn. and Va. in moist or dry open places and thin woods.

TALL GOLDENROD   *Solidago altissima* L. (*S. canadensis procera*)

Considered a variety of Canada goldenrod by Scoggan who calls it var. *scabra.* A stout hairy

stem 1-2 m tall in good soil. Leaves with three nerves and hairy. The less than 20 flowers on one side only of their bending branches.
Range. Me., sw. Que., s. Ont. to N.D., Kans., Tex. and Fla. in woods and dry soil.

STIFF GOLDENROD   *Solidago rigida* L.

Plants 25-150 cm tall, hoary with thick flat leaves rough on both sides, large and stalked at the base of the plant, smaller and stalkless above, the middle ones 2-6 times as long as wide. The flowering branches spread out equally to give a rounded effect to the top of the plant.
Range. Mass., Conn., N.Y., s. Ont., to Alta. s. to Colo., n. Mex., Tex., La. and Ga. in dry open sandy places.

FRAGRANT GOLDENROD   *Solidago odora* L.

A slender smooth stem 60-160 cm tall. The leaves stalkless or the basal ones with stalks, smooth, one nerved with rough margins. Covered with oil containing dots so that the plant when crushed smells of anise. The large spreading flowering head is showy, the flowers on one sides of their branches only.
Range., Vt., Mass., s. N.H., N.Y., to s. Ohio and Mo., s. to Fla., La. and e. Tex. in dry open woods especially in sandy soil.
Common names. Blue mountain tea, sweet or anise scented goldenrod, true goldenrod.
Goldenrods crossbreed and are difficult to identify. Other goldenrods will be referred to below in the quotations but these six are widespread and in many cases the most common native golden-rod was probably used. The word 'solidago' means to make whole and was given to the golden-rod because of its use as a wound herb from at least the times of the Crusades when it was known as the Sarracen's wound herb and was brought to Europe by the crusaders.
1633 Gerarde-Johnson 439-40. "Of Golden rod. Goldenrod provoketh urine, wasteth away stones in the kidneys, and expelleth them. . .It is extolled above all other herbes for the stopping of bloud in sanguinolent ulcers and bleeding wounds; and hath in times past beene had in greater estimation and regard than in these dayes: for in my remembrance I have known the dry herbe which came from beyond the sea sold. . .for halfe a crown an ounce. But once it was found in Hampstead wood. . .no man will give half a crown for a hundred weight of it. . .esteeming no longer of anything, how pretious so ever it may be, than whilest it is strange and rare."
1708 Sarrazin-Vaillant, Quebec-Paris, Boivin 1978 183-191. Sarrazin sent specimens to Paris and labeled all these numbers *Virga aurea* followed by various descriptions. Some are goldenrods in Boivin's estimation. But the words virga aurea were applied to all goldenrods at that time apparently.
1788 Schoepf. "Here we were introduced to still another domestic tea plant, a variety of *Solidago*. The leaves were gathered and dried over a slow fire. It was said that around Fort Little-ton Penn. many one-hundred pounds of this Bohea tea, as they call it, had been made as long as the Chinese was scarce. Our hostess praised its good taste, but this was not conspicuous in what she brewed" (Ben Charles Harris 1973: 139).
1791 Lewis Mat. Med. ed. Aitkin 455. "*S. virgaurea*, the leaves and flowers are recommended as corroborant and aperient; in urinary obstructions, nephritic cases, ulceration of the bladder; beginning dropsies. . .promise considerable medical activity."
1814 Clarke Consp. 178. "*Virga aurea*, common golden rod. Astringent tonic. In diarrhoea, atony of the viscera, &c. they are very rarely made use of."
1817-20 Bigelow 190. "*Solidago odora*. The claims of the Solidago to stand as an article of the Materia Medica are of a humble, but not despicable kind. . .An essence made by dissolving the essential oil in proof spirit, is used in the eastern States as a remedy in complaints, arising from flatulence, and as a vehicle for unpleasant medicines of various kinds. I have employed it to allay vomiting, and to relieve spasmodic pains in the stomach of the milder kind, with satisfactory success. . .Mr. Pursh informs me. . .that it has for some time been an article of exportation to China, where it fetches a high price."
1830 Rafinesque 265. "*S. odora*, Sweet Goldenrod. Prolific genus, we have nearly 70 sp. This eas-ily known by its sweet scent near to aniseed. Essential oil of it has the same sweet scent, much used for head ache, in frictions. Whole plant aromatic, stimulant, diaphoretic, carminative, use-

ful in flatulence, nausea, spasms of the stomach, chiefly used as a grateful tea. Leaves prepared like tea, have been sent to China, much used in some parts of our country, used in fevers by Cherokees. Some other sp. also medical, but more astringent, aperient, corroborant, useful in gravel, ulceration of the bladder, fevers, dropsy, cachexy, lax bowels, *S. virgaurea* (wild) and the subodorous sp. chiefly used. A species said by Schoepf to be used for wounds and bites of rattlesnakes in decoction, also in tumors, angina, pains in the breast and viscid tumors."

1868 Can. Pharm. J. 6; 83-5. Leaves of the sweet scented goldenrod, *Solidago odora*, included in list of Can. medicinal plants.

1876 Jackson Can. Pharm. J. 235. "In the genus *Solidago* which includes the goldenrod of our thickets [England] (*Solidago virgaurea*), several species have reputed medical properties. The British species itself was formerly considered a useful medicine in diarrhoea and dysentery. The goldenrod of North America (*S. odora*) is used as an aromatic stimulant and diaphoretic; it is said to lessen nausea, allay pain arising from flatulence, and to cover the taste or correct the operation of irritating or unpleasant medicines. It is said, when applied outwards, to have the power of relieving pain arising from headache. The flowers, when dried, have been used as a wholesome and not unpleasant substitute for tea. . .Other species, such as *S. sempervirens* and *S. procera*, have reputed medicinal properties."

1884 Holmes-Haydon CREE Hudson Bay 303. "*Solidago Viraurea* taken as a tonic." [Here again Holmes in England is applying the name of an English plant, see Jackson above, to a plant sent him from Hudson Bay. Several goldenrods could have been used at Hudson Bay such as Canada Goldenrod.]

1926-27 Densmore CHIPPEWA 336. *S. juncea* [early goldenrod] one root in one quart of water taken internally for convulsions. . .340. *S. rigidiuscula* [Showy goldenrod] one root in one quart of water taken cold. This remedy was used to check sudden hemorrhage from the lungs, also for pain in the back and chest with a tendency to consumption. A decoction made from a double handful of the pulverized roots in 2 quarts of water taken for lung trouble. A decoction of the root of *S. graminifolia* [grass leaved goldenrod], was particularly good for pain in the chest. . .342. *S. flexicaulis* [zigzag goldenrod] the dried root chewed for sore throat. . .344. Goldenrod root decoction, one root in one quart of water, applied hot externally for cramps. . .348. *S. rigida*, [Stiff goldenrod], 1 root steeped in ½ pint water. Dose was 'a swallow occasionally' for stoppage of urine. Pulverised root of *S. altissima*, [tall goldenrod], was moistened, not cooked, and applied as a poultice for boils. The flowers of this plant were used for burns. . .354. *S. altissima* [tall golden rod], the flowers dried, moistened with cold water and applied to ulcers. . .352. *S. rigidiuscula* [showy goldenrod] one root in one quart of water taken cold. This remedy is used to check the hemorrhage when a person has been wounded and blood comes from the mouth. *S. altissima* [tall goldenrod], the flowers dried and combined with the dried flowers of coneflower and giant hyssop. A small sunflower was combined with these. When needed the flowers were moistened, applied to bites of poisonous reptiles, and covered with a bandage; when this became dry it was not removed but was moistened with cold water. "This combination of medicine was very strong and was called Wabunowuck (eastern medicine). It is said that if a small handful of the flowers of the plants were steeped in a quart of water and a person 'washed their hands' in this decoction they could thrust their hands in boiling water and not be scalded. . ."354. A decoction was made of the dried leaves of a goldenrod, species doubtful, and taken for fever. . .358. *S. rigidiuscula* [showy goldenrod], one root was steeped in 1 pint of water and taken in three doses about 2 hours apart from difficult labor. . .363. Either the stalk or root was boiled and applied as a warm compress on sprains or strained muscles. This was especially useful when a sprain was followed by swelling. . .364. The roots and stalks were taken in decoction as a tonic and stimulant. . .350. Either the root or stalk was combined with bear's grease as an ointment for the hair. . .364. *S. rigida*, [stiff goldenrod] a decoction made of a handful of the root used as an enema.

1928 H. Smith MESKWAKI 217. "Canada goldenrod. The Meskwaki say that sometimes a child does not learn to talk or laugh. Then the medicine man must secure the bone of an animal that died when the child was born, and cook it together with this plant, then wash the baby with this liquid. This insures that the baby will grow up with its faculties intact. The daughter of Wm. Davenport was cited as an instance in which this practice was necessary, and none can say that she is not cheerful and full of fun now. Stiff goldenrod. . .The flowers are used to make a lotion for bee stings, also to cure swollen fauces. The leaves are also used as a beverage. Showy goldenrod, is used to make a tea that heals burns or scaldings from steam. Elm-leaved goldenrod (*S. ulmifolia*) is smudged and the smoke directed up the nostrils as a reviver of consciousness."

1932 H. Smith OJIBWE 366. "Fragrant goldenrod, the flowers in infusion were used by the Flambeau Ojibwe for a pain in the chest. . .429. Used the flowers to add to their hunting medicine, which is smoked to simulate the odor of a deer's hoof."

1933 H. Smith POTAWATOMI 53. "Canada goldenrod. Several of the goldenrods are used by the Forest Potawatomi for medicine. They usually take the flowering tops as a tea and treat special kinds of fevers with it. Fragrant goldenrod used the same way, also broad leaved goldenrod, *S. latifolia.* and *S. serotina.* Bog goldenrod, *S. uliginosa* has a root like a turnip which is used to make a poultice to bring a boil to a head."

1945 Rousseau MOHAWK transl. 65. "Canada goldenrod for pains in the side, use an infusion of the root and the flowers."

1950 Wintemberg German Canadians 10. "Dyes. Yellow was obtained from the flowers of some species of goldenrod, probably *Solidago canadensis.*"

1955 Mockle Quebec transl. 92. "Canada goldenrod, plant aromatic and astringent, used as a tea."

There are reports of the death of sheep and other livestock that have eaten large quantities of goldenrod in the west. The leaves appear to be toxic at the time of flowering apparently from irritant resins. Symptoms consist of vomiting, faster breathing and death if much has been eaten. The fungi which infect goldenrods are also suspected of causing abortion in cattle (Kingsbury 1964: 436-7).

1968 Adrosko 35-6. "Many professional dyers acknowledged the clarity and fastness of goldenrod yellows, but for some unknown reason this native American plant was used mainly by home dyers. Its abundance and reliable colors should have made it popular with professionals, yet they paid comparatively little attention to this excellent source of yellow. Goldenrod was applied to alum-mordanted wool and was suggested as a substitute for weld in calico printing as well. It is mentioned by the naturalist Peter Kalm. . .but was certainly used by American colonists before that time."

Solidago spp. appear to be toxic to sheep. The toxic principles have been identified as diterpenes (Lewis and Elvin-Lewis 1977: 58).

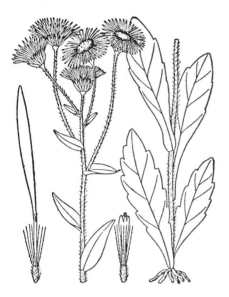

PHILADELPHIA FLEABANE

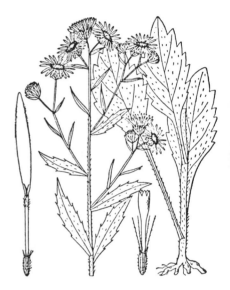

SWEET SCABIOUS

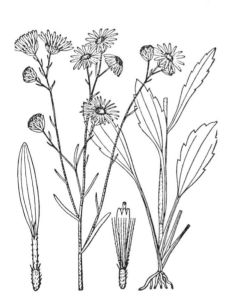

DAISY FLEABANE

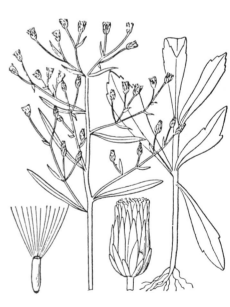

CANADA FLEABANE HORSEWEED

PHILADELPHIA FLEABANE *Erigeron philadelphicus* L. Compositae (Asteraceae)
A slender, soft hairy stem 20-70 cm tall, branched, may be almost smooth. The lower leaves broader near the tip, tapering towards the stem, seldom over 15 x 3 cm with few teeth, the upper leaves clasp the stem. There may be one or many flowers consisting of 150 or more rays (petals) each 0.5 mm wide or less and 5-10 mm long, deep pink to white with a gold center. The buds droop on their stalks.
Range. Nfld., N.B., P.E.I., N.S., Que., Ont., to Yukon and B.C., s. to Fla. and Tex. but locally rare in various habitats in moist places.
Common names. Daisy fleabane, sweet scabious.

SWEET SCABIOUS *Erigeron annuus* (L.) Pers. (*E. heterophyllum a, Aster a.*)
A hairy stem 60-150 cm tall with many leafy branches. The lower stalked leaves 10 x 7 cm with coarse teeth. The upper leaves without stalks or teeth at the very top. The many white flowers have 80-125 rays (petals) 4-10 x 0.5-1 mm.
Range. A weed over most of the U.S. and s. Canada in fields.

DAISY FLEABANE *Erigeron strigosus* Muhl. (*E. ramosus*)
A sparse plant the stem 30-70 cm tall with short close hairs. The bottom leaves not over 15 cm long their stalk included, the upper smaller without teeth. The flowers white or sometimes purplish with 50-100 rays to 6 mm long and 0.4-1 mm wide.
Range. A weed over most of Canada and the U.S. in fields.

CANADA FLEABANE HORSEWEED *Erigeron canadensis* (L.) (*Conyza c.*)
The usually hairy stem is 10-150 cm tall with many branches. The leaves at the bottom are large, toothed and stalked, and progressively smaller to the top of the plant. Numerous 3-5 mm yellow-green tight heads in which are contained the inconspicuous white rays (petals). When mature the white down holding the seeds spreads everywhere.
Range. A common weed throughout America, in fields.
1828 Rafinesque 164-67. "These weeds are valuable medicaments, possessing very active powers. . .Their Oil is so powerful that two or three drops dissolved in Alcohol, have arrested suddenly uterine hemorrhagy, in the hands of Dr. Hales of Troy, N.Y. who employs the oil of *E. canadensis*. This kind is most used in New England and New York, the others in Pennsylvania and New Jersey. . .The whole plants are used fresh or dried, in infusion, decoction or tincture. . .the Oil is one of the most efficient vegetable Styptics. This extract and a syrup of the plant have been given usefully in dry coughs, hemoptysis, and internal hemorrhages. . .As a diuretic the infusion, decoction and tincture are preferable and more active; they have increased the daily evacuation of urine from 24 to 67 ounces. A pint or two of the former may be taken daily; they agree well with the stomach. . .They are beneficial in all diseases of the bladder and kidneys, attended with pain and irritation, in which they give speedy relief. Also in all compound cases of gravel and gout. In rheumatism they have not been tried. . .In chronic diarrhoea are astringent and have cured it without auxiliary. They are even useful externally in wounds, also in hard tumors and buboes, which a cataplasm of the fresh plants dissolve as it were. But the most valuable property is the stringent and styptic power of the Oil, which has saved many lives in parturition and uterine hemorrhagy. A saturated solution of the oil in alcohol is applied and a little given in a spoonful of water; and an instantaeous stop takes place in the bloody flow. . .I highly recommend these plants to medical attention. They were known to the northern Indians by the name of Cocash or Squaw weed as menagogue and diuretics, and are often employed by Herbalists. They may be collected for medical use at any time when in blossom. . .1830 218. *E. canadensis* is called Horseweed in Kentucky and used for the strangury of horses."
1859-61 Gunn 790. "*Erigeron canadensis* known as the Canada fleabane, colts-tail and butterweed. The leaves, when rubbed, have a feeble, but disagreeable odor, and a bitterish taste. It yields its properties to both water and alcohol, but is injured by boiling, as its volatile oil escapes. . .There is an oil made from this herb, by distillation, which is considered a valuable astringent, both externally and internally, applied to small wounds, bleeding piles and the like to

stop bleeding. . .There are two other species of the fleabane—the *E. philadelphicus* and *E. heterophyllum* (*E. annuus*)—both very similar in appearance and properties to the Canada species."

1868 Can. Pharm. J. 6; 83-5. Fleabane the plant, *E. canadensis* and *E. philadelphicus*, included in list of Can. medicinal plants.

1876 Jackson Can. Pharm. J. 235. "Two or three species of Erigeron are used in North America as tonic and diuretic medicines, foremost amongst these is the fleabane (*E. canadensis*). It is an annual plant, common in waste places in many parts of England. . .having been introduced from the United States. . .It is frequently used in cases of dropsy and diarrhoea as a stimulant, tonic, diuretic and astringent. The plant is much used by herb doctors, who administer it in the form of an infusion. An infusion of the powdered flowers is considered antispasmodic, and is used in cases of hysteria and affections of the nerves. An oil is also obtained from the plant, which is said to possess remarkable styptic properties. The frost root (*E. philadelphicus*). . .has similar properties. . .and has a great reputation for the cure of calculus and dropsy. Other species of reputed medicinal value in North America are *E. strigosum* and *E. pusilum*." [the western *E. pusilus*?]

1876 Can. Pharm. J. 146. "Oil of *Erigeron canadensis* in Gonorrhoea.—Dr. G.A. Stark (Can. Med. & Surg. Rep.), gives several instances where this agent has been used with marked success. Before using the medicine, a liberal dose of fluid citrate of magnesia. U.S.P. was taken and followed by: Oil of Erigeron Canadense, two drachms; Syr. simplicis, two ounces. The mixture, of course, requires shaking before being administered. The dose is a teaspoonful every four hours. With due attention to diet a cure was generally effected in about a week, though sometimes a longer treatment was necessary."

1884 Holmes-Haydon CREE Hudson Bay 313. "*Erigeron canadensis* in diarrhoea."

1892 Heebner Pharm. Toronto 188. Oleum Erigerontis, oil of fleabane, distillation of fresh flowering herb of *Erigeron canadensis*.

1892 Millspaugh 80. *Erigeron canadensis*, Canada fleabane. The applicability of a decoction of this herb to many forms of diarrhoea was well known to the Aborigines. . .The decoction has been found useful in dropsies and many forms of urinary disorders. . .The oil of the plant. . .was introduced by Eclectic practice."

1926-7 Densmore CHIPPEWA 342. A decoction made from 2 roots and some leaves of *E. canadensis*, horseweed, in one quart of water drunk for pain in the stomach. . .356. The entire plant steeped and the water drunk for female weakness.

1925 Wood & Ruddock. For chronic diarrhoea make a tea by boiling 2 or 3 handfuls of Canada fleabane in sweet milk. Take ½ cup two or three times a day.

1930 American Medical Plants. *Erigeron canadensis* in limited demand for use in Michigan and Indiana where the oil is distilled.

1928 H. Smith MESKWAKI 213. "Horseweed (*E. canadensis*).The Meskwaki use it as a steaming agent in their sweat bath, but McIntosh did not know of any medicinal virtues in it, hence did not use it. . .The Phildalphia fleabane. The disk florets are powdered and sniffed up the nostril to make one sneeze and thus break up a cold in the head or cattarh. Specimen 3622 of Dr. Jones collection contains the disk florets along with the leaves of horsemint and another plant. . .The mixture is snuffed up the nose to relieve a sick headache."

1932 H. Smith OJIBWE 364. "Philadelphia fleabane. The Pillager Ojibwe use the flowers to make a tea to break fevers. The smoke of the dried flowers is inhaled to cure a cold in the head. The disk flowers, pulverized, were snuffed up the nostrils to cause a patient to sneeze and thus loosen a cold in the head. . .The Daisy fleabane, (*E. strigosus*) *E. ramosus*, The Flambeau Ojibwe use this plant as a perfume for curing a sick headache. . .399. The Pillager Ojibwee say that deer and cows eat the Philadelphia fleabane and that they use it in their smoking tobacco or kinnikinnik mixture. . .429. The disk florets of this plant are smoked to attract the buck deer."

1933 H. Smith POTAWATOMI 51. "The Potawatomi have no Indian name as far as we have found, for this plant (*E. canadensis*) but know it as a medicine for horses."

1945 Rousseau MOHAWK transl. 65 *E. canadensis*. An infusion of the entire plant is used for convulsions and fevers in children.

1955 Mockle Quebec transl. 89. "*E. canadensis*. This plant is known as an astringent, hemostatic and diuretic. Its extract is praised for use in anginas and chronic urititis."

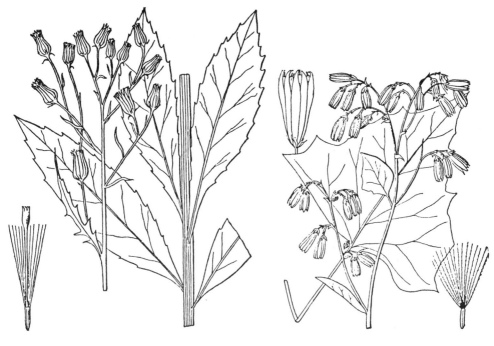

FIREWEED

WHITE LETTUCE
RATTLESNAKE ROOT

FIREWEED   *Erechtites hieracifolia* (L.) Raf. Compositae (Asteraceae)
Stem 0.1-2.5 m tall, smooth or hairy, succulent, light green with alternate long, unstalked, narrow leaves with deep teeth that have callous tips, sometimes lobed, often sticky hairy on veins beneath. Often there are reddish lines running up and down the stem. The flower heads consist of red tipped green overlapping leaflets (sepals) in a tight sheath 1.5-2 cm long swollen at the base. The yellowish white tips of the petals can just be seen above the edge of this sheath. Each flower is the end of a tube that is carrying pollen to the seed at the broadened base of the sheath. Each tube is surrounded by white silky hairs that when the sheath opens will float away with the seeds. A miserable looking weed that resembles Canada fleabane.
Range. N.B., P.E.I., N.S., Que., Ont. s. to La., Fla. an Tex. on shores, in waste places, common after fires, may be found anywhere.
1830 Rafinesque 262. "Vulnerary, acrid, tonic, astringent, useful in hemorrhage, wounds, headache, inflammations, salt rheum, herpes, diseases of the skin, chiefly externally. . .Emetic in large doses, smell strong."
1859-61 Gunn 793-4. "Fireweed (*Erechtites hieracifolius*). The whole plant is medicinal, but the leaves are principally used. . .Considered valuable in all affections of the mucous tissues, as of the stomach, bowels, lungs, and urinary organs. It is highly recommended by some in dysentery, cholera and cholera morbus, and in the summer complaints of children. As. . .a purifier of the system, it is probably an important article. . .The Fireweed is, beyond doubt, the basis of 'Kennedy's Medical Discovery,' a medicine which is, just now, quite popular."
1868 Can. Pharm. J. 6; 83-5. Root and herb of fireweed, *Erechtites hieracifolius*, included in list of Can. medicinal plants.
1872 Diary William V. Havens Ontario mss. "Take 3 bushels of firewood, boil it three hours, take it out and boil the juice into 6 or 7 gallons. Three pounds of logwood [S. America] boiled and strained out quite clean, 5 oz. of blue vitriol, ¼ spirits of salts. The above compounded and the cloth put in liquor quite warm and let it remain in it 20 minutes & take it out and partly dry it. Then put it in the liquor again and let it stand 30 minutes and that will produce an infallible blue. The above quantity will coller 16 lbs. of cotton or 20 lbs. of wool."

1892 Millspaugh 90. "The whole plant is succulent, bitter, and somewhat acrid, and has been used by the laity principally as an emetic, alterative, cathartic, acrid tonic, and astringent, in various forms of eczema, muco-sanguineous diarrhoea, and hemorrhages. The oil, as well as the herb itself, has been found highly serviceable in piles and dysentery."

1915 W.R. Harris ALGONQUIN 50. "For poison ivy and poison sumach poisoning they used fireweed. The poisoned parts were rubbed with leaves of the plant, bruised and crushed so that the sap moistened the skin freely. . .Fireweed (*Erechtites hieracifolia*)."

1933 H. Smith POTAWATOMI 51. "The Potawatomi claim that this plant has come into their territory in historic times and they have no name or use for it to our knowledge. By the whites. . .it has been used in the treatment of fevers, bowel troubles, and for curing night sweats. As a gargle. . .to heal ulcerated mouth, throat troubles and spongy and bleeding gums."

WHITE LETTUCE RATTLESNAKE ROOT   *Prenanthes alba* L. Compositae (Asteraceae)
(Nabalus albus)

A stout, smooth stem 40-150 cm tall with leaves of many different shapes, from those broad and arrowshaped, often found on seedlings to deeply cut and lobed leaves often hairy beneath. The flowers droop, are fragrant, 11-14 mm long, purplish with white waxy petals showing at their ends, 8-15 on each flowering stem. The silk at the end of the seeds is cinnamon brown. Plant has a white milky juice.

Range. Lab., New Engl., Me., w. Que., Ont., to Man., Sask. to S.D., Mo. and Ga. in woods.

Common names. Gall of the earth, Lion's foot, white cankerweed, milk weed, cancer-weed, joy-leaf.

1830 Rafinesque 253. "Root and milk very bitter, used in dysentery and to cure snakebites in men and cattle in poultice."

1868 Can. Pharm. J. 6; 83-5. The plant of lion's foot, *Nabalus alba* included in list Can. medicinal plants.

1888 Delamare Island of Miquelon transl. 22. "The pigs are avid for the roots, called on the Island 'navet de montagne'. These give an excellent flavor to their meat. The stem, hollow from one end to the other and longer than one meter, is used by hunters to drink from streams."

1892 Millspaugh 94. "As Gall-of-the-Earth, it has been known in domestic practice from an early date, and is said to be an excellent antidote to the bite of the rattlesnake and other poisonous serpents,—one who searches through the domestic literature of medicinal plants, wonders why the bite of snakes ever has a chance to prove fatal.—As an alexiteric [an antidote to poison], the milky juice of the plant is recommended to be taken internally, while the leaves steeped in water, are to be frequently applied to the wound; or a decoction of the root is taken. A decoction of the root has been found useful in dysentery, anemic diarrhoea, and as a stomachic tonic."

1926-27 Densmore CHIPPEWA 360. The root, dried and powdered was put in the broth a woman drank after childbirth to produce a flow of milk.

1932 H. Smith OJIBWE 365. "The Flambeau Ojibwe use the milk of the White Lettuce as a diuretic, especially in female diseases. The root is also used as a female remedy. White men have used the root decoction internally for dysentery. Old time herb doctors gave the milk of the plant internally, and used the leaves, steeped in hot water, as a poultice for the bite of a snake."

1942 Fenton IROQUOIS 521. Modern Senecas of Allegheny maintain that the 'rattlesnake killer' is either *Prenanthes alba* or *P. altissima*, designating the latter the male and the former the female of the species.

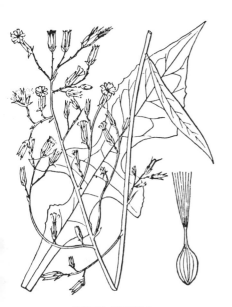

WILD OPIUM

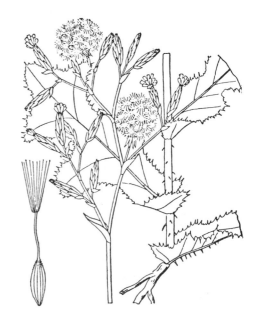

PRICKLY LETTUCE

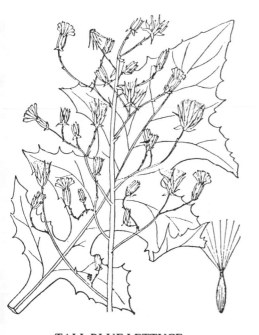

TALL BLUE LETTUCE

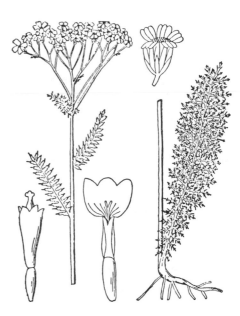

YARROW

WILD OPIUM   *Lactuca canadensis* L. Compositae (Asteraceae) (*L. elongata*)
A 30-250 cm tall stem that varies from smooth and shiny to sometimes coarsely hairy. The leaves
10-35 x 1.5-12 cm are very variable, with or without teeth and or lobes. There are 13-22 tiny yellow flowers on each flowering stalk. The thing to watch for is the seed case, black, very flat with a
line in the middle of each side, and the narrow neck about as long as the seed case holding the
white silk. See illustration.
Range. N.B., P.E.I., N.S., Que., Ont., e. Man. s. to Fla. and Tex. in fields and woods usually in
moist soil.
Common names. Devil's weed, trumpet weed, fireweed, butter and horse weed.

PRICKLY LETTUCE   *Lactuca scariola* L. (*L. serriola* the original spelling)
The 30-150 cm tall stem often prickly below or may be smooth and shiny all over. Leaves prickly
toothed on the midrib beneath and on their margins, usually twisted at their base and clasping
the stem with lobes on both sides. The flowers yellow often drying blue. See illustration of seed
case with very long narrow neck equal or longer that the seed case itself, holding the white silk.
Range. Eurasian found N.B., P.E.I., N.S., Que., Ont. to B.C. and over the United States. The
forma *integrifolia* has been called *L. virosa* in America. *L. virosa* is the European species. There
are several variations of leaf form found in Prickly Lettuce.

TALL BLUE LETTUCE   *Lactuca biennis* (Moench) Fern. (*L. spicata*)
Strong 60-200 cm tall stem smooth with much cut leaves. The seeds cases without necks holding
brown silk. All varieties of Lactuca ooze a white milky juice when cut.
Range. Lab. Nfld., N.B., P.E.I., N.S., Que., James Bay, Ont. to Yukon, Alaska and s. to Calif.,
Colo., and N.C. in thickets and clearings.
1475 Bjornsson Icelandic mss Larsen transl. 74. "Lactuca. It is very cold and wet. If one eats it,
that is good for overheating. It is also good for the stomach and lets one sleep well and purges
the bowels. And yet it is best when boiled. Lactuca seed is good for bad dreams. If one drinks
lactucam with wine, it is good for loose bowels. If a mother eats lactucam she gets sufficient milk
in her breasts. If one eats it regularly, he gets dim eyes."
1541-42 Cartier-Hakluyt 254-55. Canada. "To bee short, it is as good a countrey to plow and
mannure as a man should find or desire. We sowed seedes here of our Countrey [France] , as
Cabbages, Naveaus, Lettises and others which grew and sprang up out of the ground in eight
dayes."
1633 Gerarde-Johnson 309. Describing the prickly lettuce of Europe. . ."Some (saith Dioscorides) mix the milkie juice hereof with opium. . .beaten and applied with woman's milk it is good
against burnes and scaldes. . .It procures sleepe, aswages paine, moves the courses in women,
and is drunke against the stingings of scorpions and bitings of spiders. The seed taken in
drinke. . .hindreth generation of seed and venerous imaginations."
1785 Cutler. The milky juice is said to possess the properties of opium. It may be collected in
shells, dried by a gentle heat and made into pills.
1799 Lewis Mat. Med. 168. "*L. virosa* the milky juice is said to quench thirst, to be greatly laxative, powerfully diuretic, somewhat diaphoretic, and not disagreeable to the stomach. Recommended in dropsies."
1814 Clarke Consp. 86. "*Lactuca virosa*. Strong scented lettuce. In dropsies, visceral obstruction;
the inspissated juice is generally employed."
1820's Materia Medica Edinburgh-Toronto mss. 3. "*Lactuca virosa* narcotic, diuretic, in dropsy
in the form of inspissated juice. . .53. It is never used in this country [Great Britain]."
1830 Rafinesque 234. "Lettuce. Several sp. all equivalents. *L. elongata[canadensis]* most commonly used. . .Bitter milk of all affords the Lactucarium or Tridace, or lettuce opium. Useful and
powerful anodyne, diaphoretic, laxative and diuretic. The extract very efficient in pills for dropsy
and ascites. . .Garden lettuce is milder. Eaten in Sallad, boiled or cooked it acts as a good
refrigerant. . .sedative and anodyne: good topical sedative and a good diet in many
diseases. . .nervous complaints. . .producing a propensity to sleep, and allaying pain. The milk of
it easily collected by incisions, on cotton or a sponge, is similar to opium when inspissated. The
extract of the whole plant, although less pure, is quite equivalent, 24 lbs. of lettuce gives 1 lb. of it.
The tincture is also equal to that of opium. A better equivalent in all cases for opium, although

the doses must be double, because inducing sleep without delerium or irritation: it holds no narcotine nor morphine, but some elastine, water, extractive and salts."

1842 Christison 57. "Lactucarium is collected by cutting across the stem not long before the flowers begin to blow, scraping off the milky fluid that issues, cutting off a fresh slice as often as the surface ceases to yield juice, and allowing the product to dry spontaneously. . .nor is there any reason for dreading the narcotic properties of the wild lettuce, the scientific name of which has given rise to exaggerated notions of its activity. The value of the lactucarium is deteriorated after the middle of the period of inflorescence. . .in composition this substance is very complex. . .The investigations hitherto made on its actions and uses are not precise or satisfactory. It appears, however, to be a narcotic poison to the lower animals in moderate doses. . .it is therefore applicable in special diseases whenever a calmative, anodyne or hypnotic is desired. . .in some circumstances it is preferred over opium. . .Francois maintains that its energy is greatly weakened by giving it in any other form than its original state."

1892 Millspaugh 96."Lactucarium, or Lettuce Opium being of the same nature no matter from what species it is obtained, consists of the inspissated milky juice. . .The yield varies greatly with the species; greatest in *L. virosa*, and diminishing as follows. . .*L. Canadensis, L. sativa*, [garden lettuce] . . .Lactucarium or Thridace. . .yields Lactucerin. . .Lactucin. . . Lactucic acid. . .Lactucopicrin."

1926-7 Densmore CHIPPEWA 350. Gather the white liquid which oozes out when the stalk is broken and rub this on the wart. This remedy is used only from the fresh plant of *Lactuca canadensis* .

1923 H. Smith MENOMINI 31. "Although no Menomini had a name for this plant (*L. canadensis*), my informant said that it is used to cure poison ivy."

1928 H. Smith MESKWAKI 215. "*L. scariola*. The leaves are brewed into a tea taken in convalescence after childbirth to hasten the flow of milk from the breasts. The milk-juice of *Lactuca* was formerly used in this country [by whites] as a soporific and sedative, but it is little used now. It was given in the form of substance or syrup to babies during the course of certain infantile diseases."

1932 H. Smith OJIBWE 364. "*Lactuca spicata*. Tall Blue Lettuce. The Flambeau Ojibwe employ this plant to make a tea given to women with caked breasts to render lactation easier. A dog whisker hair is used to pierce the teat . . .429. Use this plant to make a hunting lure and say that they cut off the roots and nibble at them when hunting. The roots are milky like the stem and the hunter wanting a doe will pretend he is a fawn trying to suckle and thus attract a doe close enough to shoot with a bow and arrow."

1933 H. Smith POTAWATOMI 52. "Tall blue lettuce. The Potawatomi say that this is used for a medicine but my informant could not tell me in what manner."

1935 Jenness Parry Island Lake Huron OJIBWA 89. "For bee and wasp stings apply crushed leaves of *L. spicata [biennis]*. For colds drink or rub the throat with a decoction made by boiling the stem, leaves and flowers of *L. spicata*, tall blue lettuce."

1955 Mockle Quebec transl. 91. "*L. canadensis*, wild lettuce diaphoretic and diuretic."

1976 Palaiseul transl. 179. "Garden lettuce has been known since remote antiquity for its sedative action on the genital organs. Galen is reputed to have said that when in old age he could not sleep the best remedy he found was to eat lettuce in the evening. In the Middle ages it was used to augment the milk of nursing mothers, and to dampen sexual ardour. So well known has its reputation for sapping the power of conception and hurting fecundity become, that it is called the destructor of pleasure and the poison of love. To-day doses of lactucarium are presribed by doctors for priapism and involuntary sexual excitement. The leaves contain vitamin E. For insomnia boil one lettuce in ½ litre of water for 15-20 minutes on a lowfire. Drink a large cup in the evening before going to bed. This tea is also good for gastric spasms, palpitations, hepatic congestion, nervous coughs, take 3 cups a day between meals. Or use the seeds, 20-30 gr. to a l. of water, boil 10-15 minutes. A decoction of the fresh plant or seeds as a lotion or compress against acne, erisipalis or general inflammation of the skin, a beauty water for the skin and sunburn."

Lactuca virosa is cultivated in France and the lactucarium extracted. It is reputed to be a mild sedative and is used in cough mixtures to replace opium. Garden lettuce shows experimental hypoglycemic activity (Lewis and Elvin-Lewis 1977).

YARROW   *Achillea millefolium* L. Compositae (Asteraceae)
A feathery, gray-green plant with a strong aromatic smell, the 20-100 cm tall stem is more or less hairy. The very finely cut leaves consist of many segments that stand out around the centre stalk of the leaf. The cluster of white flowers is usually less than 10 cm across and round topped. There are varieties with flowers varying from pink to red.
Range. This is the native form. Lab., Nfld.?, P.E.I., N.S., Que. Ungava Bay, northernmost Ont., to Yukon, Alaska and the Aleutian Is. s. to Calif., Mex., Tex. and Fla. in meadows and gravelly or sandy slopes and shores. The Eurasian form which has flat topped flower clusters, white or pink, up to 30 cm across has an almost smooth stem. It is found along roadsides and waste places in the south part of the N. American range.
Common names. Thousand-leaf, millefolium, nosebleed, old-man's pepper, sneezewort, soldier's woundwort, gordaldo.
1633 Gerarde-Johnson 1073. "The leaves of yarrow doe close up wounds, and keep them from inflammation, or fiery swellings: it staunches bloud in any part of the body, and it is likewise put into bathes for women to sit in: it stoppeth the laske, and being drunke it helpeth the bloudy flixe. Most men say that the leaves chewed, and especially greene, are a remedy for the tooth-ache. The leaves being put into the nose, do cause it to bleed, and ease the paine of the megrim. . .One dram in powder of the herbe given in wine, presently taketh away the paines of the colicke."
1704 Anon ILLINOIS-MIAMI mss. 224. "The plant of a thousand leaves for all sorts of cuts."
1799 Lewis Mat. Med. 183. "The leaves are a very mild astringent in haemorrhages both internal and external, diarrhoea, debility and laxity of the fibres and in spasmodic and hysterical affec-tions. It is best given in proof spirits. Plants growing in moist rich soils, give on distillation, an essential oil of an elegant blue colour."
1830 Rafinesque 185. "Yarrow, common to Europe and America. Whole plant used. Bitter. . .tonic, restringent, and vulnerary, but subnarcotic and inebriant. Used for hemmor-rhoids, dysentery, hemotysis, menstrual affections, wounds, hypochondria, and cancer. The infu-sion and extract are employed. The American plant is stronger than the European, and has lately been exported for use: this often happens with our plants, our warm summers rendering our medical plants more efficacious. . .Used as an errhine in Europe."
1859-61 Gunn 885. "Yarrow. . .useful in tea or infusion in spitting of blood, bleeding from the lungs, from the urinary organs, in leucorrhea, diabetes, bleeding piles, and dysentery. Dose of the infusion from a gill to half a pint, three or four times a day."
1868 Can. Pharm. J. 6;83-5. Yarrow, the herb, included in list of Can. medicinal plants.
1892 Millspaugh 85. "Yarrow seems to have a decided action upon the blood vessels, especially in the pelvis. It has been proven of great utility in controlling haemorrhages, especially of the pelvic viscera. . .Millefolium causes burning and raw sensations of the membranes with which it comes in contact, considerable pain in the gastric and abdominal regions, with diarrhoea and enuresis."
1915 Speck MONTAGNAIS 315. "Yarrow is steeped for fever medicine. . .319. MOHEGAN. Tansy and yarrow are soaked together in cold water and taken as an appetizer and for the stom-ach.
1916 Waugh IROQUOIS 148. "Yarrow was used for medicine, or as a medicinal ingredient, formed a very agreeable drink when an infusion of suitable strength was made."
1922 W.D. Wallis MICMAC 25. Boiled the plant one hour and drank in warm milk to cure colds as a sweat herb.
1924 Youngken 488. "The Winnebago employed an infusion of this herb to bathe swellings. A wad of leaves as well as some infusion was placed in the ear for earache. . .1925 159. The Zuni southwestern U.S. ground up the entire plant and mixed with cold water and applied to burns. The secret fraternities who performed with fire chewed the flower heads and roots and rubbed this mixture on their limbs and chests previous to passing hot coals over their bodies. Those who danced in fire employed this same mixture for bathing prior to the exhibition. They also placed some in their mouths before taking live coals. It is said that the medicine enabled them to hold the hot coals in the mouth for as long as a minute. The Cheyenne tribe drank an infusion of the plant for coughs and a tea made from the leaves for colds and nausea."
1926-27 Densmore CHIPPEWA 336. Decoction of the leaves sprinkled on hot stones and the fumes inhaled for headaches. . .350. A decoction of the root applied externally for

eruptions. . .364. The root was dried, chewed and spit on the limbs for sprains, or strained muscles. . .366. A decoction of the leaves and stalks was given to a horse as a stimulant.

1923 H. Smith MENOMINI 29. "This plant is used in the treatment of fevers, a hot tea being steeped from the leaves. The Menomini also used the fresh tops to rub eczema sores to cure them. The leaves were used as a poultice for the rash of children."

1928 H. Smith MESKWAKI 210. "The leaves and flowers are both used to make a tea that cures fever and ague. Specimen 5183 of the Dr. Jones collection is the stem and leaves of *A. millefolium*. . .It is boiled and used 'to bathe some place on the body that is ailing.' "

1932 H. Smith OJIBWE 362. "The Flambeau Ojibwe. . .use the leaves of this plant as poultice to cure the bite of a spider. The dried flowering heads are smoked in mixture with other things, much as kinnikinnik, not for pleasure, but more for ceremonial purposes. . .The Pillager Ojibwe used the florets for ceremonial smoking and placed them on a bed of coals inhaling the smoke to break a fever."

1933 H. Smith POTAWATOMI 47-8. "The Forest Potawatomi place the flowers upon a plate of live coals to create a smudge which is used for two purposes. First it is to keep any evil spirits away from the patient and second it is to give the proper sort of scent to revive the patient who may be in a state of coma. The medicine man will sing while he fumigates the patient in a way to suggest that the patient will recover. . .Among the whites a decoction of the flowers has been used to stop falling hair. . .117. The Yarrow is one of the plants that is used as a medicine and also as a witch charm. When the seed heads are placed upon a pan of live coals, a smoke is produced which is supposed to keep the witches away."

1945 Rousseau MOHAWK transl. 64. "For cramps in the stomach drink a decoction of fragments of the plant steeped in cold water. With certain docks it is used for diarrhoea. With meadowsweet it is drunk to prevent nausea and vomiting."

1945 Rousseau Quebec transl. 103. "For a fever, place the macerated plant with the seeds removed on the limbs of the patient. It is also used in infusion."

1945 Raymond TETE DE BOULE transl. 118. "The leaves and flowers boiled and the water drunk cures the sickness of the head. The people in the country of Iberville drink the infusion for colds to procure a sweat."

1955 Mockle Quebec transl. 85. "The plant is used as a bitter tonic, inebriant, and hemostatic in hemorrhages, wounds, hemorrhoids. It is also a vulnerary and anthelmintic. The flowering tops are used as a febrifuge in a concentrated decoction. It has recently been found that an aqueous solution possesses a certain antibacterial activity against *Staphylococcus aureus* 'in vitro'. Sneezewort yarrow (*A. Ptarmica*) the tops are used as sternutatory and sialagogue."

1959 Mechling MALECITE of maritime provinces of Canada used yarrow for colds, swelling, bruises.

1970 Bye IROQUOIS mss. Yarrow drunk in infusion for diarrhea and summer complaints.

Yarrow contains chamazulene, which is its most effective therapeutic constituent. Some plants lack this substance, which is found in the flowering tops. They should be dried during the flowering period at less than 40°C. The drug is helpful drunk as an infusion for lung or kidney hemorrhage and excessive menstrual flow. It helps the circulation of the blood and stimulates the flow of gastric juices. Externally it is used for rashes and as a gargle in inflammation of the gums (Stary & Jirasek 1973:48).

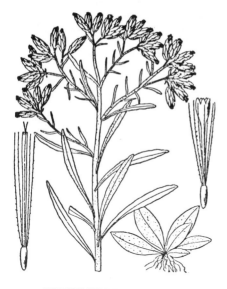

SWEET WHITE BALSAM

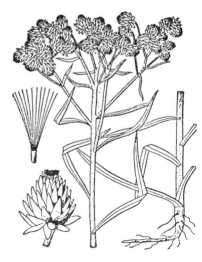

PEARLY EVERLASTING

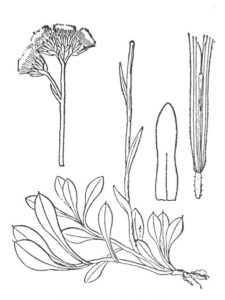

LESSER CAT'S FOOT

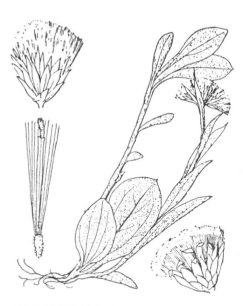

PLAINTAIN LEAVED EVERLASTING

SWEET WHITE BALSAM *Gnaphalium obtusifolium* L. Compositae (Asteraceae) (*G. polycephalum*).

An erect, fragrant, annual plant (sometimes biennial) 10-80 cm tall, the stem thinly white woolly, may be glandular near the base. Leaves numerous, 10 x 1 cm stalkless, white woolly beneath and green or slightly woolly and perhaps glandular above. Many branches bearing bisexual flowers, each surrounded by a tightly furled series of whitish to brown or purple stiff petals (bracts), the outer shorter than the inner ones, with rough, rounded sometimes dark spotted tips, woolly at the bottom.

Range. N.B., P.E.I., N.S., s. Que., s. Ont., s. to Tex. and Fla. in open sunny places.
Common names. Sweet or fragrant life everlasting, old field balsam, rabbit-tobacco, moonshine, Indian posy, fussy-gussy, poverty weed, life of man.

PEARLY EVERLASTING   *Anaphalis margaritacea* (L.) Clarke (*Gnaphalium m.,Antennaria m.*)
Perennial with a 30-90 cm tall stem covered with loose white wool, sometimes turning rusty when old. Stalkless leaves 12 x 2 cm often curling over their white woolly undersides, those at the base soon falling off. Numerous unisexual flowers consisting of a golden centre surrounded by shiny, stiff, white outer petals (bracts) that while tightly furled when young open out when old, not woolly at the base. The plant not fragrant.
Range. Lab., Nfld., New Engl., N.B., P.E.I., N.S., Que., Ont. to Alaska and Aleutian Is. s. to Calif., N. Mex., S.D. in dry open places.
Common names. Silver leaf, life everlasting, cotton weed, none so pretty, moonshine, Indian posy, ladies tobacco, poverty weed, silver button.
1633 Gerarde-Johnson 640-44. "There is a kinde of Cotton-weed, being of greater beauty than the rest, that hath strait and upright stalks 3 foot high or more, covered with a most soft and fine wooll, and in such plentifull manner, that a man may with his hands take it from the stalke in great quantitie. . .many small floures of a white colour. . .consisting of little silver scales thrust close together. . .which floure being gathered when it is young, may be kept in such manner as it was gathered (I meane in such freshnesse and well liking) by the space of a whole yeare after, in your chest or elsewhere: wherefor our English women have called it Live-long or Live for ever. . .Clusius received this plant out of England, and first set it forth by the name of *Gnaphalium Americanum*." [Raleigh may have brought it back to England from Virginia, before 1600. Clusius published his history of rare plants in Antwerp in 1601 and was in constant correspondence with botanists and growers in England. Gerarde goes on to discuss the European gnaphaliums]. 644. "Gnaphalium boyled in strong lee cleanseth the haire from nits and lice: also the herbe being laid in ward-robes and presses keepeth the apparell from moths. The same boyled in wine and drunken, killeth wormes and bringeth them forth, and prevaileth against the bitings and stinging of venomous beasts. The fume or smoke of the herbe dried, and taken with a funnell, being burned therein, and received in such a manner as we use to take the fume of Tobaco, that is, with a crooked pipe made for the same purpose by the Potter, prevaileth against the cough of the lungs, the great ache or paine of the head, and clenseth the brest and inward parts." [Johnson, ed. 1633 remarks about the *G. Americanum* described above that "Bauhinus affirms that it grows frequently in Brasill." Bauhinus in his book (1620) states that the specimen "*Gnaphalium latifolium Americanum Bauh.*" that he is listing came to him from Burser who had it from an unamed apothecary in Paris with the statement that it was collected in Brazil. See Pitcher Plant for probable name of this apothecary. Juel (1931) contends that twenty seven of the specimens described by Bauhinus actually came from New France as they were all north American species. Rousseau speculated (1964) that these specimens might have been sent by Louis Hebert from Port Royal, Acadia. This is a reasonable hypothesis as Portugese fishing boats came regularly to the Acadian coast and if Herbert sent his letters back to France by them it is understandable how any plant coming from Portugal would have been assumed to have come from Brazil. Juel considers Bauhinus's specimen to be that of *Anaphalis margaritacea*. Perhaps we have here two different plants, one from Virginia and one from Acadia both being labelled *Gnaphalium americanum* by Johnson in 1633].
1663 Josselyn Voyages New England 78. "The fishermen when they want tobacco, take this herb: being cut and dryed." [*Anaphalis margaritacea*].
1687 Clayton Virginia Indians 5-6. "They are generally most famed for curing of wounds, and have indeed various very good wound-herbs. . .They use also the *Gnaphalium Americanum* commonly called there white Plantain." [The genus is principally represented in Virgina by *Gnaphalium obtusifolium* according to Gray].
1748 Kalm Philadelphia September the 29th. 70. "The *Gnaphalium margaritaceum* grows in astonishing quantities upon all uncultivated fields, glades, hills and the like. . .It has a strong but agreeable smell. The English call it 'life everlasting' for its flowers, which consist chiefly of dry, shining, silvery, leaves, do not change when dried. . .The English ladies are accustomed to gather great quantities of this life everlasting and to pick them with the stalks. . .English ladies in general are much inclined to keep flowers all summer long about or upon the chimneys, upon a table

or before the windows, whether on account of their beauty or because of their sweet scent. . .*Gnaphalium* was one of those which they kept in their rooms during the winter because its flowers never altered. . .Mr. Bartram told me another use of this plant: a decoction of the flowers and stalks is used to bathe pained or bruised parts of the body, or they may be rubbed with the plant itself tied up in a thin cloth or bag."

1830 Rafinesque 224. "*Gnaphalium.* Cudweed. The *G. margaritaceum* also called Silver leaf, None so pretty, is anodyne and pectoral, used in colds and coughs, pains in the breast, also mild astringent and vermifuge, used in dysentery and hemorrhage in powder or decoction. Externally used in tumors, contusions, sprains, in a wash. Also in diseases of sheep. One of the good substitutes for tobacco in smoking. Many other sp. of the genus are equivalent."

1868 Can. Pharm. J. 6;83-5. White balsam, *Gnaphalium polycephalum* the herb, and *Antennaria margaritacea* the leaves, included in list of Can. medicinal plants.

1879 Can. Pharm. J. 322. "Old field balsam looks a good deal like boneset, only it don't grow so high, it is used for the same purpose (used for colds)."

1885-6 Mooney CHEROKEE 325. "*Gnaphalium decurrens,* winged cudweed, Life everlasting. Decoction drunk for colds; also used in the sweat bath for various diseases and considered one of their most valuable medical plants." [*G. decurrens* is *G. viscosum,* like *G. obtusifolium* except that the stalkless leaves run down into the stem. Range. New Engl., N.B., P.E.I., N.S., Que., Ont., s. to Oreg., Tenn., Pa. in dry places.]

1892 Millspaugh 89. "*Gnaphalium obtusifolium.* The Everlastings formed part of aboriginal medication, and from there they descended to the white settlers, who, in conjunction with the more or less botanic physicians, used them about as follows. The herb, as a masticatory, has always been a popular remedy, on account of its astringent properties, in ulceration of the mouth and fauces and for quinsy. A hot decoction proves pectoral and somewhat anodyne, as well as sudorific in early stages of fevers. A cold infusion has been much used in diarrhoea, dysentery, and hemorrhage of the bowels, and is somewhat vermifugal; it is also recommended in leucorrhoea. The fresh juice is considered anti-venereal. Hot fomentations of the herb have been used like *Arnica* for sprains and bruises, and form a good vulnerary for painful tumors, and unhealthy ulcers. The dried flowers are recommended as a quieting filling for the pillows of consumptives."

1894 Household Guide Toronto 135. "The plant called 'white everlasting' botanical name *Gnaphalium polycephalum,* is one of the best remedies for diarrhoea. . .Take a handful of the herb, flowers and leaves included, and boil in one pint of water. Strain the decoction and boil down to one-half pint. Add an equal quantity of milk and bring to a boil so as to scald the milk. Dose for adults, one-half teacupful; for children, accordingly. If desired, it may be sweetened with white sugar."

1915 Speck MONTAGNAIS 314. "The plant of *Gnaphalium polycephalum* or *Anaphalis margaritacea* furnishes a decoction for coughing and consumption, and stomach sickness."

1915 Speck-Tantaquidgeon MOHEGAN 319. "Indian posy (*Gnaphalium margaritacea*) is steeped and drunk for colds."

1925 Youngken CHEYENNE 161. "*Anaphalis margaritacea* var. *subalpina.* The leaves of this herb represent the 'strong medicine' of the Cheyenne. They were dropped on hot coals and the smoke used to purify gifts which were left on a hill for the sun or the spirits. In former times, before going into battle, each man chewed a little of it and rubbed it over his body, arms and legs because of its supposed property of imparting strength, energy and dash and hence protection from danger."

1926-27 Densmore CHIPPEWA 362. *Anaphalis margaritacea,* pearly everlasting, the flowers steeped in decoction used in combination with wild mint, sprinkled on hot stones, said to be good for paralysis.

1923 H. Smith MENOMINI 30. "*Gnaphalium polycephalum.* The leaves of this plant furnish a very important sorcerer's medicine. It is used separately or with. . .gall from the beaver's body, to make a smudge as a reviver. When one has fainted this is used to bring him back to consciousness again, the smoke being blown into his nostrils. Then again, when one in the family has died, his spirit or ghost is supposed to come back to trouble the living. Bad luck and nightmares will result to the family from the troublesome ghost. This smudge discourages and displeases the ghost which, after a fumigation of the premises with this smudge, leaves and never returns. Burning of these herbs gives off a peculiar characteristic odor, reminding one of the smell of elm bark, dried medick flowers, and colts foot herb."

1928 H. Smith MESKWAKI 214. "*G. polycephalum*, This is one of the best of this type of medicines and is sure to heal. It is smudged to bring back a loss of mind or to revive consciousness."

1932 H. Smith OJIBWE 362. "*Anaphalis margaritacea*, Pearly everlasting. The Flambeau use the flower of this plant, calling attention to the fact that it smells like acorns, reducing them to a powder which is sprinkled on live coals as a perfume. This is inhaled by a party who has had a stroke of paralysis and is said to revive him."

1933 H. Smith POTAWATOMI 48. "Pearly everlasting, *Anaphalis margaritacea*. The Forest Potawatomi dry the flowers of this species and smoke it in a pipe or smudge it on coals to drive or keep evil spirits out of the room, which might prevent a patient from recovering. . .117. Pearly everlasting is also used as a witch charm to drive or keep evil spirits out of the house. The top is dried and placed upon a pan of live coals because it is supposed to hurt the eyes of the evil spirits and cause them to stay away from the house."

1945 Rousseau MOHAWK transl. 63. "*Anaphalis margaritacea*, immortelle. For asthma drink an infusion of the flowers with the roots of the mullein."

1945 Raymond TETE DE BOULE transl. 119. "*A. margaritacea* the boiled flowers are applied to burns and dermititis."

1950 Walpole Island CHIPPEWA mss. *Gnaphalium* used to protect houses from witches. The dried plant burned until smoke is all through the house.

1955 Mockle Quebec transl. 86-7. "*A. margaritacea* is used for coughs and chest colds as well as a feeble astringent and vermifuge. It has a certain popularity for use for burns."

LESSER CAT'S FOOT   *Antennaria neglecta* Greene Compositae (Asteraceae)
The Antennarias are difficult to divide into species and there is little agreement on this subject among the taxonomists. This species, according to Scoggan 1979, is a very plastic one, he lists 19 others included within it. The basal rosette of leaves that lie on the ground in this species sometimes have obviously one nerve, a pointed tip and are at most about 2 cm broad. The leaves can be white wooly, glandular or green and smooth. The flowering stem can have up to ten heads. The scales around the flowers are brownish with white tips.
Range. Nfld., N.B., P.E.I., N.S., Que., Ont. Hudson Bay, Man. to s. Yukon, s. to Calif., Ariz. and Va. in dry fields, rocky barrens and open woods. Often forms fair sized patches.

PLANTAIN LEAVED EVERLASTING   *Antennaria plantaginifolia* (L.) Hook.
The rosette leaves to 4 cm broad, rouded at their ends with a minute sharp tip. They are silvery beneath with a fine wool on top. The flowering stem from 10 to 40 cm tall with several leaves and the flowers crowded together. The scales greenish white, the hair on the seeds to 5.5 mm long.
Range. N.S., s. Que., s. Ont., se. Man., s. to e. Tex. Tenn. and Va. in fields, clearings and open woods.
Common names. White plantain, pussy toes, love's test, Indian or woman's tobacco.
1830 Rafinesque 224. "White plantain, poor robin or Rattlesnake plantain, Squirrel ear, [the two plants described above] Scinjachu of some Indians. Both pectoral, used in coughs, fevers, bruises, inflammations, debility: also against the negro poison and rattlesnake bites: Indians will for a trifle allow themselves to be bitten and cure themselves at once."

1868 Can. Pharm. J. 6;83-5. *Antennaria plantaginifolia*, plantain, the leaves included in list of Can. medicinal plants.

1928 H. Smith MESKWAKI 210. "Plaintain-leaved everlasting. The tea is made of the leaves and drunk every day for two weeks after childbirth and then the woman does not get sick. Eclectic practitioners [white] have recognized the volatile oils contained in this species and have employed them as soothing expectorants."

1932 H. Smith OJIBWE 363. "Lesser cat's foot. The Flambeau Ojibwe use the whole herb as a valued remedy to make a tea to be given to the mother after childbirth. Eclectic practitioners [white] have used this plant as a hemostatic."

1955 Mockle Quebec transl. 87. "Plaintain leaved cut-weed. Used for coughs and colds and pulmonary inflammations."

1950 Wintemberger German Canadians 12. "A tea from the leaves of the plaintain leaved everlasting (*Antennaria plantaginifolia*) was used for dysentery."

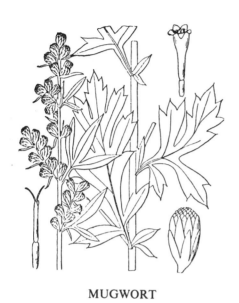

MUGWORT

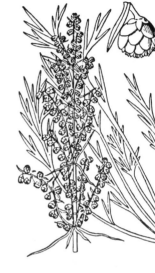

CANADIAN WORMWOOD

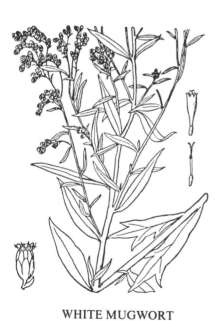

WHITE MUGWORT

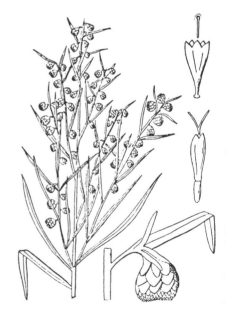

LINEAR LEAVED WORMWOOD

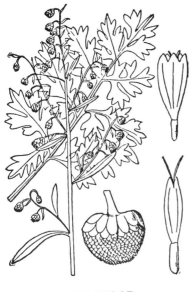

WORMWOOD

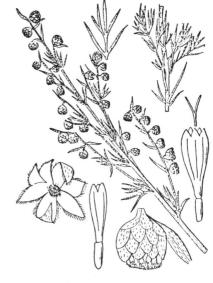

PASTURE SAGE

MUGWORT   *Artemisia vulgaris* L. Compositae (Asteraceae)
A plant 0.5 to 1.5 m tall with a rough, reddish stem. The leaves 5-10 x 3-7 cm are cut into large
segments. They are white furry beneath and usually dark green above. The grayish flowers are on
stalks growing from the stem, their central disk flowers fertile. Taste bitter and leaves when
crushed are aromatic.
Range. Native of Eurasia and possibly arctic Canada. "Either the species or its varieties have
been reported across Canada and the United States, but it is more common in the eastern part of
the area" (Montgomery 1964:175). Dry open places.
Common names. Sailor's tobacco, fellon-herb, bulwand, motherwort, green ginger.

CANADIAN WORMWOOD   *Artemisia canadensis* Michx. or *A. campestris* spp. *canadensis*
Michx.
Plant with a smooth or hairy stem 30-60 cm tall. The bottom leaves lie on the ground in a rosette.
They are divided into two, the upper into 3-7 long sections, rather rigid, smooth or sparingly
hairy. The over 45 florets are smooth, yellow and placed tightly up the stem. They have leaflets at
their base with narrow green centres and broad white rough edges (bracts). The flowers in the
centre of the disk are sterile. The plant is aromatic when crushed. Ssp *caudata* is of a more southern distribution.
Range. Alaska, Baffin Island, near Arctic circle to Nfld. and through all the provinces except
Labr., P.E.I. and N.S. s. to New Engl., Mich., Colo., Ariz. and Calif. in open sandy soil and dry
slopes.

WHITE MUGWORT   *Artemisia ludoviciana* Nutt. (*A. gnaphalodes*)
Plant 30-100 cm tall with a white woolly stem. Leaves long and narrow 3-11 cm x 4-15 mm, with
or without lobes, white woolly on both sides or can become smooth. Flowers small on slender
branches, the disk flowers fertile with normal ovary. Leaves aromatic when crushed, taste bitter.
Range. B.C., Alta., Sask., Man., apparently introd. to Ont., Que., N.B., P.E.I., s. to Mich., Ill.,
Tex., Mex. and Calif. in dry open places.
1475 Bjornsson Icelandic mss Larsen transl 141. "Artemisia is mugwort. If a woman drink it who

has a dead child in her, it will fare from her. This grass allows a man to urinate well and loosens stone in the bladder. It is also good for jaundice if a man drinks it with wine. If it is crushed with paunch-fat, it is good to bind upon tumors. If one drinks it with wine, neither leechdom [sorcerers] nor bite of beasts will harm him. If it is crushed in wine or boiled in oil, it gives forth a good smell and fragrance and helps for the illnesses which have been mentioned. It strengthens the stomach and cures the heart-roots and is useful for many other things."

1633 Gerarde-Johnson 1104. "Mugwort. Pliny saith that Mugwort doth properly cure womens diseases. Dioscorides writeth, that it bringeth downe the termes, the birth, and the after-birth. And that in like manner it helpeth the mother, and the paine of the matrix, to be boyled as baths for women to sit in; and that being put up with myrrh, it is of like force that the bath is of. And that the tender tops are boiled and drunk for the same infirmities; and that they are applied in manner of pultesse to the share, to bring downe the monethly course. Pliny saith, that the travel-ler or wayfaring man that hath the herbe tied about him feeleth no wearisomnesse at all; and that he who hath it about him can be hurt by no poysonsome medicines, nor by any wilde beast, neither by the Sun it selfe; and also that it is drunke against Opium, or the juice of blacke Poppy. Many other fantasticall devices invented by Poets are to be seene in the Works of the ancient Writers, tending to witchcraft and sorcerie, and the great dishonour of God; wherefore I do of purpose omit them, as things unworthie of my recording, or your reviewing. Mugwort pound with oyle of sweet almonds, and laid to the stomacke as a plaister, cureth all the paines and griefes of the same. It cureth the shakings of the joynts, inclining to palsie, and helpeth the con-tractions or drawing together of the nerves and sinews."

1830 Rafinesque 196. "Mugwort. Common to both continents. . . Antiseptic, stomachic, deter-gent, deobstruant, laxative, diuretic, diaphoretic, menagogue, corroborant, antispasmodic and vermifuge. Useful in hysterics, spasms, palpitations of the heart, worms, obstructions, &c. in tea, infusion or powder. The leaves, tops and seeds are used, these last and their oil equal to Santonic seeds as vermifuge. Warm fomentations of the leaves are an excellent discutient and antiseptic. Many equivalent species grow in the West . . .All species make the milk of cows bitter when grazed upon. Moxa made with them."

1892 Millspaugh 87. "*Artemisia vulgaris* mugwort. . . Hippocrates very frequently mentions Artemisia as of use in promoting uterine evacuations. . .it has nevertheless fallen entirely into disrepute, being now very seldom, if ever used in any disease. . .The Mexican Pharmacopoeia is now we believe, the only one recognizing this drug."

1902 Chesnut California 392-3. "*Artemisia heterophylla* [B.C. to Calif.]. . .No native plant is more highly esteemed for its medicinal value. A decoction of the leaves is considered by both Indians and whites as a specific for colic and for colds. Its efficiency in the cure of bronchitis is recog-nized by one of its common names, bronchitis plant. A decoction is used internally by the Indi-ans for stomach ache, headache, diarrhoea, and some kinds of fever. Externally it is used as a head wash to relieve headache and as a wash for sore eyes. The juice is reputed by one individual to be a specific against the effect of poison oak (*Rhus diversiloba*). Bruised leaves are frequently placed in the nostril to relieve the effects of a cold, and are tied in bundles around the body to cure rheumatism, and after childbirth to promote the circulation of the blood. In the sweat-bath cure for rheumatism the leaves are considered invaluable. The method of treatment consists essentially in binding the dampened leaves in large bundles to the limb and then subjecting it to heat. The heat is sometimes applied by piling heated dirt upon the bandage or by wrapping the limb or even the whole body in a blanket and lying down in a hole which has previously been heated by a small fire. It requires many hours to obtain the desired relief. The Yokin name for the plant is Ka-blu."

1926–27 Densmore CHIPPEWA 366. *A. gnaphalodes*. The flowers, dried and placed on coals and the fumes inhaled as an antidote for 'bad medicine'.

1923 H. Smith MENOMINI 29. "*A. canadensis*. This is the true herb known by this Menomini name and is a very important leaf medicine. It is used in combination with angelica root for sup-pressed menstruation. When the patient has a cold or the menstrual flow is stopped for any rea-son, tea of these two make it easy again."

1928 H. Smith MESKWAKI 211. "*A. canadensis*. The leaves of this plant are used as a poultice to cure bad burns. Specimen 5186 in Dr. Jones collection is the flowering head of *Artemesia canadensis*. . .His informant said that it was boiled and made into a drink. It was used as a poul-tice on a burn, caused by hot water. . .*A. ludoviciana*. . .The leaves of this plant are used as a poultice to cure sores of long standing. A tea is made of the leaves to cure tonsilitis and sore throat. A smudge of the leaves drives away mosquitoes. It is also used to smoke ponies when they have the distemper. Specimen 5130 of Dr. Jones collection is the leaves of *A. ludoviciana*. . .used in a tincture to heal old sores, especially those made by scrofula. According to the white man it has the same properties as *A. canadensis*."

1932 H. Smith OJIBWE 363. "*A. ludoviciana*. White Cloud. . .and John Peper, another Bear Islander. . .said the Pillager Ojibwe used it as horse medicine, but the Sioux smoked it. Miners and frontiersmen prized it in their treatment of 'mountain fevers'."

1955 Mockle Quebec transl. 88. "*A. canadensis*, stomachic, diuretic and vermifuge. *A. vulgaris* mugwort, the leaves and flowering tops, in infusion, are antispasmodic and emmenagogue. Other *Artemisia* found in Canada and which have the same properties are: *A. annua; A. biennis; A. caudata; A. frigida* and *A. ludoviciana*."

1961 Claus Pharm 512–3. "Arikari women took an infusion of the big wild sage (*Artemisia gnaphalodes* or the roots of little wild sage *A. frigida*, a bitter tonic considered useful as an aid to the physiologic functions. [menstruation].

An experimental hypoglycemic activity has been shown in *A. vulgaris* (Lewis and Elvin-Lewis 1977:218).

PASTURE SAGE
Artemisia frigida Willd.

A slender, woody stem to 50 cm often lying on the ground. The leaves to about 12 mm long and at the most 1 mm broad covered with fine hair giving the plant a silvery silky lace like appearance. Flowers at the end of the stems yellow and give off clouds of pollen.

Range. Alaska, Yukon, Alta., Sask., Man., s. to Ariz., Kans., Tex., Wis and Minn. in dry plains and prairies. Introduced eastward to Ont., Que. and N.B. In Eurasia also.

1926–7 Densmore CHIPPEWA 336. *Artemisa frigida* the root mixed with those of the wild rose, the ground plum and the seneca snakeroot in decoction drunk for convulsions. . .The leaves and flowers of *A. frigida* instead of the root in this same decoction used for hemorrhage from wounds, applied externally. . .364. The roots of these same plants were dried and that of seneca snake root kept separately. Equal parts of the others are pounded together until powdered, [see seneca snakeroot for preparation of this medicine] drunk as a tonic. . .The leaves of *A. frigida* were burned and the vapors inhaled or a decoction of them drunk for biliousness. . .366. The leaves of *A. frigida* dried, crumbled and placed on a hot stone. The necessary quantity was said to be 'about as much as 4 willow leaves.' Hold the hands and head over it so the fumes get thoroughly into the clothing as a disinfectant. This was used frequently in cases of contagious disease, the smoke filling the room.

1933 H. Smith POTAWATOMI 49. "*A. frigida*. This plant was evidently not native to the Forest Country, but had been planted by the Indians for its medicinal properties. They use it as a fumigator to revive a patient who is in a coma. The foliage and flowers are fumed upon a pan of live coals and often a cone of paper is made to direct the smoke into the nostrils of the patient."

1973 Campbell Best & Budd 93. "*A. frigida*. The common low growing sage of the prairies has been called pasture sage for many years. . .It has a wide range, occuring naturally in Northern Europe and Asia and throughout Western North America. . .The forage value of pasture sage as determined by chemical analyses is very high. Protein, phosphorus, and fat content are well above those for the associated grasses in all stages of growth, in fact protein content will equal that of good alfalfa. However the presence of aromatic oils apparently limits its palatability because only during the autumn and winter will cattle graze the plant to any degree. Sheep eat it more readily and will pasture it from early autumn through the winter and until late spring."

LINEAR LEAVED WORMWOOD
Artemisia dracunculus L. (*A. dracunculoides*)

A woody much branched stem up to 1.5 m tall, may be slightly hairy. The leaves 3-4 cm long and 2-3 mm broad but may be up to 8 cm long and 1 cm broad. Green and smooth on both sides with one or two lobes on each side at their base. But can also be finely hairy all over. The flowers small, to 4 mm tall, numerous, brownish on drooping stems. The disk flowers are sterile, the ovary abortive.

Range. s. Alaska, Yukon, B.C., Alta., Sask., Man., an isolated station near Toronto. Introd. eastward into New Engl. s. to Mo., Tex., N.Mex. and Baja Calif. Prairies and rocky slopes.

1926–27 Densmore Chippewa 338. [Possibly the White Earth Reservation in Minn. on the edge of the prairies. An unusual variety of plants grow there so that the Chippewa living on other reservations were accustomed to go there for many of their medicinal plants.] The leaves and flowers of the flowering plant of *A. dracunculoides* dried; a handful steeped in 1½ pints of water and administered when partly cooled for palpitations of the heart. Dose, ½ cup, after which the patient reclined; dose repeated every half hour until patient was relieved or the fresh leaves chewed. . . 344. The leaves and top of the flowering plant dried and steeped and drunk for chronic dysentery. . .350. The root, with that of *Dirca*, in decoction used as a wash to strengthen the hair. . . 356. The leaves and flowers, fresh or dried, chewed and used as poultice for hemorrhage from wounds. The root of a sterile plant, decoction made from 8 roots to 1 quart of water, all of which could be drunk in one day for stoppage of periods. Same remedy was used for excessive flowing. This root must be pulled, not dug. The informant stated this was the only root which must be pulled, not dug. Another informant stated that she used 4 dried chopped roots in about 3/4 cup of water. These were not boiled but steeped thoroughly, and the tea taken at frequent intervals. This remedy was considered so important that its native name is Ogima wuck, meaning 'chief medicine'. A decoction of the leaves and stalk, varying in strength according to cases, was also drunk for stoppage of periods. The leaves, stalk and root in decoction was drunk for difficult labor. . .362. Root, the best part was the fine fibers, in a strong decoction as a strengthening bath for a child, also used for 'steaming old people to make them stronger'.

TARRAGON   *Artemisia dracunculus* L. var. *sativa*
This is a variety that has the taste of anis and that leaves a sharpness in the mouth when chewed fresh. As it does not set seed it must be propagated by root divisions or cuttings and so is a cultivated plant. The leaves are long, narrow, and green on both sides. [not illustrated]
1633 Gerarde-Johnson 249. "Of Tarragon. Tarragon the sallade herbe hath long and narrow leaves of a deepe greene colour. . .with slender brittle round stalkes two cubites high: about the branches whereof hang little round flowers, never perfectly opened, of a yellow colour mixed with blacke. . .The root is long and fibrous, creeping farre abroad under the earth. . .by which sprouting forth it increaseth, yeelding no seede at all, but as it were a certain chaffie or dustie matter that flieth away with the winds. Tarragon is cherished in gardens, and is increased by the young shootes: Ruellius and such others have reported many strange tales hereof scarce worth noting, saying that the seed of flaxe put into a radish roots or sea onion, and so set, doth bring forth this herbe Tarragon. . .It is called in latin. . .Dracunculus hortensis. . .Tarragon is hot and drie in the third degree, and not to be eaten alone in sallades. . .neither do we know what other use this herbe hath."
1650 Representation of the New Netherlands 298. "The medicinal plants found in the New Netherlands up to the present time, by little search, as far as they have come to our knowlege, consist principally of: [There follows a list of 33 common names of plants and 'many sorts of fern' and 'wild lilies of different kinds'." Among the 33 plants listed is tarragon].
What fascinating questions this raises? It does seem certain however that tarragon was there and probably planted in Dutch gardens even though the other plants in the list are not garden plants. Interestingly too it is listed as a medicinal plant. Fenton 1942 commenting on this list of plants in this 1650 report implied that they were plants used by the Indians at that time. The text does not bear this interpretation. The paragraph just quoted ends by saying:–"It is not to be doubted that experts would be able to find many simples of great and different virtues, in which we have confidence, principally because the Indians know how to cure very dangerous and perilous wounds and sores by roots, leaves and other little things." The only other mention of the Indian use of plants for medicine in this report is on p.301. "The natives. . . understand how to cure wounds and hurts, or inveterate sores and injuries, by means of herbs and roots, which grow in the country, and which are known to them." This does not support Fenton's statement on p.515:–"A reporter on New Netherlands in 1650 (The Representation of New Netherlands 1650 p.298) without professed skill in medical botany found with little effort over 30 plants which he thought might convey a notion of the valuable plants that were known to the Indians."
Artemisia dracunculus, or linear leaved wormwood is a perennial, native of European Russia, Siberia, Mongolia, northern China, west coast of north America to Colorado and Texas. The var. *sativa*, called Tarragon, is rarely found growing wild. This variety contains an essential oil in which glycosides of the coumarin type have been found. It stimulates the digestive juices and bile. Its use is prohibited in pregnancy. It is used in the food and perfumery industries (Stary & Jirasek 1973:82).

That *Artemisia dracunculus* [*dracunculoides*], the native plant of the west coast of America could have been found growing near New York in 1650 and mistaken for tarragon creates even more problems. Certainly Densmore found it to be an important medicinal plant for the Chippewas in the 1920's. We have a few small pieces of an intriguing puzzle.

WORMWOOD   *Artemisia absinthium* L Compositae (Asteraceae)

Plant or near shrub 40-150 cm tall, the stem finely silky or smooth, much branched. The leaves 3-7 cm long cut into largish segments, silvery or turning green, often narrow and uncut near the top of the plant. The flowers on short stalks, drooping, fertile, yellow. Whole plant very bitter taste, strong bitter odour when crushed.

Range. Eurasian introd. along roadsides B.C., Alta., Sask., Man., Moose Factory (where found by Macoun 1884 near the old Hudson Bay Factor's garden), Ont., Que., and the Martimes, and all over the United States.

1475 Bjornnson Icelandic mss Larsen transl. 140. "Absinteum, wormwood. . .It strengthens the stomach of whoever eats or drinks it. Yet it is best that it be boiled in rain-water, and that it be cleared and cooled for a day before it is drunk. In this fashion it drives away intestinal worms and loosens a man's bowels. In this way it helps various sicknesses which he has in the stomach. It also lets a man urinate well. If a man crushes it with vinegar and rubs himself with it, flies and fleas shun its odor. If one mixes it with celery and gives it thus tempered, unboiled, it helps against jaundice. . .If a man mixes vinegar and wormwood and drinks it, that is good for the kidneys. Wormwood also helps the poison which a man gets from the cicuta [hemlock] weed which is called thus and for poisonous bites. If one mixes honey with wormwood and rubs in the eyes, that brightens them. Water from boiled wormwood is good for sore eyes. Wormwood is good for new wounds if crushed and applied. It is also good for the itch if one bathes in water it has been boiled in. Nor does one spew from seasickness if he drinks this first. If one crushes wormwood and applies to swollen testicles, that will help. If a man puts wormwood in his bed it helps sleep. If one places wormwood among clothes, moths will not harm them. If one crushes wormwood in honey, it helps for swelling of the tongue or for the blueness that comes in the eyes. . .If one's kidneys are hard apply wormwood. If one boil wormwood with new oil and rub the belly about the stomach, that helps. And mice will not eat the book written with ink in which wormwood is boiled."

1830 Rafinesque 184. "Common wormwood. In our gardens, sometimes spontaneous. Taste intensely bitter, smell strong, contains an essential oil and bitter extractive. Very valuable medical plant. Two scruples of the extract cure intermittents. Useful in cachetic, hydropic and hypochrondriac affections, in jaundice, against worms. Essential oil dark green, a powerful stimulant, antispasmodic, and vermifuge. The wormwood wine is an excellent tonic; wine, ale and beer are medicated by it. Sometimes substituted for hops in brewing. Leaves excellent topical resolvent, applied to swelled breast and tumors. The ashes produce the salt of *Absynthium*, useful in gravel, and to dissolve the stones as formerly believed. Many other properties, very early known. It is said the continued use of this plant has cured the gout, increased the milk of nurses, removed dropsy and hepatitis."

1859–61 Gunn 884. "Wormwood is an herb cultivated in our gardens, very bitter and unpleasant to the taste, but in many cases very good medicine. The herb is the part used. It is a stimulant tonic, and anthelmintic. Good for worms, and, in moderate doses, promotes the appetite, strengthens the digestive organs, and the whole system. Used in dyspepsia, intermittent fever, suppressed menses, and chronic diarrhoea. Dose of powdered leaves, ten to twenty grains; of the infusion, half to a wineglassful two or three times a day."

1868 Can. Pharm. J. 6;83-5. Top and leaves of wormwood, *Artemisia absinthium*, included in list of Can. medicinal plants.

1892 Millspaugh 88. "Absinthium, wormwood. . .This European synonym of bitterness has escaped from gardens in many places in North America especially, however, at Moose Factory, Hudson's Bay, . . .The famous 'Portland powder', once noted for its efficacy in gout, had this drug as its principal ingredient. A decoction has ever been found a most excellent application for wounds, bruises, sprains, relieving the pain nicely in most cases; every reader will recall 'wormwood and vinegar' in this connection. Latterly it has been found diuretic, discutient, and antispasmodic in epilepsy. . .Brewers are said to add the fruits to their hops to make the beer more heady; and rectifiers also to their spirits. Absinthe forms one of the favorite drinks. . .According to Dr. Legrand, the effects prominent in absinthe drinkers are: Derangement of the digestive organs, intense thirst, restlessness, vertigo, tingling in the ears, and illusions of sight and hearing. These are followed by tremblings in the arms, hands, and legs, numbness of the extremities, loss of muscular power, delirium, loss of intellect, general paralysis, and death."

1926–27 Densmore CHIPPEWA 362. "Wormwood, *A. absinthium,* entire top of plant boiled and used as a warm compress for sprain or strained muscles. This was especially when a sprain was followed by swelling."

The essential oil of *A. absinthium* contains thujone [see cedar] which is poisonous. It can cause convulsions, intoxication, and degeneration of the central nervous system. It must not be taken during pregnancy. It is used to flavor liquers, wines and apertifs (Stary & Jirasek 1973:80).

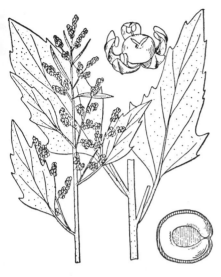

LAMB'S QUARTERS

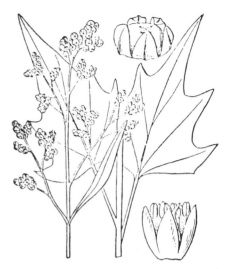

MAPLE LEAVED GOOSEFOOT

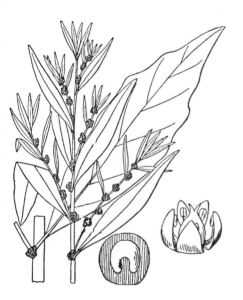

AMERICAN WORMSEED

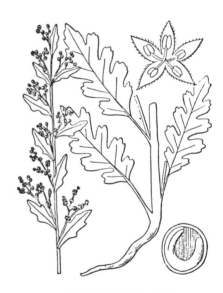

JERUSALEM OAK

LAMB'S QUARTERS   *Chenopodium album* L. Chenopodiaceae
Erect usually much branched annual plant covered with a white meal, turning reddish in the fall.
The leaves relatively thin, chiefly less than twice as long as broad, toothed. The inconspicuous
flowers in groups on spikes up the flowering stems, covered with meal. The seeds black, shining,
mostly 1-1.5 mm wide, smooth or with sculptured markings according to the variety.
Range. Greenland, Lab. all provinces of Canada, N. to L. Athabasca, Yukon and Alaska and the
whole of the U.S., also Eurasia in waste places.
Common names. Wild spinach, frostblite, bacon weed, fat-hen.

MAPLE LEAVED GOOSEFOOT *Chenopodium hybridum* L. var. *gigantospermum* (Aellen) Rouleau.

Erect bright green annual plant to 1.5 m tall. Leaves 5-20 cm long with 1-4 large teeth on each side, on long stalks. Seeds shining black, sharp edged, faintly lined, 1.5-2.5 mm wide.

Range. N.B., N.S., s. Que., s. Ont., Man., to Yukon, s. to Calif., N. Mex., Mo. and Va. Circumboreal, in woods and thickets, sometimes in waste places.

1000 B.C.-300 B.C. Chenopodium seeds found archeologically at Cowan Creek and Florence sites in Ohio (Yarnell 1964:70).

300B.C.-800 A.D. Chenopod seeds found archeologically at Kettle and Ash cave sites in Ohio and at Goessens site Ontario Canada (Yarnell 1964:70).

800 A.D.-1320 A.D. Juntunen site Michigan Yarnell 1964 41. "Perhaps the most interesting plant remains found, at least from a strictly botanical point of view, were the *Chenopodium* seeds. These are referable to two species, *C. album* and *C. hybridum* L. var *gigantospermum*. . .according to my identifications. Dr. E.H. Moss. . .Univ. of Alberta, examined the same seeds. . .The larger chenopod. seeds occured in only one collection from the Juntunen site. . .with fire cherry and blackberry seeds. . .The most significant aspect of the occurence of the seeds of *C. album* is that this species was thought to be naturalised from Europe. . .E.H. Moss states. . .'Although this species is commonly thought to be introduced, it is probably also native to Alberta, Canada'. . .Cache of four quarts of seeds recovered from a late archeological site there."

1380 Crawford Lake site Ontario McAndrews, Byrne and Finlayson. 1974:3. Of the wild plant seeds recovered. . .2.5% were *Chenopodium*.

1749 Kalm Albany April 18th. 285. "In some places hereabout there was a plant, the *Chenopodium album* L., which grew in great quantities in rich soil and was the second plant used as kale. Only the young plants, a few inches in height were used [as food]."

1330 Rafinesque 208. "Lamb's quarter, Pig weed, Sow bank. Several species, native or naturalized, eaten boiled as greens, such as *Ch. album, Ch. bonus*, &c. cooling; vulnerary externally useful in gout, pleuritis, oedema, fistula."

1870 Dodge USDA Rep. 419. The young and tender plants of the Lamb's quarter. . ."are collected by the Navajoes, the Peublo Indians of New Mexico, all the tribes of Arizona, the Diggers of California, and the Utahs and boiled as herbs alone, or with other food. Large quantities also are eaten in the raw state. The seeds of this plant are gathered by many tribes, ground into flour after drying, and made into bread mush. They are very small, of a gray color, and not unpleasant when eaten raw. The peculiar color of the flour imparts to the bread a very dirty look, and when baked in ashes, it is not improved in appearance. It resembles buckwheat in color and taste, and is regarded as equally nutritious." [Millspaugh 1898:140.]

1901 Chesnut 346. "*Chenopodium album*. No [N. Calif.] Indian name was obtained for the pigweed or lamb's quarters which is a common weed about houses. This plant was unknown to the Indians originally, and but few of them have any use for it. One Indian informed me that the old leaves were good to relieve stomach ache, several stated that they had been taught to use the young leaves for greens. The first boiling water is always thrown away on account of its bad taste."

1916 Waugh IROQUOIS 117. "Extensive use was made by the Iroquois of the vegetative parts of various plants, trees, shrubs. They were in many cases considered great delicacies and were usually collected in the earliest part of the season, while young and tender. Many of them are still in use and include the following, which are cooked like spinach and seasoned with salt, pepper or butter. . .Lamb's quarters."

1931 Grieve England 366. "This nutritious plant is grown as food for pigs and sheep in Canada, where it is called 'Pigweed'."

1923 H. Smith MENOMINI 28. "Lamb's quarters. . .used as greens in the spring."

1928 H. Smith MESKWAKI 209. "Lamb's quarters. Specimen 5096 of Dr. Jones collection is the root of *Chenopodium album*. . .tea made from it used for allaying itching at the place of the passage of urine. . .young plants used for food."

1933 H. Smith POTAWATOMI 47. "Lamb's quarters. The Forest Potawatomi consider this a medicinal food which is used to cure or prevent scurvy. . .98. It is supposed to be specific in the cure of scurvy or in its prevention. Therefore the Forest Potawatomi feel rather duty bound to include it in their diet."

The whole young plants of *Chenopodium album* collected in the early spring and tested the next day contained 130 mg of Vitamin C and 14,000 Vitamin A units per 100 grams of plant, oranges contain 50 and spinach 51 mg of Vitamin C per 100 grams of fruit or plant. The tops of older plants collected later in the year contained from 66 to 71 mg of Vitamin C and 16,000 Vitamin A Units per 100 grams of plant. (Zennie and Ogzwalla 1977.) [Was it the inclusion of the seeds that gave the higher Vitamin A content?]

1964 Yarnell 42. "The Ojibwe used chenopod seeds to make flour (Stowe 1940:12)."
[Huron Smith gives no Ojibwe use of Chenopod either as greens or as seed. Densmore gives no Chippewa use].

AMERICAN WORMSEED   *Chenopodium ambrosioides* L. var. *anthelminticum* (L.) Gray
Strong scented erect plant to 1 m, smooth or slightly sticky. Leaves to 12 cm long covered with minute yellow glands. The flowers and seeds on leafy spikes. The seed dark brown, shining, 0.7-1 mm wide, the embryo inside it shaped like a horse shoe.
Range. Native of tropical America, and a weed in waste places northwards to Me., Wis., N.S., sw. Que., s. Ont., Alta.
Common names. Jesuit's tea, Mexican tea, American wormseed, Jerusalem oak.

JERUSALEM OAK   *Chenopodium botrys* L.
Annual 20-60 cm tall covered with short gland tipped hairs, aromatic. Leaves lobed, to 8 cm long. The flowers on side branches, covered with gland tipped hairs. Seeds dull dark brown, 0.6-0.8 mm wide.
Range. Eurasian, introduced as a weed in waste places in N.B., P.E.I., N.S., sw. Que., Ont., s. to U.S. and Mexico.
Common names. Feather Geranium, hindheal, ambrose.
1672 Josselyn New England 178-9. "Oak of Hierusalem for stuffing of the lungs upon colds, shortness of wind and the ptisick,—maladies that the natives are often troubled with."
1828 Rafinesque 105-6. "*Chenopodium anthelminticum*, jerusalem oak. If the seeds are wanted October is the best time to collect them. The plant is now sometimes cultivated for medical use both in America and Europe. . .A powerful vermifuge. . .It expels speedily the Lumbrics and other worms of the intestines. It must be given in repeated small doses and the most palatable form; the seeds and their essential oil are the most efficacious, 8-10 drops of the oil mixed with sugar are a common dose for a child. . .265. It is antispasmodic. . .useful in hysteria, and a tolerable substitute for Assafetida. Called sometimes Sowbank in New England. . .Used in Europe for hemoptysis, and to help parturition. . .105-6. *Chenopodium Botrys* pectoral, resolvent, carminative, and emmenagogue, useful in asthma, suppressed menstruation."
1859–61 Gunn 812. "Jerusalem oak (*Chenopodium anthelminticum*). . .It is also known as Wormseed, and is sometimes cultivated in gardens, as a remedy for worms. . .the volatile oil. . .exists in great abundance in the seeds. This oil may be had in the drug-stores, known as Worm-seed oil, or oil of Chenopodium. This is a valuable, very certain, and always safe anthelmintic. . .It is also antispasmodic."
1868 Can. Pharm. J. 6;83-5. *Chenopodium Botrys*, Jerusalem oak, the seeds included in list of Can. medicinal plants.
1892 Heebner Pharm. 188. Officinal Volatile Oils, Oleum Chenopodii, oil of American wormseed, fruit of *Chenopodium anthelminticum*.
1892 Millspaugh 140. "*Chenopodium ambrosioides* var. *anthelminticum*, wormseed. The American aborigines used the whole herb in decoction in painful menstruation, especially of the older women, but its principal use has been the leaves and seeds as a vermifuge; as such it was noticed by Kalm, Clayton, and Schoepf, and is to-day considered one of the best expellants of lumbricoids known. The principal method of administration is in doses of from three to ten drops of the oil on sugar, three times a day for several days, the last dose being followed by a cathartic. The plant is also considered antispasmodic, antihysteric, emmenagogue, and a useful remedy in chorea. . .a narcotico-acrid poison. . .A man aged thirty took an ounce and a half of the oil and thirty drops of turpentine. . .death during a comatose state followed. . .on the fifth day from the ingestion of the drug. . .The European and Asiatic Jerusalem oak (*C. ambrosioides*), a French expectorant." [Should be *C. Botrys*].
1904 Henkel 42. "*Chenopodium ambrosioides, anthelminticum*. The entire leafy part of the plant is sometimes employed for the distillation of the oil, although the fruit alone is listed in the Phar-

macopoeia of the United States. . .Wormseed is cultivated to a considerable extent in parts of Maryland, where the distillation of the plant for oil is carried on. In ordinary seasons the price paid for chenopodium or wormseed ranges from 6-8 cents per pound. The oil distilled from wormseed is at present selling for $1.50 a pound."

1931 Grieve England 856. "Chenopodium has become the specific remedy against the Hookworm. . .The freshly distilled oil in cases of overdoses has been known to cause symptoms of poisoning. . . Chenopodium oil has also been shown to be of great service against the tapeworm and is employed in veterinary practice in a worm mixture for dogs, combined with oil of turpentine, aniseed, caster oil and olive oil. . .Carbon tetrachloride recently introduced as a remedy for hookworm, has proved most efficient. . .The European and Asiatic *C. Botrys*, Jerusalem oak, or feather geranium, is considered an expectorant in France."

1955 Mockle Quebec transl. 38. "*C. Botrys*, the plant is used in infusion as a tea as a pectoral and stomachic." [No mention of *C. ambrosioides* var. *anthelminticum*].

Chenopodium ambrosioides var. *anthelminticum*, wormseed contains ascaridol which is suspected of causing dermititis on contact with the skin. . .The dose of the oil for worms is close to the level at which the oil is toxic to man and any overdose can result in convulsions, and cardiac and respiratory problems (Lewis and Elvin-Lewis 1977; 84,291).

The confusion caused by using the common name Jerusalem oak for the *C. ambrosioides* var. *anthelminticum*, a native American plant, as well as for the European *C. Botrys* points up the value of depending only upon the botanical name of a plant.

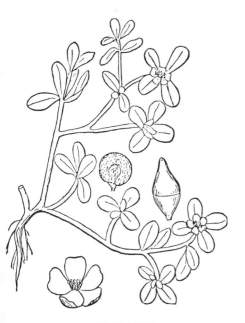

PURSLANE

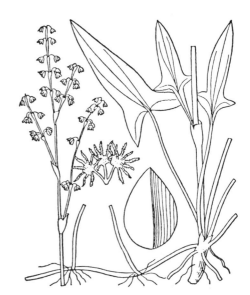

SHEEP SORREL

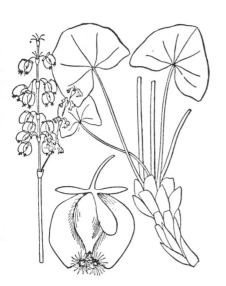

MOUNTAIN SORREL

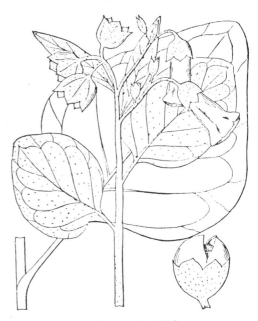

WILD TOBACCO

PURSLANE   *Portulaca oleracea* L. Portulaceae
A fleshy creeping plant with a watery juice growing from a deep central root, sending many reddish branches in all directions. Leaves flat, 1-3 cm rounded at the top. The flowers are yellow, 5-
10 mm across followed by a seed capsule that comes apart in the middle releasing large rough
seeds.
Range. Found all across Canada and the U.S. A native plant.

6000-4500 B.C. Niederberger Zohapilco site Mexico Science 1979;136. "In the type of excavation we carried out, settlement features are limited essentially to hearth areas. . .mention can be made of unit A21. . .an area with a high concentration of charcoal and fire cracked andesite rocks was exposed. Around it were scattered different artifacts and chipped stone discards. . .nearby, and in the same level, were uncovered an oblong andesite mano with a flat grinding face and, on its top surface, a small concave passive working area. . .Other identified plant remains include seeds of *Portulaca*—a plant with fleshy edible leaves—and a seed of *Cucurbita* [Pumpkin]." [This evidence, along with that of McAndrews, makes it difficult to accept *Portulaca* only as an adventitive weed, as stated by Skoggan 1978 and others.]

1380 Byrne & Mc.Andrews 1975 726. "Asa Gray even went so far as to suggest that the Vikings may have introduced it during their occupation of Greenland and Newfoundland. We now present conclusive evidence that purslane was present in the New World in pre-Columbian times. Purslane pollen and seeds were found in the sediment of Crawford Lake, which is some 35 km south-west of Toronto, Ontario. . . Routine pollen analysis of contiguous 10-year intervals indicated that purslane pollen was deposited in the lake during the period. . . from 1350 to 1539 but not to the present. . .The mechanism proposed here is that the pollen and seeds were deposited in the lake by man. More specifically, that agricultural Indians, who lived in the immediate vicinity of the lake, gathered purslane in their corn fields and washed it in the lake before eating it as a potherb. . .That agricultural Indians were in the area at this time is also indicated by the presence of maize pollen. . .Indian village site less than 1 km from the lake."

1475 Bjornsson Icelandic mss transl. Larsen 112. "Portulaca is cold in the second degree and wet in the third. Its juice is good to drink for jaundice. If one drinks it or eats it, that binds greatly a flux of blood from the stomach and other harmful things. Crushed, it is good to apply for toothache and sore eyes. It is good to eat in the heat of summer. Mixed with salt and wine it softens the bowels. It is also good to eat for stone, and for those that spit blood. This herb and sorrel have almost the same power."

1500 Draper Site Ontario Finlayson 1975 225. Recovered archeologically eight purslane seeds.

1609 Lescarbot-Erondelle Port du Mouton 1606. We found the cabins and lodgings, yet whole and unbroken, that Monsieur de Monts made two years before, who had sojourned there by the space of one month. . .We saw there, being a sandy land. . .purslane. . .We brought back to our ship wild peas, which we found good."

1612 Capt. John Smith Virginia 92. "Many hearbes in the spring time there are commonly dispersed throughout the wood, good for brothes and sallets, as Violets, Purslin, Sorrell, &c. Besides many we used whose names we know not."

1613 Champlain Voyages fac. ed. 1605 transl. 77. Indians of Boston harbour "The men who we had sent to them, brought us little squashes the size of a fist, which we ate as a sallad like cucumbers, which were very good; & some purslain, which grows in quantity amongst the corn, of which they make no more account than of weeds."

1619 Champlain-Macklem 1617 Quebec 115. "I inspected the whole place, including the farms, which were planted to corn, and the [French] gardens, where they had all sorts of vegetables growing—cabbages, radishes, lettuce, purslain, sorrel, parsley, squash, cucumbers, melons, peas and beans, among others. The vegetables were as big as those in France."

1624 Sagard HURON 239. "Any more account than all other kinds of herbs of which they make very little account, although purslane is very common and grows naturally."

1637 Le Mercier Jes. Rel. 13 HURON 93. "Gave our sick some broth of wild purslane stewed in water with a dash of native verjuice [green grape juice]."

1663 Boucher Quebec transl. 85. "Portulaca grows naturally in abandoned fields without being sown: but it is not as good as that we cultivate."

1698 Hennepin near Utica Ill. 1669 148. [writing of the buffalo.] "And the Ground where they use to lie is covered with wild purslain, which makes me believe, that the Cows Dung is very fit to produce that herb. . .295. The Cabbage and things which I had sown were of prodigious growth. The stalks of the Purslain were as big as Reeds [Speaking of the garden he had planted when held as a slave by Indians in Minn.].

1748 Kalm Philadelphia October the 7th. 90. "The *Portulaca* which we cultivate in our gardens grows wild in great abundance in the loose soil amongst the corn. It was there creeping on the ground, and its stems were pretty thick and succulent . . .It is plentiful in such soil in other places of this country. . . 1749 Albany 338. Portulacca (*Portulaca oleracea*) grows spontaneously here in great abundance and looks very well."

1768 Wesley. Poultice of purslane used for warts. [Hartwell 1970:390].

1785 Cutler, Purslane blossoms yellow. It is eaten as a pot herb and esteemed by some little inferior to asparagus.

1830 Rafinesque 252. "Esculent in salad or boiled. Diluent, cooling, corroborant, antiscorbutic, diuretic, vermifuge, subastringent, anti-syphilis, &c. Very mild, used in gravel, strangury, scurvy, gonorrhea, ulcers of the mouth. Good for children with worms. A cool salve made with it for sore lips and nipples."

1846 Cobbett Amer. Gard. 157. "A mischievous weed that Frenchmen and pigs eat when they can get nothing else. Both use it in salad, that is to say, raw." [Sturtevant 1919:451.]

1880 Claypole 177. "Every one who has owned or worked a garden in America has made the acquaintance of the ubiquitous Purslane. . .This, the only *valuable* (start not, American gardner, it is even so) plant of its order, is cultivated as a salad and pot-herb; but, transplanted into our soil and under our skies, it has squatted on the land until nothing save constant watchfulness and the hoe can prevent its complete monopoly of the garden. . .The writer would like to suggest to the Horticultural Society of Montreal the desirability of offering a prize for the best illustrated essay on the means of turning this European immigrant to account in the Canadian and American kitchens. Possibly the surest way to get rid of it would be to make it useful."

1916 Waugh IROQUOIS 116-8. Use was made by the Iroquois of. . .Purslane, *Portulaca oleracea* (partridge toes) as a food. Still in use. . .cooked like spinach and seasoned with salt, pepper, or butter.

1950 Wintemberg German Can. 15. "The leaves of the purslane (*Portulaca oleracea*) were used as a poultice for wounds."

1955 Mockle Quebec transl. 40. "The properties attributed to it are those of being an antiscorbutic, diuretic and coolant."

1970 Willaman & Li 3823. *Portulaca oleracea*, norepinephrine found in the whole plant above ground.
Portulaca widely used as a poultice or ointment for warts or tumors in folk medicine, including that of the Pennsylvania Germans (Hartwell 1970).

1974 Chapman, Stewart and Yarnell Ec. Bot. 28 411. *Portulaca oleracea* and *Molluga verticillata* were present in temperate eastern north America 2500–3000 years ago and were spread due to Indian use.
The overground plant of portulaca prior to flowering in the spring contains 8,300 Vitamin A unit per 100 grams of plant and old plants that have gone to seed contain 26 mg per 100 grams of plant of Vitamin C (Zennie and Ogzewalla 1977).

1977 Barefoot Doctor's Manual, Hunan Province, China 203. "*Portulaca oleracea*, conditions most used for: (1) Dysentery, enteritis (2) urinary tract infections, leucorrhea (3) hemorrhoids, erysipelas, boils and ulcers (4) snake and insect bites. The whole plant is used. . .taken as decoction. Or fresh plant may be crushed for external application."

1979 Globe and Mail Toronto, Wed. March 21 SB10. "The World Health Organisation Research team according to Julian Gold, U.S. Centre for Disease Control, is studying *Portulaca Oleracea*, a Chinese plant, used to make a tea which is given for diarrhea."

SHEEP SORREL   *Rumex acetosella L.* Polygonaceae
An erect stem, 10-40 cm tall from roots that run just underneath the soil. The lowest leaves on the stem have two large 'ears' at their stalk end, their tips are pointed. The flowering stem may have either male or female flowers, the latter are reddish, giving the whole plant a red look when in flower. The seeds are brownish red also. Usually growing in large patches.
Range. Native of Eurasia, naturalized throughout most of N. Am. and highly variable. In waste places, rocky and acid soil. May-Sept.

1475 Bjornsson Icelandic mss Larsen transl. 19. "Acidula, sorrel. It is cold and dry in the third degree. It is good for poor appetite, and drives away erysipelas. If crushed, it is good for swollen eyes and burns. Its juice mixed with roses is good for an old cough. If one drink it with wine, it is good for all kinds of purgation. If one eats it regularly, it is good for poison. Its juice put in the eyes makes them bright. If one puts its juice in his ear, it makes him hear well. If one wears it, a scorpion will not hurt him."

1633 Gerarde-Johnson 398. "Sorrell doth undoubtedly coole and mightily dry; but because it is sour it likewise cutteth tough humours. The juice hereof in Sommer time is a profitable sauce in many meats, and pleasant to the taste: it cooleth an hot stomacke, moveth appetite to meate, tempereth the heat of the liver, and openeth the stoppings thereof. The leaves are with good success added to decoctions which are used in Agues. The leaves of Sorrell taken in good quantitie, stamped and strained in some Ale, and a posset made thereof, cooleth the sicke body, quencheth the thirst, and allayeth the heate of such as are troubled with a pestilent fever, hot ague, or any great inflammation within. The leaves, sodden, and eaten in the manner of a Spinach tart, or eaten as meate, softneth and loosneth the belly, and doth attemper and coole the bloud exceedingly. The seed of Sorrell drunke in grosse red wine stoppeth the laske and bloudy flix."

1830 Rafinesque 259. "Laxative, refrigerant and antiscorbutic. . .but subastringent."

1842 Christison 800. "*R. Acetosa* and *R. Aquaticus*, the roots and leaves of various species of Rumex have been used in medicine, but are now almost abandoned in British practice. . .*R. Acetosella*. . .Its leaves have a pleasant and powerful acidity, which they owe to the binoxalates of potash. Till a few years ago they were the principal source of this salt and of its acid; but they are in no request now on that account as both the salt and the acid may be obtained more cheaply from the action of nitric acid on sugar."

1868 Can. Pharm. J. 6;83-5. The leaves of sheep sorrel, *R. Acetosella* and the leaves of the common sorrel, *R. Acetosa* are included in the list of Can. medicinal plants.

1916 Waugh IROQUOIS 115. "Cucumbers are said to have been preserved by washing and placing them in a brine made with salt and sheep sorrel, the sorrel being placed at the top and bottom. Quite a bit of the latter was used. A board with a stone on it was placed on top of the contents, which were allowed to stand for a couple of weeks. Pickles prepared this way were considered a great delicacy. This was probably a European recipe. . .118. the Iroquois name means paint like, red. The leaves were eaten raw in some cases with salt."

1945 Rousseau Quebec transl. 85. "The ripe seeds were used in infusion for hemorrhages."

1955 Mockle Quebec transl. 38. "The bitter and astringent roots are used as a diuretic and depurative. The leaves, rich in oxalate, are refreshing and antiscorbutic."

1968 Forsyth England 78. "The taste of the leaves and stems of both common sorrel and sheeps' sorrel, is extremely acid, due to the large amount of oxalic acid and soluable oxalates they contain. The leaves of common sorrel were used in many home made remedies of the past and are still included in salads by many people. Livestock eat small quantities of both plants without harm, but if they are forced to eat them in large amounts, or over a long period, the effects are similar to those caused by other plants which contain oxalates."

There is a long history of the use of *R. Acetosella* as a folk remedy for cancer in Europe and America. In 1926 the U.S. Nat. Canc. Inst. received a letter from Canada citing an "old Indian cure" for cancer by using a plaster made with bread and the juice of sheep sorrel (Hartwell 1970).

1972 C.A. 156770x Hungary. Researchers found that the leaves of *R. Acetosella* had a total carotinoid content of 8-12% [Vitamin A.]

1972 C.A. 76 139264b. Avin W. Hofer in Australia found that the nitrogen content of the whole plant equalled that of alfalfa when cut or ungrazed. Grazing increased the benefit.

1972 Assiniwi 101. "It is good in salads. If it is simmered for 15 minutes, it also makes a delicious lemonade drink. No Algonquin Ojibway child can ever forget 'jiwisi' the sour leaf."

[See under Woods for the clover leaved wood sorrel]

MOUNTAIN SORREL   *Oxyria digyna* (L.) Hill. Polygonaceae (*Rumex d.*)
Stem 10-40 cm with kidney shaped leaves 3-5 cm long and wide, with veins all running from the long slender stalk end. Flowers small, red or green up a spike. The fruit turns red. Related to Rhubarb.

Range. Circumboreal, in America s. to N.S. and n. N.H.

1616 Bylot and Baffin Greenland 28th.29th.July. "We therefore determined to go for the coast of Greenland to see if we could get some refreshment for our men. Master Herbert and two more had kept to their cabins above eight days, besides our cook, Richard Waynam who died the day before [of scurvy]. And diverse among our company were so weak that they could do but little labour. . .The next day, going ashore on a little island, we found great abundance of the herb called scurvy grass which we boiled in beer, and drank thereof, using it also in salads with sorrel and orpin, which here grow in abundance. By means of these, and the blessings of God, all our men were in perfect health within the space of eight of nine days."

1830 Rafinesque 51-2. "It grows in. . .Greenland, Labrador and Canada. It blossoms in the spring. The whole plant has a sour austere taste, like sheep-sorrel. . .and the same medical properties . . .They contain oxalate of lime and owe their properties to it; also to a little sulphur. They are useful in scurvy, sores, and ulcers, cutaneous eruptions, diarrhoea, putrid and inflammatory disorders. They have also been used in itch, wens, ring-worms, and even cancer. The juice or decoction is used externally and internally. Chiefly good in scorbutic disorders and equivalent of *Oxalis* in other respects."

1945 Porsild 17. "The succulent, juicy leaves and stems are edible. When raw they are somewhat acid but very refreshing, when cooked their flavour and appearance resemble spinach. A very pleasant dish, resembling stewed rhubarb, may be prepared from the sweetened juice thickened with a small quantity of flour. Because of its habit of growth the fresh and green leaves of mountain sorrel may be found throughout the summer. The mountain sorrel is found throughout the barren grounds and on the higher mountains, south of the limit of trees. It prefers somewhat shaded slopes and ravines where the snow accumulates during the winter, providing moisture that lasts throughout the growing season."

1955 Mockle Quebec transl. 37. "Plant refreshing, antiscorbutic and antiseptic."

1971 Swales 33. "The most important edible plant of the Arctic is the Mountain Sorrel, *Oxyria digyna*, whose stems and leaves may be eaten raw or cooked. I saw the Eskimo children filling plastic bags to capacity with them and taking them home where they were left on the table and the whole family nibbled at them as we would candy, but supplying them with Vitamin A,B and C. The leaves of this herb are often preserved in seal oil as well, for winter use."

WILD TOBACCO
Nicotiana rustica L. Solanaceae

Stem slender to 1½ m tall, the leaves alternate, oval. The flowers short yellow tubes 1.5-2 cm long, dilated. The whole plant slightly sticky.

Range. Cultivated by the Indians and escaped to old fields Ont. to N.Y., westward and southward.

Tropical american tobacco, *Nicotiana Tabacum* L. Brazil tobacco, has flowers with long pink, red or white tubes. It is our cultivated tobacco and does not grow in the wild.

The tobacco of the Indian tribes north of the Great Lakes, *Nicotiana rustica*, is discussed here because many native plants were smoked instead of tobacco. The ceremonial and medical smoking of tobacco is therefore, related to the smoking, for the same reasons, of other plant materials. Tubular stone pipes have been found in archeological sites of about 1000 B.C. in our range. It is doubtful that tobacco was cultivated north of the Great Lakes earlier than seven hundred years ago. It is the tradition of the Menomini that native plants were smoked before they obtained tobacco. Indian tobacco (*Lobelia inflata*), labrador tea, bearberry, poison water hemlock seeds, as well as other plants can be considered narcotic when smoked in the manner tobacco was taken by the Indians, as described by Daniel Wilson below. The evidence from Champlain in 1603 to Daniel Wilson, is that the pipe or its stem was sacred as well as the smoking of what was in it. The defeat of the Hurons, Neutrals and Tobacco (Petun) tribes by the Iroquois meant the abandonment of the Indian cultivation of tobacco north of the Great Lakes. By that time, the 1650's, the Algonkians had learnt to depend on the French and English to supply the stronger *Nicotiana tabacum*, cultivated in the French West Indies and English Virginia. The Indians preferred to mix this strong tobacco with the various other plants that they smoked.

1380 Crawford Lake site Ontario Finlayson 1975.225. "Of considerable interest is the recovery of the nine carbonized tobacco seeds (probably *Nicotiana rustica*) possibly the first evidence for their recovery on an archeological site in eastern north America."

1527-37 Cabeza de Vaca ed. Covey southern U.S. 41. "Everywhere they [Indians] produce a stupor with smoke (of presumably, peyote cactus, imported from the tribes of the Rio Grande valley and southward), for which they will give whatever they possess."

1535-6 Cartier St. Lawrence Iroquois Stadacona transl. 182-85. "They have also a herb, of which they harvest a lot during the summer for winter use, which they greatly esteem, and it is used only by the men, in the following fashion. They dry it in the sun, and carry it in a little animal skin hung at their neck, with a pipe of stone, or of wood. Then, at all hours, they powder the said herb, and putting it in one end of the pipe; they then put a hot coal on top of it and suck from the other end of the pipe, so that they fill their body with smoke, so much, that it comes out of the mouth and the nostrils, like smoke from a chimney pot. They say that this keeps them healthy and warm; and you never see them without these things. We experimented with the said smoke after it was put in our mouths, it seemed like the powder of pepper, it is so hot. . .241-245. Here follows the language of the country and kingdoms of Hochelaga and Canada, otherwise called the New France. . .They call the herb which they use in their pipes during winter QUYEC-TA."

1590 Harriot Virginia Indians 16. "There is an herbe which is sowed a part by it selfe & is called by the inhabitants Uppowoc. In the West Indies it hath divers names, according to the severall places & countries where it groweth and is used: The Spaniards generally call it Tobacco. The leaves thereof being dried and brought into powder: they use to take the fume or smoke thereof by sucking it through pipes made of claie into their stomache and heade; from whence it purgesh superflous fleame & other grosse humors, openeth all the pores & passages of the body: by which meanes the use thereof, not only preserveth the body from obstructions; but also if any be, so that they have not been of too long continuance, in short time breaketh them: whereby their bodies are notably preserved in health, & know not many greevous diseases wherewithall wee in England are oftentimes afflicted. This Uppowoc is of so precious estimation amongst them, that they thinke their gods are marvelously delighted therewith: Whereupon sometime they make hallowed fires & cast some of the powder therein for a sacrifice: being in a storme upon the waters to pacifie their gods, they cast some therein and into the aire: also after an escape from danger, they cast some into the aire likewise: but all done with strange gestures, stamping, sometime dancing, clapping of hands, holding up of hands, & staring up into the heavens, uttering therewithal and chattering strange words & noises. We ourselves during the time we were there used to suck it after their maner, as also since our returne, & have found maine rare and wonderful experiments of the vertues thereof; of which the relation would require a volume by itselfe: the use of it by so manie of late, men and women of great calling as else, and some learned physitions also in England, is sufficient witness."

1604 Champlain-Hakluyt St. Lawrence 1603 Northern Algonquins, telling him a legend. "There was a man which had store of Tobacco (which is a kind of hearbe, whereof they take the smoake). And that God came to this man, and asked him where his Tobacco pipe was. The man tooke his Tobacco pipe and give it to God, which tooke Tobacco a great while: after hee had taken store of Tobacco, God broke the said pipe into many peeces: and the man asked him, why hast thou broken my pipe, and seest that I have no more? And God tooke one which hee had, and gave it to him, and said unto him; loe here I give thee one, carry it to thy Great Sagamo, and charge him to keepe it, and if he keepe it well he shall never want any thing, nor none of his companions. . .The said man tooke the Tobacco pipe, and gave it to his great Sagamo, which as long as he kept, the Savages wanted nothing in the world. But after that the said Sagamo lost this Tobacco pipe, which was the occasion of great famine."

1609 Hudson Hudson River 48-9. "When I came on shore, the swarthy natives all stood and sang in their fashion. . .They always carry with them all their goods, as well as their food and green tobacco, which is strong and good for use. . .The people had copper tobacco pipes."

1609 Lescarbot-Erondelle Nova Francia 298-99. "They [the Indians of Port Royal] also plant great store of tobacco, a thing most precious with them. . .They will sometimes suffer hunger eight days, having no other sustenance than that smoke. And our Frenchmen who have frequented with them are so bewitched with this drunkenness of tobacco that they can no more be without it than without meat or drink, and upon that do they spend good store of money. For the good tobacco which cometh out of Brazil doth sometimes cost a French crown a pound."

1613 Champlain fac. ed. Ottawa transl. 33. "Then each of those who remained began to fill his pipe, and one after the other offered it to me; and they spent a good half hour in this exercise, without saying a single word, as is their custom. After having smoked sufficiently during this long silence I told them, through my interpreter, that the reason of my voyage was only to assure them of my affection. . .46. Kettle Falls [Ottawa River], where the savages made their accustomed ceremony, which is this. After having carried their canoes to the bottom of the falls, they gather in one place, where one of them has a wooden plate which he passes, & and each of them puts a bit of tobacco into it; having gone around, the plate is put in the middle of the group, & all dance around it, singing in their fashion; then one of the Captains makes a speech, stating that they have long been accustomed to make this offering, & by this means they are protected from their enemies, who otherwise would do them ill, so they are persuaded by the devil, & live in this superstition, as in several others, as I have said in other places. This done, the speaker takes the plate, & and throws the tobacco into the middle of the whirlpool, & they all make a great cry together. These poor people are so superstitious, that they do not believe their voyage will be a success if they have not held this ceremony at this place, all the more as their enemies lie in wait for them at this place not daring to go further because of the bad trails, so surprise them there, which they have sometimes done. . .35. They also trade furs for tobacco, grown farther downstream in the Saguenay country."

1624 Wassenaer New Netherlands 71. "In the woods are found all sorts of fruits;. . .Tobacco is planted in abundance, but much better grows in the wild parts of Brazil; it is called Virginian."

1624 Sagard HURON 26. "Our Hurons make incisions and cuts with small sharp stones.. . .With these stones they also draw blood from their arms for the purposes of joining and sticking together the broken pieces of their pipes or earthenware tobacco-burning tubes. This is an excellent discovery, and a secret that much more admirable, as the pieces glued with this blood are afterwards stronger than they were before. . .112. Sometimes the Indians held festivals at which nothing was consumed except the tobacco smoked in their pipes, which they call anondahoin. . .317. In order to get good fishing they also sometimes burn tobacco, uttering certain words which I do not understand. With the same object they also throw some into the water for certain spirits, which they suppose have authority, or rather for the soul of the water. . .88. When the Indians wished to entertain someone and demonstrate their friendship for him, they presented him with a lighted pipe after having smoked it themselves."

1626 Jes. Rel. 4: 207. "An Old Man told me he had seen as many as twenty ships in the port of Tadoussac. But now since this business [fur trade] had been granted to the association. . .we see here not more than two ships. . .These two ships bring all the merchandise which these Gentlemen use in trading with the Savages. . .[including] tobacco; and what is necessary for the sustenance of the French in this country besides."

1633 Gerarde-Johnson 356. "Of the Yellow Henbane or English Tobacco. . .[it] is sowen in gardens, where it doth prosper exceedingly, insomuch that it cannot be destroyed where it hath once sowen itselfe, and it is dispersed into the most parts of England. . . is called. . .of some Petun: of others, Nicotiana, of Nicot a Frenchman that brought the seeds from the Indies, as also the seed of the true Tabaco, whereof this hath beene taken for a kinde; insomuch that Lobel hath called it Dubius Hyoscyamus and it is used of divers instead of tobacco, and called by the same name, for that it hath beene brought from Trinidada. . .as also from Virginia and Norembega, for Tobacco, which doubtlesse taken in smoke worketh the same kinde of drunkenesse that the right tobacco doth. . .It is used of some in stead of Tobaco, but to small purpose or profit, although it do stupifie and dull the senses, and cause that kinde of giddinesse that Tobaco doth, and likewise spitting; which any other herbe of hot temperature will do, as Rosemary, Time, winter Savorie, sweet Marjoram, and such like: any of which I like better to be taken in smoke than this kinde of doubtfull henbane. This herbe availeth against all apostumes, tumors, inveterate ulcers, botches, and such like, being made into an ungent or salve as followeth: Take of the greene leaves three pounds and an halfe, stampe them very small in a stone mortaer; of Oyle Olive one quart; set them to boyle in a brasse pan or such like, upon a gentle fire, continually stirring it until the herbes seem black and will not boyle or bubble any more: then you shall have an excellent green oyle; which being strained from the feces or drosse, put the clear and strained oyle to the fire again; adding thereto of wax halfe a pound, or rosen foure ounces and of good Turpentine two ounces: melt them all together, and keepe it in pots for your use, to cure inveterate ulcers, aposthumes, burnings, greene wounds, and all cut and hurts in the head; wherewith I have gotten both crowns and credit. . .Tobaco or Henbane of Peru. . .358. These were first brought into Europe out of America. . .in which is the province of countrey of Peru. . .Nicolaus Monardus names it Tabacum. . .the forme being like to yellow henbane, but the qualities also; for it bringeth drowsinesse, troubleth the senses, and maketh a man as it were drunke by taking of the fumes only as Andrew Thevet testifieth, (and common experience sheweth). . .for they say that the use is not safe in weake and old folkes; and for this cause, as it seemeth, the women in America (as Thevet sayeth) abstayne from the hearbe Petun or Tobaco, and doe in no wise use it."

1634 Journey into the Mohawk country from New Netherlands December 18th. 143. "Three women of the Sinnekens [Oneida] came here. . .they brought, also a good quantity of green tobacco to sell; and had been six days on the march. . .December 19th. We received a letter from Martin Gerritsen [roughly 48 miles away through the forest in New Netherlands] dated December 18th. . .and with it we received paper, salt, tobacco for the savages, and a bottle of brandy."

1636 Brebeuf HURON Jes. Rel. 10; 215-21. "They believe that there is nothing so suitable as

Tobacco to appease the passions; that is why they never attend a council without a pipe or calumet in their mouths, the smoke, they say, gives them intelligence, and enables them to see clearly through the most intricate matters. . .30. I admired the ingenuity of one Savage- he did not put himself to any trouble to run after these flying pieces of fur but, as there had been nothing so valuable in this Country, this year, as Tobacco, he kept some pieces of it in his hands which he immediately offered to those who were disputing over a skin, and thus settled the matter to his own advantage."

1640 Tooker [1964] HURON 9. "By this time the Huron were firmly entrenched as the important middlemen between the French and Algonquian tribes to the west and north. . .The Huron controlled this trade to the extent that the Petun (the Tobacco nation) and the Neutral supplied them with corn, tobacco, and hemp, all products that the Huron could and did produce. . .After some years of trade the two important Iroquoian leagues, the Huron and the Iroquois, found themselves in similar positions. Both had to obtain furs from sources outside their territories by trade and both had the same goods, corn and tobacco, to trade the Algonquians for these furs."

1663 Boucher Quebec Indians transl. 101. "The men. . .grow the tobaco and make their pipes which they use for smoking."

1683 Radisson Hudson Bay 63-4. "The Indians with whom we had traded. . .came to see me to ask for tobacco, because I had not given them any of what was in the ship, on account of its not being good, but having excused myself, saying that it was in the hold, I made them a present of that which my nephew had left, with which they were satisfied, but I was surprised, when walking around the house with the governor, to see on the sand a quantity of pieces of tobacco of another kind which had apparently been thrown away indignantly. . .Captain of the Indians came to tell me that some of the young men of his band, still annoyed at the remembrance of what the Englishmen had said. . .had led to the throwing away in contempt the tobacco which had come from the English, and which the young men would not smoke. . .. But as my principal design was to discover that of the English. . .sent three [of my men] to inform themselves. . . [they] met fourteen or fifteen Indians loaded with merchandise [coming from trading with English]. . .my men asked them to come to smoke with them of Tobacco, the most highly esteemed in the country."

1685 Governor and Committee of the Hudson's Bay Co. London to Henry Sergeant, Hudson Bay May 22. "We are sorry the Tobacco we last sent you, proves so bad, we have made many yeares tryall of Engelish Tobacco by severall persons, & whiles we have traded, we have had yearly complaints thereof. We have made search, what Tobacco the French vends to the Indians, which you doe so much extoll, and have this yeare bought the like (vizt.) Brazeele Tobacco, of which we have sent for each Factorey, a good Quantety, that if approved of we are resolved in the future to supplye you with the like, as you have occasion: But be carefull to sell them, not halfe the Quantety of this, for it cost us treble the price.". . .May 1686. "Our Tobacco is also this yeare the best Brazeele, that which the Indians are so much bewitched with." (Isham 1949:86)

1698 Hennepin 125. "This Calumet is the most mysterious Thing in the World among the Savages of the Continent of Northern America; for it is us'd in all their important Transactions: However, it is nothing else but a large Tobacco-Pipe made of Red, Black, or White Marble: The Head is finely polish'd, and the Quill, which is commonly two foot and half long; is made of a pretty strong Reed, or Cane, adorn'd with Feathers of all Colours, interlac'd with Locks of Womens hair. They tie to it two Wings of the most curious Birds they find, which makes their Calumet not unlike Mercury's Wand. . .Every Nation adorns the Calumet as they think fit according to their own Genius and the Birds they have in their country. It is a Pass and safe Conduct amongst all the Allies of the Nation who has given it; and in all Embassies, the Ambassadors carry that Calumet as a symbol of Peace, which is always respected; for the Savages are generally persuaded, that a great Misfortune would befal 'em, if they violated the Publick Faith of the Calumet. All their Enterprizes, Declarations of War, or Conclusion of Peace, as well as all the rest of their Ceremonies, are sealed, if I may be permitted to say so, with this Calumet. They fill that Pipe with the best Tobacco they have, and then present to those with whom they have concluded any great Affair, and smoak out of the same after them. I had certainly perished in my Voyage, had it not been for this Calumet or pipe. . .258. Besides, he [indian chief] sent me into a neighbouring Isle, with his Wives, Children, and Servants, where I was to hough and dig with a pick-axe and shovel, which I had recover'd from those that robbed us. Here we planted Tobacco, and some European Pulse, which I brought from thence, and were highly prized by Aquipaguetin. . .295. The Tobacco which I planted before our departure, was half choak'd with

Grass. But the Cabbage and other things which I had sown, were of prodigious growth. . .304. All the rest of the Captains of this little Army came to visit us. It cost our Folks nothing but a few Pipes of Martinicao-Tobacco, which these people are passionately fond of, though their own be stronger, more agreeable, and of much better Scent. . .533. I made them a Present of two fathom of our black Tobacco; they love it passionately. Theirs is not so well cured, nor so strong as that of Martineco, of which I made them a Present."

1743 Isham Hudson Bay Indians 82-5. "They argue with Discretion Especially when they are seated with the great Callimut before them, being Chiefly the Cap't. who is for the most part an ancient man; this Callimut (alias wus Ka che) is one of their I'dols, few being admitted in a meeting but those that has a Lawfull right and title to a callimut, their Nature of itt is this. . .they give notice they want to come into the fort to smoak, in the Callimut &c. when the Ukemau enter's with the ancients after him, and a young man to each who Carry's the callimutt (and itts to be observed the women never smoak's out of these callimutts)—when they have enter'd. . .the Callimutts of Differeent shapes and Couller's, are Laid upon a Clean skin upon a table in the middle of the roome,—in this manner they sitt Very Demur'r, for some time, not speak a word, till the Ukemau, Break's Silence,—he then takes one pipe or Callimutt and presents it to the factor, who lights itt, having a young man to hold itt as before mention'd,—some of them being 4: 5: and 6 foot Long,—when Light the factor takes the Callimutt by the middle, and points the small end first to the suns's Rising, then to the Highth or midle of the Day, then at the suns setting, then to the Ground, and with a round turn presents itt again to the Leader, when they all and Everyone cry Ho! (which signifies thanks) the Chief takes 4 or 5 whiffs, according to their country, then the young man hands itt round they taking the same whiffs Each, till the pipe is Exhausted, they then Deliver itt again to the factor, who is to turn it as before observ'd according to their country three or four times round his head, by the midle of the callimutt, then Lay itt Downe upon the skin, when the whole Assembly makes the Room Ring with an Ecco of thanks,—so by Each callimutt or pipe till all is spent, when the Ukemaw makes a Speech to the factor, the Subject of which is, 'You told me Last year to bring many Indians, you See I have not Lyd, here is a great many young men come with me, use them Kindly! use them Kindly I say!—we Livd. hard Last winter and in want. . .the french sends for us go but we will not there, we Love the English, give us good (brazl, tobacco) black tobacco, moist & hard twisted, Let us see itt before op'n'd,—take pity of us, take pity."

1742 The Minister Paris to Beauharnais and Hocquart Quebec Richard 1899 151. "The ill success in the cultivation of tobacco [*Nicotiana tabacum*?] proceeds rather from a defect in the preparation of it than from any defect in its real quality. Must encourage the cultivation of it, and see that the instructions given for its preparation are adopted. The southern part of the Colony should produce a better quality."

1775 Graham Observ. Hudson's Bay BLACKFEET 313. "Some Englishmen have been sent amongst them to induce them to come down to the Forts, but they answer'd they lived very well. . .one or two had the curiosity to come to York Fort, but never repeated the visit. . .They cultivate a wild Species of Tobacco which they are fond of Smoaking."

1789 Mackenzie DOGRIB 93. "There were five families, consisting of twenty-five or thirty people of two different tribes, the Slave and the Dog-Rib Indians. We made them smoke, though it was evident they did not know the use of tobacco."

1830 Rafinesque 246. "Nauseous narcotic, poisonous weeds, digusting taste and smell; first used by priests of Indian nations to intoxicate and appear inspired, adopted by the idle savages and the vicious civilized men as a stimulant narcotic to tickle the throat and nose. . .unless we use the mild kinds or mix it with sweet herbs as the Asiatics and Indians do. . .Medically and topically a powerful anodyne, anti-spasmodic, emetic, sedative, antiherpetic, errhine, &c. Useful in all diseases of the skin, hysterics, toothache, schirrus, epilepsy, worms, &c. . .a strong injection may kill. . .juice of the green leaves instantly cures the stinging of nettles. . .The seeds equally poisonous. . .Tobacco stems, leaves and snuff destroy all kinds of insects, moths, caterpillars, &c."

1857 Daniel Wilson 336. "It is to the pipestem that the modern Indian attaches that superstitious veneration which among the Mound Builders would appear to have pertained to the pipe itself. [It is] The medicine pipe-stem. . .on which depends its [the tribe's] safety in peace and its success in war, and it is accordingly guarded with all the veneration, and surrounded with the dignity, befitting so sacred an institution. . .in its use in the war-councils, or in the medicine dance. . .254. During a visit to part of the Minnesota Territory, at the head of Lake Superior, in 1855, it was my good fortune to fall in with a party of the Saulteaux Indians-as the Chippeways of the far west are most frequently designated. . .The Indian carries his pipe stem in his hands, along with his bow, tomahawk, or other weapon, while the pipe itself is kept in the tobacco pouch, generally formed of the skin of some small animal. . .what struck me as most noticeable was that the Indians in smoking, did not exhale the smoke from the mouth, but from the nostrils. . .By this means the narcotic effects of the tobacco are greatly increased, in so much that a single pipe of strong tobacco smoked by an Indian in this manner, will frequently produce complete giddiness and intoxication. The Indians accordingly make use of various herbs to mix and dilute the tobacco, such as the leaf of the cranberry, and the inner bark of the red willow [dogwood], to both of which the Indian word Kinikinik is generally applied. . .The custom of increasing the action of the tabacco fumes on the nervous system by expelling them through the nostrils, though now chiefly confined to the Indians of this continent, appears to have been universally practised when the smoking of tobacco was introduced into the old world. It has been perpetuated in Europe by those who had the earliest opportunity of acquiring native customs. . .325. During the summer of 1855, I made an excursion. . .to some parts of County Norfolk. . .Lake Erie. . .discovered several [prehistoric] pipe-heads, made of burnt clay. . .But what particularly struck me in these, and also in others of the same type, at the Mohawk Reserve on the Grand River. . .was the extreme smallness of the bowls, internally, and the obvious completeness of most of such examples, as were perfect, without any seperate stem or mouth piece; while if others received any addition, it must have been a small quill, or straw. . .suggest by the size of the bowl, either the self denying economy of the ancient smoker, or his practice of the modern Indian mode of exhaling the fumes of the tobacco, by which so small a quantity suffices to produce the full narcotic effect of the favourite weed."

1862 Dr. Cheadle's Journal 93. "Messiter told me of his experience with scabies. . .Not being able to manufacture ung. [uentum] sulph. [ur] satisfactorily, he. . .made a decoction of tobacco boiled down to a thick paste, & rubbed this in hard for an hour, standing before the fire; soon ill, vomiting & raving delerium all night. . .towards morning better, but unable to move for a day, itch quite cured."

1868 Can. Pharm. J. 6;83-5. Leaves of *Nicotiana Tabacum* included in list of Can. medicinal plants.

1892 Millspaugh 128. "*Nicotiana tabacum*. The production of this narcotic for its specific use. . .is enormous and increasing rapidly from year to year, The United States alone raising. . .in 1880 nearly double the product for 1870. The estimated annual production of the globe. . .would furnish each inhabitant, without regard to age, sex, or condition, with over 4½ lbs. . .The important question of whether the use of tobacco in moderation is harmful or not, has been decided in the negative by many of the highest authorities."

Spaniards with Columbus in 1492 saw the Indians in Cuba smoking rolls of leaves they called tobacos. "Within a few decades there were more Spaniards converted to smoking than Indians converted to Christianity." Nicotine is generally treated as a nerve poison. "If these toxins were to be isolated from one cigar and given directly to a human being, death would result almost instantly." (Emboden 1973:108-110).

1975 Janiger and Dobkin de Rios 150. "We agree with Heiser that the tobacco used in pre-European contact times literally knocked the Indians out. Tobacco was used for magico-religious activity, divination, to treat disease, for pleasure, social interaction and to obtain fortitude. . .As with Cannabis, it is possible that novitiates who smoke tobacco must learn to recognize its effects through observation, imitative behaviour and actual instruction."

Nicotine when inhaled inhibits hunger contractions of the stomach and slightly increases blood sugar levels, deadens the sense buds in the mouth. Nicotine is more addictive than alcohol, shortens life, causes lung cancer, makes heart disease worse, increases risk of dying of other diseases, hurts the child in the womb of the mother who smokes, and lowers the skills of those who smoke. (Lewis and Elvin-Lewis 1977).

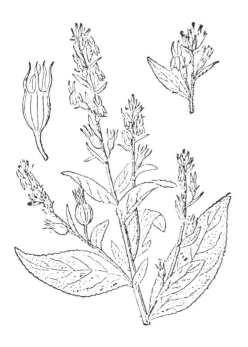

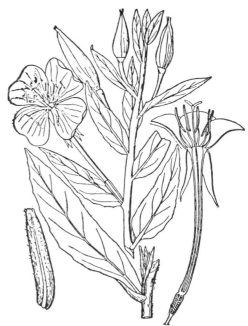

INDIAN TOBACCO LOBELIA   EVENING PRIMROSE

INDIAN TOBACCO LOBELIA   *Lobelia inflata* L. Lobeliaceae
A hairy branched stem up to 100 cm tall, somewhat angled or winged, the leaves stalkless, irregu-
larly toothed, 5-8 x 1.5-3.5 cm. The pale blue 7-10 mm flowers are inconspicuous in their long
green cups. These cups inflate as the seeds mature and the flowers fall off, they become ridged
and roughened pods that may contain up to 500 seeds of a brilliant brown color, covered with
fine lines. The whole plant has a milky juice. A biennial.
Range. N.B., P.E.I., N.S., Que., Ont. to Minn. s. to e. Kan., Ark. and Ga. in fields, roadsides and
waste places. Common names. Gag root, puke-weed, asthma weed, emetic weed, bladderpod
lobelia.
1830 Rafinesque 23. "In its effects it acts very much like tobacco, but the action is more speedy,
diffusible, and short; besides, affecting even those who are accustomed to tobacco. The herbalist,
Samuel Thompson, claims in his guide of health to have discovered the properties of this plant
towards 1790; but the Indians knew some of them; it was one of their puke weeds, used by them
to clear the stomach and head in their great concils.. . .It is now extensively used, although many
physicians consider it as a deleterious narcotic, uncertain and dangerous in practice; while
Thompson denies it, and considers it as harmless, depending almost altogether upon it in his new
and singular practice of medicine, borrowed chiefly from the steaming and puking practice of the
Indian tribes. The whole plant is used but the most powerful part are the seeds, as in *Hyosciamus*.
The medical effects are speedy and very powerful, but various, according to the preparations,
doses, and temperaments. In large doses, it is a deadly narcotic, like tobacco and henbane, producing alarming symptoms, continual vomiting, trembling, cold sweat, and even death. It
appears to act upon the brain rather than the stomach, as usual with narcotics, and is therefore
dangerous in practice unless prescribed with great care and caution. . .It has been recommended
in some shape or other for almost every disease; but those for which it is most efficient are spasmodic asthma, bronchial cough, tetanus or lock jaw, and strangulated hernia. In asthma particularly, it appears to be almost a specific, although it has failed in some cases when the disease was
not spasmodic; it has lately been introduced in Europe as a remedy for this complaint,. . .for hernia, it is given in injection, like tobacco, which produces a complete relaxation, when the hernia

can be easily reduced. . .The practice of Thompson to use it in everything, fevers, consumption, measles, jaundice, &c. is preposterous. It is not even a proper emetic for common use, as we have so many much milder. In consumption it is baneful, because it prostrates the patient without relieving the symptoms. It is however, the base of many quack medicines for consumption, which are violent and dangerous; they are erroneously called Indian specifics, the Indians having no specific for the disease, but only palliatives. This plant loses its active properties by boiling or even scalding. . .The seeds and young leaves are strongest; the whole plant is commonly collected in the fall when in seed and pulverised. One single grain is sometimes sufficient to produce emisis,"

1842 Christison 602. "The *Lobelia inflata*, or Indian tobacco, was introduced into medical practice in the civilized world after the beginning of the present century, in consequences of the representations of Dr. Cutler, a clergyman of Massachusetts in the United States; but it had been long used previously by the savages and empirics of North America. . .It is commonly imported into this country [England] compressed into small rectangular cakes, as prepared by the Shakers of New Lebanon in the State of New York. . .Lobelia had not yet been carefully analyzed. . .in large doses a narcotico-acrid poison, and in medicinal doses an emetic, sedative, diaphoretic, expectorant, and antispasmodic. As a poison it occasions violent vomiting, a peculiar acrid sensation in the throat, and subsequently anxiety, prostration, stupor, and convulsions. It is said that a teaspoonful of its powder may prove fatal in five hours, if not vomited. . . .It has been used in the United States as an emetic for general purposes, as a sedative antispasmodic in the form of injection in strangulated hernia and other intestinal obstructions, and as an expectorant antispasmodic in hooping-cough, catarrh, and asthma. Its chief application however in America, and the only use made of it hitherto in Britain, is as an antispasmodic for arresting the paroxysm of asthma. I may add my testimony to that of others. . .The breathing is commonly relieved by it in the course of five or ten minutes."

1859-61 Gunn 819. "This is the plant so much used by Botanic Doctors, called Thompsonians, supposed to have been discovered by Samuel Thompson, whose followers employ it for almost every disease as a puke; but this indiscriminate use of the plant is wrong. . . .The Penobscot tribe of Indians from traditionary evidence, used it in the form of a tea to produce vomiting, and as their unfailing remedy in colic, and hence the name of Colic Weed. The New England people obtained this information from the Indians and used it in various complaints, but particularly in colic, and considered it perfectly safe and harmless. I have traced it back to the year 1772, and with the exception of the Penobscots, I find the American aborigines had no knowlege of its properties or virtues. . .medical men have, for the last fifteen or twenty years, prejudiced the public mind against the use of it, by saying it was a poison."

1860 Trans. Lit. &. Hist. Soc. Quebec IV: 4-45. "Indian tobacco, a plant of some medicinal value, is also now in flower."

1868 Can. Pharm. J. 6-83-5. *Lobelia inflata*, lobelia, the leaves and seeds included in list of Can. medicinal plants.

1879 Can. Pharm. J. XIII;10;322. "Another herb is lobelia, and I get 10 cents a pound for it, but the price is falling. If yer ever want to get rid of what's inside yer, jist make a tea of lobelia leaves, and I'll bet my team of hosses out there it'll accomodate yer."

1890's Dr. James Richardson Toronto mss. "In the early thirties 'Thompsonianism' prevailed in the town [Toronto] as well as over the country [Canada] and neighbouring United States. . .cypripedium [moccasin flower] lobelia and a few other vegetables were the principle remedies. Thompsonians were the fathers of the Eclectics who still prevail."

1892 Millspaugh 99. "The name Indian Tobacco might have arisen from the peculiar tobacco-like sensation imparted to the tongue and stomach on chewing the leaves, or from the fact that the American Indians often smoked the dried leaves to produce the effect of the drug. . .Lobelia in large doses is a decided narcotic poison, producing effects on animals generally bearing great similitude to smaller doses of tobacco. Its principal sphere of action seems to be upon the pneumogastric nerve, and it is to the organs supplied by this nerve that its toxic symptoms are mainly due, and its 'physiological' cures of pertussis, spasmodic asthma, croup and gastralgia gained. Its second action in importance is that of causing general muscular relaxation, and under this it records its cures of strangulated hernia (by enemata), tetanic spasms, convulsions, hysteria, and, mayhap, hydrophobia. Its third action is upon the mucous surfaces and secretory glands, increasing their secretions. The prominent symptoms of its action are; great dejection, exhaustion, and mental depression, even to insensibility and loss of consciousness; nausea and vertigo;. . .death is usually preceded by insensibility and convulsions."

1894 Household Guide Toronto 120. "Lobelia is a common plant and is given as a remedy for asthma, lockjaw and coughs. It is violent in its action and a fatal poison. Care should be taken in reference to the quantity used. It is better and safer to allow the physician to prescribe it."

1904 Henkel 27. "The leaves and flowering tops are used in medicine, and there is also a good demand for the seeds. The leaves and tops should be gathered after some of the pods have become inflated, should be dried in the shade, and when dry kept in covered vessels. The dried leaves and tops have a rather disagreeable, somewhat sickening odor, and the taste, mild at first, soon becomes strongly acrid and nauseous. . .Lobelia is expectorant, acts upon the nervous system and bowels, causes vomiting and is poisonous. The price paid for the dried leaves and top range from 3 to 8 cents a pound, and that of the seed from 15 to 20 cents per pound."

1926-27 Parker SENECA 10. Among the remedies once common among the Indians that were passed on to the settlers and found to be potent. . .*Lobelia inflata*, lobelia. . .11. Use for an emetic and for coughs.

1925 Wood & Ruddock. For asthma *L. inflata* tincture take 2 tablespoonfuls. It is an antidote to poisons of all kinds whether animal or vegetable.

1949 Hobart & Melton England 72. "Lobeline is the principal alkaloid of lobelia herb. It exerts a selective and powerful stimulating action of short duration on the respiratory centre, and the hydrochloride is injected parenterally to stimulate the respiration of new-born infants, in partial suffocation (drowning, etc.), overdosage of narcotic drugs, and in other conditions where there is respiratory failure. The injection may be repeated several times at fifteen-minute intervals. Preparations of lobelia are sometimes used as antispasmodics in bronchial asthma but the action is variable. Stimulation followed by depression of the ganglia of the autonomic nervous system is said to be produced. In this respect lobeline resembles nicotine. Bronchial dilation is produced by stimulation of the sympathetic ganglia. Compound powders containing lobelia are ignited and the fumes inhaled for the relief of asthmatical paroxysms, *but the inhalation of these irritant fumes tends ultimately to exacerbate the disorder by causing bronchitis.*"

1955 Mockle Quebec transl 83. "The plant is used in dyspneic and asthmatic affections. The leaves contain 0.50 to 0.60% total alkaloids of which the principal is lobeline. Other species found in Canada are *L. Dortmanna* L. (traces of alkaloids), *L. Kalmii* L.; *L. spicata* Lam. and *L. syphilitica* L. (o.50% alkaloids.)." [and *L. cardinalis*. See wet open places.]

Lobeline has an action closely allied to that of nicotine, it first excites the nerve-cells and then paralyses them. (T.E. Wallis 1967).

Lobeline resembles coniine in its action (Forsyth 1968). [See Conium].

There is uncertainty as to the hallucinogenic properties of lobeline (Emboden 1972).

Lobeline included in Lobidan and other antismoking materials producing effects in the body similar to nicotine. It may cause nausea, vomiting, coughing, headache, dizziness, trembling and rapid heart beat. That it helps patients reduce the amount smoked has not been proved (Parish 1976).

Overdoses of the plant or its extracts will cause death in man (Lewis and Elvin-Lewis 1977).

EVENING PRIMROSE   *Oenothera biennis* L. Onagraceae

The 15-60 cm stem is four angled, red to green and can be very hairy or only sparsely hairy. The leaves are long, narrow and hairy, with hairy edges. The yellow, 4 petaled flowers are 1-2.5 cm across at the ends of long tubes which sit on a 3-6 cm hairy seed box. The flowers open one after the other in the evening, The plant is biennial, although it may persist for some years. The first year there is just a rossette of long leaves on the ground. Scoggan lists five varieties.

Range. Nfld., N.B., P.E.I., N.S., Que., James Bay, Ont., Man. to B.C. s. to Wash., Mont., Id. Tex. and n. Fla. in dry open soil, meadows, and roadsides.

Common names. Night willow-herb, tree primrose, scurvish or scabbish, King's cure-all, four o'clock, coffee or fever plant, large rampion.

The roots of the first year plants are fleshy and succulent and have been eaten in Europe since the plant was introduced there from North America in the seventeenth century. It is now extensively cultivated in gardens there. Boil the roots for 2 hours to remove the peppery taste, then french fry or eat as is with butter, pepper and salt.

1749 Kalm Quebec October the 2nd. 538. "The biennial oenothera (*Oenothera biennis* L) grows in abundance on open woody hills and fallow fields. An old Frenchman, who accompanied me as I was collecting its seeds, could not sufficiently praise its property of healing wounds. The leaves of the plant must be crushed and then laid on the wound."

1830 Rafinesque 247. "Young roots edible boiled or pickled. . .Leaves vulnerary bruised and applied to wounds. Flowers fragrant and phosphorescent at night."

1868 Can. Pharm. J. 6;83-5. The bark of the stem and twigs of tree primrose, *Oenothera biennis* included in list of Can. medicinal plants.

1892 Millspaugh 60. "That the petals do emit light on a dark night is not fanciful; still it is not due to a property of giving out spontaneous light (phosphorescence), but to a process of storing up sunlight during the day, and retaining it at night—a property identical with that exhibited by *hephar sulphuris calcarea* and the sulphides of barium and strontium.. . .About the only previous use of this plant in medicine was a strong decoction of the dried herb as an external application in infantile eruptions and as a general vulnerary. Dr. Winterburn states it to be a curative in spasmodic asthma, pertussis, gastric irritation, irritable bladder, and chronic exhaustive diarrhoeas. . .Plant contains Oenotherin."

1925 Wood & Ruddock This is an efficient remedy as a nervine and sedative to quiet nervous sensibility, well adapted to neuralgia, pains of the lungs, stomach, heart, liver, bowels and womb. Also used in whooping cough and asthma very successfully.

1932 H. Smith OJIBWE 376. "While the Flambeau Ojibwe have no Indian name for this, still they use the whole plant soaked in warm water to make a poultice to heal bruises."

1933 H. Smith POTAWATOMI 66. "The tiny seeds of the Evening Primrose are used for medicine among the Forest Potawatomi. Mrs. Spoon said they were a valuable medicine, but did not say for what particular ailment."

1955 Mockle Quebec transl. 65. "The plant is used to soothe gastrointestinal disturbances and as an antispasmodic in whooping cough and asthma. As a lotion it is used in skin diseases."

1969 C.A. 69-21863y Yugoslavia. Seed oil from the wild plant of *Oenethera biennis* contains Vitamin F. The oil was considered to be an important biologically active raw material for the preparation of medicinal preparations for the treatment of burns, wounds and skin lesions. The possibility of the utilisation in pharmacy is pointed out.

1977 Observer [newspaper] England April. "A chemical extracted from the seed of a wild flower called the evening primrose may soon be used to prevent heart attacks. . .the chemical being produced by a one-man factory at Nantwich, in northwest England, has a remarkable ability to reduce blood clotting even in low doses. The seeds from the flowers of this plant. . .contain a rare fatty acid called gamma-linolenic acid in addition to the more common linoleic acid."

1978 Hollobon Globe and Mail Sept. 20th. The first step is from linoleic acid to gamma-linolenic acid but this step can be blocked by other fats in the diet. The amount of linoleic acid being converted can also be reduced by aging and by diabetes. . .The oil from evening primrose seeds contains 9% gamma-linolenic acid and 72% linoleic acid. . .Dr. David Horrobin of the Clinical Research Institute of Montreal has been conducting an experiment using the oil from evening primrose seeds as a dietary supplement for forty multiple sclerosis patients. It is said to have helped some patients in Britain and Europe. It does not help all patients but there is good evidence it helps at least 15 percent while another 15 percent 'may be marginally improved.' The oil is also being tried as a dietary supplement for chronically hospitalized schizophrenic patients. In Britain it is being given kidney transplant patients.

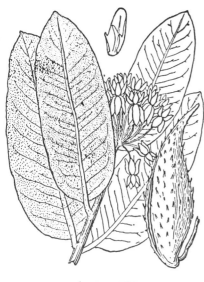

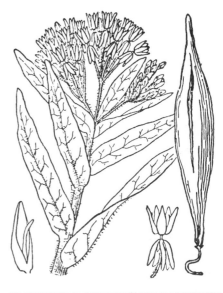

MILKWEED   PLEURISY ROOT BUTTERFLY WEED

MILKWEED   *Asclepias syriaca* L. Asclepiadaceae (*A. cornuti*)
A strong, stout stem 1-2 m tall. The leaves thick, 10-15 cm long and opposite each other, softly hairy beneath, on stalks 5-15 mm long. Flowers in numerous bunches, each with many flowers on stalks 3-10 cm long. The flowers purple to nearly green, 8-10 mm across. The pods that follow are on stems that curve sharply, they are covered with warty bumps and are softly hairy. The seeds have a parachute of fine silk attached to each one. The whole plant exudes a milky juice.
Range. N.B., P.E.I., N.S., s. Que., s. Ont., s. Man., s. to Ga., Kan, and Va. June-Aug. in fields, meadows and roadsides.
Common names. Wild cotton, silky swallow wort, Virginia silk, wild asparagus.
Aesculapius the first Greek physician is said to have named the plant after himself.
1000-300 B.C. Fiber identified in Ohio rock shelter fish net and in a Sauk-Fox bag, and a Kickapoo string by Whitford 1941:10, Yarnell 1964:164.
1609 Lescarbot-Erondelle Nova Francia 296. "They of Canada and Hochelaga. . .the Souriquois also. . .both the one and the other nation have yet at this time excellent hemp, which the ground produceth of itself. It is higher, finer, whiter, and stronger than ours in these our parts. But that of the Armouchiquois beareth at the top of the stalk thereof a pod, filled with a kind of cotton, like unto silk, in which lieth the seed. Of this cotton, or whatsoever it be, good beds may be made, more excellent a thousand times than of feathers, and softer than common cotton. We have sowed of the said seed, or grain, in divers places of Paris, but it did not prove."
1613 Champlain Voyages fac. ed. transl. 86. New England coast. "None of the savages this side of the Island Cape wear dresses, or furs, except rarely, when they do they are made of grasses and of hemp, and barely cover the body, coming just to their thighs. . .78. Cape St. Louis. . .They fish with hooks made of a piece of wood, to which they attach a bone that they form into the shape of a harpoon and tie it very well, from fear of loosing it: the whole is in the form of a little hook: the cord which is attached to it is made from the bark of a tree. They gave me one, which I took out of curiosity, where they had attached the bone on with hemp, in my opinion, like that of France, and they told me that they gathered the plant in their land without cultivating it, showing us its height as 4 to 5 feet." [See dogbanes.]
1628 de Rasieres New Netherlands Indians. "In April, May and June, they follow the course of these [the fish], which they catch with a drag-net they themselves knit very neatly, of the wild hemp, from which the women and old men spin the thread. . .106. In the winter time they usually wear a dressed deer skin; some have a bear's skin about the body; some a coat of scales; some a

covering made of turkey feathers which they understand how to knit together very oddly, with small strings. . .108. The grain being dried, they put it in baskets woven of rushes or wild hemp and bury it in the earth, where they let it lie, and go with their husbands and children in October to hunt deer, leaving at home with their maize the old people who cannot follow." [See dogbanes.]

1633 Gerarde-Johnson 898. "There groweth in that part of Virginia, or Norembega, where our English men dwelled (intending there to erect a certain Colonie) a kinde of Asclepias, or Swallow-woort, which the Savages call Wisanck. . .This plant, which is kept in some gardens by the name of Virginia Silke Grasse. . .The silke is used of the people of Pomeioc and other of the Provinces adjoyning, being parts of Virginia, to cover the secret parts of maidens that never tasted man; as in other places they used a white kinde of mosse Wisanck: we have thought *Asclepias Virginiana,* or *Vincetoxicum Indianum* fit and proper names for it: In English, Virginia Swallow-wort, or the silke wort of Norembega. We finde nothing by report, or otherwise of our own knowlege, of his physical vertues, but onely report of the aboundance of most pure silke wherewith the whole plant is possessed. The leaves beaten either crude, or boyled in water, and applied as a pultesse, are good against swellings and paines proceeding of a cold cause. The milky juyce, which is very hot, purges violently; and outwardly applied is good against tetters, to fetch haire off skins, if they be steeped in it, and the like. . .Of our Gentlewomen it is called silken Cislie. . .and now called in the shops Hirundinaria."

1640 13 Sept. Marie de l'Incarnation Quebec in a letter to Superior of the Ursulines of Tours, Mother Ursule de Sainte-Catherine-85. "I have a commission from Monsieur the Governor [Montmagny] and the Reverend Father Le Jeune to send you a certain filament, which is like cotton, so you may try by various means to find out what can be made from it. I believe it will have to be threshed and carded to see whether it could be spun. It is finer than silk or beaver. I beg you, then, to have it seen by some skilled person and, if it can be worked and put to use, to let us see some samples. We will be able to cultivate it here if it is found that it could be useful for something."

1707 June 30th. Letter from the King, Versailles to Mdme de Repentigny Quebec; Richard

1899 403. "Has received the samples of linen and the little tablets of sirop of silk-weed. . .Was pleased to get her information as to the making of sugar at Montreal." [See nettles for further correspondence].

1708 Sarrazin-Vaillant Quebec-Paris Boivin 1978; transl. 19. "This plant furnishes a sirop with which sugar is made in Canada, for this purpose the dew which is found in the bottom of the flowers is gathered."

1749 Kalm Fort St. Frederic 387. "The *Asclepias syriaca,* or, as the French call it, *le cotonnier,* grows abundant in the country, on the sides of hills which lie near rivers, as well as in a dry and open place in the woods and in a rich loose, soil. When the stalk is cut or broken it emits a lactescent juice, and for this reason the plant is reckoned in some degree poisonous. The French in Canada nevertheless use its tender shoots in spring,preparing them like asparagus, and the use of them is not attended with any bad consequences, as the slender shoots have not yet had time to suck up anything poisonous. Its flowers are very fragrant, and when in season, they fill the woods with their sweet exhalations and make it agreeable to travel in them, especially in the evenings. The French in Canada make a sugar of the flowers, which for that purpose are gathered in the morning, when they are covered with dew. This dew is pressed out, and by boiling yields a very good brown, palatable sugar. The pods of this plant when ripe contain a kind of wool, which encloses the seed and resembles cotton, whence the plant has gotten its French name. The poor collect it and with it fill their beds, especially their children's, instead of feathers. . .The horses never eat this plant."

1778 Carver 377. Tribes that inhabit the borders of Canada. "It is said that the young women who admit their lovers on these occasions, take great care, by an immediate application to herbs, with the potent efficacy of which they are well acquainted, to prevent the effects of their illicit amours from becoming visible; for should the natural consequences ensue, they must forever remain unmarried." [See Rousseau below]

1785 Cutler. The silk may be carded and spun into an even thread, which makes excellent wick yarn. The candles will burn equally free, and afford a clearer light than those made with cotton wicks. They will not require so frequent snuffing and the smoke of the stuff is less offensive. The texture of the down is weak, but sufficiently strong for dipped candles. If greater strength is necessary, a small quantity of cotton wool may be mixed with the down."

1792 Simcoe 140. "I send you some seeds of the wild asparagus. It may be eaten when very young; afterwards it becomes poisonous. The milky cotton in the seed vessels is very pretty, and makes excellent pillows and beds. I hope it will grow enough to stuff a muff."

1817-20 Bigelow 188 Note A. "A memoire on the cultivation and use of *Asclepias Syriaca*, by J.A. Moller, may be found in Tilloch's Philosophical Magazine, Vol. viii. p. 149. Its chief use was for beds, cloth, hats and paper. It was found that from eight to nine pounds of the silk occupied a space of from five to six cubic feet, and was sufficient for a bed coverlet and two pillows. The shortness of the fibre prevented it from being spun and woven alone. It, however, was mixed with flax, wool, &c. in certain stuffs to advantage. Hats made with it were very light and soft. The stalks afforded paper in every respect resembling that obtained from rags. The plant is easily propagated by seeds or slips. A plantation containing thirty thousand plants yielded from six hundred to eight hundred pounds of silk."

1828 Rafinesque 76. "The flowers produce a honey by compression. . .264. Has lately been employed as an anodyne in asthma, and a powerful diuretic in dropsy, Ives states many cures performed in New York, but it fails sometimes and relapses often happen. . .1830 196. The Oregon and Western tribes call many species Nepesha, they use the roots in dropsy, asthma, dysentery, and as emetics, chiefly the *A. syriaca*, *A. incarnata*, and *A. obtusifolia*."

1859-61 Gunn 829. "The root of this plant is regarded as a powerful diuretic, and a valuable remedy in dropsy, retention of urine, and the like. It is also an emmenagogue, and alterative. Used generally in decoction by boiling half a pound of the dry root, bruised, in six quarts of water, down to two quarts, and take half a teacupful three or four times a day. In drops it may be combined with gin. . .The tincture is a good form to use it in as an emmenagogue, to be taken three times a day."

1860 Trans. Lit. & Hist. Soc. Quebec, IV; 441. "In the spring the Habitants bring into town a vegetable called wild asparagus."

1867 Kirkwood Toronto Treatise on *Asclepias* and *Urtica* [nettles]. Advocating that these plants be turned to industrial use. Kirkwood was chief clerk in the lands sales section of the government of Upper Canada (Lambert 1967:165).

1868 Can. Pharm. J. 6;83-5. The root of *A syriaca* (*A. cornuti*) included in list of Can. medicinal plants.

1879 Can. Pharm J. 322. "Yarb digger' silk weed root is used in ager medicine, but it is scarce in my part of the country [Cincinnati]; it is worth 10 cents a lb."

1881 Can. Pharm J. 89. "In remarking on the intoxicating effect produced on bees by the flowers of *Asclepias cornuti* (*A. syriaca*), a correspondent. . .says that this is not the only apian dram-shop that is to be found, but that many plants appear to contain the intoxicating principle."

1892 Millspaugh 134. "The juice when applied to the skin forms a tough, adhesive pellicle; this has led to its use by the laity as a covering for ulcers and recent wounds to promote cicatrization. . .the root is a diuretic (increasing the solid constituents as well as the watery portion of the urine) and diaphoretic, not by stimulating but by lowering the action of the heart."

1915 Harris HURON 50. "For the cure of dysentery, dropsy, and asthma the Hurons drank a decoction of the milk-weed (Ne-pe-sha). It was also employed as an emetic. . .56. Milkweed or milkweed plants of the genus *Asclepias*, of which there are at least twenty species in America being very common in Ontario. I have identified five species around Toronto. . .It was thought fifty years ago, that the milkweed, on account of its fiber, might replace flax, but experiments failed to realise the expected results."

1916 Waugh IROQUOIS 117. "Usually collected in the earlier part of the season, while young and tender. Many of them are still in use and include the following, which are cooked like spinach and seasoned with salt, pepper, or butter. Milkweed (*Asclepias syriaca*). . .1. The young plants, stem and leaves. 2. When the stem becomes a little more mature, the leaves only are used. 3. The immature flower clusters. Plants with white leaves should not be used. These are oygo (witch)."

1926-27 Densmore CHIPPEWA 320. The flowers were cut up and stewed, being eaten like preserves. . .It is said that this plant was sometimes eaten before a feast, so that a man could consume more food. . .360. During confinement take ½ a root, break it up and put it in a pint of boiling water, let it stand and get cold. Whenever a woman takes any liquid food, put a tablespoon of this medicine in the food. This remedy was used to produce a flow of milk. . .Note at bottom of 360. "A young Chippewa women whose husband was unable to support a large family said that her mother told her of an herb to prevent childbearing and that she took it. In this connection it is interesting to note that a physician of more than 20 years experience in the Indian service told the writer that on all the reservations where he had been stationed he was aware that the Indian women used such a herb and that he had not seen any injurious results from its use." [Densmore does not say what the herb was, see Rousseau below]. . .376. The root combined with root fibres of *Eupatorium perfoliatum* [boneset] applied to whistle for calling deer.

1928 Parker SENECA 11. Diuretics, milkweed. . .12. For dropsy give a treatment of milkweed juice alternated with plantain decoction.

1923 H. Smith MENOMINI 74. "This and other milkweeds are used in the same way that spreading dogbane is used, for sewing thread and making cords for fishlines etc."

1928 H. Smith MESKWAKI 256. "When these milkweeds are in bloom, or even better, when they are in bud, the Meskwaki gather them for their soups. They are cooked with meat of some kind, generally pork, and taste very much like okra. They are sometimes added to cornmeal mush. There are two or three varieties used in the same way, but they do not use the buds of the Butterfly Weed (*Asclepias tuberosa*). They are also gathered and dried and stored away in paper bags for winter use. . .267. The bast fiber used in same manner as the bast of the dogbane family, but was considered a bit coarser than the dogbane fiber."

1932 H. Smith OJIBWE 357. "Although the Pillager Ojibwe used this chiefly for food, the root was also used as a female remedy, but for what phase of illness, we were not able to discover. . .397. The Pillager Ojibwe eat the fresh flowers and tips of the shoots in soups. . .gather and dry the flowers for refreshening in the winter time, to make into soup. . .428. Use the milk along with the milk of Canada Hawkweed to put on a deer call, thinking that it will better imitate the call of a fawn that is hungry or in distress."

1933 H. Smith POTAWATOMI 42. "The root is used as a medicine but we were unable to find out for what ailments. . .111. Not only this but other species of the Milkweed have been used for thread materials in the same manner as the spreading dogbane. . .96. One always finds a riot of milkweed close to the wigwam or house of the Indian, suggesting that they have been cultivated. Meat soups are thickened with the buds and flowers of the Milkweed and it imparts a very pleasing flavor to the dish."

1939-45 Univ. Toronto Botany Dept. "An active group took part in the general search for native rubber plants, and concentrated on one of these, milkweed, and on the Russian dandelion. Research on milkweed was directed partly toward finding and improving strains with a relatively good yield of rubber. But milkweed has a second use. Its floss made a good substitute for kapok in Mae Wests' and in Air Force clothing. Mr. D.G. Hamly invented a machine for separating seeds from floss, patented by the National Research Council. The legacy to the Botany Department was bits of milkweed floss in nooks and crannies throughout the building for years to follows." (Forward 1977).

1945 Rousseau MOHAWK transl. 59. "The silk attached to the seeds is used as a dressing for wounds. To make women sterile, a fistful of milkweed and three rhizomes of *Arisaema*, [Jack-in-the-pulpit] dried and pulverized, in infusion in a pint of water during 20 minutes. Drink a cup once every hour. The sterility is however temporary. . .16. Among the seven plants mentioned above for the genital organs of the woman, two, common milkweed (*Asclepias syriaca*) and the Indian turnip, [jack-in-the-pulpit (*Arisaema atrorubens*)] are considered anticonceptual. Their effectiveness is not questioned. . .this practice reveals a continuing preoccupation by the Indian woman with birth control." [Perhaps it was this use of milkweed by the Ojibwe and Potawatomi women that Huron Smith's informants were unable to tell him about, and that Densmore either did not know of or did not report. See pleurisy root under Mockle].

1955 Mockle Quebec transl. 74. "Plant anti-catarrhal and antiasthmatic. The silk of the seeds is used to cover wounds. Marion found in the root 1-nicotine."

1977 Nielsen et al Science 198 942-4. It has been suggested that certain plants. . .might be cultivated and grown as renewable sources of highly reduced photosynthetic products. . .we can tap latex containing plants. . .*Asclepias* sp. . .Although the results of this research are still fragmentary the possibility of future 'petrochemical plantations' is becoming apparent."

New method of extracting oil from Asclepias for use in manufacturing reported on CBC Radio, Quirks and Quarks, Suzuki October, 1978.

PLEURISY ROOT BUTTERFLY WEED   *Asclepias tuberosa* L. Asclepiadaceae

A stout, green or red, round stem, 30-70 cm tall, covered with stiff coarse hairs. The leaves are alternate, 5-10 cm long, narrow, curled, hairy, without stalks or only very short ones. There are several branches at the top of the plant. The leaves on these may be opposite. Many, or a few bunches of bright orange flowers are at the end of these branches. Occasionally the flowers may be greenish yellow to yellow. The pods stand up on U-curved stems. They do not have warty bumps but do have fine hair. The plants have scarcely any or no milky juice.

Range. New Engl., sw. Que., s. Ont., to Minn. s. to Ariz., Colo., Tex., Fla. and Mex. June-Aug. in open woods, sandy soil, fields.

Common names. Canada root, butterfly root, Indian posy, orange swallow-wort.

700 B.C.-1000 A.D. Fibers found in an Ohio mound textile. Whitford 1941:10 Yarnell 1964:53.

1817-20 Bigelow 63. "This fine vegetable is eminently entitled to the attention of physicians as an expectorant and diaphoretic. It produces effects of this kind with great gentleness and without the heating tendency. . .relieving the breathing of pleuritic patients in the most advanced stages of the disease."

1828 Rafinesque 76. "*A. tuberosa.* The root is brittle when dry, and easily reduced to powder. It is a valuable popular remedy, and a mild sudorific. . .It is supposed to act specifically on the lungs. . .It often acts as a mild cathartic, suitable for children. . .In the low state of typhus fever, it has produced perspiration when other sudorifics had failed. It restores the tone of the stomach and digestive powers. It has been given in rheumatism, asthma, syphilis, and even worms. All these valuable properties, many of which are well attested, entitle it to general notice, to become an article of commerce, to be kept in shops, &c. . .1830 264. The Southern Indians employ it in dysentery, dropsy and asthma, also as an emetic in large doses, and they use the powder exter- nally in venereal chancres as well as fungus ulcers. They make a kind of hemp with the stem. . . and use it in strings to bows. . .Mease says that our *A. tuberosa* is a safe and powerful diuretic."

1859-61 Gunn 389. "It is a very popular remedy for pleurisy in many places. . .It is used in the form of an infusion or tea to be drank freely, warm."

1868 Can. Pharm. J. 6;83-5. The root of *A. tuberosa* included in list of Can. medicinal plants.

1870 Dodge 405. Some of the Canadian tribes use the young shoots as a pot-herb after the man- ner of asparagus. (Millspaugh 1892:135).

1871 Palmer 405. Used for food by 'some Indians of Canada.' Yarnell 1964-53. [These seem to refer to the same source. I have not been able to find any record of the use of *A. tuberosa* for food by Indians in Canada. The Meskwaki ate other Asclepias blossoms but not those of *tuberosa.* Fyles regards the leaves and stems as poisonous. There may be a mistaken identification here that has been perpetuated].

1892 Millspaugh 135. "The pleurisy root has received more attention as a medicine than any other species of this genus. . .Schoepf first brought it before the medical profession. . .Barton esteemed it as one of the most important of our indigenous remedies. . .Other and more recent writers as usual have looked with doubt upon all its given qualities, except maybe its utility as an expectorant and diaphoretic."

1920 Fyles 82. "The leaves and stem are poisonous. They contain the amorphous, bitter gluco- side, asclepiadin. Horses and cattle avoid eating the plant, but sheep are sometimes poisoned when driven over dry districts where other herbage is scarce. The swamp milkweed, the common milkweed, the showy milkweed and the oval-leaved milkweed. . .are said to be more or less poi- sonous and must be viewed with suspicion until more is known of them."

1924 Youngken 490. "The Penobscot Indians employed the root as a diaphoretic and cold medi- cine. The root was eaten raw by other tribes for pulmonary trouble. It was also chewed and put into wounds or pulverized, when dry, and blown into wounds, and also applied as a remedy to old obstinate sores. In the Omaha tribe a certain member of the Shell society was the authorized keeper of this medicine. It was his duty to dig the root and distribute bundles of it to the mem- bers the society. The ceremonials connected with the digging, preparation, consecration and dis- tribution occupied four days."

1923 H. Smith MENOMINI 25. "This is one of the most important Menomini medicines. The root is pulverized and used for cuts, wounds and bruises. It is also used in mixing with other roots for other remedies. One of the most important of these compounds consists of this root, ginseng, man-in-the-ground (*Echinocystis lobata*) and sweet flag. This is considered by the Menomini to represent four Indians in power. The 'deceiver' is half boiled, then pounded to strings, to get out the substance, in this case. When a Menomini cuts his foot with an axe, this is the first remedy that comes to mind."

1928 H. Smith MESKWAKI 256. "When these milkweeds are in bud, the Meskwaki gather them for their soups. . .but they do not use the buds of the Butterfly weed, *A. tuberosa*. . .205. McIntosh considered this a great medicine antidote for poison taken internally. The Meskwaki did not know it as a medicine, but as a dye. They say it is a permanent red dye, used long ago to color basketry fibers."

1955 Mockle Quebec transl. 75. "The root is prescirbed as a tonic, and the fruits as emetic and cathartic. Recently American authors have found that the fluid extract of the roots exerts an appreciable oxytocic action at once 'in vitro' and 'in vivo' and that it contains an oestrogene substance that is biologically active." [Oxytocic. To produce a quick delivery in childbirth].

[Pleurisy root or butterfly weed, common milkweed, swamp milkweed among other milkweeds contain cardiac glycosides. These are the product of special metabolic processes in certain plants. The best known is digitalis extracted from the foxglove. In heart failure this drug causes the heart muscles to work more efficiently. Cardiac glycosides from plants are irreplaceable in current medical therapy. They are very potent even in small doses, and extremely poisonous. Plants containing these glycosides have been used since prehistoric times as arrow and ordeal poisons. Their use, described below, by the monarch butterfly is a nice example, among others, that it isn't only man who uses plants for their chemical effects.]

1972 Brower, McEvoy, Williamson, Science 177;426-29. Variation in cardiac glycoside content of monarch butterflies from natural populations in eastern north America. This cardiac glycoside content results from the fact that the monarch larvae feed exclusively upon milkweed. Brower's research at Amherst College showed that birds that eat such a monarch are poisoned, suffering nausea and vomiting for up to half an hour. Some birds, after this experience, when they catch a monarch, taste the tip of its wing and if they detect the glycoside, let the butterfly go. The female monarchs contain 24% more of these cardiac glycosides than the males.

1975 Urquhart of the University of Toronto working since 1937 finally solved the puzzle of where the monarchs, who feed on the eastern north American milkweeds, winter. They cannot tolerate cold and fly to Mexico returning to the milkweeds in the spring.

The milkweed that contains one of the highest cardiac glycoside contents is *Asclepias curassavica* [a native of Mexico]. It is being tested as a possible cancer chemotherapeutic drug (Lewis and Elvin-Lewis 1977;134, 184).

Study of 5 overwintering sites of monarch butterflies in Mexico resulted in the finding that from one site 29% of the monarchs were palatable by birds who fed on them as their bodies did not contain enough cardiac glycosides to make the birds sick. The birds, including orioles and grosbeaks had learned which parts of the butterflies contained the largest amount of the glycosides and ate only the palatable parts. They attacked the butterflies hanging on the edges of the enormous colonies. The butterflies in the centre were safe from attack, which might be one reason for the dense packing of these colonies. (Calvert, Hedrick and Brower, Science 1979 204;847-851)

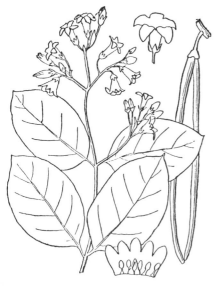

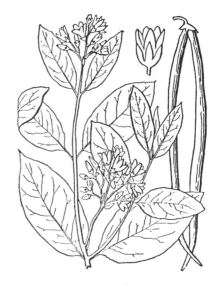

DOGBANE   INDIAN HEMP

DOGBANE   *Apocynum androsaemifolium* L. Apocynaceae
Several branches spread in all directions from the reddish, woody main stem which is 20-50 cm
tall. The stalked, 3-8 cm long leaves are opposite at intervals on these branches. The flowering
stems grow from the top of the plant or near it. The tubular, 6-10 mm pinkish flowers hang
slightly down, they have four recurring lobes at their ends. The pea pod like seed pods hang two
from each stalk, long and thin. Each seed has a parachute of silky down attached to it. It is easy
to see the pith in the root.
Range. Nfld., N.B., P.E.I., N.S., Que., Ont., Hudson Bay, to Yukon, Alaska, s. through B.C., to
Calif., N. Mex., Tex. and Ga. in Dry thickets and fields. A western var. has erect pods.
Common names. Wild Ipecac, bitter-root, rheumatism root, fly trap, honey bloom. All parts of
the plant contain a milky juice which may cause blisters on the skin of sensitive people when
handled.
1541-42 Cartier St. Lawrence Hakluyt 254-5. "And beyond the said Vines the land groweth full
of Hempe which groweth by itself, which is as good as possibly may be seene, and as strong."
[Rousseau (1937) considers this reference to hemp in Cartier's account of his voyage to be certainly an *Apocynum*].
1590 Harriot Virginia 8. "The trueth is that of Hempe and Flaxe there is no great store in any
one place together, by reason it is not planted but as the soile doth yeeld it of it selfe; and how-
soever the leafe, and stemme or stalke doe differ from ours; the stuffe by the judgement of men
of skill is altogether as good as ours. . .24. [Indians] Neither have they any thing to defend themselves but targets made of barcks; and some armours made of stickes wickered together with
thread." [References to Indian thread that follow could refer to other plants, see Indian hemp,
milkweed, basswood].
1609 Lescarbot-Erondelle 296. "They [Indians] of Canada and Hochelaga. . .The Souriquois
also. . .both the one and the other nation have yet at this time excellent hemp, which the ground
produceth of itself. It is higher, finer, whiter, and stronger than ours in these parts. [The French
had sowed at Port Royal seeds of hemp, *Cannabis*, and gathered the plants].
1632 Champlain-Bourne IROQUOIS Lake Champlain (1609) 212. "The Iroquois were much
astonished that two men [Iroquois] had been so quickly killed, although they were provided with
armour woven from cotton thread and from wood, proof against their arrows. This alarmed
them greatly."

1634 Journey to MOHAWK country New Neth. 146. "Some of them [Mohawk] wore armour and helmets that they themselves make of thin reeds and strings braided upon each other so that no arrow or axe can pass through to wound them severely."

1633 Gerarde-Johnson 902-3. "Dogbane. They grow naturally in Syria and also in Italy. . . my loving friend John Robin Herbarist in Paris did send me plants of both the kinds for my garden, where they floure and flourish, but whether they grow in France, or that he procured them from some other region [Canada?], as yet I have not certaine knowledge. . .Dogs-bane is a deadly and dangerous plant, especially to some foure footed beasts; for as Dioscorides writeth, the leaves hereof being mixed with bread and given, killeth dogs, wolves, foxes and leopards, the use of their legs and huckle-bones being presently taken from them, and death itself followeth incontinent, and therefore not to be used in medicine. . .except there be in readiness an Antidote or preservative against poison and given, which by probabilitie is the herbe described in the former chapter, called Vincetoxicum." [see *Asclepias*, milkweed].

1635 Cornut 90. Plate of Le Chanvre Indien, Apocynum Maius Syriac Rectum, drawn from plants in the garden of the Faculty of Medicine, Paris, curator, J. and V. Robin.

1642 De Vries's Notes on New Netherlands 219. "And the savages use a kind of hemp, which they understand making up much stronger than ours is, and for every necessary purpose, such as *notassen*, (which are their sacks, and in which they carry everything); they also make linen of it."

1964 Yarnell 92. *Apocynum androsaemifolium* was extensively used by the Indians for both food and medicine as well as a source of fine strong fibre to make thread and cordage for sewing, weaving fish lines. Women carried the seeds with them when they married to other tribes, particularly the Algonquin women.

1687 Clayton Virginia Indians 9. "When they design to give a *Purge* they make use of the following herbs. . .They also use some sort of the *Apocinum's*, particularly that which I think Gerarde calls Vincetoxicum Americanum [Asclepias], for there are several sorts of Apocinum's, I think thirteen or fourteen, but they are not all purgative. For having got some of the root from an Indian which he assured me was the *Rattlesnake root*, I thought the root was an *Apocinum*. . .Wherefore I gott some quantity thereof, and carrying it in my pocket, I ventured to eat thereof little by little, till I believe I have taken a dram at a time, to observe if it had any particular operation on the body, but could never find that it had." [See Bigelow below].

1749 Kalm Fort St. Francis July 11th. 386. "The *Apocynum androsaemifolium* grows in abundance on hills covered with trees, and is in full flower about this time. The French call it Herbe a la puce [fleaherb]. When the stalk is cut or torn, a white milky juice comes out. The French attribute the same qualities to this plant as the poison tree, or *Rhus vernix* has in the English colonies; that its poison is noxious to some people and harmless to others. The milky juice, when spread upon the hands and body, has no bad effect on some persons, whereas others cannot come near it without being blistered. I saw a soldier whose hands were blistered all over, merely by plucking the plant in order to show it me; and it is said its exhalations affect some people, when they come within reach of them. It is generally allowed here that the lactescent juice of this plant, when spread on any part of the human body not only swells that part but frequently corrodes the skin, at least there are few examples of persons on whom it has no effect. As for my part, it has never hurt me, though in the presence of several people I touched the plant and rubbed my hands with juice till they were white all over, and I have often rubbed the plant in my hands till it was quite crushed without feeling the least inconvenience or change on my hands. Cattle never touch this plant."

1799 Lewis Mat. Med. 164. "To what species of plant the ipecacuanha belongs, has not yet been determined. Geoffroy, Neumann, Dale and Sir Hans Sloane inform us, that the roots of a kind of Apocynum (dog's bane) are too frequently brought over [to England] instead of it: and instances are given of all the consequences following from use of these roots."

1817-20 Bigelow 150. "*Apocynum androsaemifolium*. . . In various parts of the Eastern States this plant has been shewn to me by country practitioners under the name of *Ipecac*. This name is applied to it from its power of acting on the stomach in the same manner as the Brazilian emetic. In my own trials it has appeared to me much less powerful than the latter substance; and though it produces vomiting, yet this power is diminished by keeping. . .recently powdered root should be used. The sensible and chemical qualities of the root seem to promise a good effect when given in small doses as a tonic medicine to the stomach."

1828 Rafinesque 262. "There are several varieties of this plant. . .The milk of this plant is acrid; when dried it forms a kind of gum elastic, very inflammable. It bears also the vulgar name of

Snake's milk, and is called Houatte in Canada and Louisiana like Asclepias. The roots are creeping: the bark of these roots is the only active part, being two thirds in weight of the whole. This bark is soluble in water and alcohol; as a tonic the dose is fifteen to twenty grains, as an emetic thirty to forty, it acts like Ipecac without inducing vertigo. It is also employed as a cathartic, to purge the bile, and cure costiveness. . .1830 193. Very valuable, affording hemp and cloth from the stems, cotton in the pods, sugar in the blossoms, shoots edible like asparagus, root very powerful emetic. . .All the species nearly equal, and deserving attention."

1859-61 Gunn 748. "The Bitter root. . .as a restorative after fever and ague. The root should be gathered in the fall, and the bark of the root or outside part, after being thoroughly washed and scraped clean, should be stripped off and dried, when it may be easily powdered in a mortar. It may be given in fine powder, in doses of ten grains, two or three times a day, as a laxative and alterative, to act on the liver; and also for dyspepsia."

1868 Can. Pharm. J. 6;83-5. The roots of *A. androsaemifolium*, bitter root, included in list of Can. medicinal plants.

1892 Millspaugh 132. "The only previous use of this herb is said to be that of the Indians, who employed it in syphilis. . .The drug has been dismissed from the U.S.Ph. on account of lack of knowledge of its action. . .When desired as a tonic, diaphoretic or laxative agent, a decoction prepared as follows is the most effectual: Take an earthern. . .vessel and place in it one oz. of the sliced plant, roots, stems and leaves, to which add one pint of pure cold water; place the vessel in a pot of water and let it come to the boil, and remain so for at least an hour, replenishing as fast as it evaporates, with hot water, then strain the decoction from the inner vessel before it cools. It should be covered with a tight lid while heating, and after bottling should always be kept tightly corked; even then it is worthless after standing a few days. Dose, a tablespoonful three times a day. . .[It] is an emetic without causing nausea, a cathartic, and quite a quite powerful diuretic and sudorific; it is also expectorant and considered antisyphilitic."

1926-27 Densmore CHIPPEWA 326. "In dogbane the part preferred was the elbow of the root. The plant having a root which descends straight downward for 15-18 inches and then turns sharply to one side. . .336. Four pieces of dried root about the size of a pea were pulverized and the dry powder snuffed up the nostrils for a headache. Or the powdered root was put on hot stones, the patient covered his head and inhaled the fumes. Or the powdered root was moistened with lukewarm water and applied to an incision on the temple by means of soft duck down [see cinquefoil]. This herb was not simply for a pain in the head but for a serious affection of the nerves of which the headache was the symptom. It was given for excessive nervousness as when the mouth twitched, for dizziness, and with one herb added, for insanity. As an instance of its successful use Gagwin said that a certain woman said someone threatened to poison her. Gagwin told her to steep this root, keep it in a bottle and drink some occasionally, and if this did not have the desired effect he would give her something else to take with it. This remedy was however sufficient and she did not return". . .The root is used with *Lathyrus venosus* for convulsions. . .338. Take 4 pieces of the dried root and boil about 2 minutes. Take a good drink of this decoction when desired for heart palpitations. The root was said to grow to a great length, and usually to be found running north and south. A weaker decoction was used as a remedy for earache, and a very weak decoction was said to be good for a babies cold. . .356. A decoction of 1 arm length of the root and a very little boiling water, moisten cotton in this and stuff up the nose for hemorrhage or in severe cases use the mashed root as a plug. . .360. A decoction made of about 1 inch of root poured into a sore ear with a scoop. . .376. The root is chewed to counteract evil charms.

1923 H. Smith MENOMINI 73. "The outer bark or rind of this herb furnished the finest Menomini thread material. The smallest divisions of this bast fibre are finer than our finest cotton thread and stronger. Just before the fruit has ripened the outer bark is peeled. By using three strands it is plaited so that a very strong cord is obtained. In the old days this was the way the Menomini made their bow strings. It was also by further combining and plaiting, made into heavier rope. . .79. This plant stalk is used as a helper to call up deer. It becomes a magnet. The hunter has a regular deer 'squacker' and keeps this plant or cynthia in his mouth, sucking it as he proceeds, making believe that he is a fawn, wanting to call the doe because he is hungry. When he is hunting deer he must not eat pepper, onions or any sweet. After he has killed the deer, he may eat whatever he chooses."

1928 H. Smith MESKWAKI 267. "The outer rind or bark of this particular species was considered the best because it grew on the uplands and was therefor tougher than that of *A.*

cannabinum which grew on the bottom lands. . .201. The root is used in medicine for dropsy. Specimen 5092 of the Dr. Jones collection is a mixture containing the rind of spreading dogbane together with the wood of sugar maple, the stem of angelica, the bark of crab apple, the root of swamp dock and the flower base of blue-eyed grass. It was used by a woman with an injured womb." 193. It is one of 9 ingredients in a poultice for snake bites and as a tea to cure dropsy.

1932 H. Smith OJIBWE 354. "Bearskin, Flambeau medicine man, said that the stalk and root of this plant are steeped to make a tea for women to drink. It keeps the kidneys open during pregnancy. Under the Ojibwe name of 'medicine lodge root' the Pillagers declare it to be one of the sacred roots that is eaten during the medicine lodge ceremony. They also use it for throat trouble. When one has a coated tongue and is afflicted with headache, the root is also used. In case of headache, the root is placed upon live coals and the incense inhaled. . .428. The Pillager say that this is one of the roots the use of which is taught in the fourth degree of the medicine lodge, and that it is not only eaten during the medicine lodge ceremony, but it is also chewed to keep other witch doctors from affecting one with an evil charm."

1933 H. Smith POTAWATOMI 38. "Called 'woman's breast weed' by the Forest Potawatomi. . .Use the root of Spreading Dogbane as a diuretic and urinary medicine, although Mrs. Spoon and the Prairie Potawatomi informant called it a heart and kidney medicine and used the green fruits, which they boiled to extract the active principle. . .111. Just about the time the pods are green, and before they open, the rind or bast fiber of the bark is very strong and tough. By twisting the stalk in opposite directions and pulling upon it they can determine just when the bast fiber has matured to suit their purposes. They then cut down the entire stalk and remove the bark, which is bound into braids for future use. It is usually then thrown into a kettle of hot water and this also renders it more readily separable and tougher. The fine divisions of this fibre are very strong and also quite slender. A strand no thicker than no. 200 D.M.C. cotton will be many times stronger. They use it as a thread for sewing on the fine beadwork that is put upon buckskin, such as moccasins and coat work."

1925 Wood & Ruddock. "Bark of the root, this is celebrated among the Indians for the cure of venereal diseases and is regarded as almost infallible. . .A wash made by steeping the root in water is good for scald head and ulcers.. . .The extract has lately been employed by some practitioners for nervous headaches."

1931 Grieve 108. "One of the digitalis group of cardiac tonics, *apocynum* is the most powerful in slowing the pulse, and its action on the vaso-motor system is also very strong. Being rather irritant to the mucous membranes, it may cause nausea and catharsis, so that some cannot tolerate it. . .The dosage and the patient must be carefully watched and guarded. . .It should not be substituted for *A. cannabinum*."

1935 Jenness OJIBWA Parry Island Lake Huron 89. "Sores from poison ivy, boil the leaves of the dogbane, *A. androsaemifolium* for half an hour and rub over the sores. They should disappear in two or three days."

1955 Mockle Quebec transl. 74. "The plant is toxic and vesicant. Simply touching it can provoke eruptions and redness all over the body. The root contains heterosidic cardioactive principles: apocynine, apocyneine, apocynamarine."

1954 de Lazlo and Henshaw Science 3097 626-31. The Indians used the boiled roots as an oral contraceptive, thought to excite temporary sterility.

INDIAN HEMP   *Apocynum cannabinum* L.

The strong, erect main stem is 30-45 cm tall. The leaves on 5-10 mm stalks are opposite, smooth or hairy beneath and 5-11 cm long. The shape of the flower is different from that of spreading dogbane. Indian hemp's flower stands upright, is only 3-6 mm long, is without lobes that bend outward and is greenish white. The seed pods are 10-15 cm long. The roots have very little if any pith in them.

Range. Nfld., N.B., N.S., Que., Ont., Man. to B.C., s. to Calif., Tex. and Fla. in rocky or gravelly shores, borders of woods and thickets. Local in the east, more abundant from N.Y. to N.D.

1000-300 B.C. Fiber identified in Ohio Hopewell fabric and Adena fabric, and in a Sauk-Fox bag by Whitford 1941:9, Yarnell 1964:191.

1609 Juet Hudson River 18. "This day many of the people came aboord, some in Mantles of Feathers, and some in skinnes of divers sorts of good Furres. Some women also came to us with Hempe."

1612 Capt. John Smith Virginia Indians 100. "We have seen some use mantles made of Turky feathers, so prettily wrought and woven with threads that nothing could be discerned but the feathers, that was exceedingly warme and very handsome." See Zeisberger below.

1749 Kalm Delaware 27th. March 272. "The Swedes. . .when they first settled. . .sowed flax here, and wove linen cloth. Hemp was not to be had; they made use of linen and wild hemp for fishing tackle. . .April the 9th. 277. *Apocynum cannabinum* grew plentifully in old grain grounds, in woods, on hills, and in high places. The Swedes have given it the name of Indian hemp, because the Indians formerly and even now apply it to the same purposes as the Europeans do hemp; for the stalk may be divided into filaments, and is easily prepared. When the Indians were still living among the Swedes in Pennsylvania and New Jersey, they made ropes of this *Apocynum*, which the Swedes bought and used them for bridles, and for nets. These ropes were stronger and kept longer in water than such as were made of common hemp. The Swedes usually got thirty feet of these ropes for one piece of bread. Many of the Europeans still buy such ropes because they last so well. The Indians also make several other articles of this hemp, such as various sizes of bags, pouches, quilts and linings. On my journey into the country of the Iroquois I saw women employed in the manufacture of this hemp. They made use neither of spinning wheels nor distaffs, but rolled the filaments upon their bare thighs, and made thread and strings of them, which they dyed red, yellow, black, etc. and afterwards worked them into goods with a great deal of ingenuity. . .Sometimes the fishing equipment of the Indians consists entirely of this hemp. The Europeans made no use of it that I know. . .1748 September 29th. 71. Instead of flax several people made use of a kind of dog's bane or Line's *Apocynum cannabinum*. The people [English in Philadelphia] prepared the stalks of this plant in the same manner as we prepare those of hemp or flax. It was spun and several kinds of stuffs were woven from it. The savages are said to have had the art of making bags, fishing nets, and the like from it many centuries before the arrival of the Europeans."

1779 Zeisberger DELAWARE 16. "They train their daughters in this and also in such other work as will be expected of them, as cooking, bread-making, planting, making of carrying-girdles and bags, the former used to carry provisions and utensils on their backs while journeying and the latter to hold the provisions. Both are made of wild hemp which they gather in the fall and use for various purposes, for mending shoes and making the thread with which they sew amongst the rest. . .Wild hemp is much tougher than that cultivated by the whites. . .24. These carrying girths are made by the women of wild hemp which is first spun. The part of the girths which passes across the breast and over the shoulders is three fingers (inches) broad and decorated with various figures; from it depend long, plaited, durable bands to which the burden is bound. [Note by A.B. Hulbert 1909 that this is *Apocynum cannabinum*]. . .29. The women make blankets of turkey-feathers which are bound together with twine made of wild hemp. Of such many are to be found even at the present day among the Indians, and these in winter are better protection against the cold than the best European blanket. The women also made themselves petticoats of wild hemp."

1828 Rafinesque 51. "The *A. cannabinum* has been used by the Americans to make a kind of hemp; the fibrous tough bark of all the species are calculated to afford it by maceration. All have a bitter milky juice, and yet the flowers smell of honey and produce that sweet substance. . .The root when chewed has an intensely bitter and unpleasant taste. . .This is a very active plant, highly valued by the Southern Indians. It is tonic, emetic, alterative and antisyphilitic. The root is the most powerful part: but it must be used fresh, since time diminishes or destroys its power. At the dose of thirty grains of the fresh powdered root, it acts as an emetic, equal to ipecacuana; in smaller doses, it is a tonic, useful in dyspepsias and fevers. The Chickasaw and Choctaw Nations employ it in syphillis and consider it a specific, they use the fresh root chewed, swallowing only the juice. This later use has been introduced into Tennessee and Kentucky as a great secret."

1863 Porcher 484. "The decoction affords a permanent dye, black or brown, according to the mordant used.

1868 Can. Pharm. J. 6;83-5. The root of Indian hemp, *A. cannabinum*, included in list of Can. medicinal plants.

1915 Speck PENOBSCOT 310. "Several of the roots of worm-root (*Apocynum cannabinum*). . .are steeped in water and administered to expel worms."

1928 H. Smith MESKWAKI 201. "The bast is used for sewing where very fine thread is needed. The root medicine is a universal remedy for many things. It is specially used by these Indians in dropsy and ague. . .This grows in the bottom lands and is not considered as strong as dogbane which grows on the uplands."

1926-7 Densmore CHIPPEWA 340. *Apocynum* species, the root dried and pulverized and snuffed up the nostrils. Used for a heavy cold in the head, and was said to cause sneezing and relieve the head.

1955 Mockle Quebec transl. 74. "This species is used as a hydragogue, diaphoretic, diuretic, febrifuge and drastic purge. The rhizome contains principally cymaroside.

1964 Kupchan, Hemingway & Doskotch, J. Med. Chem. 7;803. Tumor Inhibitors IV. The entire plant of *Apocynum cannabinum* contains the glycosides cymarin and apocannoside which have shown anti tumor activity.

1975 Trevor Robinson 159. The cardiac glycosides are found in several quite unrelated plant families such as Apocynaceae, Liliaceae, Moraceae and Ranunculaceae. Plants containing them have been used since prehistoric times as arrow and ordeal poisons. The glycosides have specific cardiotonic effect.

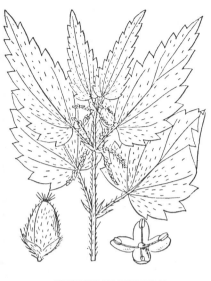

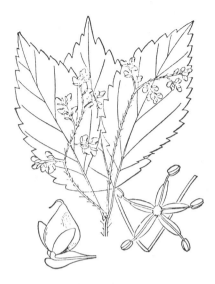

STINGING NETTLE   WOOD NETTLE

STINGING NETTLE   *Urtica dioica* L. ssp.*gracilis* (Ait.) Sel. Urticaceae (*U. Lyallii*)
Erect four angled stem to 2 m covered with stinging hairs. The 5-15 cm leaves are opposite on
long stalks with 2-3.5 mm teeth, sparsely hairy on both sides. The female and male flowers are
usually on separate branches, both are inconspicuous, on short drooping stalks growing from the
axils of the leaves. There are several erect shiny 1.5 mm seeds on each stalk. The European variety of *U. dioica* usually has the male and female flowers on separate plants. This variety has been
introduced in America and is here along with our native *U. dioica*.
Range. Lab., N.B., P.E.I., N.S., Que., Ont. Hudson Bay to Yukon and s. Alaska s. to Mexico and
S. Am. in thickets, shores and waste places.

WOOD NETTLE   *Laportea canadensis* (L.) Wedd. (*Urticastrum divaricatum*)
The 50-100 cm stem often bends, the leaves are alternate and wide, 8-15 cm long, sharply
pointed and coarsely toothed. The fertile flowers are on stalks growing from long branched
stems. The whole plant is sparsely hairy, each hair can sting. The seeds are 0 shaped 3-4 mm
long.
Range. St. Pierre & Miqu., N.B., N.S., Que., Ont., s. Man., se. Sask., s. to Okla., Ala., and Fla. in
moist woods and streambanks.
300 B.C. Ohio Hopewell and rock shelter fabrics. Whitford (1941:13) identified *Urtica gracilis*
and *Laportea canadensis* in the facbrics. Yarnell 1964:189. *Boehmeria cylindrica*, stingless nettle.
Its fiber was used for bowstrings by the Ojibwa. (Whitford 1941:12. Yarnell 1964:189.)
The principle plants used for hemp by the St. Lawrence Iroquois were nettles, basswood, dogbane and milkweed. The quotations that follow, if the plant is not named, could refer to any of
these plants. However, as later writers say the Hurons used the nettle as hemp, they are grouped
here. See the other plants. Although found in wet places, Nettle is placed here to be with the
other main fiber plants.
1475 Bjornsson Icelandic mss transl. Larsen 134. "Urtica, nettle. It is very hot. It is good for
jaundice if one crushes it with wine and drinks it. If one boils the seed in wine, that is good for
diseases of the testicles. It cures, too, old cough if one drinks it often, and drives away cold from
the lungs, and it is good for swollen stomach. For all this, nettle seed is good together with honey, or if one drinks green nettle juice. If one crushes salt with nettle leaves, it is good for boils and
foul sores. It is good for teeth and dog-bite. With this too, flesh is put on the bare bones, and all
dangerous humor is dried. But if nettle roots are crushed with vinegar, that is good for swelling

of the spleen and of the feet. If a man places nettle leaves in his nose it bleeds. If one anoints his face with nettle, then flow of blood is stopped. Nettle seed crushed with honey is good for swellings of the ribs, for ache of the side and pustules of the lungs. Green nettle-kale loosens the bowels. If one rinses his mouth long with nettle juice, it is good for swollen uvula. Ointment made of nettle makes a man sweat if he rubs himself with it."

1534 Cartier Voyage Gaspe transl. 62-3. "We found great quantity of mackerel, which the Indians had caught with nets made of the cord of hemp which grows in their country, where they ordinarily live; for they come to the sea only at the time of fishing."

1535 Cartier St. Lawrence IROQUOIS transl. 123-4. "It is called Stadacona, there is as good earth here as it is possible to see. . .other trees underneath which grows hemp, as good as that of France, growing without being planted or cultivated."

1624 Sagard HURON 332. "In marshy and humid places there grows a plant named Anonhasquara, which makes very good hemp; The Indian women gather and pluck it in season and prepare it as we do ours, without my being able to learn who gave them the invention of it other than necessity, mother of inventions. After it is prepared they spin it on their thighs, as I have said; then the men make snares and fishing nets of it. They use it also for various other things, but not to make cloth, for they have not the use nor the knowledge of that."

1632 Champlain-Bourne (1616) HURON 81. "Their clothing is made from skins of all sorts. Some of they get by skinning their own game; others they get in exchange for corn, meal, beads and fish nets from the Alkonkins and Nippissings, who are great hunters. . .83. The women do much of the work around the house. . .stripping and spinning hemp, making fishnets. . .98. The men also make their own nets and fish right through the winter."

1600's HURON ALGONQUIN Tooker 1964; 9. "By this time, the Huron were firmly entrenched as the important middlemen between the French and the Algonquian tribes to west and north. . .The Huron controlled the trade to the extent that the Petun [Tobacco]. . .and the Neutral provided them with corn, tobacco, and hemp, products that the Huron themselves could and did produce. (Hunt 1940:59 and passim probably overemphasizes the amount of hemp traded by the Petun to the Huron). The Huron reaped a profit from these transactions."

1633 Gerarde-Johnson 707. "The downe of it [European nettle] is stiff and hard, piercing like fine little prickles or stings, and entering into the skin; for if it be withered or boyled it stingeth not at all, by reason of the stiffnesse of the downe is fallen away. . .Being eaten. . .it maketh the body soluble, doing it by a kinde of cleansing qualitie: it also provoketh urine, and expelleth stones out of the kidneys: being boyled with barley creame it bringeth up tough humours that sticke in the chest, as it is thought. . .The seed of Nettle stirreth up lust, especially drunke with Cute. . .878. That liquor which we call in English Cute, which is made of the sweetest must [juice pressed out of grapes used in wine making] by boyling it to a certain thicknesse, or boyling it to a third part. . .707. Nettle is good for them that cannot breathe unless they hold their necks upright, and for those that have the pleurisie, and for such as be sick of the inflammation of the lungs, if it be taken in a looch or licking medicine, and also against the troublesome cough that children have, called Chin-cough [whooping cough]."

1642-44 Jes. Rel. HURON 203. "About forty persons went to gather some wild plants of which they make a kind of twine for the nets they use in fishing."

1663 Boucher Quebec transl. 34-5. "There grows in the woods a prodigious quantity of nettles good for making hemp; the savages, Hurons & Iroquois use them to make many things, such as bags, nets, necklaces & armor; there is a great quantity growing in many places in this country. . .86. Nettles with which thread and very good cordage is made."

1670 Marie de l'Incarnation Quebec. 372. "They [Indians] also make thread of nettles, which they spin without a spindle, twisting it on their knees with the palm of the hand. With this they make their embroidery, ornamenting it with black and white porcupine quills, combined with others boiled in roots, which makes them as beautiful as cochineal makes scarlet in France."

1698 Hennepin 522. "The Iroquois in the fishing season sometimes make use of a Net of forty or fifty fathom long, which they put in a great canow; after they cast it in an oval Form in convenient places in the Rivers. . .They sometimes catch four hundred white fish, besides many sturgeon, which they draw to the Bank of the River with Nets made of Nettles.. To fish in this manner, there must be two Men at each end of the Net, to draw it dexterously to the shoar. They take like wise a prodigious quantity of Fish in the River of Niagara, which are extremely well tasted. . .528. [The women] make Thred of Nettles, and of the Bark of the Line Tree [basswood,], and of certain Roots, whose Names I know not."

1709 Raudot Quebec 369. "These savages of the northern regions [ALGONQUINS]. . .are as skillful at fishing as at hunting; they have on this subject a story that a certain Sirakitehak, who they say created heaven and earth and who is one of their divinities, invented the way of making nets after having attentively considered the spider when she worked to make her web to trap flies. They make these nets of nettles or wild hemp, of which there is much in moist places, and the women and girls spin and twist these on their bare thighs. . .It is with these nets that they take all sorts of fish."

1913 Short 495. "In 1705 a French armed cruiser, escorting a fleet of small French vessels bringing to Canada the greater part of the annual supplies. . .was taken by the English. . .Great loss and suffering ensued. Among the wants most severely felt was that of cloth. This was so extreme. . .that the inhabitants were driven to manufacture rough cloth out of whatever fibres they could obtain. The chief of these was the Canadian nettle and the inner bark of the bass-wood. Naturally this experience had considerable influence in developing domestic industry in several important lines, which remained features of Canadian produce long after the close of French rule."

1705 Letter Vaudreuil Quebec to the King Versailles 210. "Dame de Repentigny makes herself very useful by her manufacture of blankets from nettle thread and woollen stuffs."

1706 Letter from Versailles to Raudot Quebec 202. "Would like samples of the linen made from nettles and the bark of trees, by Dame de Repentigny, and which she claims is better than that made with flax or hemp."

1707 June Letter from Versailles to Raudot 203. "His Majesty received the articles manufactured by Dame de Repentigny. His Majesty continues his gratuity to her."

1707 June 30 Mem. from the King to Vaudreuil 209. "They have not informed him whether the English employed by Madame de Repentigny have become Catholics."

1707 November Vaudreuil to Versailles 215. "The English employed by Dame de Repentigny have gone back to Boston."

1708 Raudot Mem. 227. "There is a great lack of clothing. . .the people will work only for high wages, saying that they wear out more clothes when working, than they earn by their labor."

1712 25th. June Versailles to the son of Madame de Repentigny 456. "As the King does continue in favour of the widows the pensions granted to their husbands, could not recommend what he asks for his mother. . .27 June. Cannot send coats for the soldiers this year. They must clothe themselves as best they can. They could work for the settlers during the winter and earn their clothes. . . 29th June to Dame de Repentigny. "Will represent her son's claims to an ensigncy, in view of his service. Urges her to devote herself with still greater energy to developing her manufacturing industry."

1695 List of important men in the colony prepared by the Governor for the King. [Richard 29] De Repentigny the elder. A Canadian gentleman. A native of Normandy. Aged 65 to 66 years. A worthy man. Married to the daughter of a settler. Has had at one time 10 children in the service, two of whom were killed by the Iroquois.

1709 July Died Sr. De Repentigny.

[All the above quotations from Richard 1899 Suppl. Rep. to Can. Arch. 1901.]

1722 La Potherie IROQUOIS 34. "Fiber of nettle were spun by the Iroquois women into cords, with which they made fish nets."

1830 Rafinesque 272. "Nettles, Native sp. all nearly equal, *U. dioica* best known as medical. . .The property of stinging when fresh, called urtication, formerly used as a powerful stimulant and rubefacient in palsies and to cause revulsions. When dry no longer stinging. Cultivated in Sweden for fodder, cows fed on it give much milk and yellow butter. Makes horses smart and frisky. Stimulates fowls to lay many eggs. Spring shoots are boiled in Europe for pot herbs. The stems of all afford a kind of tow, hemp, flax, cloth and paper. . .Our *U, procera* and *canadensis* once began to be cultivated as fine perennial hemp. Seeds vermifuge, laxative, good food for fowls and turkeys, said to cure goitre and reduce excessive corpulence."

1833 Howard Quebec mss.1. "For vomiting blood take 2 spoonfuls of Nettle Juice. . .58. To cure Hoarseness. Dry nettle roots in an oven. Then powder them finely and mix them with one quantity of treacle. Take a spoonful twice a day. . .86. To cure the Bleeding Piles Lightly boil juice of Nettles with a little sugar take 2 ounces of it. It seldom needs repeating. . .89. To cure Pleurisy Boil Nettles and apply them as a poultice as hot as can be bourn. Mr. Wesley says 'He never Knew it to Fail'. . .105. To cure an old running sore. Take every morning 2 or 3 spoonfuls of Nettle juice and apply nettles bruised in a mortar to the part. This cures any old sore or ulcer. . .116.

To cure the tooth ache. . .lay bruised nettles to the cheek."

1859-61 Gunn 832. "It is astringent, tonic and diuretic. A decoction of the root is highly valuable in diarrhoea, dysentery, in all bowel affections, and in hemorrhages from the lungs, and other organs. A strong decoction of the Nettle root, Wild Cherry bark, and Blackberry root, made into a sirup, is an extremely valuable remedy for the bowel complaints of children, as well as for grown persons. A decoction of the root is also one of the best remedies in bleeding from the urinary organs. The seeds and flowers of the Nettle, tinctured in wine or spirits, and given in teaspoonful doses three or four times a day, is said to be an excellent remedy for intermittent fever and ague; the seeds, taken in doses of 12 or 15, three times a day, are reputed a sovereign remedy for goitre, or bigneck. An infusion of the leaves is a good remedy for bleeding at the lungs or stomach; the expressed juice of the fresh leaves, in teaspoonful doses, still better."

1868 Can. Pharm. J. 6;83-5. Common nettle *Urtica dioica*, root and leaves included in list Can. medicinal plants.

1892 Millspaugh 153. "The most ancient use of the Nettle is flagellation or urtication, a practice of whipping paralyzed limbs, to bring the muscles into action. This practice extended also to a stimulation of impotent organs, and to bring into action dormant energies. It was also resorted to in apoplexy, general cerebral and portal congestion, to bring blood to the surface and thus relieve more vital organs. . .The Nettle was afterwards found to be styptic and anti-hemorrhagic. . .Their decoction was found to be diuretic. . .The young shoots are considered excellent 'greens' on their appearance in the spring. . .A strong decoction of the plant, salted, is said to coagulate milk very quickly, and the product to prove devoid of any unpleasant taste. . .Constituents Formic Acid. This volatile acid is found in a free state in the stings of this species; it is also found in the poison bags of the red ant. . .in pine needles, turpentine and many plants."

1916 Waugh IROQUOIS 118. Nettles, *U. dioica*, eaten in the spring as greens, cooked like spinach and seasoned with salt, pepper or butter.

1926-7 Densmore CHIPPEWA 344. *U. gracilis* [*dioica*] a decoction of the root drunk for dysentery. . .346. A decoction of the root drunk for stoppage of urine. . .348. Cut the root of the lady fern into bits and take a small handful. The nettle root has lobes on it. Take 4 of these lobes with the first named root and boil them up quickly. Use as soon as cool enough to drink for stoppage of urine. This is known as a Winabojo remedy as it is supposed to have been received from him. . .378. Twine was also made from the dry stalks of the false nettle, *Laportea canadensis*. This was used in sewing and, in two grades of fineness, was used in making fish nets. It is said that a cloth was once made of this fiber and used for women's dresses.

1923 H. Smith MENOMINI 56. "Wood nettle, it is strange that this is not regarded as an aboriginal medicine by the Menomini, for it possesses peculiar diuretic properties. Notable quantities of ammonia have been distilled from this plant. . .77. Both this nettle and *U. gracilis* are retted to obtain the Indian hemp twine, which is used in making fiber bags called anup minuti."

1928 H. Smith MESKWAKI 251. "Wood nettle, the root is used by the Indians as a diurient and cures the incontinence of urine. . .270. The inner bark of this nettle is comparable to the China grass fiber, for it is fine and strong. It is probably fifty times as strong as the same diameter of cotton string. The fibers are gathered in about three foot strips and braided into a large hank until wanted. Then it is twisted together, [as shown in plate XXXLX of the original publication,] in the same manner as other fibers to make a cord. This cord is kept in a round ball and, when using from the ball, an end is tied fast to some solid support, and this forms the central core around which the weaving of the edge of a cat-tail mat is done. The same string is used in the binding."

1932 H. Smith OJIBWE 391. "Wood nettle, the Pillager Ojibwe used the root to make a medicinal tea for its diuretic properties. It is said to cure various urinary ailments. . .423. They say that their old people used the rind of this nettle as a sewing fiber. . .*U. dioica* (*U. Lyallii*) in aboriginal times, the Flambeau Ojibwe used the bark or rind of this nettle to give them a fine, stout sewing fiber."

1933 H. Smith POTAWATOMI 87. "The Forest Potawatomi make a medicinal tea from the leaves of this plant (*U. dioica*) and use the roots also to make a tea for the treatment of intermittent fevers. . .115. They gather the outer rind of the nettle for its textile strength."

1931 Grieve England 574. "Each sting is a very sharp, polished spine, which is hollow and arises from a swollen base. In this base, which is composed of small cells, is contained the venom, an acrid fluid, the active principle of which is said to be bicarbonate of ammonia. When, in consequence of pressure, the sting pierces the skin, the venom is instantly expressed, causing the resultant irritation and inflammation. The burning property of the juice is dissipated by heat, enabling the young shoots to be eaten as a pot herb. . .The length of the nettle fibre varies from 3/4 of an inch to 2½ inches: all above 1 3/8 inch is equal to the best Egyptian cotton. It can be dyed and bleached in the same way as cotton, and when mercerized is but slightly inferior to silk. It has been considered much superior to cotton for velvet and plush. . .A decoction of nettle yields a beautiful and permanent green dye. . .the root boiled with alum yields a yellow colour. . .seeds yield a burning oil."

1935 Jenness OJIBWA Parry Island Lake Huron 16. "Nets made of false nettle (*Urticastrum divaricatum*) [*Laportea canadensis*] with floats of cedar or other light wood and with sinkers of stone."

1949 Emmelin and Feldberg New Phytologist 48;143-48. Hairs and leaves contain histamin and acetylcholine. C.A. 43;8455.

1955 Mockle Quebec transl. 36. "Wood nettle, the seeds laxative and anthelmintic. *Urtica dioica*, an astringent and diuretic remedy. The nettle is used in decoction in nephritis, gravel, jaundice and hemoptysis. It is also used as a revulsive externally. In certain countries the leaves are used for the industrial preparation of chlorophyll: they obtain from 5 to 6 grams for each kilogram of dried leaves."

The seeds of nettles taken in wine and cooked excite to games of love according to Galen who advised for impotence a tablespoon of powdered seeds mixed with jam or honey. (Palaiseul 1972 transl.)

An extract of nettle containing the volatile oils has long been used in Europe as a nettle hair rinse. The root is used in commercial preparations to stimulate hair growth and the seeds are used at home for general hair troubles (Lewis and Elvin-Lewis 1977;340).

1979 Niederberger Zohapilco site Mexico Science 203;134. "The presence of certain plants, such as *Urtica*, in the floristic community of Playa [6000-4500 B.C.] is of archeological interest to the degree that it indicates, together with other evidence, human interference in the occupied area." Docks [Rumex] generally grow near nettles, crush the dock leaves and rub on the nettle sting.

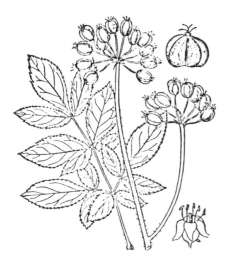

BRISTLY SARSAPARILLA

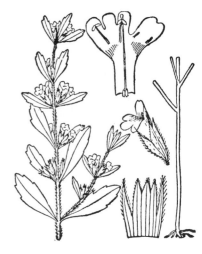

AMERICAN PENNYROYAL

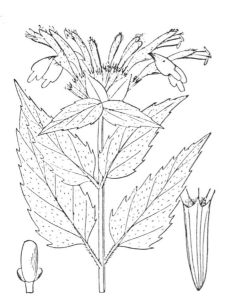

WILD BERGAMOT

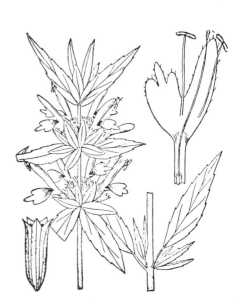

HORSEMINT

BRISTLY SARSAPARILLA   *Aralia hispida* Vent. Araliaceae
There are long sharp bristles on a sheath at the base of this plant. The reddish, woody, up to 1 m
tall, stem has bristles here and there as do the leaf stalks. The leaflets are longer than wide,
sharply pointed at the end with sharply pointed teeth around their edges, 5-7 on each of the three
stalks. The long flower bearing stems grow from near the top of the plant with loose balls of
white flowers, followed by dark blue berries.
Range. Lab. Nfld., N.B., P.E.I., N.S., Que., James Bay, Ont., Man. Sask., s. to Minn., Ill., Ohio,
and N.C. in rocky or sandy sterile soil.
Common names. Dwarf elder, wild elder, rough sarsaparilla, pigeon berry, There is a shrub or
small tree *Aralia spinosa* or Hercules' club found further south.

1828 Rafinesque 54. *Aralia hispida* has the same properties as *Aralia nudicaulis*, wild or American sarsaparilla, and may be used in the same way. [See under woods, for what Rafinesque writes about *A. nudicaulis*].

1859-61 Gunn 789. "The bark, and especially the root, is diuretic and alterative, and considered quite valuable in dropsy, supressed urine, gravel, and all affections of the kidneys and urinary organs. Used in decoction; dose from half to a teacupful, three or four times a day."

1868 Can. Pharm. J. 6;83-5. Bristly sarsaparilla, the bark of the roots included in list of Can. medicinal plants.

1925 Wood and Ruddock. The best preparation is an extract of the bark of the root mixed with vaseline. This makes one of the best healing salves.

1933 H. Smith POTAWATOMI 40. "This medicine seems known only to Mrs. Spoon and she said the root is used as an alterative and tonic, that it is nowhere common in the Forest country. . .Most of the other Indian tribes consulted had never noticed the difference between this species and sarsaparilla."

1970 Bye IROQUOIS mss. "Used as a medicine."

AMERICAN PENNYROYAL   *Hedeoma pulegioides* (L.) Pers. Labiatae (Lamiaceae)
A slender annual plant with a stem 10-40 cm, usually branching and hairy. The leaves 1-3 cm long, thin and with few teeth, the main one with stalks. The flowers are in the axils of the leaves, only a few in each cluster. Their cups are hairy, their tubes bluish purple. This tiny mint has a very strong odor.

Range. N.B., N.S., Que., Ont. to Minn. to S. Dak. s. to e. Kans., Ark., Tenn. and Fla. in dry soil.

Common names. Squaw mint, tick-weed.

1475 Bjornsson Icelandic mss transl. Larsen 106. "Pulegium [*Mentha pulegium* of Europe] is dry and hot in the third degree. If a pregnant woman eats it frequently, there is danger that her child die. If she drinks it with warm wine, it purges the afterbirth. If one crushes it with salt and mixes it with honey, it is good for crippled limbs. If it is crushed with honey and drunk or eaten, it is good for that secretion, which comes in man's chest like glue. If one drinks it with wine, it is good for poisonous bites and for cold and dry blood. If one crushes it with vinegar, it is good to put in the nose of the man that faints from some illness or from loss of blood, or for some other reason. If it is crushed fine when dry, it is good to put in the mouth for loose gums. If it is applied to swellings of the feet or other puffed places, then it is good together with other poultice. If one crushes it with salt it is good to apply for the spleen. If one washes in its broth, it is good for the itch. It is good to drink with warm wine for a cough. It also greatly provokes urination. . .If one drinks it with water, it is good for poison; and it gives desire for women. . .S18. Item for the breath of a man if it smells from lung trouble and is spoiled in a man, take pulegium and mint and make a drink and mix it with honey and drink every day; then he will improve."

1624 Sagard HURON 239. "We use them for putting into our sagamite to give it a flavor, and also a certain small herb, which in taste and shape resembles wild sweet marjoram, and which they call ongnehem. [This may be pennyroyal as there is no wild sweet marjoram in n.e. America. See Gerarde]

1633 Gerarde-Johnson 671-2. "Of Pennie Royal or pudding grasse. . .the male kinde groweth upright of himselfe without creeping, much like in shew unto wild Marjerome."

1698 Hennepin HURON 579. "Our common Food was the same with the Savages, viz. Sagamite, or Pottage made of water and Indian Corn with Gourds: To give it a Relish, we put into it Marjoram, and a sort of Balm, with wild Onions which we found in the Woods and Fields."

1748 Kalm Philadelphia October the 14th 103. "Pennyroyal is a plant which has a peculiar strong scent, and grows abundantly on dry places in the country. Botanists call it *Mellisa pulegiodes*. An extract from it is reckoned very wholesome to drink as a tea when a person has a cold, as it promotes perspiration. I was likewise told that on feeling a pain in any limb, this plant, if applied to it, would give immediate relief."

1820's Materia Medica Edinburgh-Toronto mss 30. *Mentha pulegium* [English pennyroyal] likewise resembles the peppermint in its qualities & used for the same purposes but less agreeable & pungent."

1828 Rafinesque 232. "[American pennyroyal] is as yet commonly blended, even by medical writers, with the European Pennyroyal or *Mentha pulegium* which does not grow in America; the shape, smell, and properties being somewhat similar, whence the same vulgar name; but our plant appears to be more effecient. . .the whole plant is scented; but the smell far from agreeable, being strong and graveolent: many persons, however, like it and call it pungent, reviving and pleasant: females are sometimes fond of it. . .It is a popular remedy throughout the country for female complaints, suppressed menstruations, hysterics &c. . .Eberle. . .deems its menagogue property problematical. . .that he is mistaken, is proved by daily experience. It promotes expectoration in whooping cough, it alleviates spasms, pains in the hips, and spasmodic or dyspeptic symptoms of menstruation. Schoepf mentions it for palpitations, fevers and gout; but it is too stimulant in fevers. . .Some herbalists in the north, employ it extensively for colds, cholics of children, to remove obstructions, warm the stomach and promote perspiration. . .The plant is also frequently used to kill Ticks. . .By rubbing the legs or boots with this plant or its oil, these insects will avoid you, or if they have taken hold, the oil kills them. A strong decoction of the plant is equally convenient."

1833 Howard Quebec mss 21. "To cure the Hooping Cough. Take a spoonful of the Juice of Penny Royal mixt with brown sugar candy twice a day. . .73. To Cure Obstructed menses or Courses. Take half a pint of strong decoction of pennyroyal every night going to bed. . .22. To Sett away Musquites. Take one oz. of pennyroyal. Saturate a rag with it and hang it on the bedpost, they will never bother you and when you go fishing rub a little on your face and they will never trouble you."

1859-61 Gunn. 839. "This well known herb needs no description; it grows almost everywhere, and is known by everybody. It is a pleasant, aromatic diaphoretic, diuretic and emmenagogue. May be used freely in the form of a tea, as a sweating and cooling drink in fevers; in diseases of the urinary organs, and suppressed menses, and in cold's generally."

1868 Can. Pharm. J. 6;83-5. *Hedeoma pulegioides*, pennyroyal the whole plant included in list of Can. medicinal plants.

1879 Can. Pharm. J. 322. "Yarb digger. . .Pennyroyal and peppermint brings 10 cents a pound, but when dry it takes a heap to make a pound."

1892 Millspaugh 118. "Hot pennyroyal tea. . .combined with a gill of brewer's yeast, frequently acts well as an abortivant should the intender be not too late with her prescription. The oil is anti-emetic, anti-spasmodic, and rubefacient in rheumatism; with raw linseed oil, it makes an excellent dressing for recent burns. The oil has been recommended as an ointment to keep off gnats, ticks, fleas, and mosquitoes; many who have camped in the northern woods, have anointed their hands, neck, and face with this body, to guard against the pests of that region, but with only partial success. . .a case of poisoning by the oil is reported by Dr. Toothacker, of a woman who took at intervals, doses of a teaspoonful of the oil; she presented the following symptoms; severe headache; difficult deglutition; great nausea, severe retchings but inability to vomit; intolerable bearing down, labor-like pains, with tenderness of the abdomen; constipation; dyspnoea; semi-paralysis of the limbs; nervous weakness and prostration."

1896 Sir Charles Roberts Toronto 24. "The flies and mosquitoes were swarming, but we inflicted upon them a crushing defeat by the potent aid of 'slitheroo'. This magic fluid consists of Stockholm tar and tallow spiced with pennyroyal, and boiled to the consistency of treacle. It will almost keep a grizzly at bay."

1902 Beauchamp ONONDAGA 97. Called it smelling weed and made a tea for a headache medicine.

1915 Speck NANTICOKE 321. Pennyroyal a sudorific.

1925 Youngken PENOBSCOT 177. Used this herb as a remedy for suppressed menstruation.

1925-26 Tantaquidgeon MOHEGAN 265. Made a tea to warm the stomach.

1979 Walter H. Lewis speaking in Ottawa described the case of a woman who took one ounce of pennyroyal oil. Within two hours she vomited blood and bled from the vagina and the eyes. By the third day her liver was damaged. On the sixth day she sank into a coma and died on the seventh day.

WILD BERGAMOT   *Monarda fistulosa* L. Labiatae (Lamiacea) (*M. mollis*)
The square stem is hairy and branched, 50-120 cm tall. The leaves on stalks that are 1-1.5 cm long. The larger leaves are 6-10 cm long and can be smooth, slightly hairy to very hairy, always with teeth. The flowers are in a tight bunch at the end of the stem in deep hairy cups (calyx) 7-10 mm long. The flowering tube is pale to deep lavender, 2-3 cm long and very hairy on its upper lip.

Range. sw. Que., s. Ont., s. Man. to N. Mex. n. Mex., Ariz., Tex., La., and Ga. in dry soil, thickets, borders of woods. There is a var. *menthaefolia* whose leaves have stalks that are rarely longer than 5 mm which grows further north, from Man. to B.C.

Common names. Oswego tea, horsemint.

1885 Mooney OJIBWA 201. "*Monarda fistulosa* The root is used, making a decoction and drinking several swallows, at intervals, for pain in the stomach and intestines."

1916 Waugh IROQUOIS 149. "Monarda, or Oswego tea, as it is variously called, *Monarda fistulosa*, represented the mint family, as a tea."

1926-7 Densmore CHIPPEWA 350. *M. mollis* [*fistulosa*,] Horsemint, the flowers and leaves steeped. "Bathe child with the tea and then rub it with tallow, venison tallow if possible. Used especially for children with eruptions". . .346. Decoction of root and flowers for worms. . .354. The flowers and leaves, dried, powdered in the hand, moistened with water and applied to a burn. Especially good for a scald.

1923 H. Smith MENOMINI 39. "*M. fistulosa* This is the universal remedy of the Menomini for catarrh. The leaves and inflorescence are the parts employed, and are used alone or in combination with others to form a tea."

1928 H. Smith MESKWAKI 225. "*M. fistulosa*, used this plant in a combination for making a cold cure. . .*M. punctata* snuffed up the nostrils to relieve a sick headache. . .Monarda was also used in a medicine to revive a patient on the point of death and to sniff for catarrh and cold in the head as well as with other plants in a medicine for cramps in the stomach."

1932 H. Smith OJIBWE 372. "*M. fistulosa* The Flambeau Ojibwe gather and dry the whole plant, boiling it in a vessel to obtain the volatile oil to inhale to cure catarrh and bronchial affections."

HORSEMINT   *Monarda punctata* L. Labiatae (Lamiaceae)

The 30-100 cm tall stem is finely hairy. The leaves 2-5 cm long on very short or no stalks are usually hairy. The flowers cluster in the axils of the leaves, they are pale yellow spotted with purple and brown or may be all white. A ruff of brilliant pink, lavender or white leaflets (bracts) surround the flowers. The cup holding the flowers is nearly as long as they are and is hairy.

Range. Vt. to Minn. and Kans. s. to Fla. and Tex. in dry sandy soil.

Common names. Rignum, from Origanum.

1830 Rafinesque 37. "The whole plant has a grateful smell. . .much stronger when bruised. The taste is pungent, warm, bitterish & c. . . .Schoepf long ago recommended this plant in intermittent fevers:. . .The oil become an officinal article, kept in shops, as an excellent rubefacient. The monarda oil is chiefly made from the *M.punctata*, as strongest and most pungent, but all other species yield it. . .it is very active, producing heat, redness, pain, and vesication when applied to the skin; Dr. Atlee in 1829 had used it with much advantage as a rubefacient liniment in chronic rheumatism, paralytic affections, cholera infantum, difficulty of hearing, periodical headache, and typhus. It must be dissolved in alcohol and rubbed. A liniment made with camphor and opium, cured the periodical headache. The simple liniment rubbed on the head, cured one hard of hearing. . .It relieves the gastric irritability in cholera infantum, by bathing the abdomen and limbs. . .Internally, two drops of oil in sugar and water, act as a powerful carminative, and stop emesis or profuse vomiting. The plant is used in New Jersey in cholic, and in gravel as a diuretic, being often united to onion juice in gravel and dropsy. The root of *M. coccinea* is said to be a stronger diuretic yet, and also emmenagogue, the Indians use it as such in strong doses, it acts sometimes as a cathartic on the bowels."

1859-61 Gunn 805. "*M. punctata.* This well known and very grateful smelling herb, common all over the country. . .a good. . .emmenagogue in painful menstruation. It may be used freely and should be taken warm. There is an essential oil made by distilling the herb, which can be had at the drug stores, and which may be used for the same purpose as the infusion. . .and is good applied externally over the region of the kidneys, in affections of these organs."

1868 Can. Pharm. J. 6;83-5. *Monarda punctata*, horsemint, the whole plant included in list of Can. medicinal plants.

1931 Grieve England 545. "The American Horsemint (*M. punctata*) is of considerable importance, as it may before long be available as a regular source of Thymol. . .It yields from 1 to 3% of a volatile oil which contains a large proportion of Thymol, up to 61% having been obtained. Carvacrol also appears to be a constituent.

1949 Hobart & Melton 96. "Thymol is a powerful antiseptic resembling phenol in its action. It is more slowly absorbed from wounds than the latter, and is also less irritating and less toxic. It has received extensive trials as an intestinal antiseptic, but with dubious benefit, and, internally, its principal use is as an anthelmintic. It is employed externally as a parasiticide and to mucuous surfaces as an antiseptic. Listerine is the liquor of thymol used as a mouthwash diluted with one

or two parts of warm water. It is applied undiluted as a deodorant. Karvol. This preparation, containing chlor-carvacrol, is used as a mouth wash and gargle."
See other mints under Wet Open Places.

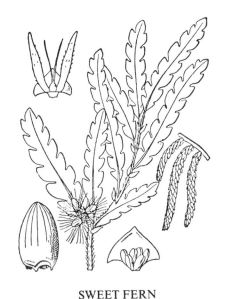

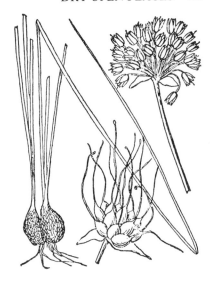

SWEET FERN

WILD GARLIC

SWEET FERN   *Myrica asplenifolia* L. Myricaceae (*Comptonia peregrina, C. asplenifolia*)
A woody reddish brown stem covered with conspicous long white hairs and with many branches,
up to 1.5 m. tall. The leaves are 6-12 x 1 cm with scalloped edges, fragrant when crushed, covered
with resinous glands containing oil. The undersides have a conspicuous vein with brownish hair
on it. Male catkins 1-3 cm long, clustered at the ends of the branches, hanging down. The female
catkins are bur-like in fruit.
Range. N.B., P.E.I., N.S., Que., nw. Ont. s. to Minn., Ill., Tenn. and n. Ga. in open sandy fields,
woodlands. See under shrubs, Sweet Gale, a closely related species.
Common names. Canada sweet gale, fern-gale, meadow or shrubby fern, spleenwort.
1748 Kalm Philadelphia December 31st. 228. "Among the Iroquois. . .on the Mohawk River, I
saw a young Indian Woman. . .had gotten a violent toothache. To cure it she boiled the *Myrica
asplenii folia*, and tied it, as hot as she could bear it, on the whole cheek. She said that remedy
had often cured the toothache before."
1828 Rafinesque 117. "It possesses all the properties of the tonic and astringent balsams. Barton
recommends it for diarrhea, loose bowels, and summer complaints of children, or cholera infantum, in the form of a weak decoction; but it is used in Pennsylvania and Virginia for many other
diseases, such as all children's bowel complaints, (where it forms a grateful drink for them) in
rachitis, in debility, in fevers as a diluent tonic, in rheumatism and contusions it is less available.
The root chewed stops blood-spitting. . .266. The root is styptic, and the Indians chew it for
hemoptysis. . .They make a tea of the leaves for female complaints. The Herbalist, Whitlow,
employs it for scrofula in his vapour baths. Other herbalists use the buds, blossoms or leaves simmered in cream or butter for the itch and sores. A syrup is also made with it. . .1830 212. Can
make ink. Boiled in milk good for all fluxes, tooth ache and sore mouth."
1855 Trail 137. "There is a species of fern, known by the country people by the name of sweet-
gale and sweet fern. . .When it is boiled, it has a slightly resinous taste, with a bitter flavour, that
is not very unpleasant. This sweet-fern is in high repute among the Yankee and old Canadian
housewives, as a diet-drink: they attribute to it many excellent virtues, and drink it as we do tea.
It grows only on very light, sandy soil, by waste on the road side, or at the edge of pine woods.
At dewfall, at night, or early in the morning, this shrub gives out a delightful perfume: it is very
elegant in form, and in quality tonic and astringent: it has been recommended as a specific for
ague."
1959-61 Gunn 868. "Astringent, tonic and alternative. The leaves and branches used in decoction, in diarrhoea, dysentery, and the bowel complaints of children; also leucorrhea, bleeding

from the lungs, and as a restorative in recovery from fevers. May be given in ordinary doses, three or four times a day."

1879 Can. Pharm. J. 12;302. Tannin value of various vegetable substances. . .sweet fern leaves, Mass. 9.42%.

1892 Millspaugh 160. "The American Sweet Fern. . .is in constant domestic use in some localities for checking diarrhea, and is a fomentation in rheumatism and bruises."

1915 Speck PENOBSCOT 309. "'Antwood', leaves steeped and rubbed on skin will cure the effects of poison ivy. It gets its name from its abundance in dry fields where ant-hills are common."

1915 Speck-Tantaquidgeon MOHEGAN 318. Leaves are steeped and liquid rubbed on skin to cure toxic effects of poison.

1923 H. Smith MENOMINI 42. "Sweet Fern is used as a seasoner as well as a potent medicine for childbirth. A tea is made from it. Sweet Fern and mullein leaf together are sometimes used by Menomini medicine women to kill someone they hate. The two leaves are pulverized and peppered upon the medicine that they give to the sick person. Sweet fern is also used to keep berries from spoiling."

1932 H. Smith OJIBWE 375. "Sweet Fern is called a 'coverer', because it is used to line blueberry pails and cover the berries to keep them from spoiling. . . .The Flambeau Ojibwe consider the leaves too strong for a beverage tea, but make a medicine tea to cure the flux and cramps in the stomach."

1933 H. Smith POTAWATOMI 65. "The Forest Potawatomi make a tea from the leaves of the Sweet Fern to cure the itch. . .121. Gather the leaves of the Sweet Fern to throw on the fire to make a smudge to keep away the mosquitoes. They also use it to line their berry pails, to keep the berries fresh."

1928 Parker SENECA 12. Tea of sweet fern used as a body deodorant.

1955 Mockle Quebec transl. 33. Astringent, balsamic, expectorant.

1959 Mechling MALECITE of maritime provinces of Canada use sweet fern for sprains, swellings and catarrh.

1974 Lawrence & Weaver 385-8. The fresh leaves of *Comptonia peregrina* were obtained from a wet bog area near Barry's Bay, Ontario. . .Steam distillation of the leaves produced an oil that contained 36.2% caryophyllene and 11.1% myrcene, as well as many other compounds. [Interestingly, caryophyllene is a component of the oil from cloves which is also used for toothache.]

WILD GARLIC   *Allium canadense* L. Liliaceae

From a conical bulb 1-3 cm long an erect, stout 20-60 cm tall stem grows with leaves only on the lower third. These are long and flat and only 2-4(7) mm wide. At the top of the stem there are most often no flowers, just bulblets to 1 cm across with fine filaments sticking out of their ends. When there are flowers they are pink or white.

Range. s. Ont. to N.D., s. to Fla. and Tex. in the open in rocky crevices or dry meadows.

1749 Kalm Fort Sarotoga 25th. June. Dore 1970. and communication to him from Rousseau. Kalm found *Allium rupestre*. . ."growing on the rocky pavement near rapids on the upper Hudson, right where they, like other wilderness explorers before them had to land and pull up their canoe. At that date in the season, the plant is at the peak of growth and its bulblet-heads are well developed; later on, the stalks become dry and fallen over, hard to see. . .In the northern part of its range, Canada onion is invariably found in crevices of otherwise bare and exposed rock. . .always along the shores of major rivers, and especially at rapids and waterfalls where portages would be necessary, leaves little to the imagination as to how it got around."

1830 Rafinesque 187. "Wild garlic, several species, *A. canadense* most common, gives a bad taste to the milk and butter of cows feeding on them. The tincture used for the gravel. The Cherokees use them in cockery."

1916 Waugh IROQUOIS 118. Cooked and eaten.

1923 H. Smith MENOMINI 69. "The smaller wild onion is sweeter in flavor and is much sought after by the Menomini for food. It is too small to be a very large addition to their menu."

1928 H. Smith MESKWAKI 262. "It is the favorite food of the Indians and the tiny size is their only regret. . .it is gathered and dried for winter cookery and seasoning." Both the Ojibwe tribes like the wild onion and wild leek in the spring as an article of food.

1933 H. Smith POTAWATOMI 104. "While the flavor of this plant is very strong, the Indians use it in soup and have always accounted it a valuable wild food."
1939 Medsger 176. "In places, the bulbs that grow on top are highly appreciate for pickles."
1955 Mockle Quebec Transl. 27. "The bulbs are given in a tincture for gravel."

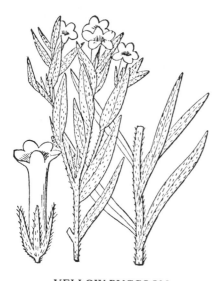

YELLOW PUCCOON

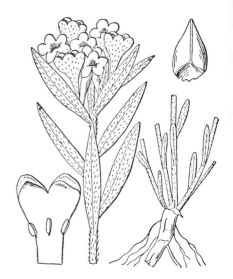

HOARY PUCCOON

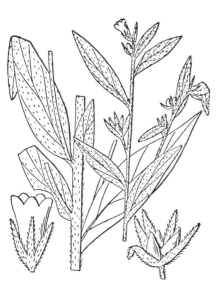

GROMWELL

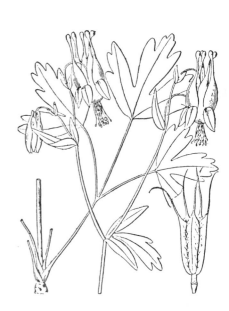

WILD COLUMBINE

YELLOW PUCCOON   *Lithospermum caroliniense* (Walt.) MacMill. Boraginaceae (*Batschia c.*) A stout, many branched, very leafy and hairy plant 30-60 cm tall. The stalkless leaves are 3-6 cm long with stiff hairs all over. The orange yellow flowers have 7-14 mm long tubes with lobes 8-11 mm at their ends. The seeds are ivory white, smooth and shining against this grey green plant. **Range**. s. Que., sw. Ont., Okla., Nev., Ill., se. Va. to Fla., Tex. and Mex. May-July in upland woods, shores, in sandy soil. Roots dye red.

In the following quotations where no plant is named the references could be to other plants than the puccoon. See dogwood, bloodroot, and index.

1590 Harriot Virginia Indians 11. "Dyes of divers kindes. . .little small rootes called Chappacro. . .which Dies are for divers sortes of red. . .The inhabitants use them only for the dyeing of hayre and colouring of their faces, and Mantles made of Deare skinnes; and also for dying of Rushes to make artificial workes withall in their Mattes and Baskettes; having no other thing besides that they account of, apt to use them for."

1609 Lescarbot-Erondelle Nova Francia 208. "Now our savages. . .for as much as when they are merry and paint their faces, be it with blue or with red, they paint also their hairs with the same colour. . .212. The maids and women do make matachias with the quills or bristles of the porcupine, which they dye with black, white, and red colours, as lively as possibly may be, for our scarlets have no better lustre than their red dye."

1612 Capt. John Smith Virginia Indians 93. "Is a small root that groweth in the mountains, which being dryed and beate in powder turneth red; and this they use for swellings, aches, annointing their joints, painting their heads and garments. . .100. Their heads and shoulders are painted red with the roote Pocone braied to powder mixed with oyle; this they hold in somer to preserve them from the heat, and in winter from the cold. Many other formes of painting they use, but he is the most gallant that is the most monstrous to behold.. . .108. And at night where his lodging is appointed, they set a woman fresh painted red with Pocones and oile to be his bed-fellow."

1613 Champlain fourth voyage fac. ed. Ottawa river transl. 24. "The earth is sandy, & here is found a root which dyes a crimson color, with which the savages paint their faces, & the little decorations they use."

1619 Champlain-Macklem 82. "Some of the tribes are more skilful in dressing skins than others, and more ingenious in decorating them. The Montagnais and the Alkonkins take more pains with it than any of the others. They decorate their skins with bands of porcupine quills, which they dye a bright scarlet. They prize these trimmings and when they discard a skin they take the trimmings off and use them over again. They even use them to adorn their faces when they want to look their best. Usually they paint their faces black and red, mixing the pigment with vegetable oil (sometimes made from sunflower seeds) or animal fat. They also dye their hair, which some of the men grow long; others grow it short, while still others grow it on one side of the head only. The women and girls all do their hair the same way, keeping it well combed, oiled and dyed."

1653 Bressani Jes. Rel. HURON 38;253. "This painting serves them in winter as a mask against the cold and the ice; in war, it prevents their countenances from betraying them by revealing inward fear, makes them more terrible to the enemy, and conceals extremes of youth or age, which might inspire strength and courage in the adversary. It serves as adornment at the public feasts and assemblies. They also paint the prisoners destined to the flames, as victims consecrated to the god of war, and adorn them as the ancients adorned theirs. They do the same also to their dead, for the same reasons for which we adorn ours."

1670 Marie de l'Incarnation Quebec 372. "With this (thread of Nettles) they [Indians] make their embroidery, ornamenting it with black-and-white porcupine quills, combined with others boiled in roots, which makes them as beautiful as cochineal makes scarlet in France."

1830 Rafinesque 199. "*Batschia*, Puccoon, Red Paint. . .several species. . .Red root, used as a die and paint by the Indians, also as a vermifuge."

1926-27 Densmore CHIPPEWA 370-1 Formulae for dyes, red dye second formula. *Lithospermum caroliniense.* Nine inches of the dried root or an equivalent amount of the pulverized root. Hot water, 1 quart. Ochre one teaspoonful. If this is being used for dyeing porcupine quills, let it boil a little, then put in the quills, which have previously stood for a while in hot water. Let the quills boil half an hour to an hour, keeping the kettle covered, then remove from the fire and let the quills stand in the dye for several hours. If they are not bright enough they may be redyed, letting them stand in the dye as before. The process is substantially the same in dyeing other materials.. . .377. Used for face paint, Puccoon, *Lithospermum caroliniense.*

1662 Montgomery 119. "The root, a thick perennial producing a purple stain."

HOARY PUCCOON   *Lithospermum canescens* (Michx.) Lehm. Boraginaceae (*Batschia c.*) Several stems covered with soft whitish hair grow from 10-40 cm tall. The stalkless leaves are 2-6 cm long on the upper part of the stem. The yellow 7-14 mm long tubular flowers are close together. The lobes at their ends are 3-6 mm wide. The nutlets are yellowish white, smooth and shining.

Range. Ont. to Sask., s. to Ga. and Tex. April-May in prairies and dry open woods.
1858 Barnston Can. Nat. & Geol. Montreal 3;29. "Sanguinaria. . .Lindley in his system has called it the 'Puccoon', which I suspect is a mistake, that name being given to another plant, the *Batschia canescens*, the root of which is used to dye a red by the native tribes. The root of Sanguinaria bloodroot having a red juice may have led the compiler to consider it the Puccoon. [*Batschia* an old name for *Lithospermum*].
1923 H. Smith MENOMINI 80. "It is very difficult for a white man to get any information about the sacred objects of the Menomini. The white ripened seed of this plant is supposed to be a sort of sacred bead used in the 'mita win' ceremony."

GROMWELL   *Lithospermum officinale* L. Boraginaceae

The stem is hairy with many branches, up to 30 cm tall. The hairy stalkless leaves, 6-15(20) cm wide, partially clasp the stem. The whitish flowers are 5-7 mm long and are spaced apart on the upper parts of the stem. They are followed by seeds that are hard, shining, white to pale brown nutlets, 3-3.5 mm long attached at their base to the stem.
Range. Native of Eurasia, intr. as a weed of waste places from Que. to Minn. s. to N.J. and Ill. May-Aug. Lots around Toronto.
Common names. Graymile, littlewale, pearl plant.
1741 Farrier's Disp. "Gromwell, these are powerful Diuretics and force very much by the Urinary Passages, and therefor are given with good success in all Stoppages in those Parts."
1791 Lewis ed. Aitkin 73. "Long been discarded from practice."
1945 Rousseau MOHAWK transl. 56. "The ripe seeds are mixed with those of the gourd (bottle shaped) (*Cucurbita Pepo*) dried in a saucepan and pulverized. An infusion of a pinch of this powder in boiling water is given to children whose 'urine does not come out'. This is an introduced species. Ancient medicine of Europe by virtue of the doctrine of signatures recommended using the seeds, hard as stones, to dissolve calculus. Was the recipe given by the informer, borrowed from the French?"
1955 Mockle Quebec transl. 76. "The fruits are prescribed in infusion to dissolve calculus."

WILD COLUMBINE   *Aquilegia canadensis* L. Ranunculaceae

The smooth or slightly hairy stem can be up to 200 cm tall. The smooth leaves are compound, three leaflets on a long stalk, each leaflet divided into three other leaflets, the ends each having three lobes. The flowers nod at the ends of their stalks. They are scarlet outside and yellowish inside with five nectar tubes standing up in the centre like a crown.
Range. Nfld., N.B., N.S., Que., Ont. to se. Sask. s. to Tex. and Fla. in rocky woods and open places, April-June.
Common names. Rock lily, honeysuckle, cluckies, bells, meeting-houses.
1558 Belon Paris described *Aquilegia canadensis* from Canada. [Ewan 1978].
1633 Gerarde-Johnson 1095 *A. vulgaris*, [the European columbine]. "Notwithstanding that what temperatures or vertues Columbines have is not yet sufficiently known, for they are used especially to decke the gardens of the curious, garlands, and houses. . .Most in these daies following others by tradition, do use to boile the leaves in milk against soreness of the throat, falling and excoriation of the uvula. . .Clusius saith, that Dr. Francis Rapard, a physition of Bruges in Flanders, told him that the seed of this common columbine very finely beaten to powder, and given in wine, was a singular medicine to be given to women to hasten and facilitate their labour, and if the first taking it were not sufficiently effectuall, then they should repeat it again."
1830 Rafinesque 194. "A beautiful native flower, adorning our rocks, cultivated for beauty. Equivalent of *Aq. vulgaris*, which is diuretic, emmenagogue, sudorific, antiscorbutic, and aperative. The roots, flowers and seeds are used in Europe; the seeds are acrid oily, taken in vinous infusions for jaundice."
1928 H. Smith MESKWAKI 238. "The root of this plant is chewed for stomach and bowel troubles. The ripe capsules are mixed with smoking tobacco by the young beaux among the Indians, to make it smell good and refined. Specimen 3674 of the Dr. Jones collection is the seed of *A. canadensis* and is called. . .love perfume. This is used with love medicine and also without as for smoking. Specimen 5082. . .the root and leaves are boiled and made into a drink to cure diarrhoea. It is also used as a power of persuasion at trade or council. Specimen 5167 is the root of *A.*

canadensis and, in connection with the bark of *Zanthoxylum americanum*, [prickly ash]. . .is taken when the contents of the bladder are thick, according to the Meskwaki."

1932 H. Smith OJIBWE 383. "The root is considered good medicine for stomach trouble. Eclectic practioners [white] consider it diuretic, diaphoretic, and antiscorbutic, using it in jaundice, in smallpox to promote eruption, and in scurvy."

1955 Mockle Quebec transl. 41. "*A. canadensis* stems and leaves antiscorbutic and diuretic; seeds diaphoretic. *A. vulgaris*, seeds depurative, diaphoretic and diuretic."

1968 Forsyth England *A. vulgaris* 38. "They are not likely to be eaten in any quantity, but Cornevin (1893) points out that their poisonous properties are similar to those of aconite, and that an infusion of the seeds, used medicinally in several countries, is dangerous to children."

1970 William & Li 3878. The root of *A. canadensis* contains aquileginine, berberine, magnoflorine and 2 unamed alkaloids.

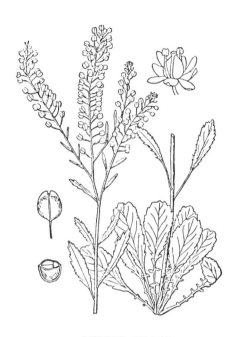

PEPPER GRASS

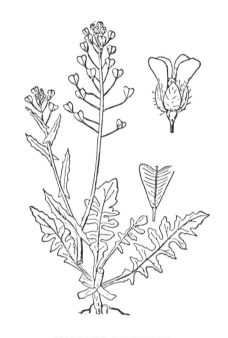

SHEPHERD'S PURSE

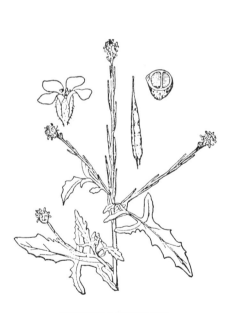

HEDGE MUSTARD

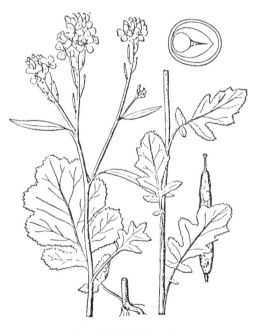

BLACK MUSTARD

PEPPER GRASS *Lepidum virginicum* L. Cruciferae (Brassicaceae)

An erect shiny 10-50 cm stem, its leaves smaller and often without lobes while those growing from the roots have one large and many smaller sharply toothed lobes. The flowering stems up to 10 cm long with inconspicuous white petaled flowers on slender stalks followed by flat seed pods, 2.5-4 x 2-3.5 mm the top with a notched edge.

Range. Nfld., N.B., P.E.I., N.S., sw. Que., s. Ont., Minn., s. to Fla. and Tex. in moist or dry soil in the open, tastes peppery.

Lepidum densiflorum Schrader, Common paper grass is very similar but has smaller or no white petals and the seed pods are only 2-3.3mm.

1475 Bjornsson Icelandic mss Larsen transl. 95. "Cress. Hot and dry in the first degree. It lessens the desire for women. If cress is crushed with sorrel and applied to a boil, it draws the matter out and lessens the pain. Its juice is good for toothache if it is put in the mouth in which the toothache is. . .Cress seed is stronger than the herb itself. . .If one crushes cress seed in wine and drinks it, that is good for poison. If snakes notice the smoke or smell of burning cress, they flee. . .If one crushes cress with paunch fat of a goose, it is good to apply for sore flesh and itch."

1830 Rafinesque 237. "From Canada to Guyana. . .eaten as cresses. All acrid, diuretic, antiscorbutic, antiscrofulous: used in scurvy, dropsy, asthma, scorfula, hernia, gravel, &c. as a diet."

1923 H. Smith MENOMINI 33. "This was the first plant to be pointed out to me as a cure for poison ivy. It is steeped in water to compound a liquid wash. My informant said the freshly bruised plant is just as efficacious. The white man uses *Lepidum* infusions as a cure for scurvy."

1955 Mockle Quebec transl. 49. "Antiscorbutic."

Seed pods are a good seasoning for soups stews etc. put in just before eating, not cooked.

SHEPHERDS PURSE *Capsella bursa-pastoris* (L.) Medic. Cruciferae (Brassicaceae)

The basal leaves grow from all around the stem at the bottom, they are 5-10 cm long with many lobes. The stem is 10-60 cm and its leaves clasp it with an ear on each side at their base, they are pointed and may or may not be toothed. The flower stalks are 1-2 cm long standing out from the stem. The white flowers minute and followed by seed pods shaped like hearts, or old fashioned purses.

Range. Probably a native of s. Europe now a cosmopolitan and ubiquitous weed from Greenland, Lab., Hudson Bay to Alaska and south across the continent.

1633 Gerarde-Johnson 276. "Shepherds purse stayeth bleeding in any part of the body, whether the juices or the decoction thereof be drunke, or whether it be used pultesse-wise, or in a bath, or any other way else. In a Clyster it cureth the bloudy flix: it healeth greene and bleeding wounds: it is marvellous good for inflammations new begun, and for all diseases which must be checked backe and cooled. The decoction doth stop the laske, the spitting and pissing of bloud, and all other fluxes of bloud."

1892 Millspaugh 25. "The Shepherd's Purse has been used in English domestic practice from early times, as an astringent in diarrhoea; it was much used in decoction with milk to check active purgings in calves. Later its value here was much doubted,. . .It has been used in fresh decoction in hematuria, hemmorrhoids, diarrhea and dysentery, and locally as a vulnerary. . .application in rheumatic affections. The juice on cotton, inserted in the nostrils, was often used to check hemorrhage. . .It has been found curative in various uterine hemorrhages, especially those with which uterine cramp and colic are associated; also in various passive hemorrhages from mucous surfaces."

1915 Speck-Tantaquidgeon MOHEGAN 319. "'Peppergrass' seed pods are made into tea for general benefit of the stomach. Its pungency is thought to kill internal worms." (*Capsella bursa-pastoris*)

1923 H. Smith MENOMINI 33. "This plant seems to hold equal favor with the Virginia Peppergrass as a cure for poison ivy. The plant is steeped and the water when tepid is used as a wash. Next to mustard, horseradish and scurvy grass, this is the most important drug of the family according to white man's uses, on account of a peculiar acid. Among the eclectics it is used as a diuretic, emmenagogue, and anti-rheumatic, and is an excellent healing agent for unhealthy sores."

1928 H. Smith MESKWAKI 219. "While this had no Indian name, the Meskwaki claimed that they used it as a medicine."

1939 Medsger 164. "Shepherd's-Purse is found as a weed in fields and waste places nearly all over the world. It has the peppery flavor of other members of the mustard family and was formerly used as a potherb. . .A good substitute for spinach. Delicious when blanched and served as a salad. Tastes somewhat like cabbage, but is much more delicate."

1931 Grieve England 738. "When dried and infused, it yields a tea which is still considered by herbalists one of the best specifics for stopping haemorrhages of all kinds. . .Its haemostyptic properties have long been known and are said to be equal to those of ergot and hydrastis. During the Great War, when these were no longer obtainable in German commerce, a liquid extract of *Capsella bursa-pastoris* was used as a substitute.

1955 Mockle Quebec transl. 48. "Diuretic, febrifuge and hemostatic. This plant has enjoyed as well a certain popularity as a uterine stimulant."

The basal leaves of first year plants picked in late winter and early spring contain 91 mg of Ascorbic acid or Vitamin C in each 100 grams of leaves. Oranges contain 50 mg of ascorbic acid per 100 grams of orange. 5,000 Units of Vitamin A Units are found in each 100 grams of the leaves of shepherd's purse. (Zennie and Ogzewalla 1977).

1979 Susuki CBLT Science Magazine February. Report on the seeds of shepherd's purse. When soaked in water they emit a gelatine-like substance as they germinate. If put in the water containing the larvae of fever carrying mosquitoes this gelatine trapped the larvae disintegrating them.

BLACK MUSTARD   *Brassica nigra* (L.) Koch Cruciferae (Brassicaceae) (*Sinapis nigra*)
The stiff, branching stem is rough hairy below and smooth above, up to 150 cm tall. The lower, dark green, stalked, toothed leaves have a large lobe at their ends and 2-4 smaller ones. The flowers are 1 cm wide, bright yellow, on 3-4 mm stalks followed by smooth, 1-2 cm long four-sided pods that are upright and tend to lean in towards the stem. Their beak is slender, 2.5-4 mm long.

Range. Eurasian naturalised as a weed throughout our range in fields and waste places.

Common names. Cadlock, warlock, kerlock scurvie senvie.

White mustard, (*Sinapis alba, Brassica hirta*) and Charlock (*Sinapis arvensis, Brassica Kaber*) are also found introduced in our range. White mustard has bristly pods, Charlock's pods have beaks nearly a third as long as the pod.

1475 Bjornsson Icelandic mss. Larsen transl. 122. "Mustard whets men's wits. And it loosens the belly, breaks stone and purges the urine. . .If one eats mustard, that strengthens the stomach and lessens its sickness. Crushed mustard in vinegar heals viper's bite. With mustard one may cauterize."

1633 Gerarde-Johnson 264. "The seed of these herbes be so extreame hot and vehement in working, that being taken in too great a quantitie, purgeth and scoureth even unto bloud, and is hurtfull to women with child, and therefore great care is to be taken in giving them inwardly."

1820's Mat. Med. Edinburgh-Toronto mss 42. "*Sinapis alba.* The powder given in the dose of a large teaspoonfull mixed with water acts as an Emetic. It is used externally as a Rubefacient & vesicatory. . .50. Emmenagogues from the class of Cathartics. . .*Sinapis alba* is a popular remedy in amenorrhoea & Chlorosis & may have some effect by its stimulating action on the intestinal canal.. . .69. The flour of mustard forms what is called a sinapisne when mixed with equal parts of wheat flour or crumbs of bread, which acts as a powerful Rubefacient applied to the soles of the feet in typhoid fever where there is extreme debility."

1830 Rafinesque 263. "Leaves acrid antiscorbutic. Seeds very active, contain fixed oil, acrid oil, sulpher &c. Oil by expression similar to rape oil, good for lamps. . .flour of mustard much used as a condiment, but the abuse produces dyspepsia, atrophy and palsy. It is errhine, rubefacient, in topical use; applied to the feet. . .very useful revulsion in fevers. . .The milder white mustard seeds chiefly used whole in large doses. . .merely laxative, nearly inert. Larger doses still or infusions are emetic by irritating the stomach; may cause convulsions in children when mixed with bread."

1868 Can. Pharm. J. 6;83-5. The seeds of black and white mustard, *Sinapis nigra* and *alba* included in list of Can. medicinal plants.

1892 Millspaugh 23. "The unground seeds of white mustard have held a high place in former practice. . .but proved dangerous, as they are liable to become impacted in the bowel and set up a fatal inflammation. . .24. The fresh plants of black mustard, soon after they make their appearance, while the leaves are yet young and tender are used by the laity in many parts of the country as a pot-herb."

1894 Household Guide Toronto 120. "Mustard is an excellent household remedy. In cases of poisoning, when taken in large quantities, it will produce vomiting. A tablespoonful of white mustard seed mingled with syrup, and taken once a day, will act gently on the bowels and is a beneficial remedy in dyspepsia and constipation."

1904 Henkel 44. Black and white mustard seeds collected when most of the tops are nearly mature, but before they are ready to spring open. They should then be placed on a clean dry floor or shelf, allowing the pods to ripen and dry out, when they will burst open and the seeds can be readily shaken out. . .In medicine mustard seeds are used principally in the preparation of plasters and poultices. They are used also in dyspepsia, and in large doses act as an emetic. The imports into the United States of black and white mustard together during the fiscal year ended June 30th, 1903, amounted to 5,302,876 pounds. The price ranges from 3 to 6 cents per pound for both the black and white mustard seeds."

1915 Speck- Tantaquidgeon MOHEGAN 318. "Wild mustard (*Brassica nigra*) leaves are bound on the skin to relieve toothache or headache."

1916 Waugh IROQUOIS 117. "Mustard, various species, more particulary *B. nigra* were collected in the earlier part of the season, while young and tender. . .cooked like spinach."

1928 H. Smith MESKWAKI 219. "Black mustard. The seed of this mustard is ground up and used as a snuff to cure a cold in the head, reminding one of the inhalants formerly offered on the American market. The oil is quite pungent and penetrating."

Black mustard seed contains about 29% protein, about 4% of a glycoside, sinigrin, an enzyme, myrosin and a small amount of acid sinapine sulphate. White mustard seed contains about 25% protein, a crystalline glycoside, sinalbin and mucilage (T.E. Wallis 1967: 200-201).

Fish stuffed with wild mustard leaves tastes marvelous (Assiniwi 1972).

Powdered seeds of black and white mustard act as stimulants to gastric mucosa and increase pancreatic secretions. The mustard seed powder is a useful home emetic for children and is especially valuable in treating narcotic poisoning. (Lewis and Elvin-Lewis 1977: 273, 278).

HEDGE MUSTARD
Sisymbrium officinale (L.) Scop. Cruciferae (Brassicaceae)

A grey green plant, the stem erect, 30-80 cm tall. The lower, stalked leaves with one very long, toothed lobe and several smaller ones, the upper without stalks or lobes. The tiny 3 mm flowers bright yellow on 2-3 mm stalks followed by pods 10-15 cm long, tapering to their tops and closely pressed to the stem.

Range. Native of Europe commonly established as a weed throughout most of north America. There are two varieties, one finely hairy on top, the other smooth.

Common names. St. Barbara's hedge mustard, singer's plant, scrambling rocket.

1681 Culpeper 246. "It is good in diseases of the chest and lungs, and hoarseness; by use of the decoction lost voice has been recovered. The juice made into a syrup with honey and sugar, is effectual for the same purpose, and for coughs, wheezing, and shortness of breath. The same is profitable for the jaundice, pleurisy, pains in the back and loins, and colic. The seed is a remedy against poisons and venom, and worms in children. It is good for sciatica, and in joint-aches, ulcers, cankers in the mouth, throat, or behind the ears, and for hardness and swelling of the testicles, or of women's breasts."

1868 Can. Pharm. J. 6;83-5. The seeds and plant of hedge mustard, *Sisymbrium officinale* included in list of Can. medicinal plants.

1923 H. Smith MENOMINI 33. "Three *Sisymbriums* were found, of which one was suspected of Menomini importance, the Tall Sisymbrium (*S. altissimum*)"

1955 Mockle Quebec trans. 49. "The plant is diuretic and expectorant, recommended for pulmonary catarrh and to dissipate hoarseness. . .*S. sophia* is antiscorbutic, apertive, antiputrid and vulnerary." [This plant is now called *Descurainia sophia*, flixweed, a grey, hoary plant with finely dissected leaves and long upright pods, naturalised from Europe and found N.B. to Ont. to Oregon, s. to Utah, Neb., Ill. N.Y.]

Hedge mustard is a specific for the vocal cords. . .Take 40-60 gr. of dried leaves in a litre of warm water, left overnight and drunk next day, 4 or 5 cups between meals, warming it and adding honey. Or take the juice of fresh plant with milk and honey (Palaiseul 1972:139 transl.).

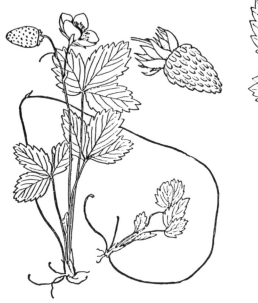

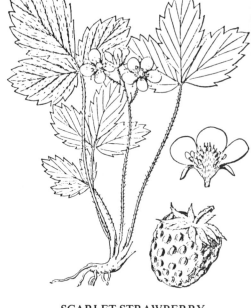

STRAWBERRY   SCARLET STRAWBERRY

STRAWBERRY   *Fragaria vesca* L. var *americana* Porter *Rosaceae*
Three leaflets without stalks join at the top of the hairy leaf stem. The leaflets have sharp, spread
out teeth, and are usually silky beneath. The flowering stem mostly has several branches, is hairy,
and the five white petals of the flowers are each 5-7 mm long. The fruit's seeds are on its surface.
Range. Nfld., N.B., N.S., Que., James Bay, Ont. to B.C. s. to Calif., N. Mex., Nebr., Mo., Ill. and
Va. in open woods and meadows. There are many variations of this strawberry in the wild, some
very hairy. Runners from the roots produce new plants.

SCARLET STRAWBERRY   *Fragaria virginiana* Duchesne
The leaflets are stalked, can be silky beneath or smooth, the teeth blunter and not as wide apart.
The many white flowers have petals mostly 7-10 mm long and the flowering stalk usually stands
above the leaves. The fruit has its seeds sunk in pits on its surface.
Range. Lab. Nfld., Que., northernmost Ont. to Yukon Alaska, s. to Calif., Colo., Okla. Tenn. and
Ga.
1500 Draper site Ontario Finlayson 1975: 225. Found archeologically 670 strawberry seeds.
1590 Harriot Virginia 18. "Strawberries there are as good & as great as those which we have in
our English gardens."
1619 Champlain-Macklem HURON (1615): 41. "They also grow. . .strawberries."
1624 Sagard HURON 237-8. "Berries, particularly strawberries, rasberries, and blackberries
were plentiful. . .Fruits were dried for winter use, to be used in preserves for the sick, to give taste
to sagamite, and to put into the small cakes that were baked in the ashes."
1634 Narr. of journey into MOHAWK country from New. Neth. 146. "December 23rd. . .This
day we were invited to buy bear meat, and we also got half a bushel of beans and a quantity of
dried strawberries, and we bought some bread, that we wanted to take on our march."
1637 Le Mercier HURON Jes. Rel. 227-31. A description of a curing ceremony among the
Huron where a blind man, Tscondacouane having dreamed it was necessary for him to fast for 6
days, resolved to fast for 7. . .in order to stop the epidemic which prevails. . .the spirits
said. . ."we can do nothing more to you, you are associated with us, you must live hereafter as we

do; and we must reveal to you our food, which is nothing more than clear soup with strawber-ries." In order not to get sick, the Huron ate dried strawberries as it was January.

1643 Roger Williams Narragansett. "This berry is the wonder of all the fruits growing naturally in these parts. It is of itself excellent; so that one of the chiefest doctors of England was wont to say, that God could have made, but God never did make, a better berry. In some parts where the Indians have planted, I have many times seen as many as would fill a good ship, within a few miles compass" (Sturtevant 1919:282).

1653 Bressani Huron Jes. Rel. 38:243. Use by the Huron of strawberries of two sorts.

1680 Bacqueville de la Potherie Michilimackinac. "A general meeting place for all the French who go to trade with stranger tribes; it is the landing place and refuge of all the savages who trade their peltries...When they choose to work, they make canoes of birch bark which they sell two at three hundred livres each. They get a shirt for two sheets of bark for cabins. The sale of their French strawberries and other fruits produces means for procuring their ornaments...They make a profit on everything." (Blair 1911:282).

1785 Cutler. "The fruit in its uncultivated state, if the soil be rich, is large and well tasted, but may be greatly improved by culture. The white fruited, double flowering and other varieties are produced by cultivation. It is subacid, cooling...Dr. Withering says, they promote perspiration, impart a violet smell to the urine, and dissolve the tartarous incrustations upon the teeth. People afflicted with the stone or gout have found great relief by using them very freely. Hoffman says he has known consumptive people cured by them."

1828 Rafinesque 193. "Although strawberries have been commonly considered as an article of food, they highly deserve a place among medicaments, which are not the worse I should think for being palatable. Linnaeus introduced them in his Materia Medica, as well as Schoepf, &c...They are useful in fevers, Gravel, Gout, Scurvey, and Phthisis. They are cooling, promote perspiration, give relief in diseases of the bladder and kidneys, upon which they act powerfully, since they impart a violet smell and high color to urine. Hoffman and Linnaeus have long ago extolled them in gout and phthisis [consumption]; persons labouring under these chronic complaints ought to eat them frequently when in season, and use at other times their Syrup. An excessive dose of either is however liable to produce emesis or a painful stricture in the bladder, with red urine, as I have experienced myself...They possess also the property of curing chill-blains, their water is used in France for that purpose as a wash. A fine wine can be made of them and some sugar. The plant and leaves have nearly the same properties, although they are less cooling and more astringent. Both have been employed, like Cinquefoil and Agrimony for sore throat, swelled gums, bowel complaints, jaundice and fevers in infusion and decoction...1830 221. Dried for use in Europe."

1855 Trail 73. "On summer fallows on these plains, and in the first and second year's ploughed lands, the strawberries attain a size that is remarkable for wild fruits of this kind, and quantities are gathered for home consumption, and also carried into the towns for sale."

1859-61 Gunn 864. "Strawberry leaves and roots are an excellent astringent, and useful in bowel complaints, expecially for children. A strong decoction or tea may be made of them, or of the leaves alone, and used freely; or a sirup or cordial may be made...the roots alone are also said to be diuretic. The berry is a very delicious fruit and to most persons healthy."

1868 Can. Pharm J. 82. Woodruff, Bentley & Co. Wholesale Dealers and Manufacturers of Patent Medicines, Brougham, Ontario. Established 1844. We are the sole manufacturers and Proprietors of the following medicines:- Dr. Fowler's Extract of Wild Strawberry. [Advertisement]

1879 Can. Pharm J. 303. "Dr. T.L. Philson has recently been engaged in an examination of the constituents of the root of the strawberry plant, and finds it to contain several substances which are closely allied to some which are yielded by cinchona [quinine]. One of these, which he terms *fragarianine*, is a kind of tannin allied to quinotannic acid, but instead of yielding cinchona red it gives another substance, to which the name fragarine has been applied."

1885 Hoffman OJIBWA 200. "Referred to in the ceremony of the 'Ghost Society'. The fruit is highly valued as a luxury."

1892 Millspaugh 55. "The previous medical uses of Fragaria were few; the berries were ordered to be freely eaten of in various calcareous [stone] disorders. Many early writers considered the fruit as beneficial in gouty affections; Linnaeus extols their efficacy in preventing paroxysms of gout in his own case; and Rousseau claims that he was always relieved of calcareous afflictions by eating freely of them. The root in infusion has been used in England for dysuria and gonorrhoea. The dried leaves yield a slightly astringent infusion used in domestic practice as an excitant, and as an astringent in diarrhoea and dysentery."

1916 Waugh IROQUOIS 125. "Among the earliest berry to ripen is the strawberry. . .These welcome events are celebrated by longhouse ceremonies in which thanks are given, while quantities of the fruit are eaten in the feasts which follow. . . .145. Berries were evidently quite frequently used in the preparation of drinks. . . .blackberries or thimbleberries and water sweetened with maple sugar is common both for home consumption and in longhouse ceremonies. . .and the making of. . .medicine, as are also similar concoctions of strawberries. . .at their respective festivals. At certain of these functions the juice is sometimes sprayed from the mouth upon the heads of those desiring health and prosperity for the coming season. In such cases the liquid must be made by those undergoing the ceremony. . .An active medicinal value, aside from the ceremonial uses, is ascribed to several varieties of the berries and other fruits or to beverages made from them."

1926-27 Densmore CHIPPEWA 346. Steep 2 or 3 roots in 1 quart of boiling water. Let the child drink freely until the effect is evident for cholera infantum.

1928 Parker SENECA 11. Strawberry root astringent. . .strawberry runners used for tuberculosis.

1932 H. Smith OJIBWE 384. "The root is used to make a tea good for the stomach ache and especially for babies."

1933 H. Smith POTAWATOMI 77. "Use the root for the treatment of stomach complaints. . .107. Gather large quantities for food. . .They sometimes dry them and at other times preserve them for winter food." [Gathered, eaten and preserved by Menomini, Meskwaki and Ojibwe, also].

1955 Mockle Quebec transl. 59. "*Fragaria vesca* L. the roots are given as an astringent and diuretic; the fruits as a depurative and for gout. . .*Fragaria virginiana* Duchs. The roots astringent, much used in decoction or as a tea for diarrhea; the fruits in refreshing drinks."

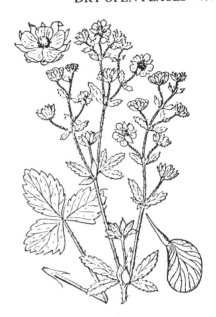

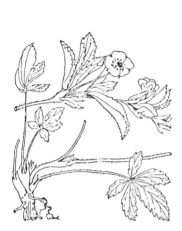

CANADA CINQUEFOIL

ROUGH CINQUEFOIL

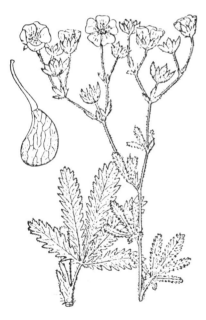

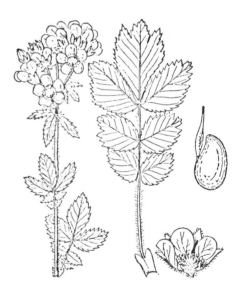

SULPHER CINQUEFOIL

TALL CINQUEFOIL

The Cinquefoils
The cinquefoils are members of the rose family, *Rosaceae*, and their botanical name is *Potentilla*. This is the diminutive of *potens*, meaning powerful because of their long use in medicine and magic.

CANADA CINQUEFOIL
Potentilla canadensis L.

From a stout underground root there rises a weak, hairy stem. The leaves have five leaflets that are hairy beneath. The middle leaflet is usually more than half as wide as long with teeth around the top half of the leaflet only. The five petalled yellow flowers are 10-15 mm wide, each on its own stalk.

Range. Nfld., N.S., P.E.I., Me., s. Que. and Ont. to Minn., s. to Ala., Mo., Okla., Tenn. and Ga. in open woods or their borders.

Common names. Wild or barren strawberry, sinkfield, running buttercups. The very similar *P. reptans* has smooth leaves. It is an eurasian plant introduced along roadsides, waste places in N. Am. Cinquefoil means five leaved.

1748 Kalm Phildalphia October 30th. 197. "Others boiled the leaves of the *Potentilla reptans* or of the *Potentilla Canadensis* in water and make the patients drink it before the chill came on [of the ague], and it is well known that several persons recovered by this means."

1830 Rafinesque 253. "All sp. mild astringent, tonic and vulnery. *P. reptans, P. canadensis* and *P. fruticosa* mostly used in weak bowels, hemorrhage, agues, menorhea, &c."

1868 Can. Pharm. J.6;83-5 The roots of *P. canadensis* included in list Can. medicinal plants.

1925 Wood & Ruddock. The root of *P. canadensis* for treatment of bowel diseases, excessive menstruation, hemorrhages from the womb. Drink the decoction three times a day for night sweats. It is an excellent gargle for sore throats.

1928 Riddell 119. "Our Canadian cinquefoil or fivefinger is *P. canadensis*: it was used in a mouthwash."

1955 Mockle Quebec transl. 60. "The root is very rich in tannins. It is used as an astringent in diarrheas and chronic catarrh."

TALL OR GLANDULAR CINQUEFOIL *Potentilla arguta* Pursh. Rosacea (*Drymocallis agrimonoides, D. arguta*)

The 30-100 cm straight stem is covered with gland tipped hairs, as is the whole plant, making it sticky. The leaves consist of 7 to 11 leaflets or only 5 in the uppermost leaves. The many flowers are 12-18 mm across and white.

Range. e. Que. to Mack., s. to D.C., Ind., Mo. and Ariz. June-July in dry woods or rocky soil.

1926-27 Densmore CHIPPEWA 332. "The letting of blood was a remedial measure frequently used among the Chippewa and was resorted to for numerous causes. The principle instrument used in this treatment was a small pointed blade set in a handle about 3 or 4 inches long. By means of this instrument the part to be cut was firmly stroked downward, forcing the blood to the extremity; a bandage was then applied above the point at which the incision was to be made. In making the incision the instrument was held close to the flesh and lightly snapped with the thumb and finger of the right hand, thus inflicting a slight incision of the vein. If too much force was applied, the result might be fatal; thus an instance was related in which the vein was severed and the man died. It is said that about 'half a basin' of blood was usually taken. A medicine to check the bleeding was then applied and the upper bandage removed. The root commonly used for this purpose was identified as *Drymocallis arguta* (Pursh.) Rydb. The prepared root was either used dry or was moistened with warm water, placed on soft duck down, and laid over the incision. It was said by three informants that this treatment was used especially for persons who had met with an accident, as a fall or injury to the back, and that the medicine 'prevented' the blood from settling in one place. This treatment was also used for 'persons who seemed to have too much blood'". . .338. The dried and pulverized root was applied to an incision in the temple for convulsions, or the moistened root was inserted in the nostril. . .344. Decoction was drunk for dysentery. . .350. The dried and pulverized root was moistened and applied to cuts.

ROUGH CINQUEFOIL
Potentilla norvegica L. Rosaceae

A hairy, branched stem, 20-50 cm tall with long stalked leaves consisting of three leaflets. These may be as broad as long, or only a third as wide as long. They are green on both sides, deeply toothed all around. There are several inconspicuous 6 mm across, yellow flowers at the end of their stems.

Range. Circumboreal, s. in Am. to N.C., Tex. and Calif. June-Aug. in a wide variety of sites. Also the European variety introduced in part of the range.

1926-27 Densmore CHIPPEWA 342. "Root and stalks chewed or used in decoction for a sore throat.

1932 H. Smith OJIBWE 384. "This plant seems to be known to all the Pillager Ojibwe, even the eight-year-old girls, as a physic."

1933 H. Smith POTAWATOMI 77. "The root of this plant is known to be a medicine to the Forest Potawatomi but our informant was not able to tell us the malady it was supposed to cure."

SULPHUR CINQUEFOIL   *Potentilla recta* L. (*P. sulphurea*)

Many stout, hairy stems, 20-80 cm tall, bear leaves at intervals. Each leaf consists of five leaflets joining their stalk at the same spot and spread apart like the fingers of a hand. The leaflets, green on both sides, are 3-4 cm long and about half as wide, sparsely covered with long white hairs, these stand out on the underside and are pressed to the surface on the upper. There can be only 3 or as many as 7 leaflets to each leaf. The flowers, 2-2½ cm across, are conspicuous. The five deep yellow petals grow from a ridge like ring which secretes honey. The seeds are ridged, the young seedlings can be deceptive, consisting only of tiny single toothed leaves a cm wide, the whole plant 3 cm tall. There may be clumps of 100 seedlings near old sulphur cinqefoil plants.

Range. Native of Europe, found as a weed in dry soil throughout our range. *P. erecta* (*P. tormentilla, Tormentilla erecta*) The European tormentil is found in e. Mass. and in mossy places in se. Nfld. Possibly left there by the early fishing fleets because of its importance as a medicinal herb. Many of its uses have been carried over to both the introduced and native potentillas of America.

1633 Gerarde-Johnson 992. "Tormentil is not only of like vertue with Cinkefoile, but also of greater efficacie: it is much used against pestilent diseases: for it strongly resisteth putrifaction, and procureth sweate. The leaves and roots boiled in wine, or the juice thereof drunken provoketh sweat, and by that means driveth out all venome from the heart, expelleth poison, and preserveth the bodie in time of pestilence from the infection thereof, and all other infectious diseses. The roots dried made into pouder and drunke in wine. . .or in the water of a Smiths forge, or rather water wherein hot steele hath often been quenched of purpose, cureth the laske and bloudy flix, yea although the patient have adjoined unto his scouring a grievous fever. It stoppeth the spitting of bloud, pissing of bloud, and all other issues of bloud, as well in men as in women. The decoction of the leaves and rootes, or the juice thereof drunke, is excellent good for all wounds, both outward and inward: it also openeth and healeth the stoppings of the liver and lungs and cureth the jaundice. The root beaten into pouder, tempered or kneaded with the white of an egge and eaten, stayeth the desire to vomit, and is good against choler and melancholie."

1799 Lewis Mat. Med. 255. *P. erecta.* Root is one of the most agreeable and efficacious of the vegetable astringents and is employed with success in all cases where medicines of this class are proper. It is more used, both in extemporaneous prescriptions and in officinal compositions than any other strong vegetable astringent. . .given in substance, and in large doses, either by itself or joined with gentian, it has been said to cure intermittents.

1820's Edinburgh-Toronto Mat. Med. mss. 35. "*Tormentil erecta* is strongly astringent with little flavour or bitterness. Has been used in decoction in Diarrhoea & in substance in intermittents."

1841 Trousseau & Pidoux Paris transl. *P. erecta.* "A strong astringent used in Theriaque & Diascordium, powdered infusions and decoctions for hemorrhage, fluxes. . .Theriaque is a mixture of opium and bitter and digestive substances. Diascordium is a mixture of opium and astringents used in diarrhea." [These were two of the most important medicines of the 17th. and 18th. centuries].

1842 Christison 925. "Take of root, bruised, 2 ozs., distilled water a pint & half, boil to a pint and strain. The root of tormentil is a very old article of Materia Medica. . .It has a tuberous root about the thickness and length of the upper joint of the forefinger, tough, woody. . .The infusion contains 17.5% tannin. A powerful astringent and one of the most active indigenous drugs, although now scarcely ever used. . .Applicable to treatment of chronic mucous discharge and chronic dysentery."

1864 Dr. Chase 258. "Looseness or scouring in horses and cattle- In use for over seventy years- Tormentil root, powdered. Dose for a cow or horse 1 to 1½ oz. It may be stirred in 1 pt. of milk and given, or it may be steeped in 1½ pts. of milk and then given from 3 to 5 times daily until cured. It has proved valuable also for persons. Dose for a person would be from one-half to one teaspoon steeped in milk. . .An English gentleman from whom it was obtained, had been familiar with its use nearly eighty years, and never knew a failure, if taken in any kind of seasonable time. The tormentil or septfoil, is an European plant and very astringent."

Tormentil has been used since the middle ages in Europe in the folk treatment of cancer (Hartwell 1971).

See Wet Open Places for other cinquefoils.

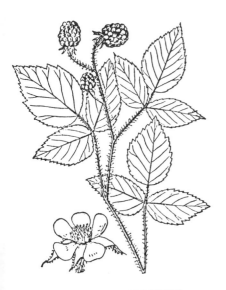

WILD RED RASPBERRY

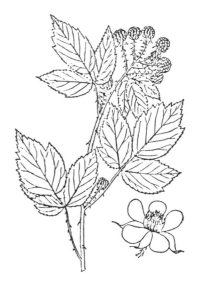

BLACK RASPBERRY

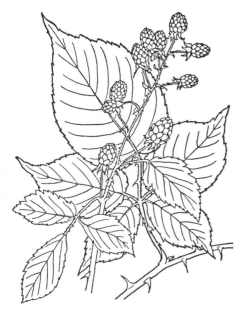

BLACKBERRY

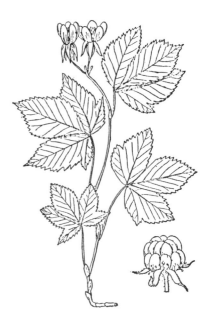

DWARF RED BLACKBERRY

WILD RED RASPBERRY   *Rubus idaeus* L. var. *strigosus* Michx. Rosaceae
Stems to 2 m erect, spreading or lying down, with few slender thorns and stiff bristles. The bristly
stalked leaves usually have three leaflets that are whitish beneath. The flower stalks have gland
tipped hairs and usually 2-5 white flowers followed by red berries that pull off their cores.

Range. Lab., Nfld., N.B., P.E.I., N.S., Que., Ungava Bay to Yukon, Alaska, s. to Calif., N. Mex., n. Mex., Tenn. and N.C. and Eurasia in thickets, open woods and fields.

1380 Crawford Lake site Ont. McAndrews, Byrne and Finlayson 1974 3. "The largest number of seeds were those of *Rubus*, which totalled 54.5% (1052) of the wild plant remains. *Rubus* occurs in all the feature types and 53.9% (48) of the features sampled. . .92 seeds recovered from the earth oven, 72 from the midden, 539 from natural depressions filled with refuse."

1500 Draper site Ont. Finlayson 1975 225. "3,000 samples processed. . .An examination of 200 of these samples. . .recovery of. . .716 raspberry seeds."

1534 Cartier voyage St. Lawrence transl. 43. On the coast of Prince Edward Island. "The land that was not wooded was very beautiful and full of. . .raspberries". . .North coast of baie des Chaleurs. . ."Gooseberries, red and white, strawberries, raspberries and red roses."

1619 Champlain-Macklem Ottawa river 1616 34-5. "We also found-it was almost as if God had wished to bestow a gift of some sort on this barren and unfriendly country for the succour and support of its people—that in season the riverbanks were thick with berries of all sorts, including raspberries and blueberries. . .The savages dry the berries for use during the winter, much as we in France dry prunes for use during Lent. . .Lake Huron . . .37. By this time we had little left, though for some time we had been eating only one meal a day. Luckily, there was also plenty of blueberries and raspberries. Without them we might have starved to death. . .40-41 Cahiague is largest of all the villages. . .most of the land is cleared of trees. . .The savages grow. . .grapes and plums, raspberries, strawberries, crab-apples and nuts. . .74. The lakes are full of fish and dotted with islands, some of which have been cleared and planted with vines and small fruits. . .78. The staple of their diet is Indian corn. . .to make bread they boil the dough, as if they were making corn soup. This makes it easier to whip. After it is thoroughly boiled they sometimes add blueberries or dried raspberries."

1681 Culpeper 290. "The fruit. . .strengthens the stomach, stays vomiting, is somewhat astringent, and good to prevent miscarriage. The fruit is very grateful as nature presents it, but made into a sweetmeat with sugar or fermented with wine, the flavour is improved. . .It dissolves the tartarous concretions on the teeth, but is inferior to strawberries for that purpose."

1830 Rafinesque 258. "Nearly 30 wild species. . .Roots of all more or less astringent, subtonic, much used in cholera infantum, chronic dysentery, diarrhea, &c. The Cherokis chew them for cough; a cold poultice useful in piles; used with Lobelia in gonorrhea. . .Ripe fruits, preserves, jam, jelly or syrup, grateful and beneficial in diarrhea, gravel, hemoptysis, phthsis, sorethroat, putrid and malignant fevers, scurvy. . .Raspberries afford delicious distilled water, beer, mead and wine. Said to dissolve tartar of teeth. Twigs dye silk and wool."

1859-61 Gunn 848. "The leaves are the part used as medicine and those of the red species are considered the best. They are one of the most valuable astringents—to be used in decoction or strong tea, in looseness of bowels, especially in the summer complaint of children. A strong tea of raspberry leaves is also an excellent article to be drank freely, in painful and profuse menstruation, and to regulate the labor pains of women in child-birth. . .A tea is good to wash and clean old sores, ulcers, scalds, and excoriated or raw and irritable surfaces."

1885 Hoffman OJIBWA 199. The roots are sometimes used as a substitute for the black raspberry.

1901 Morice DENE 24. "As most of the drudgery of the daily life. . .still falls to the lot of the woman, accidents, oftentimes quite serious, follow as a matter of course. . .frequently enough occasion displacement. . .of the womb. In such cases, the treatment observed is quite rational, and therefore, it is ordinarily crowned with success. The patient is immediately laid in a recumbent position with the head rather lower than the womb, and. . .by dint of external manipulation, the injured organ is pressed up to its normal place, after which strong bandages covering a plaster-like padding, added to copious draughts of the decoction of the stems of the raspberry bush, help to neutralize the effects of the accident. But I am bound to confess that, in the more severe cases, sterility ensues even in otherwise healthy women."

1916 Waugh IROQUOIS 119. "The fresh shoots are peeled and eaten. . .145. Berries were evidently quite frequently used in the preparation of drinks. These were not only noted historically, but are popular at present. . .berries and water sweetened with maple sugar. . .This drink is employed as a refreshment at meetings. . .and the making of medicine, as are also concoctions of strawberries and raspberries at their respective festivals. . .148. The young twigs of red raspberry according to Barber Black, Tonawanda, N.Y., were stripped of the leaves, placed in hot water and steeped, then sweetened with sugar in the usual way."

1926-27 Densmore CHIPPEWA 344. A decoction of the root for dysentery. . .360. The inner bark of red raspberry root and that of a rose (species doubtful). These two remedies are used successively, the rose for removing inflammation, and the second for healing the eye. They are prepared in the same way, the second layer of the root being scraped and put in a bit of cloth. This is soaked in warm water and squeezed over the eye, letting some of the liquid run into the eye. This is done three times a day. It was said that these would cure cataract unless too far advanced, and that improvement would be shown quickly if the case could be materially helped.
1923 H. Smith MENOMINI 50. "Root is used as a seasoner for other medicines. Berries also eaten fresh."
1932 H. Smith OJIBWE 386. "The root bark makes a tea for healing sore eyes, the berries used as a seasoner. . .When the red raspberry is not readily available the black cap raspberry is used in the same manner. . .410. Favorite fresh fruit of the Flambeau Ojibwe and is also used for making jams for winter use."
1933 H. Smith POTAWATOMI 79. "The root is made into an infusion to use as an eye wash. . .A decoction of the leaves has been combined with cream by [white] eclectic practioners to suppress nausea and vomiting. It has also been sometimes used as an aid to labor to promote uterine contractions where ergot has failed."
1945 Rousseau MOHAWK transl. 48. "A mixture of the roots of bracken with the leaves of the red raspberry and wheat flour is given to cows in labor."
1945 Rousseau Quebec transl. 48. "The purple flowering red raspberry, *R. odoratus*, leaves placed in their leather shoes by the coureurs de bois to protect their feet."
1945 Raymond TETE DE BOULE transl. 130. "The roots, steeped in boiling water, and the water drunk in cases of blood in the urine."
1971 Jolicoeur Quebec 5. Used for diarrhoea.

BLACK RASPBERRY   *Rubus occidentalis* L.
Long straight upright stems that curve over and root at the tips where they touch the ground, prickly. The berries are raspberrys that are black in color when fully ripe.
Range. Que. to N.D. and e. Col., s. to Ga. and Ark. in dry or moist woods and fields.
Common names. Black cap, purple raspberry.
1741 Farriers Disp. The leaves are said to be cooling and strengthening and may therefor be given to such Horses as are troubled with too much inward heat, chopped amongst his hay.
1748 Kalm Philadelphia September 20th. 47. "The ladies make fine wine from some of the fruits of the land. . .The American blackberries or *Rubus occidentalis*. are also used for this purpose."
1885 Hoffman OJIBWA 199. "*Rubus occidentalis*. A decoction made of the crushed roots is taken to relieve pains in the stomach.
1916 Waugh IROQUOIS 127. Black raspberry eaten fresh and dried.
1926-27 Densmore CHIPPEWA 356. *R. occidentalis*, black raspberry. A decoction of the root for pain in the back and female weakness.
1923 H. Smith MENOMINI 50. "Black raspberry (*R. occidentalis*). The root was used with the giant St. John's wort in curing consumption when it was in its first stages."
1928 H. Smith MESKWAKI 243. "Black raspberry (*R. occidentalis*). A beverage tea is sometimes made from the root."

BLACKBERRY   *Rubus allegheniensis* Porter Rosaceae
Stems 0.5-3 m mostly erect, prickles straight, spreading not hooked. The stalks of the flowers covered with gland tipped hairs, the flowers white, 2 cm wide. The black berry consists of many globules sticking together.
Range. N.B., P.E.I., N.S., s. Que., s. Ont. to Minn., s. to Mo., Tenn., and N.C. in thickets and clearings. Britten and Brown 1913 *R. villosus* var. *montanus*. is a synonym.

DWARF RED BLACKBERRY   *Rubus pubescens* Raf. (*R. triflorus*)
The stems without prickles trailing, rooting, or loosely ascending. The leaves with three leaflets soft and thick. The flowering stem upright 20-50 cm with stalks bearing 1-3 pale pink or white flowers and petals about 1 cm long and 3 mm broad. Berry red purple.

Range. Nfld., N.B., P.E.L., N.S., Que., northernmost Ont. Man to Great Slave Lake, s. to Wash., n. Colo., s. Dak., Pa. and N.J. in thickets, open woods and shores, conifer swamps.

Common names. Catherinettes, dewberry, running raspberry, plum-bog-swamp berry. The references that follow to *R. villosus* probably are in part to *R. argutus* a southern variety and in part to *R. allegheniensis*.

1785 Cutler Sowteat, bumblekites. [Probably *R. argutus*]. The fruit is pleasant to eat and communicates a fine flavor to red wine. It is frequently infused in brandy or rum. The green twigs are said to be of great use in dyeing woolens, silk and mohair black.

1817-20 Bigelow 162. "The bark of the root of this bramble (*R. villosus*) is the part which has been medicinally employed. It is a pure and strong astringent. . .As we continue to import and consume various foreign medicines of this kind, we ought not to exclude from attention native articles of equal efficacy. Professor Chapman of Philadelphia. . .says. . .to the declining stages of dysentery after the symptoms of active inflammation are removed, it is well suited. . .in cholera infantum. . .no remedy has ever done so much in my hands. Even two or three doses will sometimes so bind the bowels that purgatives becomes necessary. . .Useful. . .in the diarrhea of very old people. . .The fruit of the blackberry is among the most delicious productions of the uncultivated forest. To an agreeable combination of sweetness and acid it adds an aromatic fragrance. . .Low or running blackberry. . .the bark is not less astringent."

1830 Rafinesque 259. "Blackberries dye purple, are more astringent and acid."

1833 Howard Quebec 18. "To cure the Cholera. Take two quarts of Juce of Blackberrys, one pound of lofe sugar, half oz. of nutmeg, half oz. of allspice, boil all together a little, let stand till cold then add one pint of fourth proof Brandy. Take from a tea spoon full to a wine glass 2 or 3 times a day."

1859-6 Gunn 745. "[*R. villosus* probably *argutus*] Blackberry sirup. . .one of the most valuable remedies that can be found in diseases of the bowels. . .blackberry root eight ounces, finely cut up and bruised, Bayberry bark four ounces, Crane's bill two ounces [geranium root], Gum Myrrh one ounce, Cinnamon bark two ounces, Fennel seed half an ounce, Cloves one ounce. The whole should be well bruised and put into six quarts of water, and let to steep six or eight hours, simmering slowly till reduced about one half; then strain, and simmer down to two pints; add while hot one pound of loaf or white sugar; when cold add one pint of best French brandy, and it is ready for use. A tablespoonful is a proper dose for a grown person, repeated every one, two, or three hours, or every half-hour according to circumstances, or as the urgency of the case may require, in all cases of diarrhoea, cholera, and cholera morbus; for children, from one to two teaspoonfuls, according to age. Blackberry cordial. . .Take a quart of the berries, mash; add, say an ounce, of crushed Cinnamon bark; half an ounce each of Allspice and Cloves, crushed, and a pint of water; simmer slowly for an hour or two, then strain; add half a pound of loaf sugar, simmer till there is but about a pint, and add a fourth as much good French brandy. Dose for children, one or two teaspoonfuls, repeated often in diarrhea and summer complaints."

1868 Can. Pharm. J. 6;83-5. Bark of the root of the blackberry, *R. Villosus*, included in list of Can. medicinal plants.

1894 Household Guide Toronto 114. "The root is recommended for diarrhea, dysentery, and summer complaints in children. Boil the small roots in a quart of water and reduce this quantity by boiling it down one-half. One or two tablespoonfuls may be given three or four times a day."

1915 Speck-Tantaquidgeon MOHEGAN 318. "Running blackberry, berries are steeped and drunk as a vermifuge [worm medicine]."

1915 W.R. Harris 51. "In bowel complaints the Indians administered an infusion of the dewberry roots (o-ga-she-ga)."

1916 Waugh IROQUOIS 127. "Berry eaten and dried for winter use:-black raspberry, dwarf raspberry and thimbleberry. . .145. "Blackberries or thimbleberries and water, sweetened with maple sugar, is common both for home consumption and in longhouse ceremonies. This drink was called uhiagei. The fresh berries are preferred when these are obtainable, though they are also dried, or otherwise preserved and enjoyed throughout the winter. This drink is employed as a refreshment at the meetings called hadihidus and the making of. . .medicine. . .Fresh blackberries are particularly sought after for the Big Green Corn Dance in the early autumn. The drinkers in each case make an effort to get a share of the berries which settle to the bottom. An active medicinal value, aside from ceremonial uses, is ascribed to several varieties of berries and other fruits or to beverages made from them."

1926-27 Densmore CHIPPEWA 340. Blackberry root and the inner bark of the bur oak used in decoction for lung trouble. . .358. A decoction of the root for stoppage of periods. *R. frondosus* [Britten and Brown 1913 synonym *R. villosus frondosus*. Mass. to N.Y.]

1928 Parker SENECA 11. Blackberry root as an astringent. . .12. For dysentery.

1923 H. Smith MENOMINI 50. "Blackberry (*R. allegheniensis*). . .An infusion of the steeped root is used to cure sore eyes, an eye wash, and is also used as a poultice."

1928 H. Smith MESKWAKI 243. "The Meskwaki use the root extract for stomach trouble, but McIntosh uses the liquid of the root for treating sore eyes. Specimen 5070 of the Dr. Jones collection is the root of *R. allegheniensis*. This is boiled and prepared for a drink as an antidote to poison."

1932 H. Smith OJIBWE 385. "The Flambeau Ojibwe boil the canes (*R. allegheniensis*) to obtain a tea that is used as a diuretic. The roots furnish a tea for arresting flux."

1933 H. Smith POTAWATOMI 79. "The Prairie Potawatomi use the root bark (*R. allegheniensis*) for treating sore eyes. The Forest Potawatomi did not have any medicinal use for the plant."

1935 Jenness Parry Island Lake Huron OJIBWA 14. "Women gathered wild berries. . .blue berries they crushed raw and dried in the sun on sheets of birch bark; but thimble berries they cooked into cakes before drying. . .80. Women, if unwell, must not eat berries, or they will spoil all the berries on the bushes."

1945 Rousseau MOHAWK transl. 48. "The young mothers whose 'blood seems thickening' must drink an infusion of the roots of the blackberry mixed with that of black cherry. This infusion must be reduced in half by boiling. The catherinette [dwarf red blackberry] is not used medicinally. The Ojibwes use the roots to make a remedy for pregnant wives threatened with abortion from overwork."

1945 Raymond TETE DE BOULE transl. 130. A tea of the scrapings of the bark of the branches is used to cure bronchial affections.

1955 Mockle Quebec transl. 61. "Astringent. The bark contains up to 20% of tannin and a bitter substance, villosine." [High blackberry, *R. villosus* Ait].

Rubus odoratus, purple flowering raspberry is being examined as a possible cancer therapeutic agent on account of its tannin content (Lewis and Elvin-Lewis 1977:135).

GLOSSARY

Absorbent; absorbing or sucking in noxious matter.

Abstergent or detergent; cleaning foul ulcers and sores.

Allopathic; the regular physicians in practice.

Alterative; producing a change in the whole system, or altering the appearance of local disease.

Alvine; belonging to the belly or intestines.

Amenorrhea; suppression of menses, especially from causes other than age or pregnancy.

Analgesic; pain reliever that does not produce loss of consciousness.

Anodyne; soothing the nerves, allaying pain, similar to sedative and nervine.

Anthelmintic; expelling worms from the body.

Antipyretic; an agent relieving or reducing fever.

Antispasmodic; medicines which relieve spasms.

Aperient; promoting excretions.

Aphthous; an eruption, ulceration in the mouth.

Ascites; a kind of dropsy.

Astringents; substances that contract organic tissue and lessen secretion.

Atony; debility, weakness of any organ.

Balsam; the gum of the tree *Balsamodendron Gileadense* or *Opobalsamum* of Middle east.

Balsamic; a mild healing stimulant.

Bloody flix, bloody flux; morbid or excessive discharge of blood, a flowing out, or dysentery.

Cachexia; a morbid state of the body.

Cacochymia; a morbid state of the fluids of the body.

Calculus; stones in the bladder.

Calomel; mercurous chloride used as a purgative.

Cantharides; Spanish flies, blistering beetles, *Cantharis vesicatoria* put on the body externally to produce blisters, if taken internally an irritant poison.

Cardiac glycosides; substances having a stimulating effect on the heart.

Cardiacal; acting on the heart, increasing its muscular action.

Carminative; local stimulant, expelling wind from the stomach.

Catamenia; the menses.

Cataplasm; a poultice.

Catarrh; inflammation of the upper respiratory tract with mucus discharge.

Cathartic; catharsis or purgative, a medicine that cleans the bowels.

Cephalic; of the head.

Chancre; a venereal ulcer or sore.

Cholera infantum; enterocolitis of infants.

Chologogue, chologogic; purging the bile.

Cholorosis; the green sickness, a peculiar form of anemia which afflicts young women at the onset of puberty.

Chorea; a nervous disease with spasmodic, irregular movements that are uncontrollable.

Cicatrisant; process of healing in wounds.

Cinchona; bark of a south American tree of genus *Cinchona* which contains quinine.

Clyster; an injection of a liquid substance into the lower intestine.

Colophony; dark resin distilled from turpentine.

Corroborant; a medicine that strengthens the human body when weak.

Coryza; a bad cold in the head.

Cystitis; inflammation of the bladder.

Cytitis; a skin disease.

Decoction; any medicine made by boiling a substance in water to extract its virtues.

Demulcent; a mucilaginous medicine which sheaths the tender and raw surfaces of diseased parts.

Deobstruant; any medicine which removes obstructions and opens the natural passages of the fluids of the body.

Depurant, depuration; cleansing from impure matter.

Desquamation; scaling of the skin as in scarlet fever.

Detergent, detersive; a medicine that cleanses the vessels or skin of impure matter.

Diaphoresis, diaphoretics; those medicines which increase the natural exhalation by the skin, when they excite this so copiously as to produce sweat, they are termed sudorifics.

Diarrhea; a morbidly frequent evacuation of the intestines, excessive looseness of the bowels.

Diluent; that which increases the proportion of water in the blood.

Discutient; a medicine which scatters a swelling or tumor or any coagulated fluid or body.

Diuretic, diurient, diuresis; a medicine which increases the discharge of urine.

Dropsy; a morbid accumulation of watery liquid in any cavity of the body or tissues.

Dysnoe, dysneic; difficulty in breathing.

Dysuria, dysury; urination that is painful.

Eclectic; physicians who borrow treatments from all schools of medicine such as the allopaths, botanic, homeopathic etc.

Electuary; a medicine composed of sugar or honey and some powder or other ingredient.

Emmenagogue, menagogue; those substances which are capable of promoting the menstrual discharge.

Empiric; botanic physicians and others who experimented with different drugs.

Empyreumatic; pertaining to or having the taste or smell of slightly burned animal or vegetable substances.

Epipastic; local stimulant acting on the skin to produce blisters.

Ergot; the fungus *Claviceps purpurea* on grain used to accelerate childbirth.

Errhine; substances which promote sneezing and discharge from the nose.

Eructations; belching.

Erysipelas; local disease producing a deep red color in the skin.

Escharotic; substances which erode or dissolve the animal solids.

Exanthema; eruptive diseases which are accompanied by fever.

Fauces; the back part of the throat.

Febrifuge; a medicine which drives away fever by producing sweat.

Flix or flux; diarrhoe, looseness, see bloody flux or flix.

Fluour albus; see leucorrhea.

Galatogogue; a medicine which promotes secretion of milk in the breast.

Gastralgia; stomach ache.

Gravel; small stones and sand resembling gravel which form in the kidneys.

Gravid; pregnant.

Hematosis; a morbid quantity of blood.

Hematuria, haematuria; presence of blood in the urine.

Hemoptysis; spitting of blood.

Hemostatic; an agent that arrests bleeding.

Hepatic; useful in diseases of the liver.

Herpes; an eruption on the skin, produced by the herpes simplex virus.

Hipped; fungous growth on the hip joint of a horse.

Hydragogue; a purgative that causes watery discharges from the bowel.

Hydropic; a dropsical person, medicine that cures dropsy.

Infusion; medicine prepared by steeping substances in either cold or hot water.

Inspissated; a fluid substance rendered thicker by evaporation.

Laske; looseness, flux, diarrhea.

Leucorrhea; a white vaginal discharge by females, fluor albus.

Lithontriptics; medicines which are supposed to have the power of dissolving urinary stones.

Menorrhea; normal menstrual flow, menorrhagia.

Menstruum; a dissolvent, any liquid used to extract the medical virtues from soft substances.

Morbid; diseased, not sound or healthy.

Mucus; a sticky, slimy substance secreted by the mucous membranes.

Narcotic; substance inducing drowsiness, sleep, stupor or insensibility, often administered to allay pain.

Nephritic; local stimulant to the kidneys.

Nervine; acting particularly on the nerves, soothing pain, promoting sleep.

Odontalgic; allaying or curing toothache.

Officinal; herb or drug used in medicine or the arts, often made from recipes in Pharmacopoeias.

Ophthalmia; inflammation of the eye.

Opthalmic; useful in diseases of the eye.

Oxytocic; hastening childbirth.

Papillomatous; having small nipple-like protuberances in a part or organ of the body.

Parturition; the act of childbirth.

Pectoral; useful in diseases of the breast and lungs.

Pellant; or repellant; repelling morbid fluids.

Pertussis; cough.

Porrigo; excema of the scalp.

Phthisis; consumption, TB.

Pyretic; feverish of, for or producing fever.

Pyrosis; a peculiar disease of the stomach called water brash.

Pytalism; poisoning by taking too much mercury such as calomel.

Refrigerant; cooling, lessening the heat of the body, allaying local or general inflammation.

Resolvant, resolutive; promoting suppuration of ulcers or tumors.

Rubefacient; an application which produces redness of the skin with heat.

Salicin; see text, willow and poplar.

Salt Rheum; a vague, indefinite popular name applied to almost all non feverish skin eruptions which are common among adults, except perhaps ringworm.

Scorbutic; of the nature of scurvy.

Scrofulous; a scaly skin.

Scurvy; a disease now known to be due to Vitamin C deficiency. See text Spruce.

Sialogogue; medicines which incite an increased flow of saliva.

Simple; a plant that is used to treat a disease by itself and not in combination with other plants.

Specific; a medicine which acts specifically to cure one particular disease.

Sternutatory; substances which promote sneezing.

Stimulant; a medicine which acts by stimulating some part of the body.

Stomachic; a strengthening medicine for the stomach, exciting its action.

Strangury; a painful and difficult discharge of urine.

Styptic; a medicine which coagulates the blood and stops bleeding.

Strumous; scrofulous, scurfy.

Sudorific; see diaphoresis.

Suppurate; to form pus as in a boil.

Syncope; fainting or swooning.

Tetanic convulsions; convulsions and death resulting from a nervine or narcotic administered in an overdose.

Tetters; cutaneous eruption, scurf, excema, impetago, herpes.

Tincture; a medicine in which the vertue of the plant is extracted by alcohol.

Tonic; those substances which give strength to the whole system.

Topical; a remedy acting by external application.

Tympanites; dropsy of the belly.

Vermifuge; taenifuge; agent that expels worms from the intestines.

Vesicatory; raising blisters on the skin.

Vulnerary; medicines used for the cure of wounds.

SOURCES CITED

Addenda to Sources Cited — see page 511

Abbreviations

c. circa	J. Journal	pub. published
ed. editor	Jes. Rel. Jesuit Relations	publ. publication
eds. editors	Misc. miscellaneous	Rec. recherche
Edinb. Edinburgh	mss. manuscript	Res. resources
fac. ed. facsimile edition	pap. papers	Rev. revised
enl. enlarged	Pharm. Pharmacy	Sci. Science
Geol. Geologist	Philad. Philadelphia	ser. series
Ind. Industry	Phys. Physicians	supp. supplement
Inst. Institute	Proc. proceedings	surg. surgeons
intro. introduction	Prof. Professor	tr. translate or translated

Adrosko, Rita J. 1968 Natural dyes in the United States. Smithsonian Inst. Press U.S. Nat. Mus. Bull. 281. Washington D.C.

Alderson, J. 1804 An essay on the *Rhus Toxicodendron* with cases of its effects in the cure of paralytic affections and other diseases of great debility. Rawson 3rd ed. Hull.

Alex, J.F. & Switzer, C.M. 1976 Ontario weeds. Univ. of Guelph Ontario.

Alfonse, Jean. 1544 La cosmographie. Finished as mss. 1544 after Jean Fonteneau called Alfonse de Saintonge returned from accompanying Roberval as pilot of his 1542 voyage to Canada. Published Hakluyt 1600; Biggar from the original mss. 1930; reprinted in part in French by Rousseau 1937. tr. in text by author.

Aller, Wilma F. 1954 Aboriginal food utilization of vegetation by the Indians of the Great Lakes region as recorded in the Jes. Rel. Wisconsin Archeol. n.s. 35;59-73.

American medical plants of commercial importance. 1930 USDA 77 Washington D.C.

Anderson, Andrew. 1813 An inaugural dissertation on the *Eupatorium perfoliatum* of Linnaeus. Van Winkle N.Y.

Anderson, Fanny J. 1946 Medicine at Fort Detroit in the colony of New France 1701-1760. J. Hist. Med. April; 208-228.

Anderson, H.W. & Zsuffa, L. 1975 Yield and wood quality of hybrid poplar grown in two-year rotation. Forest Research Branch, Min. Nat. Res. Ont.

Anderson, James R. 1925 Trees and shrubs, food, medicinal and poisonous plants of British Columbia Dept. of Educ. Victoria B.C.

Anon. 1724 Manuscript on medical use of plants by the Illinois and Miami tribes. Printed by Kinietz 1965;223-226.

Anon. 1918 Wood and wood products, their uses by the pre-historic Indians of Ontario. 30th. Ann. Archeol. Rep. Min. Educ. Ont. 25-48. Toronto.

Assiniwi, Bernard. 1972 Survival in the Bush. Copp Clark Toronto.

Bacqueville de la Potherie, Claude Charles Le Roy. 1722, 1753 Histoire de l'Amerique septentrionale. Paris 4 vols. Parts printed in Blair 1911.

Bailey, Alfred Goldsworthy. 1969 The conflicts of European and eastern Algonkian cultures 1504-1700. 2nd ed. Univ. of Toronto Press Toronto.

Balfour, J.H. 1875 Manual of botany. 5th ed. Edinburgh.

Banting, Sir Frederick. 1939 Papers in rare books Univ. of Toronto library. Toronto.

Barefoot Doctor's Manual, 1977 Prepared by the revolutionary health committee of Hunan Province, China. A revised and enlarged version of the work originally pub. by the Fogarty International Centre, Betheda, Md. 1974 Cloudburst Press Ltd. Mayne Isle, B.C. or Seattle Washington.

Barnston, George. 1858 Remarks on the geographical distribution of plants in the British possessions of North America. Can. Naturalist & Geol. 3:1;26-32 Montreal.

Barrett, S.A. 1911 The dream dance of the Chippewa and Menomini Indians of Wisconsin. Bull. Pub. Mus. 1;357-368 Milwaukee. Not seen.

Barton, B.S. 1810 Collections for an essay towards a materia medica of the United States. Bull. Lloyd Library 1 1900 Cincinnati.

Bartram, John. 1851 Observations in travels to the Onondaga. London. Descriptions, virtues. and uses of sundry plants of these northern parts of America; and particularly of the newly discovered Indian cure for venereal disease (*Lobelia sp.* L.). Cited Fenton 1942;522.

Bartram, William. 1791 Travels of William Bartram. ed. Harper Yale Univ. Press. 1958 New Haven. First published 1791 Philadelphia. Reprinted. 1928 Dover.

Bauhin, C. 1620 Prodromus theatri botanici. Franckfurt. Describes several plants which had been sent him by Joachim Burserus who had received them from an unnamed apothecary in Paris. Specimens in Burserus Herbarium Finland. See Juel.

Benson, Adolph B. ed. 1964 Travels in North America 1748-50 by Kalm. See Kalm.

Benson, Herbert. 1979 Placebos effective in improving power of medicine. Globe and Mail 25th. June p. 14 Toronto.

Beauchamp, William M. 1902 Onondaga plant names. J. Am. Folk-Lore 15;91-103.

Beverley, Robert. 1705 The history and present state of Virginia. ed. L.B. Wright Univ. N. C. Press 1947 Chapel Hill.

Bigelow, Jacob. 1817-20 American medical botany, being a collection of the native medicinal plants of the United States. 3 vols. Cummings & Hilliard Boston. Prof. of Materia Medica at Harvard Univ.

Biggar, H.P. 1913 Les précurseurs de Jacques Cartier, 1479-1534. Collection de documents relatifs á l'histoire du Canada. Pub. Arch. Can. 5 Ottawa.

1924 The voyages of Jacques Cartier. Published from the originals with tr., notes and app. Pub. Arch. Can. 11 Ottawa.

1930 A collection of documents relating to Jacques Cartier and the sieur de Roberval. Pub. Arch. Can. 14 Ottawa.

Birkett, H.S. 1908 A brief history of medicine in the province of Quebec. 1535-1838 Am. Laryngological Ass. Trans. 13;1-27.

Bjornsson, Thorleif. 1475 An Icelandic medical manuscript tr. by Larsen 1931, who writes, p. 23. "Of course these facts do not prove that the Thorleif of the Icelandic records and the Thorleif of our mss. are one and the same. However, until the opposite is proved, it is a fair conjecture. The linguistic peculiarities show Icelandic scribes of the fifteenth century working on the basis of Norwegian originals. We have . . . one section named 'the leechbook of Thorleif Bjornsson', we have found a contemporary man of consequence, an Icelander by birth and heritage but with strong contacts with Norway and with a particular intellectual centre, the Munkeliv monastery, Bergen. We have embodied in the mss. a section, the Book of Simples, [the section quoted in this text] that clearly goes back to a west Norwegian Medical Book . . . It would seem probable that the volume was compiled by Icelandic scribes who used material already available in Iceland and also additional medical works secured by or for Thorleif Bjornsson in Norway through the aid of the monks of Munkeliv . . . 261 The source of the information in the Herbarium [Book of Simples] is ascribed to Henrik Harpestraeng, physician of the Danish King, who is identical with the Maistre Henry de Danemarche, who studied and practiced medicine in Orleans, France in 1181, and with Magister Henricus Dacus, author of the learned latin treatise, Liber de simplici medicina laxativa, or Dosis M.H. Daci, and with the canon of Roskilde, Magister Henricus Harpestraeng who died in 1244 . . . For [the Book of Simples] Herbarium of Harpestraeng, the sources have been fully established by M. Kristensen. . . to be Macer Floridus. . . not only is Macer Floridus used, but every chapter of Macer has contributed. . . Practically all chapters that do not go back to Macer are derived from the 11th. century Salernitan work De Gradibus Simplicum by Constantinus Africanus. . . the principal source of Macer." Rhode 1922:42 writes:

"The vast majority of the herbal mss. of the fifteenth century in England are merely transcriptions of Macer's Herbal." So the Icelandic medical mss. quoted in this text is based on the popular knowledge of the use of plants current in Europe from the eleventh to the sixteenth centuries but written for Scandanavians.

Blair, E.H. tr. & ed. 1911 The Indian tribes of the upper Mississippi valley and region of the great lakes, as described by Nicholas Perrot. . . Bacqueville de la Potherie and others. Arthur Clark 2 vols. 1911, 1912 Cleveland.

Blanton, Wyndham B. 1930 Medicine in Virginia in the seventeenth century. William Byrd press Richmond.

Boerhaave, H. 1755 A method of studying physick. Materia medica. Hodges London.

Boivin, Bernard. 1978 La flore du Canada en 1708. Étude d'un manuscrit de Michel Sarrazin et Sébastien Vaillant. Provencheria 9 Inst. Rech. Biosystématique Agric. Can. Ottawa. See Victorin for the discovery of this mss. and its history from 1919 until 1978 when it was pub. by Boivin, who having seen the extant copies, prepared a collated text. He has also given the contemporary botanical name for the plants listed by Vaillant. The mss. is a list kept by Vaillant in Paris of the plants sent him from Quebec by Sarrazin between 1698-1708 along with an occasional note by Sarrazin on the use of the plant in Quebec.

Bonnycastle, Sir Richard. 1846 Canada and the Canadians. 2 vols. Colburn London.

Borden, Charles E. 1979 Peopling and early culture of the pacific northwest, a view from British Columbia. Science 203;963-970.

Boucher, Pierre. 1663 Histoire veritable et naturelle de la nouvelle-France vulgairment dite le Canada. Paris. Reprinted la societie historique de Boucherville 1964 with an app. by J. Rousseau entitled La flore de la nouvelle France. tr. by the author.

Bouvet, Maurice. 1937 Histoire de la pharmacie en France des origins à nos jours. Occitania Paris.

    1954 L'apothicaire Louis Hébert, premier colon francais du Canada. Rev. d'Hist. de la Pharm. 143.

Briante, John Goodale. 1870 The old root and herb doctor. Granite books Claremont N.H.

Britton, Nathaniel Lord. & Brown, Hon. Addison. 1913 An illustrated flora of the northern United States and Canada. 3 vols. Scribner N.Y. fac. ed. Dover 1970.

Brockville Gazette. 1829 July 3rd. death of children after eating *Cicuta* Brockville Ontario.

Brooks, Harlow. 1929 The medicine of the american indians. Bull. N.Y. Acad. Med. ser. 2:5;509-537.

Brower, L.P., McEvoy, P.B. & Williamson K.L. 1972 Variation in cardiac glycoside content of monarch butterflies from natural populations in eastern north America. Science 177;426-429.

Brown, R. 1868 *Heracleum lanatum.* Edinb. Bot. Soc. Trans. 9;381.

Buchan, William. 1805 Domestic medicine or every man his own doctor. Conn. One of three medical books owned by the grandfather of Canniff Haight in Kingston in the 1790's. Malloch 1946 writes:-"It must have been the most widely read medical book in America, 21 eds. appeared in the U.S. between 1771-99." Only plants that grew in Europe and were used in the materia medica there are discussed by Buchan.

Burgess, T.J.W. 1881 On the beneficent and toxical effects of the various species of *Rhus.* A paper read before Can. Med. Ass. Ottawa printed in Can. Pharm. J. 14:6;161-168.

Bye, Robert A. Jr. 1970 The ethnobotany and economic botany of Onondaga County N.Y. unpublished thesis Oake Ames Library Harvard Univ. Boston.

Byrne, Roger., McAndrews, J.H. & Finlayson, W.D. 1974 Report on investigation at Crawford Lake. Royal Ont. Mus. Toronto.

Byrne, Roger. & McAndrews, J.H. 1975 Pre-columbian purslane in the new world. Nature 253:5494;726-7.

Cabeza de Vaca. 1527-37 Adventures in the unknown interior of America. Cyclone Covey tr, ed. 1961. Wake Forest Univ. MacMillan 1972 N.Y.

Cadillac, A. de la Mothe. c. 1695 Relation on the Indians. mss. Cadillac papers Mich. Pion. Hist. Coll. 1904-5;33,34. Lansing Mich.

Calvert, W.H., Hedrick, L.E. & Brower, L.P. 1979 Mortality of the monarch butterfly. Avian predation at five overwintering sites in Mexico. Science 204;847-851.

Campbell, Duncan. 1875 History of Prince Edward Island. Bremmer Charlottetown.

Campbell, J.B., Best, K.F. & Budd, A.C. 1966 Ninety-nine range forage plants of the Canadian prairies. Can. Dept. Agric. Ottawa.

Canadian Formulary. 1933 Canadian Com. on Pharm. Standards. Univ. of Toronto Press. Toronto.

Canadian Horticulturist. 1880-1881. ed. D.W. Beadle Pub. Fruit Growers Assoc. of Canada. St. Catherines Ontario.

Canadian Medicinal Plants, a list. 1868 Canadian Pharmaceutical Journal, ed. Shuttleworth Toronto. "This list contains over two hundred names and does not exhaust all the possibilities of medicinal plants growing in Canada. . . It is surely desirable that the bountiful stores of Materia Medica provided by nature should be made available." Prizes were offered by the Canadian Pharmaceutical Assoc. for the best collection of medicinal plants. Many articles from this Journal between its founding in 1868 until 1882 are quoted in this text.

Canniff, William Haight. 1894 The medical profession in Upper Canada 1783-1850. Briggs Toronto. fac. ed. 1979 Breezy Creeks Press Aurora Ontario.

Cantino, Albert of Lisbon. 1501 Report to Duc de Ferrara on the voyage of Corte-Real to Labrador and along the American coast. Printed in part by Rousseau in French 1937. tr. by author.

Cartier, Jacques. 1534 First voyage to Canada. 1535-6. Second voyage to Canada when he wintered over at what is now Quebec. Pub. in original and tr. by Biggar 1924 and in part in French by Rousseau 1937 in La botanique canadienne a l'epoque de Jacques Cartier. tr. in text by author. The third voyage of 1541 exists in part only in an English text published by Hakluyt in 1600 and also in Rousseau 1937.

Cartwright, George. 1792 A Journal of transactions and events, during a residence of nearly sixteen years on the coast of Labrador. 3 vols. Allin & Ridge Newark.

Carver, J. 1778 Travels through the interior part of north America in the years 1766, 67 and 68. London. Coles fac. ed. 1974 Toronto.

Champlain, Samuel. 1604 Des sauvages, ou voyage de Samuel Champlain de Brouage fait en la France Nouvelle, l'an mil six cens trois. Paris. Pub. 1625 in English by Hakluyt in Purchas his Pilgrims, London. Cited in text as Champlain-Purchas and the Hakluyt text quoted.

1613 Les voyages de sieur de Champlain Xaintongeois. Berjon Paris. Covers four voyages between 1604 and 1613 to north America. fac. ed. Univ. microfilms 1966 Ann Arbor. Cited in text fac. ed. tr. by author.

1619 Journal of Champlain for the years 1615-1618. Paris 1619. Laval Univ. Quebec has a copy of 1st ed. tr. Michael Macklem 1970 Oberon. Cited in text 1619 Champlain-Macklem.

1632 Les voyages de la nouvelle France occidentale dicte Canada, faits par le Sr. de Champlain Xantongeois..& toutes les descouvertures qu'il à faites en ce pais depuis l'an 1603, jusques en l'an 1629. Paris. tr. A.N. Bourne, ed. E. Gaylord Bourne Allerton 1904 N.Y. Cited in text 1632 Champlain-Bourne.

Chandler, R. Frank., Freeman, Lois & Hooper, Shirley. 1979 Herbal remedies of the maritime Indians. J. Ethnopharmacology 1;49-68.

Chapman, J., Stewart, R.B. & Yarnell, R.A. 1974 *Portulaca oleracea.* Economic Botany 28;411.

Chapman, L.J. & Putnam, D.F. 1966 The physiography of southern Ontario. Univ. Tor. Press Toronto.

Charlevoix, F.X. 1744 Description des plantes principales de l'Amérique septentrionale. App. à la fin du Histoire et description generale de la nouvelle-France. Nyons filles, 3 vols. Paris. Fac. ed. Elysee 1976 Montreal. Charlevoix based his description on the works of Cornut, Jussieu, Vaillant and Gaultier.

Chase, A.W. 1864 Dr. Chase's Recipes. Chase Ann Arbor. Owned by Toronto family.

Chemical Abstracts. Cited in text as C.A. with year and access number.

Chesnut, V.K. 1902 Plants used by the Indians of Mendocina county Calif. USDA Botany div. contrib. Nat. Herb. 7;3 Washington D.C. Only quoted when notes increase our understanding of the use of plant in our area.

Cheadle, William Butler. 1862-3 Journal of trip across Canada. 1931 Graphic Press Ottawa.

Chomel, P.J.B. 1761 Abregé de l'histoire des plantes usuelles. 3 vols. Veueve Damonville Paris.

Christison, Robert. 1842 A dispensatory or commentary on the pharmacopoeias of Great Britain. Black Edinburgh Prof. Materia Medica Univ. Edinburgh; Hon. Fellow Coll. Phys. and Surg. of Upper Canada, 1840; Memb. Philad. Coll. of Pharm.

Clarke, E.G. 1814 A conspectus of the London, Edinburgh and Dublin pharmacopoeias. 2nd ed. Cope London. Physician to the Forces. London Pharmacopoeia used in York 1831 for testing candidates applying for a license to practice.

Claus, Edward P. & Gathercole, Werth. 1961 Pharmacognosy 4th ed. Lea & Febiger Philadalphia.

Claypole, E.W. 1880 The migration of plants from Europe to America. Can. Pharm. J. 13:7; 173-9, 215-20, 252-55.

Clayton, Rev. John. 1687 Letter from Virginia to Dr. Grew in answer to several quaerys sent to him by that learned gentleman. Br. Mus. Addit. MS 4437 fols. 85v 97v Photostat copy in Library of Congress and the Library of Royal Ontario Museum Toronto.

Clusius, Carolus. 1601 Rariorum Plantarum historia. Antverpiae. Have not seen this.

Coats, Capt. William. 1727, 1751 The geography of Hudson's Bay-being the remarks of Captain W. Coats, in many voyages to that locality between the years 1727 and 1751. ed. John Barrow, Hakluyt Society 1852. London.

Cobbett, W. 1846 The American gardener. New York.

Coe, Michael D. 1966 The Maya. Editions Lara Mexico.

Colden, Cadwallader. 1711-1775 Letters vols. 1-7 Coll. New York Hist. Soc. 1918-1925 New York.

Copway, G. 1850 The traditional history and characteristic sketches of the Ojibway nation. Charles Gilpin London. Coles fac. ed. 1972 Toronto.

Cormack, W.E. 1822 Narrative of a journey across the Island of Newfoundland in 1822. ed. F.A. Bruton Longmans 1928 London.

Cornevin, Ch. 1887 Des plantes veneneuses. Paris.

Cornut, Jacques P. 1635 Canadensium plantarum . . . historia. Simon Le Moyne Paris. Fac. ed. J. Stannard ed. 1966 Sources of Science series. Johnson Reprints New York.

Corte Real, Caspar. 1501 sailed from Portugal to Labrador. Mention of this voyage made by Pasqualigo, Venitian Ambassador to Portugal and Cantino to Duc de Ferrara.

Coues, Elliott ed. 1799-1814 New light on the early history of the greater northwest. The manuscript Journals of Alexander Henry, fur trader of the Northwest Company, and of David Thompson, official geographer and explorer of the same company, 3 vols. Francis P. Harper New York.

Coulter, Harris. L. 1973 Homeopathic influences on nineteenth century allopathic therapeutics. Amer. Inst. Homeopathy Washington, D.C.

Creighton, Helen. 1950 Folklore of Lunenburg County, Nova Scotia. Bull. 117 Nat. Mus. Canada. Ottawa.

Culpeper, Nicolas. 1681 The English physitian enlarged. George Sawbridge London. Malloch 1946;127 writes:– "The first English medical book [in America] was Nicolas Culpeper's The English physician reprinted for Nicholas Boone 1708 Boston."

Cuming, Fortescue. 1809 Sketches of a tour of the western country. . . concluded in 1809. in vol. 4 of Thwaites early western travels, Clarke 1905 Cleveland.

Curtis Botanical Magazine. 1640;849. The pitcher plant.

Cutler, Rev. Manasseh. 1785 An account of some of the vegetable productions, naturally growing in this part of America. Mem. Am. Acad. Arts. & Sci. 1;396-493. Reprinted Lloyd Library Bull. 7 series 4. 1903 Cincinnati.

Cutter, Ephraim. 1860 *Veratrum viride* as a physiological and therapeutical agent. London n.p.

Dashwood, R.L. 1871 Chiploquorgan, or life by the camp fire in the Dominion of Canada and Newfoundland. Simpkins & Marshall London first published Dublin 1871.

David-Neel, Alexandra. 1931 With mystics and magicians in Tibet. Penguin Books 1936 London.

Davies, K.G. ed. 1819-1835 Northern Quebec and Labrador journals & correspondence. Hudson's Bay Record Soc. Publ. 24 1963 London.

de Laet, Johan. 1625-40 New World. In narratives of new Netherlands ed. Jameson 1909 Scribner New York.

Delamare, E., Renauld, F. & Cardot, J. 1888 Florule de l'ile Miquelon. Assoc. Typographique Lyon France.

Deliette, Louis. 1702 Memoire concerning the Illinois country. ed. T.C. Pease and R.C. Werner. Col. Ill. State Hist. Lib. 23 french ser. 1;302-395 1934. Parts reprinted Kinietz 1965.

Densmore, Frances. 1926-27 Uses of plants by the Chippewa Indians. Forty-fourth annual Report of Bur. Am. Ethn. Smithsonian Inst. 1926-27. Published USG Pr. Office 1928. Reprinted Dover 1974. Careful identification of each species of plant and the use of that particular plant recorded from field work at the White Earth, Red Lake, Cass Lake, Leech Lake and Mille Lac Reservations in Minnesota, the Lac Court Oreilles Reservation in Wisconsin and the Manitou Reserve in Ontario. A pleasure to use. Much of her material is in tabular form.

Department of the Interior, Canada. 1877 Annual Report Sess. Pap. 11 Ottawa.

de Rasieres, Isaack. 1628 Letter to Samuel Blommaert from New Netherlands (New York). In narratives of new Netherlands ed. Jameson 1909; 102-115. A Description of place and people.

Description of Prince Edward Island. 1818 3rd. ed. Bristol England n.p.

de Serre, C. 1822 Trans. Hort. Soc. London 4;445. On Hydrophyllum.

de Vries, David. 1642 Notes on the New Netherlands. In narratives of new Netherlands ed. Jameson 1909. The observations those of a capable and energetic trader in the New Neth.

Dictionary of Canadianisms on historical principles. 1967 Editorial board W.S. Avis, Charles Crate, Patrick Drysdale, Douglas Leechman, M.H. Scargill, C.J. Lovell. Gage Toronto.

Dictionnaire biographique du Canada. 1974 vol. 3 1741-1770. Univ. Laval Press. Quebec.

Dodge, J.S. 1870 U.S. Agric. Rep. p. 419 Washington. Lamb's quarters.

Dore, William G. 1970 The wild Canada onion. The Herbarist 34-38. Boston.

Doskotch, R.W. & Vanevenhoven, P.W. 1967 *Asarum canadense.* Lloydia 30; 141-4.

Dotto, Lydia. 1978 Lowly poplar could become gourmet sensation. Globe and Mail 22 Aug. Toronto.

Doutt, Margaret. 1970 Ramps. The Herbarist 30-33. Boston.

Drummond, A.R. 1869 The introduced and spreading plants of Ontario and Quebec. Can. Naturalist Dec. 377-387.

Dudley. 1720-21 Sugar Making in New England from the maple. Philos. Trans. Royal Soc. London.

Dufresnoy, André. 1788 Des Propreités de la plante appelée *Rhus Radicans*, de son utilite et des succes qu'on a obtenu pour la guerison des dartres, etc. Mequignon Leipzig.

Dutilly, Arthème, & Lepage, Ernest. 1963 Contribution á la flore du versant sud de la baie James. The Catholic Univ. Press Washington. D.C.

Edinburgh pharmoacopoeia medicorum 1817. This list of pharmaceutical recipes in latin has a blank page between each two printed ones. On these blank pages someone wrote lecture notes on the subject of materia medica in English. See under materia medica Edinburgh-Toronto.

Ellis, Henry. 1748 A voyage to Hudson's Bay by the Dobbs Galley and California in the years 1746 and 1747. London, Whitehead 1748. In Isham, Hudson's Bay Record Soc. 1949.

Elliot, John. 1800 Medical pocket book, London 5th ed. Copy of earlier edition one of medical books owned by Haight in Kingston 1795. Like Buchan mentions only European plants used in materia medica.

Elliott, R.W. 1868 New Lebanon. Paper read before the Canadian Pharmaceutical Society in Jan. and printed in Can. Pharm. J. 1. An account of visit to the Shakers on invitation of Benjamin Gates.. They "are extensive producers of vegetable medicines in various forms, their productions having a world-wide and well deserved reputation for purity and excellence. They cultivate many medicinal plants ordinarily found wild which by the process are greatly increased in yield. *Taraxcum* [dandelion] . . . attains the size of parsnips." Describes methods of preparation.

Emboden, William A. jr. 1972 Narcotic plants, hallucinogens, stimulants, inebriants, and hypnotics, their origins and uses. MacMillan, New York.

Ermatinger, Lawrence. 1772 Letter books. Can. Arch. S. 812. Ottawa.

Emmelin Feldberg. 1949 New Phytologist 48;143-48. Nettle. Chem Abstr. 43;8455.

Eusebii, Caesariensis. 1512 Episcopi Chronicon. in Weise 1884 p. 299.

Evans, Harold J. & Barber, Lynn E. 1977 Biological nitrogen fixation for food and fiber production. What are some immediately feasible possibilities? Science 197;332-339.

Ewan, Joseph. 1978 Seeds and ships and healing herbs, encouragers and kings. Bartonia 45; 24-29.

Farnsworth, Norman R. 1967-74 The Lynn Index. A bibliography of phytochemistry. Organized and ed. by N.R. Farnsworth, R.M. Blomster, M.W. Quimby and J.W. Schermerhorn. Pub. by Norman R. Farnsworth. Univ. Illinois Chicago.

Farrier's Dispensatory. 1741 Medicinal simples commonly made use of in the diseases of horses. 5th. ed. London.

Fell, J.W. 1857 A treatise on cancer, and its treatment. J. Churchill London.

Fenton, William N. 1941 Iroquois suicide. Bur. Am. Ethnol. Bull. 128: 14; 79-138.

1942 Contacts between Iroquois herbalism and colonial medicine. Ann. Rep. Smith. Instit. for 1941;503-526 published 1942 Washington. D.C.

Fernald, M.L. 1900 Some Jesuit influences upon our northeastern flora. Rhodora 19;133-142.

1908 Gray's new manual of botany, 7th. ed. American Book Company New York.

1910 Notes on the plants of Wineland the good. Rhodora 12;17-38.

1950 Gray's manual of botany, 8th ed. American Book Company New York.

Fernald, M.L. & Kinsey, A.C. 1943 Edible wild plants of eastern north America. Gray Herbarium of Harvard Univ. Spec. Publ. Idlewild Press Boston.

Fernie, W.R. 1914 Herbal simples. ed. J. Wright Bristol.

Finlayson, William D. 1794 Archeological investigations in the Crawford Lake region. Friends of the pleistocene Toronto. Royal Ontario Museum library. mss.

1975 The rescue excavations at the Draper site, a preliminary report. Can. Archeological Bull. 7;221-229.

Forsyth, A.A. 1968 British poisonous plants. Bull. 161 Min. Agric. Food. H.M. Stat Off. London.

Forward, Dorothy F. 1977 The history of botany in the University of Toronto. Un·v. of Toronto Press Toronto.

Fox, W.S. 1949 Survey in southern Ontario of chestnut trees, Can. Field-Naturalist 63(2);88-89.

Franklin, John. 1823 Narrative of a journey to the shores of the polar sea in the years 1819, 1820, 1821 and 1822. John Murray London.

Fracastorius, Hieronymus. 1530 De contagionibus, morbisque, contagiosis, et eorum curatione. His works on syphilis translated and annotated by Riddell, 1928.

Fyles, Faith. 1920 Principal poisonous plants of Canada. Canada Dept. Agric. Bull. 39 Ottawa.

Garrett, Blanche Powell. 1973 Fruits of the earth. Centennial Printers. Peterborough Ontario. Gives recipes for use of native plants in conserves, wines etc.

Gerarde, John. 1633 The herball or general history of plants gathered by John Gerarde of London, Master in Chirurgerie. Very much enlarged by Thomas Johnson, Apothecary of London Norton and Whitakers. This, the most famous of English herbals, was first published in 1597. Dr. Priest, a member of the College of Physicians, had almost finished his translation of Dodoens herbal, called Pemptades, from the latin, when he died. This translation Gerarde used as the basis for his herbal, without acknowlegement. For this he has rightly been censured. But Gerarde's herbal is far more than the bones of Dodoens, although these "bones" were the medical wisdom of Europe at that time, its materia medica. Gerarde really knew his plants, was a true gardener, grew them in his own garden, collected them all over England and in some parts of Europe. His friendships with the men in England and Europe who imported, grew and passed on rare and interesting plants is reflected in his herbal as is the great flowering of interest in and knowledge of the plants of the world in the seventeenth century. His loving friend Jean Robin was Curator of the Botanical Garden of the Faculty of Medicine in Paris, where so many of the plants from Canada were sent and where Cornut made the sketches for his book. Gerarde corresponded with Robin and his son and shares with us the excitement of finding a valuable new plant. He used his plants in his medical practice and tells us of their medical vertues from personal experience. He writes in a language all his own that is a joy to read and savor. In quoting from this third edition revised by Johnson after Gerarde's death, the letters s, v, and j have been printed in their modern form to make for easier reading. Rhodes 1922;98 writes;–"A copy of Gerarde's herbal in Oxford has been identified as having belonged to Dorothy Rolfe, the mother-in-law of the Princess Pocohontas." Gerarde's herbal was carried to the new world by the settlers who were much more likely to have used the plants they found there as Gerarde advised than as the Indians did. Gerarde's name is spelled here with the e at the end as it appears on the 1633 title page. Reprinted by Dover 1975.

Gibson, D. 1804-5 Observations on the internal use of *Rhus radicans*. Philadelphia Med. Physical J. 1;33-35.

Gilmore, M.R. 1933 Some Chippewa uses of plants. Papers Mich. Acad. Sci. Arts. Letters 17; 119-143.

Gleason, Henry A. & Cronquist, Arthur. 1963 Manual of vascular plants of northeastern United States and adjacent Canada. Van Nostrand Toronto. The source, with Gray and Scoggan, Flora of Canada, of the botanical nomenclature in the text.

Gosse, P.H. 1840 The Canadian naturalist. The natural history of Lower Canada. John van Voorst London. Fac. ed. Coles 1971. Toronto.

Graham, Andrew. 1775 Observations on Hudson's Bay. Parts printed as app. B in Isham 1949; 309-17. Hudson's Bay Record Soc. Publ. 12 London.

Grant, P. 1804 The Sauteux Indians. Pub. in vol. 2 of L.F.R. Masson, Les Bourgeois 1889-90.

Gray, Asa. 1908 New manual of botany, a handbook of flowering plants and ferns of the central and northeastern United States and adjacent Canada. eds. Rev. Benjamin Lincoln Robinson and Merritt Lyndon Fernald. American Book Co. 7th ed.

  1950 Manual of botany. 8th ed. American Book Company New York.

Greive, Maude. 1931 A modern herbal. 2 vols. Cape London. ed. Mrs. C.F. Leyel. Dover fac. ed. 1971 2 vols. A modern classic. The standard by which all subsequent herbals are judged. Mrs.

Grieve writes of the plants of the world, when discussing north american plants she draws on Millspaugh.

Green. 1832 An universal herbal. London. Cited Greive 1931;848.

Griffith, R. 1847 Medical botany; or description of the more important plants used in medicine. Lea and Blanchard Philadelphia.

Gunn, John D. 1861 New domestic physician or home book of health. A complete guide for families, pointing out in familiar and plain terms the causes, symptoms, treatment and cure of the diseases incident to man, women and children with directions for using medicinal plants. Moore, Wilstach, Keys Cincinnati. 1st. ed. 1857, sec rev. ed. 1859. The 1861 ed. was received by the author from Mrs. Walter Pattenden, Vandorf Ontario, who had received it from her father, who had it from his mother, who received it from her father, all resident in York County Ontario. There are illustrations and descriptions of the plants. A sensible text.

Hahnemann. 1796 Lesser writings. Cited by Coulter 1973.

Haight, Canniff. 1885 Country life in Canada fifty years ago. Hunter Rose Toronto. Sketches of early history. Paper read before Mechanics Inst. Picton 1859. Both items reprinted in one vol. by Mika 1971 Belleville.

Hakluyt, Richard. 1600 Navigations, voyages, traffiques and discoveries of the English nation in America. 3 vols. 1589-1600 London. Reprinted ed. and publisher Goldsmid 1889 Edinburgh.

Hall, Francis. 1818 Travels in Canada and the United States in 1816 and 1817. Longman, Hurst, London.

Handbook of Canada. 1897 Published by the publication committee of the British Assoc. for the Advancement of Science for the Toronto Meeting 1897. Contains a sketch of the flora and forests of Canada by John Macoun and the chemical industries of Canada by W. Hodgson Ellis.

Hansel, Rudolph. 1972 Medicinal plants and empirical drug research. Printed in Plants in the development of modern medicine. ed. Tony Swain Harvard Univ. Press Cambridge.

Hardin, J.W. & Arena, Jay M. 1974 Human poisoning from native and cultivated plants. Duke Univ. Press Durham N.C.

Harlow, William M. 1957 Trees of the eastern and central U.S. and Canada. rev. ed. Dover N.Y.

Harriot, Thomas. 1590 A briefe and true report of the new found land of Virginia. Theodor de Bry Franckfort. Dover reprint 1972. Harriot was an important scientist see J.W. Shirley ed. Thomas Harriot, renaissance scientist. Clarendon Oxford, 1974.

Harmon, Daniel Williams. 1820 A journal of voyages and travels in the interior of north America. Flagg & Gould Andover Mass.

Harris, Ben Charles. 1961 Eat the weeds. Barre. Reprint 1973 Keats Conn.

Harris, Seale. 1946 Banting's miracle. The discovery of insulin. p. 179 Lippincott Philadelphia.

Harris, W.R. 1915 Practice of medicine and surgery by the Canadian tribes in Champlain's time. Written in 1900. 27th. ann. Archeol. Rep. Min. Educ. Ontario.

Hartwell, J.L. 1967-71. Plants used against cancer. A survey. Lloydia 30; 379-436, 1967. 31;71-170 1968. 32;79-107, 153-205, 247-296 1969. 33;97-124, 288-392 1970. 34;103-160, 204-255, 310-360, 386-425 1971.

Havard, V. 1895 Food plants of the north American Indians. Bull. Torrey Bot. Club 22; 98-123.

   1896 Drink plants of the north American Indians. Bull. Torrey Bot. Club 23;33-46.

Havens, William V. 1872 Diary, typewritten pages in Toronto Public Library. Toronto.

Head, George. 1829 Forest scenes and incidents in the wilds of north America. Being a diary of a winter's route from Halifax to the Canadas and during four months residence in the woods on the borders of Lakes Huron and Simcoe. John Murray London. Coles fac. ed. 1970 Toronto.

Heagerty, J.J. 1928 Four centuries of medical history in Canada. 2 vols. MacMillan Toronto.

Hearne, Samuel. 1795 Journey from Prince of Wale's Fort in Hudson's Bay, to the northern ocean in the years 1769, 1770, 1771 and 1772. ed. J.B. Tyrrell. Champlain Soc. Publ. VI. Toronto 1911. First pub. Strachan and Cadell 1795 London.

Heckewelder, J.G.E. 1820 A narrative of the mission of the United Brethren among the Delaware and Mohegan Indians. McCarty & Davis Philadelphia.

Heebner, Chas. F. 1892 Manual of pharmacy and pharmaceutical chemistry. Carveth Toronto. Prof. Pharm. Ont. Coll. of Pharm.

Henderson, Velyien & Lusk, C.P. 1908 A text book on materia medica and pharmacy. Univ. of Toronto Press. Toronto.

Henkel, Alice. 1904 Weeds used in medicine. Farmer's bull. 188 USDA Wash. D.C.

Hennepin, Father Louis. 1698 A new discovery of a vast country in America. Bently et al London. Reprint 1903 A.C. McClurg Chicago ed. Thwaites. Reprint fac. ed. 1974 Coles Toronto.

Henry, Alexander (the elder). 1776 Travels and adventures in Canada and the Indian territories, between the years 1760 and 1776. 1809 I Riley N.Y. 1901 Morang Toronto.

Henshaw, H.W. 1890 Indian origin of maple sugar. Am. Anthrop. 3;341-351.

Heriot, George. 1807 Travels through the Canadas. 2 vols. Phillips London. Reprint fac. ed. 1971 Coles Toronto.

Hind, Henry Youle. 1860 Narrative of the Canadian Red River exploring expedition of 1857 and of the Assiniboine and Saskatchewan exploring expedition of 1858. 2 vols. Longman & Roberts London.

Hobart, F.G. & Melton, G. 1949 A concise applied pharmacology and therapeutics of the more important drugs. 3rd ed. Leonard Hill London. Dr. Hobart was head of Pharm Dept. Westminster Hospital London.

Hodge, F.W. & White, James. 1913 Handbook of Indians of Canada. Geograph. Board of Canada. App. 10th. rep. Ottawa. fac. ed. 1971 Coles Toronto.

Hofer, Alvin W. 1972 Chemical Abstracts 76 139264g *Rumex acetosella*.

Hoffman, W.J. 1885-86 The midewiwin or grand medicine society of the Ojibwa. 7th ann. rep. Bur. Amer. Ethn. Washington 1891;149-300

1892-93 The Menomini Indians. 14th. ann. rep. Bur. Amer. Ethn. 1896;3-328.

Hollobon, Joan. 1978 40 sufferers of multiple sclerosis to test oil of primrose as remedy. Globe & Mail 20th. Sept. Toronto.

Holmes, E.M. 1884 Notes on recent donations to the Museum of the Pharmaceutical Soc. London. The Pharm. J. & Trans. Oct. 302-304. Medicinal plants used by the Cree Indians at Hudson's Bay and sent by Walter Haydon from there to Holmes in London. Haydon had lived in Hudson's Bay and noted the native use of some of the plants he sent. They were identified by Holmes and often given the name of a related English species.

Hosie, R.C. 1973 Native trees of Canada. Canadian Forestry Service. Dept. Environment Ottawa.

Household Guide. 1894 A practical family physician. eds. E.G. Jefferis & J.L. Nichols. Nichols Toronto. Fac. ed. 1972 Coles Toronto.

Howard, George. 1833 A rare and choice collection of well-tried and invaluable recipes for healing human beings and likewise horses, cows, sheep, dogs &c.&c. Howard came to St. Piers Quebec from England in 1820, moved to Streetsville Ont. 1847-49. He was a blacksmith and farrier. His mss. note books were lent to author by his great great granddaughter.

Howison, John. 1821 Sketches of Upper Canada. Oliver & Boyd Edinb. Fac. ed. 1970 Coles Toronto.

Huizinga, J. 1924 The waning of the middle ages. 1st and 2nd. Dutch editions 1919-21. tr. F. Hopman English edition 1924. Penguin Books 1955 Harmondsworth England.

Hulbert, A.B. & Schwarze, G.N. eds. 1910 History of northern American Indians by Zeisberger. Ohio Archeol. Hist. Publ. 19;1-173 Columbus.

Hunt, George T. 1940 The wars of the Iroquois. Univ. of Wisconsin Press. Madison Wisc.

Hunter, John D. 1823 Manners and customs of several Indian tribes located west of the Mississippi. Maxwell Philad. Reprinted 1957 Ross & Haines Minn.

Icelandic mss. 1475 tr. Larsen 1931. See entry under Larsen and under Thorlief Bjornnson.

Innis, Harold A. 1956 The fur trade in Canada. Univ. of Toronto Press. rev. ed. 1970 Toronto.

Isham, James. 1743 Observations on Hudson's Bay and notes and observations on a book entitled 'A Voyage to Hudson Bay in the Dobbs Galley 1746-7'. Pub. 1949 eds. E.E. Rich & A.M. Johnson. Hudson's Bay Record Soc. Publ. 12 London. Isham was the factor at Fort York on Hudson's Bay for over 20 years.

Jackson, John R. 1876 Notes on some medicinal plants of the Compositae. Can. Pharm. J. 1875-76; 231-236. Reprinted from Pharm. J. and Trans. England.

James, Capt. Thomas. 1633 The strange and dangerous voyage of Captain Thomas James. I Legatt London. Parts pub. Mowat Ordeal 1960. James gave his name to James Bay where he wintered 1631-32.

Jameson, Anna Brownell. 1838 Winter studies and summer rambles in Canada. Saunders and Ottley London. Abridged and ed. McLellan and Stewart. Toronto 1965. Mrs. Jameson travelled by steamer from Detroit to Mackinaw across Lake Huron, by canoe to Sault St. Marie and along the eastern shore of the lake and Georgian Bay to Penetanguishene.

Jameson, J. Franklin. ed. 1909 Narratives of New Netherlands 1609-1664. Scribner N.Y. In Original narratives of early American history. Original accounts printed.

Janiger, Oscar, & Dobkin de Rios, Marlene 1976 *Nicotiana* an hallucinogen? Economic Botany 30;149-151.

Jaynes, Richard A. ed. 1975 Handbook of north American nut trees. Northern American Nut Growers Assoc. 1969 W.H. Humphrey Press Geneva N.Y.

Jefferys, Thomas. 1760 The natural and civil history of the French dominions in north and south America: a description of New France. 2 vols. Jefferys London.

Jenness, Diamond. 1935 The Ojibwa Indians of Parry Island, their social and religious life. Nat. Mus. Can. Bull. 78 Anthrop. ser. 17 Ottawa.

Jesuit Relations and allied documents. 1610-1791 Travel and explorations of the Jesuit missionaries in New France. Ed. Reuben G. Thwaites 1896-1901. 73 vols. Burrows Cleveland. The Relations were written for the Catholics of France and Europe as a report on the work of the Missions and as a help in raising funds. They were edited for this purpose in France. So the accounts of the details of Huron life were abridged to our sorrow and the emphasis was placed on religion and language.

Johnson, C.P. 1862 Useful plants of Great Britain. A treatise upon the principal native vegetables capable of application as food, medicine, or in the arts and manufactures. London.

Johnston, W.V. 1942 The early Canadian Indian and his medicine. 12 page pamphlet pub. privately. Based almost entirely on W.R. Harris 1915 without acknowledgement, valueless.

Jolicoeur, Catherine. 1971 Traditional use of herbs in Quebec. The Potomac Herb J. winter 3-5 Washington D.C. This information was taken from les Archives de Folklore Univ. Laval Quebec.

Jones, Volney H. 1937 Notes on the preparation and uses of basswood fiber by Indians of the great lakes region. Pap. Mich. Acad. Sci. Arts. Lett. 22;1-14

1937 Notes on manufacture of cedar-bark mats by Chippewa. ibid 32;341-63

1965 The bark of the bittersweet vine as an emergency food among the Indians of the western great lakes region. Mich. Arch. 11;170-80.

Josselyn, John. 1672 New England rarities. London.

1674 An account of two voyages to New England made during the years 1638, 1663. London. Reprinted William Veazie 1865 Boston.

Journey into the Mohawk and Oneida country. 1634-35. On foot from Fort Orange (Albany) New Netherlands possibly written by Armen Meynderts van den Bogaert, surgeon at the fort. In Narr. of New Neth. ed Jameson 1909.

Juel, J.O. 1931 The French apothecary's plants in Burser's herbarium. Rhodora 393;177-179. See under Bauhin, Juel concludes that all the plants referred to were collected in Canada that he lists. Rousseau 1964 suggests that according to Bouvet 1954 it may have been Louis Hebert who collected these plants while in Acadia. See under pitcher plant for Gerarde account of a french apothecary in Paris who received plants and passed them on.

Juet, Robert. 1610 Third voyage of master Henry Hudson. Discovery of the Hudson River. pub. in Narr. of New Neth. ed. Jameson 1909.

Jussieu, A. c. 1708 Plantes envoyées de Canada par M. Sarrazin. An mss. of 15 ff. Written by Jussieu in Paris who replaced Tournefort and Isnard as Prof. botany at the Jardin Royal in 1710. This is essentially a list of latin names with synonyms, of the plants sent by Sarrazin, with a few notes by him on the medical use of the plants abbreviated by Jussieu. A photocopy was reproduced in an unreadable form by Vallée 1927 who apparently could read his copy of this list as he reproduces some of the comments in his book on Sarrazin. The original is in the Museum of Nat. Hist. in Paris, and a microfilm is in possession of the Am. Philosophical Soc. Philad.

Kalm, Peter. 1748-51 Travels in north America. English version 1770 2 vols. Revised from original Swedish and ed. by Adolph B. Benson. 1937 Wilson-Erickson N.Y. With a tr. of new material from Kalm's diary notes in 1964 ed. This edition reprinted 1966 Dover New York. Kalm travelled by canoe and on foot from the last U.S. Fort north of Albany, Fort Nicholson, through no man's land to the first French fort, Fort St. Frederic to reach Quebec where he spent many months as a guest of the French government. Jean Francois Gaultier was his guide and companion on his botanising trips.

Kilmon, Jack. 1976 Venoms, extracting healing from the serpent's tooth. News and Comment, Constance Holden Science 193;385-87.

Kinietz, W. Vernon. 1965 Indians of the western great lakes. Univ. Mich. Press Ann Arbor. First pub. 1940. Ann Arbor. A survey of documents relating to the Indians of Michigan and the great lakes during the contact period, 1615-1760.

King, Antoine. 1901-1978 Resident of Go-Home Bay and Penetanguishene Lake Huron. Personal communication on how he used the plants of the area during that period.

King, J. 1854 The american eclectic dispensatory. Moore, Wistach, Keys Cinn. Reprinted 1866 King.

Kingsbury, John M. 1964 Poisonous plants of the United States and Canada. Prentice Hall N.J.

    1965 Deadly harvest, a guide to common poisonous plants. Holt Rhinehart & Winston N.Y. Pap. 1972 N.Y.

Kirby, E.D. 1902 Violets and cancer. Brit. Med. J. 1;55.

Kirkwood, Alexander. 1867 Treatise on milkweeds and nettles advocating that these plants be turned to industrial use. Toronto.

Kohl, J.G. 1860 Kitchi-Gami. wanderings round Lake Superior. tr. Germ. pub. Chapman-Hall Minn. Reprint 1965 Ross & Haines Minn.

Krochmal, A., Wilkin, L. & Chien, M. 1972 Lobeline content in *Lobelia*. Lloydia 35;303-04.

Kupchan, S.M., Hemingway, R.J. & Doskotch, T.W. 1964 Tumor inhibitors IV. J. Med. Chem. 7; 803. *Apocynum cannabinum.*

Kupchan, S.M., Hemingway, R.F. & Knox, J.R. 1965 Tumor inhibitors VII. Podophyllotoxin, the active principle of *Juniperus virginiana*. J. Pharm. Sci. 54;659-660.

Lafitau, Joseph Francois. 1724 Moeurs des sauvage ameriquains, comparées aux moeurs des premiers temps. Saugrain Paris 2 vols. Reprint 1977 Champlain Soc. Univ. Toronto Press Toronto.

Lahanton, L.A. Baron de. 1703 New voyages to north America. Bonwick London. tr. ed. Thwaites 2 vols. 1905 McClurg Chicago.

Lamb, Charles. 1823 In praise of Chimney-sweeps. Essays of Elia. London.

Lambert, Richard, & Pross, Paul. 1967 Renewing nature's wealth. Ont. Dept. Lands and Forests. Toronto.

Larsen, Henning. 1931 An old Icelandic medical miscellany. MS Royal Irish Academy 23 D 43. Oslo J. Dybwad. Larsen ed. and tr. See under Bjornsson.

Lawrence, B.W. & Weaver, K.M. 1974 Essential oils and their constituents. *Myrica Gale* and *Comptonia peregrina*. Planta Medica 25; 385-388.

Lawson, G. 1869 Description of the Canadian species. . . of the natural order of Boraginaceae. Can. Naturalist Dec. 398.

LeClercq, Christien. 1691 First establishment of the faith in New France. Paris. Reprinted 1881 tr. notes J.G. Shea 2 vols. Shea N.Y.

1691 New relations of Gaspesia with the customs and religion of the Gaspesian Indians. Paris. Reprinted 1910 ed. W.F. Ganong Champlain Soc. Toronto.

Leechman, D. 1956 Native tribes of Canada. Gage Toronto.

Lefroy, John Henry. 1843-44 In search of the magnetic north. A soldier surveyor's letters from the north-west 1843-44. ed. G.F.G. Stanley 1955 Macmillan Toronto.

Leising, W.A. 1959 Arctic wings. Doubleday Garden City.

Leroi-Gourhan, Arlette. 1975 The flowers found with Shanidar IV, a neanderthal burial in Iraq. Science 190;562-564.

Lescarbot, Marc. 1609 Nova Francia, a description of Acadia 1606. First pub. 1609 Histoire de la Nouvelle France Paris. tr. Pierre Erondelle 1609 into English pub. London. Erondelle tr. only chap. 31-48 of book 2 and the whole of book 3 of the Histoire. The 30 chap. of book 1 describing the voyages of Verrazano, Ribault, Laudonnière and Villegagnon as well as the first 30 chap. of book 2 describing those of Cartier, Roberval and Champlain were ommitted. Hakluyt reprinted the Erondelle text in part in Purchas his Pilgrim 1625. Reprinted in full 1745, 47. Repub. 1928 introd. notes H.P. Biggar Harper N.Y. Lescarbot spent from July 1606-July 1607 at Port Royal Acadia and writes with wit.

Letters from Hudson's Bay. 1703-1740 ed. K.G. Davies. Hudson's Bay Record Soc. Pub. 35 1965 London.

Letters Outward. 1679-94. Hudson's Bay Record Soc. Publ. 11 1948 London.

Lewis, Walter H. & Elvin-Lewis, Memory P.F. 1977 Medical botany. Wiley New York.

Lewis, William. 1791 An experimental history of the materia medica. The 4th. ed. with numerous additions and corrections by John Aitkin MD. London.

Lewis, William. 1799 The new dispensatory containing the elements of pharmacy and the materia medica. The 6th ed. in which are inserted the various improvements that have occured in medicine from the period of its last publication. London. A quite different book from the Aitkin edition and much more useful. This book was in general use in the United States at the time of its political separation from Britain. Reprinted three times in the U.S. One of the three medical books in the library of Canniff Haight's grandfather in Kingston in 1795. Copies of both editions in Pharmacy Library Univ. of Toronto.

Lindley, John. 1846 Vegetable kingdom. London.

Long, John. 1791 Voyages and travels of an Indian interpreter and trader. Long London. Fac. ed. 1971 Coles Toronto.

Loskiel, G.H. 1794 History of the mission of the United Brethren among the Indians in north America. 3 pts. tr. from German The Brethren London.

Loudon, J.C. 1854 Arboretum et Fruticetum. . . trees and shrubs of Great Britain. London.

Lower, A.R.M. 1938 The north American assault on the Canadian forest. Ryerson Toronto.

Malloch, Archibald. 1946 Medical interchange between the British Isles and America before

1801. Based on the FitzPatrick Lectures of the Royal College of Physicians of London for 1939. Published by the College London.

Marie de l'Incarnation. 1639-71 Word from New France. The selected letters of Marie de l'Incarnation founder and first Mother Superior of the Ursulin Monastery and school in Quebec city. ed. Joyce Marshall 1967 Oxford Toronto.

Marie Victorin. See Victorin, Marie.

Marker, R.E. 1942 Analysis of Trilliums, Smilacina and Clintonia. J. Am. Chem. Soc. 64;1283-5 and in 1947:69;2242.

Marten, G.C. & Anderson, R.W. 1975 Relative palatability and nutritive value of 12 weed species in comparison to oats. Crop Science 15;821-7.

Mason, John. 1620 A briefe discourse of the Nevv-found-land. Andro Hart Edinburgh.

Masson, Louis F.R. 1889-90 Les bourgeois de la comagnie du nord-ouest. Récits de voyages, lettres et rapports inédits relatifs au nord-ouest canadien. 2 vols. Coté & Cie Quebec. Most of the items are in English. Contains Grant on the Sautaux.

Masters, M.T. 1870 Contributions to the treasury of botany. ed. John Lindley London

Materia-Medica Edinburgh-Toronto 1820's. These are handwritten lecture notes on the subject of materia medica. They are written in several hands on the blank interleaved pages of the Edinburgh pharmoacopoeia medicorum of 1817. On the fly leave of the book is written "from Dr. Gilian." Below this is the name, possibly the signature, of J. Porter Daly who passed his examination in materia medica, among others given by the College of Physicians and Surgeons of Upper Canada in 1828, practised in Toronto 1835-6, leaving then for the West Indies according to Canniff 1894. After J. Porter Daly on the fly leaf appears the word York 1830. The signature of Henry H. Wright with the words Toronto U.C. 1837 is at the top of the title page. I had this signature compared with that of Dr. Henry Hover Wright and it seems to be his own writing. Wright studied medicine with Dr. Rolph and when he fled to the U.S. in 1837 followed him there to continue his medical studies. Wright passed the examinations of the College of Physicians and Surgeons of Upper Canada in 1839. He then taught medicine first at Rolph's school, now again established in Toronto, and then at the faculty of medicine of the University when it was established. What seems likely is that this complete series of notes on the subject of materia medica was made at Edinburgh, (internal evidence points to Great Britain) and taken to Canada where Porter Daly procured them. As there is no record of a Dr. Gilian in either Upper or Lower Canada at this time it must be assumed he was practising in Edinburgh. This could be regarded as one of the first texts on materia medica used in a medical school in Upper Canada. It is based, as were all others for this whole century, primarily on European plants. It seldom mentions any from north America. Nevertheless some plants were common to both continents. A photographic copy of the whole handwritten text is in the possession of the author who discovered the original in April 1977.

Mattson, M. 1845 American vegetable practice. Boston.

Maugh, Thomas H. 11 1979 An account of the isolation of prostaglandin A from onions by Moses Attrep Jr. of East Texa State University. Science 204;293.

Mechling, W.H. 1959 The Malecite Indians with notes on the Micmacs. Anthropologica 8;239-263.

Medsger, O.P. 1939 Edible wild plants. MacMillan N.Y. Reprinted 1966 N.Y.

Meijar, William. 1974 *Podophyllum peltatum* a potential new cash crop plant of eastern north America. Economic Botany 28;1.

Memoire of Medicines necessary for the King's troops in Canada 1693. List of those sent to Quebec from France printed in full in app. Vallée 1927. Mss in Can. Arch. Ottawa.

Merring, George. 1960 Walpole Island herbalism. A study of the medico-ethno-botany of the amalgamated Indian Band of Walpole Island Reservation, Ontario. A thesis, Wayne State Univ Detroit.

Meyer, Joseph. 1918 The Herbalist. Indiana Herb Gardens Hammond Ind. Many reprints.

Michaux, André. July 15th 1973– April 11th 1796 Journal of travels into Kentucky. In Vol 3 of Early Western Travels ed. R.G. Thwaites 1904 Arthur H. Clark Co Cleveland.

Millspaugh, Charles F. 1892 American medicinal plants, an illustrated and descriptive guide to plants indigenous to and naturalized in the United States which are used in medicine. 2 vols. Yorston Philad. First pub. 1887 N.Y. A one vol. unabridged republication of the 1892 ed. 1974 Dover N.Y.

Mockle, J. Auguste. 1955 Contributions a l'étude des plantes médicinales du Canada. Paris ed. Jouve. A doctoral thesis in the Faculty of Pharmacy University of Paris. Mockle writes in intro. "I am dealing with the wild plants, picked locally in Quebec and used in popular medicine." A valuable contribution to our knowledge of Canadian medicinal plants. The chemical analysis has been ommitted in most citations as outside the scope of this work. Tr. by the author.

Monardes, Nicolas. 1577 Ioyfull newes out of the newe founde worlde. 1st complete ed. in Spanish 1574. Tr. by John Frampton Norton London.

Montaigne, Michel Eyquem de. 1595 Essays. Paris. tr. E.J. Trechmann Oxford Univ. Press. n.d. London.

Montgomery, F.W. 1962 Native wild plants of eastern Canada and the adjacent northeastern United States. Ryerson Toronto.

Moody, Charles Stuart. 1910 Backwoods surgery & medicine. Outing New York.

Mooney, James. 1885-6 The sacred formulas of the Cherokees. 7th Ann. Rep. Bur. Am. Ethn. Printed 1891, 301-397. Washington D.C.

Morice, Adrian G. 1901 Dene surgery. Read Feb. 1900. Pub. Trans. Can. Inst. 15-27.

1910 The Great Dene race. Anthropos. Winnipeg.

Morton, Julia F. 1974 Folk remedies of the low county. Seeman Miami.

Mowat, Farley. 1960 Ordeal by ice. Contains parts of Abacuk Pricket's account of Henry Hudson's voyage to Hudson Bay 1610; The strange and dangerous voyage of Captain Thomas James by himself 1631-2; The letter of the Sieur de la Potherie to Monseigneur the Duke of Orleans 1697-98. McLelland and Stewart Toronto.

1967 The Polar passion. Contains parts of the Ventursome voyage of Robt. Bylot and Wm. Baffin, written by Baffin 1616.

1973 Tundra. Contains parts of Samuel Hearn's journey from Prince of Wale's Fort in Hudson Bay to the northern ocean in the years 1769, 1770, 1771 and 1772 and of Alexander Mackenzie's Voyage to the frozen ocean 1789. McClelland and Stewart Toronto.

Muldrew, W.H. 1905 Sylvan Ontario, a guide to our native trees and shrubs. Briggs Toronto.

Mackenzie, Alexander. 1801 Voyages from Montreal. . . to the frozen and pacific oceans in the years 1789 and 1793. Cadell & Davies London. Reprint 1793 voyage 1967 Citadel Press New York.

MacNutt, W.S. 1965 The emergence of colonial society, 1712-1857. McLelland & Stewart, Toronto.

MacTaggart, John. 1829 Three Years in Canada 1826-28. Colburn London.

McAndrews, J.H., Byrne, R.T. & Finlayson, W.D. 1974 Report on investigation at Crawford Lake. Canada Council grant. Royal Ontario Museum. Toronto.

McAndrews, J.H. & Boyko, M. 1974 Investigation at Crawford Lake, geological and vegetational history. Friends of the Pleistocene. Toronto. mss. Royal Ont. Mus.

McAndrews, J.H. & Byrne, Roger. 1975 Pre-Columbian purslane in the New World. Nature 253; 494;726-727.

ndrews, J.H. 1977 Personal communication one seed of *Aralia racemosa* found archeologi- Crawford Lake.

J. 1828 Historical and descriptive sketches of the maritime colonies of British Ameri- London.

McKay, Sheila Mary. 1973 A biosystemic study of the genus *Amelanchier* in Ontario. A thesis submitted to University of Toronto.

McKeevor, Thomas. 1812 A voyage to Hudson's Bay during the summer of 1812. 1819 Sir Richard Phillips London.

National Dispensatory of the United States. 1916 Hare, Caspari and Rusby.

New Dispensatory 1789 Edinburgh

Nickell, J.M. 1911 Botanical ready reference. Chicago. Cited Huron Smith 1933.

Nickle Family Book 1852 Galt. Typewritten pages in rare book room Toronto Public Library. Toronto.

Niederberger, Christine. 1979 Early sedentary economy in the basin of Mexico. Science 203;131-142. Reports finding seeds of *Portulaca* archeologically.

Nielsen, P.E. 1977 Plant crops as a source of fuel and hydrocarbon like materials. Science 198; 942-44. *Asclepias.*

Palaiseul, Jean. 1972 Nos grand-meres savaient la verité sur les plantes et la vie naturelle. Ed. de Jour Montreal. ed. Robert Laffont Paris. European plants and uses to-day. Tr. by author.

Palmer, Edward. 1871 Food products of the north American Indians. Rep. USDA 1870;404-428. Pub. 1871 Washington D.C.

Pammel, L.H. 1911 Manual of poisonous plants. Torch Cedar Rapids.

Parish, Peter. 1976 Medicines. A guide for everybody. Penguin Books Middlesex England.

Parker, Arthur C. 1928 Indian medicine and medicine men. 36th Ann. Archeolog. Rep. 1928;9-26 Min. of Educ. Toronto. Parker was a Seneca and distinguished anthropologist.

Pasqualigo, Pietro. 1501 Letter to his brother. Cited Weise 1884. Pasqualigo was the Venetian Ambassador to Portugal and wrote of the Corte-Real trips to Labrador.

Penhallow, D.P. 1887 A Review of Canadian botany from the first settlement of New France to the nineteenth century. Part 1. Trans. Roy. Soc. Canada 45-61.

1897 A Review of Canadian botany Part 11. Trans. Roy. Soc. 3-56. Valuable bibliographies and list of French Canadian sources. Penhallow was Prof. of Botany at McGill and Director of the Botanic Garden.

Perrot, Nicolas. 1660 Memoire sur les moeurs, coustumes et religion des sauvage de l'Amerique septentrionale. ed. Tailhan 1864 Paris. Reprinted in part in Blair 1911.

Perry, Frances. 1972 Flowers of the World. Royal Horticultural Society London.

Pharmacy Recipe Book. 1854 Ben Beveridge Jr. name written on first page beside an advertisement from Fredericton N.B. and a business card pasted on the first page from Cunningham Drug Stores, Robson & Thurlow St. Vancouver. Recipes for drugs and cordials written in by hands as well as hair lotions etc. Photographed copy in possession of author.

Phelps, J.W. 1840-41 Diary kept while at Mackinac. Microfilm of mss. Univ. Chicago Library.

Philosophical Trans. Roy. Soc. London England. 1684-5 An Account of a sort of sugar made of the juice of the maple in Canada.

Pike, Warburton. 1892 The barren ground of northern Canada. MacMillan London.

Porcher, Francis P. 1869 Resources of the southern fields and forests, medical, economical and agricultural; being also a medical botany of the southern states; with practical information on the useful properties of the trees, plants and shrubs. New ed. rev. and enlarged Walker, Evans & Cogswell Charleston. 1st ed. 1863.

Porsild, A.E. 1937 Edible roots and berries of northern Canada. Nat. Mus. 17 pp.

1945 Emergency food in arctic Canada. Nat. Mus. Canada Spec. Contrib. 45-1. Ottawa.

1953 Edible plants of the arctic archipelago. Arctic 6:1;15-34.

1957 Illustrated flora of the Canadian arctic archipelago. Nat. Mus. Canada Bull. 146; 1-209. Ottawa.

Provancher, abbé Leon. 1862 Flore Canadienne. 2 vols. Darveau Quebec.

Pursh, Frederick. 1807 Journal of botanical excursions. ed. T.P. James 1869 Phil Brinckloe & Merot

1815 A Catalogue of plants indigenous and exotic by the late James Donn corrected and augmented by Frederick Pursh author of the Flora of North America. Richard and Arthur Taylor London. A useful listing of the plants growing in Great Britain with their country of origin and date of introduction with references.

Radin, Paul. 1937 Primitive religion its nature and origin. Dover ed. 1957 New York.

Radisson, Pierre Esprit. 1885 Voyages of Peter Esprit Radisson; being an account of his travels and experiences among the north American Indians from 1652-1684. Transcribed and ed. by Gideon D. Scull Prince Society 1885 Boston.

1896 Relation of the voyage of P.E. Radisson esquire to the north of America in years 1682 and 1683. Both the original french and a tr. pub. in Rep. Can. Arch. 1-84 Ottawa.

Rafinesque, C.S. 1828 Medical flora or manual of medical botany of the United States vol. 1 Atkinson & Alexander Philad.

1830 Medical flora vol 2. Samuel C Atkinson Philad.

Rapson, W.H. 1977 Unlocking treasures from our forests, chemicals and energy. Ontario Forests, Ont. For. Assoc. 19:2;8-9 Toronto.

Raudot, Antoine Denis, 1709-1710 Memoir concerning the different Indian nations of north America. Tr. letters 23-41 and 45-72 pub. app. Kinietz 1965.

Raymond, Marcel. 1945 Notes éthnobotaniques sur les Tete de Boule de Manouan. In Études éthnobotaniques québécoises, Contributions Lab. Bot. Univ. Montreal 55;113-135. Montreal.

Reagan, Albert. 1928 Plants used by the Bois Fort Chippewa. Wisconsin Archeol. N.S. 7;230-248.

Reis, Mayne. 1853 The young voyageurs. Routledge London.

Report from the Select Committee on the Hudson's Bay Company. 1857 Westminster England.

Representation from the New Netherlands 1650. Document accompanying memorial to the Dutch Government on the way its representatives treated the settlers. Printed in Narratives of the New Netherlands ed. Jameson 1909. See tarragon in text.

Rhodes, Eleanour Sinclair. 1922 The old English herbals. Longmans, Green London. fac. ed. 1971 Dover London.

Rich, E.E. & Johnson, A.M. 1949 eds. James Isham's Observations on Hudsons Bay 1743. Hudson Bay Record Society 1949. See Isham.

Richard, Edouard. 1899 Supp. Dr. Brymner's Rep. Can. Min. Agric. 1901 Ottawa. Research by Richard in Paris in the colonial archives which were in the attic story of the Louvre and "anything but safe. I forthwith went to work and made on analysis of the 17 volumes of the Moreau St. Mery collection, the 12 vol. of the Raudot-Pontchartrain correspondence etc." A fascinating precis of the contents of these documents.

Richardson, Dr. James Henry. 1829-1905. Reminiscences. An mss in the Roberston collection of 'he rare book room Toronto Public Library Toronto. Richardson was the first medical graduate 'he Univ. of Toronto. Insight on medical thinking of the period.

'son, Sir John. 1852 Arctic searching expedition. Harper New York.

'e Hon. William Renwick. 1928 Hieronymus Frascatorius and his poetical and prose 'hilis. The Canadian Social Hygiene Council Toronto. With notes and comments by 'medical terms and plants used in the sixteenth century in France. A delight to

'onal communications on his contact with the Cree in Hudson Bay.

Riley, John, & McKay, S.M. 1979 The vegetation and phytogeography of coastal southeastern James Bay. (in press Royal Ont. Mus. Life Sci. Contrib.)

Rimpler. 1970 New glycoside isolated from *Verbena hastata* and *v. officinalis*. Lloydia 33:4;491.

Roberts, Sir Charles G.D. 1896 Around the camp fire. Crowell New York.

Robinson, H. 1879 The great fur land or sketches of life in the Hudson's Bay territory. Sampson, Low, Marston, Searle London.

Robinson, John & Rispin, T. 1774 Journey through Nova Scotia. In Rep. Pub. Arch. Nova Scotia. Halifax.

Robinson, Percy James. 1933 Toronto during the french regime. A history of Toronto from Brule to Simcoe. Ryerson Toronto. 2nd ed. Univ. of Toronto Press 1965 Toronto.

Robinson, Trevor 1975 The organic constituents of higher plants. Cordus Press, North Amherst Mass.

Rousseau, Jacques. 1937 La botanique canadienne à l'époque de Jacques Cartier. Contributions du Laboratoire de Botanique de l'Université de Montréal 28;1-77. Rousseau reprinted all the botanical comments made by Cartier or by whoever dictated or wrote parts of the texts of his Voyages. He used the edition of 1924 published by Biggar. The original french mss. of Cartier's 1534 voyage was discovered in 1867 in Paris. There are three french mss. of the 1535-36 voyage in existence. Rousseau kept the page numbers used by Biggar, in his publication of the original mss. of the Cartier voyages. Rousseau has comments on each plant mentioned by Cartier. He also reprints the botanical comments of Cartier's precursors and contemporaries, who visited the St. Lawrence estuary, and discusses each plant mentioned by them. A very valuable source.

1945 Le folklore botanique de Caughnawaga. Études Éthnobotaniques québécoise. Contrib. Inst. Bot. Univ. Mon. 55; 7-74. Submitted for publication 1943. The local plants growing on the Caughnawaga reservation of the Mohawk in Quebec identified by Rousseau and his informants and their uses by the Mohawks given with valuable comments by Rousseau.

1945 Le folklore botanique de l'Ile aux Coudres. Études Éthnobotaniques québécoises. Contrib. Inst. Bot. Univ. Mon. 55;75-111. Submitted for publication 1943. The information was for the most part gathered in 1940. French Canadian families had been living on the island since 1765. There had been little immigration to the Island as all the land was soon occupied and communication made visiting the island difficult, so the folklore was relatively untouched by outside influences.

1960 Movement of plants. Published in The evolution of Canadian flora, ed. Taylor and Ludwig 1960.

1964 La flore de la Nouvelle-France. In P. Boucher naturaliste, an app written by Rousseau for the 1964 edition of Boucher's Histoire published by Soc. Hist. Boucherville. It is here that Rousseau writes "Louis Hebert, during his stay at Port Royal, sent specimens of plants to France that Bauhin stated came from Brazil." Citing Bouvet, Rev. Hist. Pharm 143 1954, and Juel 1931. See Bauhin, Juel, Gerarde, and under pitcher plant in this text. All Rousseau citations above translated by the author. The contributions of Jacques Rousseau to our knowledge of the use of our native plants is inestimable.

Rudakov, I.F. 1952 Chemical Abstracts 46:2240. Protoanemonin in Clematis sp.

Rush, Benjamin. 1774 An inquiry into the natural history of medicine among the Indians of north America. . . Read before the Am. Phil. Ass. Feb. 4th. n.p.n.d. Philadelphia.

1812 Diary Dec. 15th. p. 303. Labrador Tea.

Sagard, Father Theodat Gabriel. 1624 (1632) Le gran voyage du pays des Hurons, situe en l'Amerique vers la mer douce, es dernier confines de la Nouvelle France, dite Canada. Denys Moreau 1632 Paris. Published in translation by the Champlain Soc. XXV 1939 ed. Wrong. fac. ed. 196ʳ Greenwood N.Y. Sagard spent ten months of 1623-24 among the Huron. He borrowed frc Champlain's 1615 account of his stay with them but was himself an accurate and sympath observer.

Sansom, Joseph. 1820 Travels in Lower Canada. Phillips London. Fac. ed. 1970 Coles Torc

Sarrazin, Michel. 1708 La flore du Canada. mss. ed. Boivin 1978. see Boivin.

Saunders, Charles F. 1920 Useful wild plants of the United States and Canada. McBride N.Y.

Scoggan, H.J. 1978-1979. The Flora of Canada. In four parts. A comprehensive survey of the ferns and flowering plans of Canada. Nat. Mus. Can. Ottawa.

Schoolcraft, Henry Rowe. 1851-57 History of the Indian tribes in the United States. 6 vols. Lippincott Philadelphia. Schoolcraft was the U.S. government agent in charge at Mackinaw where Mrs Jameson stayed with him and his Ojibwa wife in 1837.

Schultes, Richard Evans. 1965 The Widening panorama in medical botany. Rhodora 65;97-120.

1968 The plant kingdom and modern medicine. The Herbarist 18-26. Boston.

1972 The future of plants as sources of new biodynamic compounds. In Plants in the development of modern medicine ed. Swain. 1972.

Seigler, David S. 1975 Plants of the northeastern United States that produce cyanogenic compounds. Economic Botany 30;395-407.

Seton, E.T. 1912 The forester's manual. Doubleday New York.

Shaw, A.C. 1952 The preparation and composition of some Canadian coniferous oils. Pulp and Paper Magazine of Canada. March 53;119.

Short, Adam. 1913 The colony in its economic relations. New France Vol. 2 Canada and its Provinces. Publisher's Assn. of Canada Toronto.

Simcoe, Elizabeth P. 1792-6 The diary of Mrs. John Graves Simcoe. ed. J. Ross Robertson William Briggs 1911 Toronto.

Slippy, H.A. 1915 Chem. News 111:2-3 *Clintonia borealis*.

Smith, Huron H. 1923 Ethnobotany of the Menomini. Bull. Pub. Mus. Milwaukee 4;1-82.

1928 Ethnobotany of the Meskwaki. Bull. Pub. Mus. Milwaukee 4;189-274. "The writer is also fortunate in having available the excellent ethnobotanical data of the late Dr. Wm. Jones, collected so many years ago when the tribe was even less spoiled by contact with whites."

1932 Ethnobotany of the Ojibwe. Bull. Pub. Mus. Milwaukee 4;348-433. "The Ojibwe are probably the best informed and the strictest observers of the medicine lodge ceremonies in the country. Their knowlege of plants, both in their own environment and far away, is probably the best of any group of Indians. . . They make trips far away from their home to obtain the necessary plants."

1933 Ethnobotany of the Potawatomi. Bull. Pub. Mus. Milwaukee 7;32-127. Huron Smith collected the plants, identified them, showed them to his Indian informants who them gave him their name for that plant and their use of it. This positive identification of the species and the first hand information of the use of that species is what makes Huron Smith's ethnobotanical work so valuable, as well as his sympathetic understanding of Indian religion and life. He regretted he could not have spent more time living with each tribe he wrote about. As it is difficult to obtain copies of his work it is reproduced in full in this text. If Huron Smith wrote of one of the plants discussed here, then he is quoted. Misquotation of his work is probably due to use of secondary source or to a careless reading, another reason for quoting from the original publication.

Smith, James. 1755-59 (1870) An Account of the remarkable occurences in the life and travels of Col. James Smith, during his captivity with the Indians in the years 1755, '56, '57, '58 and '59. Reprinted with appendix Robert Clarke 1870. Ohio Valley Hist. ser., No. 5. Cincinnati.

Smith, Capt. John. 1612 Description of Virginia and proceedings of the colony. Oxford 1612. ·ded in narratives of Early Virginia ed. Tyler 1959 New York.

·ter. 1812 The Indian doctor's dispensatory. Reprinted Lloydia Bull. 2 ser. 2 1901 Cin.

⁊ S. 1975 Shanidar IV, a neanderthal flower burial in northern Iraq. Science 190;

·r of the Society of Ontario Nut Growers, ed. Douglas Campbell, Niagara on

Spalding, V.N. Fernow, B.E. 1899 The white pine. Washington D.C.

Soper, James H. 1949 The vascular plants of southern Ontario. Mss. Univ. Toronto, Toronto.

Speck, Frank G. 1915 Medicine practices of the northeastern Algonquians. Proceedings Intern Congress of Americanists. xix;303-32 Washington Pub. 1917. Gives the plants and their use by the Montagnais north of the St. Lawrence and the Penobscot south of it. "An essentially practical popular herbalism disassociated from shamanistic ritual or magic is shared by many other eastern tribes." Medicine practices of the Micmac-Montagnais of Newfoundland is taken from Cartwright and quoted in Howley The Beothucks 1915. The Mohegan medicinal practice was given by Miss G.I. Tantaquidgeon herself a Mohegan.

Speck, Frank G., Hassrick, R.B. & Carpenter, E.S. 1942 Rappahannock herbals, folk-lore and science of cures. Proc. Delaware County Inst. Sci. 10:55pps.

Stary, Frantisek, & Jirasek, Vaclac. 1973 Herbs. Tr. from Czech. Huthanova. Hamlyn London.

Stearns, S. 1801 The American herbal or materia medica. Thomas & Thomas N.H.

Stepka, W. & Winters, A.D. 1973 A survey of the genus Crataegus for hypertensive activity. Lloydia 36:4;436.

Stone, Eric. 1934 Medicine among the Iroquois. Ann. Med. Hist. n.s. 6;529-39

Stowe, C.C. 1940 Plants used by the Chippewa. Wis. Archeol. n.s. 21;8-13.

Strickland, Samuel. 1853 Twenty-seven years in Canada West. 2 vols. Bentley London.

Sturtevant, E. Lewis. 1919 Sturtevant's notes on edible plants. Lyon Albany. Reprinted 1972 Dover N.Y.

Su, K.L., Staba, E.J. & Abul-Hajj, Y. 1973 Preliminary studies of aquatic plants from Minnesota. Lloydia 36;72-79. 1973 Antimicrobial effects of aquatic plants from Minnesota. ibid 80-87.

Suzuki, David. 1979 Science magazine, CBC TV May. Quirks and quarks CBC radio Oct.

Swain, T. ed. 1972 Plants in the development of modern medicine. Harvard Univ. Press Cambridge. Includes Swain, The significance of comparative phytochemistry in medical botany.

Swales, Dorothy. 1970 Herbs and their uses in the Canadian arctic. The Herbarist 31-34. Boston.

Tantaquidgeon, Gladys. 1925-26 Mohegan medicinal practices, weather-lore and superstitions. Ann. Rep. Bur. Am. Ethnol. 43;264-79

1932 Notes on the origin and uses of plants of the Lake St. John Montagnais. J. Am. Folk-Lore 45;256-67.

Tayeau, Francis. 1950 Chemical Abstracts 45;7187c. Univ. of Bordeaux. *Polygala*.

Taylor, Roy L. & Ludwig, R.A. eds. 1960 The evolution of Canada's flora. Univ. Toronto Press Toronto.

Thévet, André. 1557-58 Les singularitez de la France antarctique. Paris. 1568 New founde worlde or Antarcticke. London.

1575 La cosmographie universelle. 2 vols. Paris. The sections of both works that mention plants growing in northeastern north America reprinted Rousseau 1937 in French. tr. by author. The 1878 edition ed. Caffarel in Paris is the one used by Rousseau. Thevet was never in the new world but is thought to have talked to both Cartier and the chief, Donnacona whom Cartier had brought to France.

Thompson, David. 1784-1812 Narrative of his explorations in western America. Ed. J.B. Tyrrell. Champlain Soc. Pub. 13 1916 Toronto.

Thomson, R.B. & Sifton, H.B. 1922 A guide to the poisonous plants and weed seeds of Canada and northern United States. Univ. of Toronto Press Toronto.

Thwaites, R.G. ed. 1896-1901 The Jesuit Relations and allied documents. 73 vols. Burrows Cleveland. See under Jesuit relations.

1905 Early western travels. Arthur Clarke Cleveland.

Tooker, Elisabeth. 1964 An ethnography of the Huron Indians 1615-1649. Smith. Inst. Bull. 190 Bur. Am. Ethnol. Washington. Reprinted Huronia Historical Developement Council and Ont. Dept. Educ. 1967. Dr. Tooker has read all the Jesuit Relations that speak of the Hurons during this period as well as Champlain and Sagard and under different aspects of Huron life refers to what each of these sources said. A very valuable book. She writes, 62 note–"The Iroquoians gathered more varieties of wild foods than the 17th-century observers noted. . . The reason for this neglect are obvious: gathering was probably not as important as hunting and fishing and, as it was done by the women, the French writers, being men, probably overlooked much of this activity. . . 84 The Jesuits probably underestimated the Huron use of medicinal plants."

Trail, Catherine Parr (Strickland). 1838 The backwoods of Canada-being letters from the wife of an emigrant officer. 3rd ed. C. Knight London. Reprinted in part by McLelland and Stewart Toronto 1966. First Published London 1836.

1855 The Canadian settler's guide. Old Countryman Office Toronto. Reprinted McClelland and Stewart 1969 Toronto.

Transactions of the Literary and Historical Society of Quebec. 1829-1861. Quebec.

Trousseau, Armand. Pidoux, H. 1841 Traité de therapeutique et de matiere medicale. Paris second edition given by Dr. James Richardson to the Academy of Medicine Library Toronto. Many editions published. Tr. by the author.

Trueblood, Emily Emmart. 1964 The Badianus manuscript. Herbarist 1-20 Boston.

Turner, Lucien M. 1894 Ethnology of the Ungava district. Smith. Inst. 1889-90 Washington.

Turner, William. 1568 The first and second partes of the herbal of William Turner doctor in phisick, Birckman Cologne.

Vallée, A. 1927 Un biologiste canadien Michel Sarrazin 1659-1735. A. Proulx Quebec. Vallée reproduced as an app. the Jussieu list (see under Jussieu) in an unreadable form.

VanWart, A.F. 1948 The Indians of the Maritime Provinces, their diseases and native cures. Can. Med. Assoc. J. 59;573-77.

Varma, S.D., Mizuno, A. & Kinoshita, J.H. 1977 Diabetic cataracts and flavonoids. Science 195; 205-06.

Victorin, Marie. 1919 Notes recueillies dans la region de Témiscamingue. Naturalist can. 45;163-69.

1935 Flore laurentienne. Montreal.

1936 Un manuscrit botanique prélinnéen. Rev. trim. can. 22;225-237. Marie-Victorin found a mss. in the Seminary of Sainte Hyacinthe which he was allowed to read and copy. He called it Histoire des plantes de Canada. The first chapter contains a list of 198 plants and the second 29. He intended to publish this mss in 1919 but decided to try and solve the problem of who had sent the plants from Quebec and to whom in Paris. He finally proved that it was Sarrazin who had sent them to Vaillant in the Jardin des Plantes in Paris. In 1934 he was in the Herbarium in Paris and to his joy found that all the plants, numbered as they appeared in the mss were in the Herbarium. He came to the conclusion that the mss. entitled Plantes envoyees du Canada par M. Sarrazin was but an abridged version of his manuscript from St. Hyacinth. See under Jussieu for this List, also Vallée. Rousseau came into possession of the St Hyacinth mss. on Victorin's death. He was able to identify the plants as well as prove that the writing was that of Vaillant. The Histoire was finally published in 1978, after Rousseau's death, by Boivin who looked at all the copies of this mss. extant and prepared the most plausible and correct copy of the lost original of 1708. What interests us in this book is the remarks made by Sarrazin on the use in Quebec of some of the plants he sent to Vaillant. tr. by author.

Vindicator. 1836 Newspaper Montreal Quebec.

Vogel, Virgil J. 1970 American Indian medicine. Univ. of Oklahoma Press Norman.

von Reis Altschul, S. 1973 Drugs and foods from little-known plants. Harvard Univ. Press. Cambridge.

Wallis, T.E. 1967 Textbook of Pharmacognosy. 5th ed. Churchill London.

Wallis, W.D. 1922 Medicines used by the Micmac Indians. Am. Anthrop. 24;24-30.

Wallis, W.D. and Wallis, R.S. 1955 The Micmac Indians of Eastern Canada. Univ. of Minn. Press 125-36. Minn.

1957 The Indians of New Brunswick. Nat. Mus. Can. Bull. 148 54 pp Ottawa.

Walpole Island Herbalism. 1960 A study of the medico-ethno-botany of the analagamated bands of the Chippewa. A thesis by George Merring Wayne State Univ. Detroit.

Wassenaer, Nicolaes. 1624-30 Historisch Verhael. Repr. in Narratives of new Netherlands 1909; 61-96 A learned scholar and physician commenting on the New Netherlands.

Waugh, F.W. 1916 Iroquois foods and food preparation. Mem. 86 Anthrop. ser. 12 Can. Dept. Mines. Ottawa. A very thorough study of the subject.

Weiner, M.A. 1972 Earth medicine-earth foods. Collier New York. Very general and western.

Weise, A.J. 1884 The discoveries of America to the year 1525. London. Reprints Alberto Cantino, Pietro Pasqualigo and Eusebii Caesariensis.

Wentsel, W.F. 1807-24 Letters to the Hon. Roderick McKenzie. in Masson Les Bourgeois.

Wesley, J. 1768 Primitive Physick. 13th edition W. Pine Bristol.

Yanofsky, Elias. 1936 Food Plants of the north American Indians. USDA Misc. Pub. 237 Washington D.C.

Yarnell, Richard Asa. 1964 Aboriginal relationships between culture and plant life in the upper great lakes region. Anthrop. Pap. 23. Mus. Anthrop. Univ. of Mich. Ann Arbor. Reprinted 1970. "This report deals with; (1) utilization of native plant products as determined from ethnographic records and the results of archaeological research; and (2) aboriginal agriculture with respect to its historical aspects. . . I located and identified, in the laboratory, most of the archaeological remains of uncultivated plant food and charcoal of the upper great lakes region."

Yarnell, R.A., Parmallee, Paul W. & Muson, P.J. 1970 Subsistence ecology of Scovil, or terminal middle woodland village. Am. Antiquary 36:4.

Youngken, H.W. 1924-25 The drugs of the north American Indian. Am. J. Pharm 96;485-502, 97; 158-185, 257-271.

Zeisberger, David. 1779 History of the north American Indians. The mss written in German by the Moravian missionary Rev. David Zeisberger in Ohio. Tr. by W.N. Schwarze and ed. A.B. Hulbert. Pub. Ohio Archeol. Hist. Publ. 19;1-189. 1910.

Zennie, Thomas M. & Ogzewalla, C. Dwayne. 1977 Ascorbic acid and Vitamin A content of edible wild plants of Ohio and Kentucky. Economic Botany 31;76-79.

Addenda to Sources Cited — see page 511

GENERAL INDEX

INDEX OF BOTANICAL NAMES

The current names appear in Roman type in this Index. Names listed as synonyms appear in italics.

The taxonomy is based for the most part on the *Manual of Vascular Plants of northeastern United States and Adjacent Canada* (1963) by Henry A. Gleason and Arthur Cronquist and the *Flora of Canada* (1978-79) by H. J. Scoggan. The synonymy (the no longer current botanical names used in old sources) were sought in Gray's *Manual of Botany* (1908 and 1950), Britten and Brown's *Flora of northern United States and Canada* (1913), as well as in the two manuals mentioned above.

ADDENDA TO SOURCES CITED

Allouez, Claude-Jean. 1670 Jesuit Relations.

Biard, Pierre. 1611 Jesuit Relations.

Brebeuf, Jean de. 1636 Jesuit Relations.

Bressani, Francesco. 1653 Jesuit Relations.

Bylot, R. and Baffin, Wm. 1616 Ventursome voyage printed in part in Mowat the Polar passion.

de Laet, Johan. The book quotes some of Henry Hudson's comments in 1609 on the Indians he met.

de Laszlo, Henry and Henshaw, Paul. 1954 Plant materials used by primitive peoples to affect fertility. Science May 7th. 626-31 No. 3097.

Gray, Hugh. 1809 Letter from Canada written during a residence there in the years 1806, 1807 and 1808, Longman London. Coles fac.ed. 1971.

Journal of Senate of Canada. 1887 Ottawa.

Lalemant, Hierosme. 1640-43 Jesuit Relations.

Le Jeune, Paul. 1634, 1639, 1656-57 Jesuit Relations.

Le Mercier, Francois Joseph. 1737 Jesuit Relations.

Mowat, Farley. 1965 Westviking. McClelland and Stewart Toronto.

Nouvel, Henri. 1672 Jesuit Relations.

Reid, Mayne. 1853 The young voyageurs. Routledge London.

Schoepf, D. 1787 Materia Medica Americana. J.J. Palm Erlangen Germany.

Stoerck, Anton. 1760 Libellus quo demonstratur:cicutam. . .Trattner Vienna.

Thomson, Samuel. 1832 The new guide to health, or the botanic family physician. Hamilton Upper Canada.

Urquhart, F.A. 1960 The monarch butterfly. University of Toronto Press.

Whitbourne, Richard. 1620 Discourse and discovery of Nevv-found-land. Felix Kyngston & F.W. Barrett London. "In a voyage to that country about 36 years since at the time of Sir Humphrey Gilbert."

Whitford, A.G. 1941 Textile fibers used in eastern North America. Am. Mus. Nat. Hist. Anthrop. Pap. 38;1-22.

Willaman, J.J. and Hui-Lin Li. 1970 Alkaloid bearing plants and their contained alkaloids, 1957-68. Lloydia 33 No. 3A. "The purpose is to assemble in one place all the scattered information on the occurrence of alkaloids in the plant world."

Williams, Roger. 1643 A key into the language. London. Reprinted Pub. Narragansett Club Vol. 1 1866 Providence R.I.

Williams, Stephen W. 1849 Report on the indigenous medical botany of Massachusetts. Trans. Am. Med. Assoc. Vol. 2;863-927. Uses Rafinesque without acknowledgement.

Willis, N.P. 1840-42 Canadian scenery. 2 vols. George Virtue London.

Wilson, Daniel. 1857 Narcotic usages and superstitions of the old and new world. Can. Journal of Industry, Science and Art, conducted by the editing committee of the Can. Inst. July and August. X;233-264 and XI;324-44. Interesting account of Indian smoking habits with a general account of tobacco smoking.

Winder, William. 1846 Indian diseases and remedies. The Boston Medical and Surgical Journal 34;9-13. Dr. Winder of Montreal quotes from Dr. Darling's report from Manitoulin Island 1841-42 then adds his own comments on the Indian use of plants for medicine, an intelligent report.

512 ADDENDA TO SOURCES CITED

Wintemberg, W.J. 1950 Folk-lore of Waterloo county, Ontario. Nat. Mus. Can. Bull. 116. Only pages 9-16 refer to the use of plants by the German-Canadian population.

Wood, G.P. and Ruddock, E.H. 1925 Vitalogy or encyclopedia of health and home adapted for family use. Chicago. Book in use in home in York county, Ontario. The last of the texts on domestic medicine, from Peter Smith in 1812, Howard in 1833, Gunn in 1859-61 to Household Guide 1894 that are quoted in this book to give a fair representation of that branch of plant use.

Wood, Horatio C. 1890 Letter on effects of *Rhus toxicodendron* or poison ivy in the Therapeutic Gazette 14;95. Cited Coulter.

Wood, William. 1764 New-England prospect. Published by Prince Soc. 1865 Boston.

Wright, J.V. 1972 Ontario prehistory, an eleven-thousand-year archaeological outline. Nat. Mus. Can. Ottawa. A beautiful, informative book.